S0-BCP-842

THE HOSPITAL RESEARCH AND EDUCATIONAL TRUST

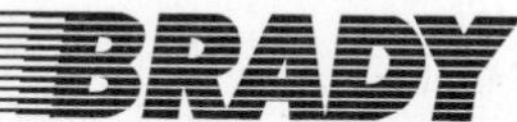

Being a Health Unit Coordinator Fourth Edition

Kay Cox, R.N., M.A.
Health Careers Specialist
Professor, Saddleback College
Mission Viejo, California

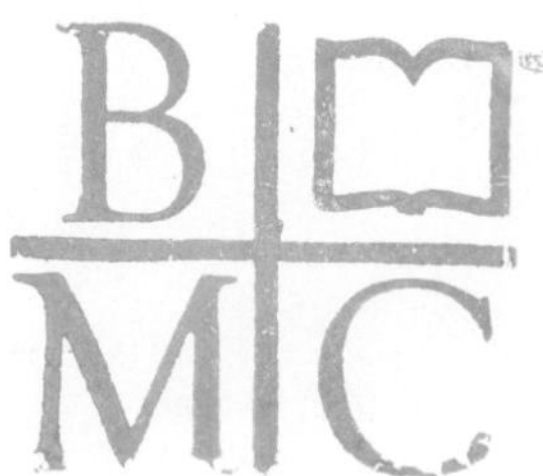

BRADY
Prentice Hall
Upper Saddle River, New Jersey 07458

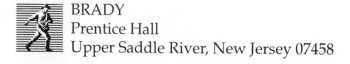

Library of Congress Cataloging-in-Publication Data

Cox, Kay, (date)
Being a health unit coordinator / Kay Cox. — 4th ed.
p. cm.
Rev. ed. of: Brady being a health unit coordinator. 3rd ed. c1991.
At head of title: Hospital Research and Educational Trust.
Includes bibliographical references and index.
ISBN 0-8359-5158-8
1. Hospital ward clerks. I. Hospital Research and Educational Trust. II. Title.
[DNLM: 1. Personnel, Hospital. 2. Medical Records. WX 159 C877 1998]
RA972.55.C69 1998
362.1'1'068—dc21
DNLM/DLC
for Library of Congress 97-34711
CIP

To my mother, Donna Priest, for her love and support. To my children, Dana, Tod, and Ryan, and to Suzanne and in memory of my dear friends: Bonnie Bach Meade, Karen Strong, and John Riling.

Publisher: Susan Katz
Acquisitions Editor: Barbara Krawiec
Editorial Assistant: Stephanie Camangian
Marketing Manager: Judy Streger
Marketing Coordinator: Cindy Frederick
Director of Production and Manufacturing: Bruce Johnson
Senior Production Manager: Ilene Sanford
Managing Editor for Production: Patrick Walsh
Art Director: Marianne Frasco
Cover Design: Bruce Kenselaar
Composition: Clarinda Company
Printer and Binder: Banta Co., Harrisonburg, VA

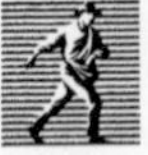

© 1998, 1991 by Prentice Hall, Inc.
A Simon and Schuster Company
Upper Saddle River, New Jersey 07458

Notice

The procedures described in this textbook are based on consultation with medical authorities. The author and publisher have taken care to make certain that these procedures reflect currently accepted clinical practice; however, they cannot be considered absolute recommendations.

The material in this textbook contains the most current information available at the time of publication. However, federal, state, and local guidelines concerning medical clerical practices can change rapidly. The reader should note, therefore, that new regulations may require changes in some procedures.

It is the responsibility of the reader to familiarize himself or herself with the policies and procedures set by federal, state, and local agencies, as well as the institution or agency where the reader is employed. The authors and the publishers of this textbook, and the supplements written to accompany it, disclaim any liability, loss, or risk resulting directly or indirectly from the suggested procedures and theory, from any undetected errors, or from the reader's misunderstanding of the text. It is the reader's responsibility to stay informed of any new changes or recommendations made by any federal, state, and local agency as well as by his or her employing health care institution or agency.

All rights reserved. No part of this book may be reproduced, in any form or by any means, without permission in writing from the publisher.

Printed in the United States of America
10 9 8 7 6 5 4 3 2 1

ISBN 0-8359-5158-8

Prentice-Hall International (UK) Limited, *London*
Prentice-Hall of Australia Pty. Limited, *Sydney*
Prentice-Hall Canada Inc., *Toronto*
Prentice-Hall Hispanoamericana, S.A., *Mexico*
Prentice-Hall of India Private Limited, *New Delhi*
Prentice-Hall of Japan, Inc., *Tokyo*
Simon & Schuster Asia Pte. Ltd., Singapore
Editora Prentice-Hall do Brasil, Ltda., *Rio de Janeiro*

CONTENTS

PREFACE

Today's sophisticated world of medicine places many demands on health care workers. Advanced technology, government regulations, and the increasingly complex nature of medical care have resulted in a critical need for competent, well-trained and responsible personnel.

The fourth edition of *Being a Health Unit Coordinator* continues to provide the basic, easy-to-understand, current information necessary to perform the duties of a health unit coordinator (unit secretary, ward clerk, and so on). It is designed for students enrolled in unit coordinating programs and as a reference for employed unit coordinators.

Organization

The text is organized into nineteen chapters and is logically arranged, moving from simple to complex. The first nine chapters provide a core of information considered necessary for all medical–clerical workers. The next eight chapters focus on subject matter more specific to the performance of health unit coordinating procedures. Chapter 18 discusses review for the national certification examination and Chapter 19 contains numerous sets of physician's orders for order transcription practice.

There are clearly stated objectives at the beginning of each chapter; key ideas are highlighted; lists of vocabulary words, medical terminology, and abbreviations are included; and there are review questions and activities at the end of the chapters.

New Features of the Third Edition

This new edition contains considerable new and updated information. Medical terminology has been expanded, as has the chapter on medications, which now includes generic terms for the drugs. The new standard precautions and isolation procedures are presented. More information has been included on the business side of health care and managed care. This new edition retains numerous sets of physician's orders (many in actual, handwritten form) and instructions for scenarios that give students opportunities for real-life practice in performing health unit coordinator procedures in the classroom.

The field of health care is one of rapid change. A textbook cannot be updated as often as new procedures or equipment are adopted by modern health care institutions, nor is it possible for this text to describe every procedure, form, or exact method your hospital will use. However, your instructor keeps informed of these changes and knows the specific way of doing things in your hospital and in your community.

Now you are ready to study, to think, and to practice. The work you will learn to do is important work. Mastering it will be an accomplishment of which you can be proud.

Acknowledgments

I would like to express my utmost gratitude to the wonderful people at South Coast Medical Center in South Laguna, California, for their generosity in helping me with this revision. My sincere thanks goes to Betsy Brewington, Education Coordinator, for paving the way and assisting me so graciously; Marianne Dickey, Information Systems Services, for providing me with so much of the information on computers; Lesa Blake, Director of Food Services and Chief Clinical Dietitian; Jan Bentley McDaniel, Epidemiology Department and President, Orange County Chapter of APAC; and to Phil Fagan, Ann O'Brien, Melissa McCourt, Maeve Delaney, Holly Bowden, and Daria Wysmierski. I would especially like to thank Kay Deol, R. N., Vice President of Patient Services, for allowing me access to the hospital. I would also like to express my appreciation to NAHUC and especially to Rosemary Boessele, President; Sandra Ayres, President Elect; and Karen Wiggins, Certification Board Director. Thanks also to the people at Brady, Barbara Krawiec, Executive Editor, Health Professions; and Stephanie Camangian, Editorial Assistant.

KAY COX, R.N., M.A.

About the Author

This edition of *Being a Health Unit Coordinator* is once again prepared by Kay Cox, R.N., M.A. Ms. Cox is a Professor of Health Sciences at Saddleback College in Mission Viejo, California, and owns a consulting business, Achiever's Development Enterprises. She is a former instructor of health unit coordinators. She is a founding member of NAHUC (The National Association of Health Unit Coordinators) and a former regional representative and Director of Education of that organization. She is the series editor for the Brady Medical Clerical Series and for the Clinical Allied Health textbook series for Career Publishing.

CHAPTER 1

Introduction to Being a Health Unit Coordinator

OBJECTIVES

When you have completed this chapter, you will be able to:

- List desirable characteristics for health unit coordinators.
- Name and state the purpose of the national association for health unit coordinators.
- State the importance of good hygiene and of a dress code.
- Discuss the importance of accuracy and dependability in your daily work.
- State the three main categories of a health unit coordinator's duties and list the basic tasks you will perform.
- Describe methods for growth and advancement in your job.

A health unit coordinator is a very important member of the health care team. The health unit coordinator performs the clerical, reception/communication, and coordination tasks for the nursing unit, leaving more time for the nursing staff to perform the clinical or patient care duties. Through your performance as a health unit coordinator, you will make a valuable contribution to the care of the patient.

As a health unit coordinator, you will be working with the medical and nursing teams doing the work of one of the most respected professions in the world: caring for the sick and promoting wellness. This is rewarding work which deserves careful attention and the determination to do a good job. During your training and while you are at work, remember that the *most important person* in the hospital is the PATIENT.

KEY IDEA: HISTORY OF HEALTH UNIT COORDINATING

Before the evolution of the health unit coordinator position, the registered nurse performed not only the clinical, but also the clerical and reception tasks necessary to render care to the hospitalized patient. During World War II, nurses were in short supply and it became necessary to train others on the job to assist the registered nurse. The clerical and reception tasks were designated to persons called ward clerks and the patient care or clinical tasks to persons now called nursing assistants. Rapid advances in medicine have resulted in an expanded role for ward clerks, and it has grown into the responsible and challenging position it is today.

In the past, the only training for health unit coordinators occurred on the job. Today there are educational programs in vocational schools and colleges throughout the nation.

KEY IDEA: NAHUC

In recognition of the importance of the health unit coordinator's role, a professional association was formed on August 23, 1980, in Phoenix, Arizona. At the invitation of Myrna Lafleur Brooks, who became the founding president, a small group of educators and practitioners from throughout the nation attended that first meeting. The founding members in addition to Myrna Lafleur Books were Kay Cox, Helga Hegge, Carolyn Hinken, Estelle Johnson, Connie Johnston, Kathy Jordan, Velma Kerschner, Jane Pedersen, and Winifred Starr. At that meeting the National Association of Health Unit Clerks-Coordinators (NAHUC) was born. At a second meeting hosted by Kay Cox in San Juan Capistrano, California, the constitution was ratified and the new association's officers were elected. In 1990 the NAHUC membership voted to change its name and drop the word "Clerk." Figure 1–1 shows the NAHUC logo.

August 23 has been named "Health Unit Coordinator Day" and it has been listed in the American Hospital Association Calendar of Health Observance Days.

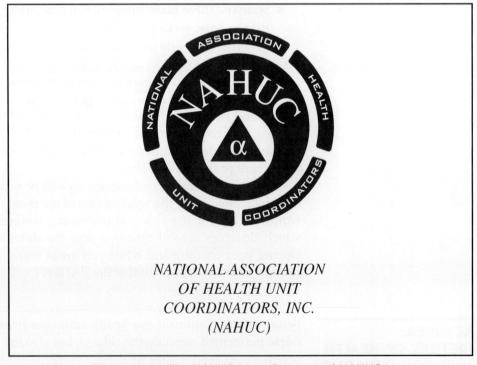

Figure 1–1 The NAHUC logo (Courtesy of NAHUC.)

The National Association of Health Unit Coordinators, as it is now known, provides opportunities for local, state, regional, and national participation. It is a professional organization that promotes the professionalism and competence of health unit coordinators. Membership includes both individual and institutional members.

Another contribution of NAHUC is the development of a national certification examination. When certified, a health unit coordinator is called a certified health unit coordinator (CHUC). There are over 9,000 CHUCs in the United States. The examination is offered throughout the nation to anyone who is a health unit coordinator, has completed health unit coordinating training, or is involved in activities related to health unit coordinating. Membership in NAHUC is not required, but applicants must have a high school diploma or a GED.

For more information on NAHUC write NAHUC, 1211 Locust Street, Philadelphia, PA 19107 or call 888-22-NAHUC (215-545-3310).

KEY IDEA: PERSONAL QUALIFICATIONS

You have chosen to become a health unit coordinator and you want to do the best possible job. What kind of a person makes a good health unit coordinator? Certain traits, attitudes, and habits are regularly seen in people who are successful in their work in the health care institution. Some of these traits are already part of one's personality. Other traits can be learned through practice and *become* part of one's *improved* personality.

Go through this list and see where you stand. Review those qualities you already have. Check those you think you could learn and actually make a part of yourself. You have the qualifications if:

- You are trustworthy and dependable
- You enjoy working with people
- You get along well with others
- You are considerate and tactful
- You want to help people
- You try to be gracious and polite at all times
- You show empathy and patience with others
- You like to communicate with others
- You are a good listener
- You like clerical work and attention to detail
- You like to be organized
- You strive for accuracy
- You have reasonably good reading comprehension
- You have good spelling ability
- You have neat and legible handwriting
- You can work under pressure
- You always try to control your temper
- You believe that you are doing important work
- You can follow rules and instructions

- You want to improve your performance
- You like to learn new things
- You don't let your private life interfere with your work
- You are interested in the medical field

Dependability

Your hospital is organized to function efficiently when a certain number of people are on the job. Your absence could deprive a patient of needed care.

Your absence may also cause your fellow workers to have an overload of work. It is essential that you arrive promptly every day unless you are ill. If you *are* sick, you must always notify the nursing office or appropriate supervisor as soon as possible so arrangements can be made for a replacement for you.

Dependability, however, means more than coming to work on time and coming to work every day. It also means that when you are asked to do something, you can be relied upon to do it at the proper time and in the proper way.

Accuracy

Accuracy and dependability are closely related. (Fig. 1–2.) In a hospital you are concerned with human lives. What might appear to you as a tiny mistake or oversight could delay the recovery of the patient. Whether you are recording a temperature, taking off doctor's orders and inputting them into the computer, or answering the telephone, it is vitally important that you stay alert, follow instructions, and be accurate. Try never to make mistakes; however, *should you make a mistake*, correct it at once and, when appropriate, report the error to your supervisor. If you do not understand, ask again. There is a reason for every step in the routine of the hospital. Remember, accuracy in this job is not just important-it is essential!

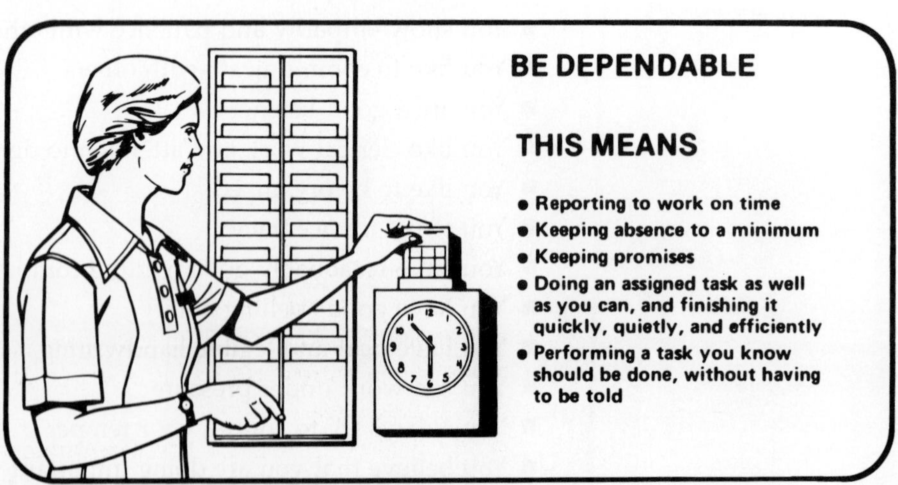
BE DEPENDABLE
THIS MEANS
• Reporting to work on time
• Keeping absence to a minimum
• Keeping promises
• Doing an assigned task as well as you can, and finishing it quickly, quietly, and efficiently
• Performing a task you know should be done, without having to be told

Figure 1–2

Following Rules and Instructions

Every business has its own rules and regulations. Rules and regulations governing a hospital are even more significant to know and follow than those of a business because life and death situations are often involved. There are *specific* policies that will guide your work or conduct in the hospital. Most of these rules are in writing. Learn the rules and, if you do not understand something, ask your instructor or the nurse in charge.

A hospital staff is concerned with human lives. Instructions may be given to you very quickly and in tense situations. You must be able to follow instructions carefully and accurately. Be ready to adjust quickly to any new situation.

Rules and regulations which relate to employment are called personnel policies. Following is a list of personnel practices and employment matters about which your hospital is likely to have rather precise instructions and regulations. As you consider employment in a hospital, you will want to become informed about these regulations.

1. Miscellaneous regulations:
   - Locker assignment and use
   - Permission to leave during working hours
   - Policy for lost and found items
2. Time assignments:
   - Tours of duty (shift rotation or working on different units) and hours
   - Off-duty days
   - Use of the time clock
3. Salary administration:
   - Wage scales
   - Payday: time and place
   - Cashing personal checks
   - Payroll deductions
   - Salary differentials for various tours of duty
   - Overtime pay
   - Increases in salary, with advancement for certified health unit coordinators (CHUC)
4. Appearance:
   - Regulations on uniforms
   - Identification badges
   - Laundering of uniforms
   - General cleanliness and good grooming
5. Meals:
   - Assigned areas for eating or snacking
   - Meal hours and breaks
   - Cafeteria and coffee shop hours and prices and employee discounts
   - Assigned coffee breaks and rest periods
6. Personal health:
   - Physical examinations including tuberculosis, hepatitis B, rubella, and other infectious disease screening and immunizations
   - Employee health service

- Use of outpatient or clinic facilities
- Sick leave
- Absence from work because of illness, including going off duty because of illness and reporting ill from home

7. Employee benefits:
   - Vacations
   - Holidays
   - Hospitalization and medical insurance
   - Pension and retirement plans
   - Social security and unemployment compensation insurance
   - Pharmacy prescriptions
   - Leaves of absence, with pay and without pay
   - Education stipends
8. Job status improvement:
   - Transfers
   - Promotions
   - Inservice education
9. Termination of employment:
   - Dismissals, including causes for dismissal and regulations concerning salary and benefits
   - Resignations, including length of notice required and whether notice must be in written form
10. Personnel records:
    - Applications
    - Incident reports
    - Performance evaluations
    - Letters of resignation
    - Changes of address, marital status, and dependents
    - Health record
11. Personnel-management relations:
    - Causes for disciplinary action
    - Grievance procedures
    - Personnel committee
    - Union affiliation
12. Personal conduct:
    - Smoking regulations
    - Confidential information
    - Hazards of noise
    - Other unprofessional behavior, such as noisiness, rowdiness, and gum chewing

There are certain general standards and regulations to be aware of. They are:

- Use of alcohol and other drugs: Consumption of alcohol or drugs or being under the influence of these substances while on duty is strictly forbidden.
- Solicitation and canvassing: Solicitation for unauthorized charitable contributions is forbidden. Authorized collections for charitable purposes,

such as that for the United Way, will be conducted by the hospital administration. In such instances, employees will be so notified. No employee is permitted to solicit other employees, patients, or visitors on hospital property to sell articles or services of any kind.

- Statements to the press: No statement or report of any kind concerning the hospital, its policies, or its patients is to be made by hospital staff to the press. All inquiries from the press are to be referred directly to the appropriate administrator. No staff member will pose for photographs at any time without first obtaining permission.
- Telephone calls: Adequate telephone service must be available for hospital purposes at all times. Employees must keep incoming calls at a minimum, both in number and in duration. Personal long-distance calls are forbidden. The use of hospital telephones for local calls of a personal nature is prohibited except in an emergency, and then only with the permission of the employee's supervisor.
- Use of hospital address: Employees, other than those living on the premises, are prohibited from using hospital mail facilities for receipt of personal mail. The messenger and mail facilities are reserved for hospital use only.
- Gifts and gratuities: Personnel are discouraged from accepting gifts from patients and visitors. Staff members are prohibited from accepting gifts in the form of money.

KEY IDEA: PERSONAL HYGIENE AND APPEARANCE

The health unit coordinator, as the receptionist of the nursing unit, regularly meets the public and must maintain a pleasant, neat, and businesslike appearance at all times. Most hospitals have a dress code for health unit coordinators. Follow the dress code of the health care institution where you work. Your clothes must be clean and neat. Wear clean clothes every day, repair rips and hems, and replace missing buttons on your clothing. Wear comfortable, businesslike low-heeled shoes with nonskid soles and heels. Keep jewelry at a minimum. Women should use makeup conservatively and men should keep facial hair trimmed. Wear your name pin and assigned hospital identification (such as your picture). Don't chew gum.

Cleanliness is the most essential ingredient of any dress code. Bathe daily and use a deodorant. Keep your hair clean and neatly combed. Keep your mouth clean and your teeth in good condition. Keep your nails short, clean, and in good repair. Because you will be working closely with others, you must avoid fragrances such as cologne, perfume, or after shave lotion.

KEY IDEA: JOB DESCRIPTION

Health care institutions use various titles for the position of health unit coordinator. These include ward clerk, unit clerk, ward secretary, unit secretary, and service coordinator. Whatever the title, the fundamental tasks and procedures you, as a health unit coordinator, will be accountable for will be found in the job description given to you by your hospital.

Working primarily at the desk on a nursing unit, you will be within easy reach of the unit telephones, computer, intercommunications system, and files. The health unit coordinator deals with both licensed and unlicensed

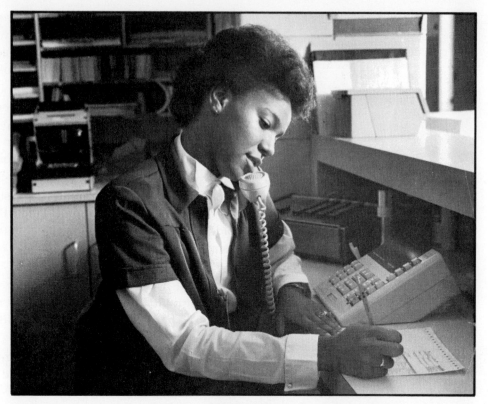

Figure 1–3

nursing personnel, members of the medical staff, personnel from the other hospital departments, patients, and with visitors to the nursing unit. The health unit coordinator's duties fall under three main categories:

- Clerical
- Reception/communication
- Coordination

Everything the health unit coordinator does will be under the supervision of a registered nurse. (Fig. 1–3.)

CLERICAL DUTIES

- Transcribes doctors' orders and uses the computer to process these orders
- Maintains an orderly office environment
- Completes admission, transfer, discharge, preoperative, postoperative, and other patient records
- Keeps daily and interval records and reports
- Maintains patients' charts including filing of patient data in the chart holder
- Orders the daily diets
- Maintains an up-to-date bulletin board

- Requisitions supplies and services from various hospital departments as required
- Operates certain equipment at the nurses' station such as the computer and imprinter (to stamp the patient's name on different forms)

RECEPTION/COMMUNICATION DUTIES

- Answers, places, and transfers telephone calls
- Answers the intercom
- Records and relays messages
- Receives and directs visitors
- Receives and assists patients within prescribed limits
- Maintains communications (by telephone, intercom, computer, mail, FAX, or messenger) within the nursing unit and between the nursing unit and other hospital departments
- Assists doctors and other health personnel as needed at the nurses' station

Coordination Duties. Through communication, requisitioning, and management of supplies and equipment, the health unit coordinator coordinates the activities of the nursing staff, the patient, the doctor, other hospital departments, and visitors to the nursing unit. (Fig. 1–4.)

The Health Unit Coordinator and the Patient. The health unit coordinator does not perform direct patient care but aids in the care of the patient by

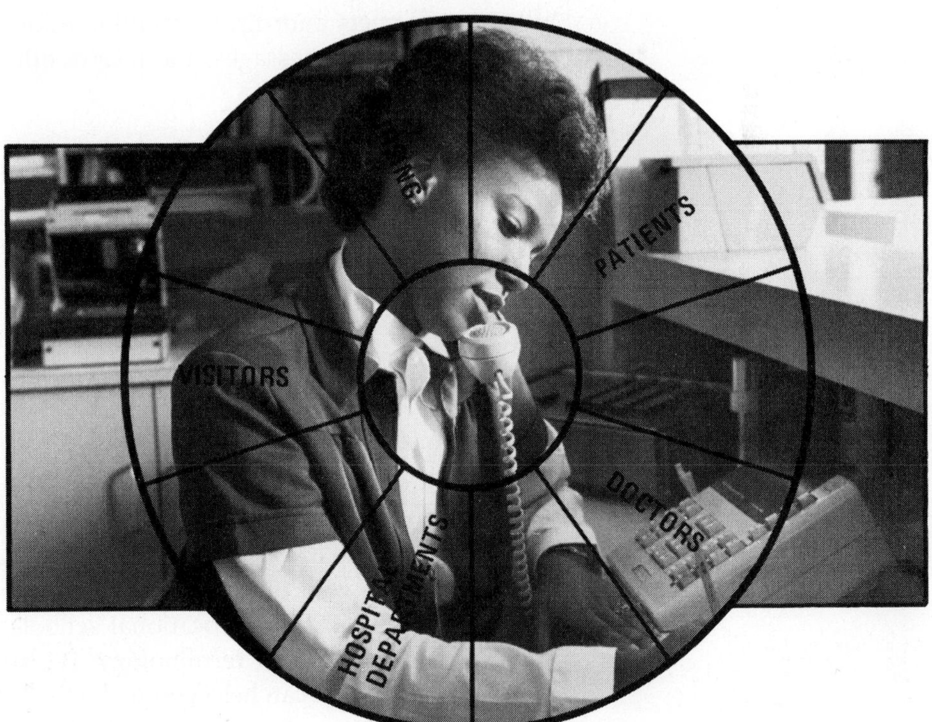

Figure 1–4

performing such procedures as requisitioning tests, treatments, medications, and supplies that the doctor has ordered.

The health unit coordinator greets new patients and relays patient requests to nursing personnel, to doctors, and to other hospital departments.

The Health Unit Coordinator and Nursing. The health unit coordinator is usually a member of the nursing department. You will be working under the supervision of a registered nurse and with other registered nurses, licensed practical or vocational nurses, nursing assistants, and other health unit coordinators.

The Health Unit Coordinator and the Doctor. The health unit coordinator has a great deal of contact with doctors both in person and by telephone. When doctors arrive on the nursing unit, the health unit coordinator greets them, handles their clerical requests, places and receives their calls, and relays messages for them to nursing personnel and other departments.

The health unit coordinator transcribes the doctor's orders. This means that after the doctor has written an order on the patient's chart, the health unit coordinator completes the necessary forms, orders the necessary equipment or services by computer, telephone, FAX, and/or in writing, and communicates the orders to nursing personnel.

The Health Unit Coordinator and Other Departments. The health unit coordinator is in frequent communication with the many other hospital departments ordering tests, supplies, equipment, and other services. Messages by telephone, by computer, and in writing are sent, received, and relayed by the health unit coordinator.

The Health Unit Coordinator and the Patient's Visitors. The health unit coordinator greets and directs visitors, informs them of hospital rules as necessary, relays messages, and locates other hospital staff as requested.

KEY IDEA: OPPORTUNITIES FOR ADVANCEMENT

To keep up with new advances in the medical field, all health care workers are expected to take refresher courses and study new medical developments that affect their employment all their working lives. As you continue to learn, your job will become more interesting and rewarding personally and professionally.

You can continue to learn while you are on the job and expand your knowledge of the health care field. You can find better ways to do your work. All of this can make you a more effective health unit coordinator. This means you will become more secure in your job.

Within the hospital, you will find many classes offered for nursing and other health care personnel through the Department of Inservice Education. You may use this department as a resource to seek out classes best suited to enhance and enrich your learning on the job.

Classes offered through vocational schools, adult education, and community colleges in medical terminology, typing, computer skills, business skills, and management can help you make the lateral and vertical moves you desire. However, if you do not have a high school diploma, that should be your first goal. Adult education programs at local high schools offer basic education programs that lead to a high school equivalency diploma. (Fig. 1–5.)

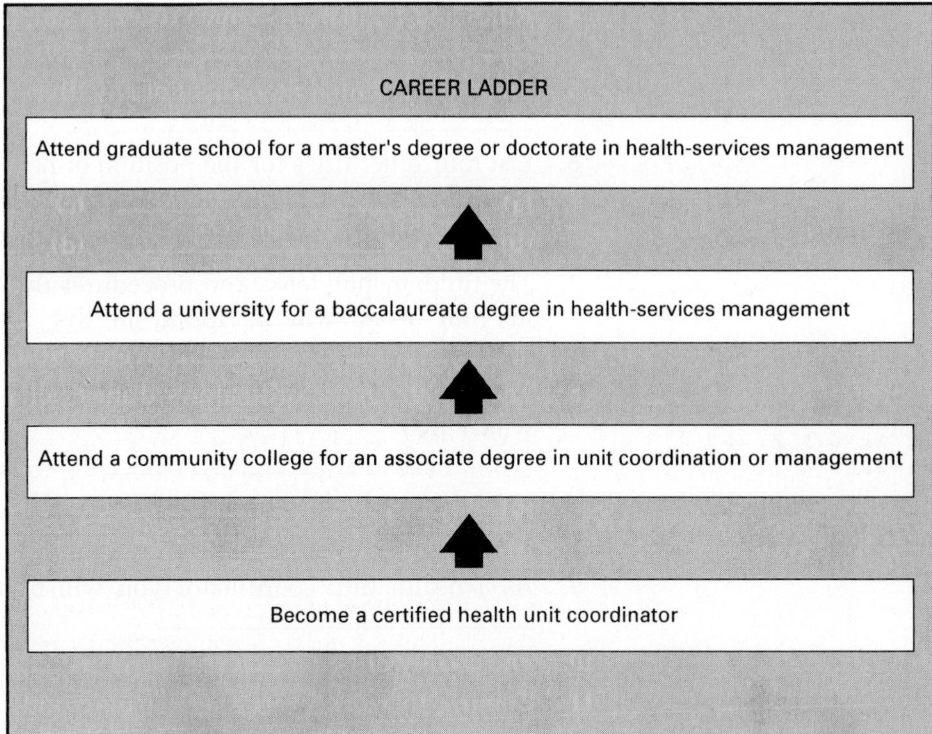

CAREER LADDER
Attend graduate school for a master's degree or doctorate in health-services management
Attend a university for a baccalaureate degree in health-services management
Attend a community college for an associate degree in unit coordination or management
Become a certified health unit coordinator

Figure 1–5

NAHUC, like other professional organizations, requires contact hours for recertification. A variety of continuing education opportunities are available through NAHUC.

LEARNING ACTIVITIES

Complete the following:

1. The most important person in the hospital is the ______________________.
2. The name of the national professional association for health unit coordinators is the ______________________.
3. List 10 qualifications of an excellent health unit coordinator.
   (a) ______________________
   (b) ______________________
   (c) ______________________
   (d) ______________________
   (e) ______________________
   (f) ______________________
   (g) ______________________
   (h) ______________________
   (i) ______________________
   (j) ______________________

4. Rules and regulations which relate to employment are called ______________________________.

5. The most essential ingredient of any dress code is ______________________________.

6. List four other titles for the position of health unit coordinator.
   (a) ______________________________ (c) ______________________________
   (b) ______________________________ (d) ______________________________

7. The fundamental tasks and procedures that you will be accountable for in your work will be found in the ______________________________ ______________________________ given to you by your employing hospital.

8. The health unit coordinator's duties fall under three main categories which are
   (a) ______________________________
   (b) ______________________________
   (c) ______________________________

9. As a health unit coordinator you will be under the supervision of a ______________________________.

10. The quality of being exact or correct is ______________________________.

11. Coming to work every day on time and doing what is asked at the proper time and in the proper way is called ______________________________.

12. A method of advancement through experience and education is called a ______________________________.

13. What does CHUC stand for? ______________________________.

CHAPTER 2
The Working Environment

THE HEALTH CARE INSTITUTION

OBJECTIVES

When you have completed this chapter, you will be able to:

- Explain the purposes, organization, and classifications of hospitals.
- Discuss the responsibilities of the medical staff.
- Define common medical specialties.
- Describe how the business side of health care is changing.
- Discuss the responsibilities of various levels of nursing personnel.
- Identify abbreviations and definitions of the various nursing units.
- Describe three ways of organizing the nursing health care team.
- Describe the primary functions of the various hospital departments.
- Discuss important practices for good staff relationships.
- Discuss the purpose and some contributions of the volunteer services.

KEY IDEA: HOSPITAL HISTORY

The history of medicine and surgery dates back to the earliest ages, since there has been some form of hospital for centuries. The word hospital stems from the Latin *hospitalis*—relating to a quest—one of the most ancient expressions of people's concern for a stranger. In ancient Greece, temples were used to house the sick, and the first church hospital was built in A.D. 369 at Ceesarea (now a part of Turkey). As Christianity spread, the sick became the concern of the church. Monasteries established hospitals for lepers, cripples, the blind, and the poor.

The first established hospitals were founded in the United States in the early eighteenth century. As medical knowledge grew, hospitals developed from the early crude establishments to our modern sophisticated institutions.

Today's hospital is a health team, a source of hope, a center for community health, an educational institution, and a laboratory; it is a provider of many different types of service—all of them important.

KEY IDEA: FUNCTIONS AND PURPOSES OF HOSPITALS

There are several basic functions and purposes of health care institutions, all of them having to do either with the immediate care of patients or with the health of the community—present and future. These purposes include:

- Giving expert care to the sick and injured
- Preventing disease
- Promoting individual and community health
- Providing facilities for the education of health workers
- Promoting research in the sciences of medicine and nursing

KEY IDEA: ACCREDITATION

Hospitals that are accredited have met a standard by complying with a variety of rules and regulations set forth by the accrediting agency.

The *Joint Commission on Accreditation of Health Care Organizations (JCAHO)* is a highly coveted accreditation. A JCAHO health care institution has been visited by a team of surveyors, evaluated, and approved as a hospital which is meeting high standards of operation.

There are several other accreditation agencies which also survey and evaluate health care institutions. Licensing of hospitals is usually a function of the State Department of Health.

Preparation for accreditation can be a stressful time for a hospital, and the health unit coordinator must appreciate the seriousness of the event and assist in any way possible. The JCAHO accredits over 16,000 hospitals and other health care facilities.

KEY IDEA: CLASSIFICATIONS

Hospitals are classified most commonly by ownership or type of service offered.

Ownership. Hospitals may be privately owned (groups of doctors-corporations) and operated for profit, community operated, owned by churches and fraternal organizations, or by the government.

Type of Service. There are many different kinds of hospitals. The most common is the general hospital which offers a variety of patient care services to persons of all ages. Specialized hospitals restrict their services to certain age groups (i.e., children or the elderly) or to those requiring a specialized type of care (i.e., orthopedic, maternal, psychiatric).

KEY IDEA: THE BUSINESS SIDE OF HEALTH CARE

Hospitals must be very business minded in their delivery of health care. In response to skyrocketing health costs the government, insurance companies, and employers have placed intense pressure on hospitals and doctors to provide health care in a cost-effective manner. There have been and will continue to be significant changes in the way health care is provided and financed in this nation.

Because cost containment is such a major concern, the government in 1983 implemented a payment system requiring that Medicare payments for hospital inpatient services be paid under a prospective payment system based on Diagnosis Related Groups (DRGs). With DRGs, patient's diseases and disorders are clustered into almost 475 groups with a payment level specified for each group. Hospitals are reimbursed a flat rate which allows both payers and the hospital to predict reimbursement before the care is provided (prospectively). This is why this type of reimbursement is called a prospective payment system (PPS). DRGs provide a basis for payment to hospitals for care of Medicare, Medicaid, and an increasing number of patients with commercial insurance. It serves as an important tool in cost containment and in hospital utilization (how long patients stay in the hospital).

Managed care is a system of health care designed to control costs. There are many types of managed care organizations (MCOs) and arrangements. Some common examples include:

- *Health Maintenance Organizations (HMOs)*—systems of health care in which a fixed sum is prepaid and after which health services are made available to the patient at a reduced rate. The kinds of services available and the reimbursement levels are outlined in the contract with the HMO. HMOs emphasize preventive medicine.
- *Preferred Provider Organizations (PPOs)*—a non-HMO type of managed care that contracts to provide care at a reduced rate that is usually more than for an HMO patient but less than regular commercial insurance would pay.
- *Independent Practice Association (IPA)*—an organization of providers who contract with payers at a discounted or capitated rate. (Money is paid based on number of enrolled patients rather than on number of services rendered.)
- *Point-of-Service Plan (POS)*—a plan that allows the patients considerable leeway in their choice of providers but provides greater reimbursement if they use a network provider.

Forty-one million or 17.4 percent of the United States population is without insurance. This has placed tremendous financial stress on hospitals who continue to provide care to the uninsured.

All health care workers must realize that cost-containment practices are an essential part of their job. The health unit coordinator should understand that because of DRGs and managed care, hospitals must do everything possible to legally obtain the reimbursement they are due. From admission to discharge great care must be taken by the hospital personnel to properly record charges and follow policies and procedures set forth by the hospital so that it can be reimbursed for the care that is given. A hospital simply cannot survive without this cooperation from its staff.

There are other trends which affect the way health care is provided. The American population as a whole is getting older. According to the American Association of Retired People (AARP), since the turn of the century the percentage of people in the United States over 65 has tripled. People over the age of 65 are expected to represent 20 percent of the population by the year 2030. The fastest-growing group of people are those over age 85 (29 times larger than in 1900). The implications of these statistics are fairly clear. The longer people live, the more health care services will be needed. This will result in more demand for community-based programs and increased public pressure for protection against the costs of long-term care. More and more emphasis will be placed on preventive health care. We have already seen the shift from inpatient to ambulatory care settings, which has resulted in a high acuity level for hospitalized patients. *Acuity* refers to how sick a patient is and/or how much nursing care is required.

There is competition for patients today, and health care workers must realize that marketing of the hospitals' services has become increasingly important. Hospitals strive constantly to identify, understand, and meet the needs of their patients and expand their visibility in the community.

The business side of health care affects health care workers who strive to provide quality care in a rapidly changing environment. The health unit coordinator must recognize that cost-containment practices are an essential part of the job and understand the importance of such procedures as coding (the assignment of numbers and letters to diagnoses and procedures for billing purposes) and utilization review (the determination of the appropriateness of care and length of service for a hospitalized patient) which are performed by other members of the hospital staff.

Changes in health care delivery systems may create new duties for the health unit coordinator with greater emphasis on business and management practices and increasing use of information systems.

KEY IDEA: ORGANIZATION

Health care institutions are comparable to business organizations in their division of functions. Most are governed by a board of directors (i.e., persons from the business and professional community who establish general policies, approve the budget, and hire the hospital administrator).

The hospital administrator is in charge of the hospital and functions much as the president of a business does. With the aid of one or more assistant administrators, often called vice presidents, the hospital administrator handles the day-to-day operation of the hospital and carries out the policies of the board.

Each hospital will have its own organizational chart which will vary somewhat depending upon the type and ownership of the facility. (Fig. 2–1.)

THE MEDICAL STAFF

KEY IDEA: RESPONSIBILITIES

The medical staff is responsible for the diagnosis and treatment of the hospitalized patient. It is the doctor who orders the laboratory tests, the radiographs, and other diagnostic examinations; the doctor also prescribes the patient's medications and other therapy.

In many hospitals you will be working with licensed physicians, residents, interns, and medical students. However, the care of all private patients is assumed by attending physicians—that is, by licensed physicians who are either family practitioners or specialists.

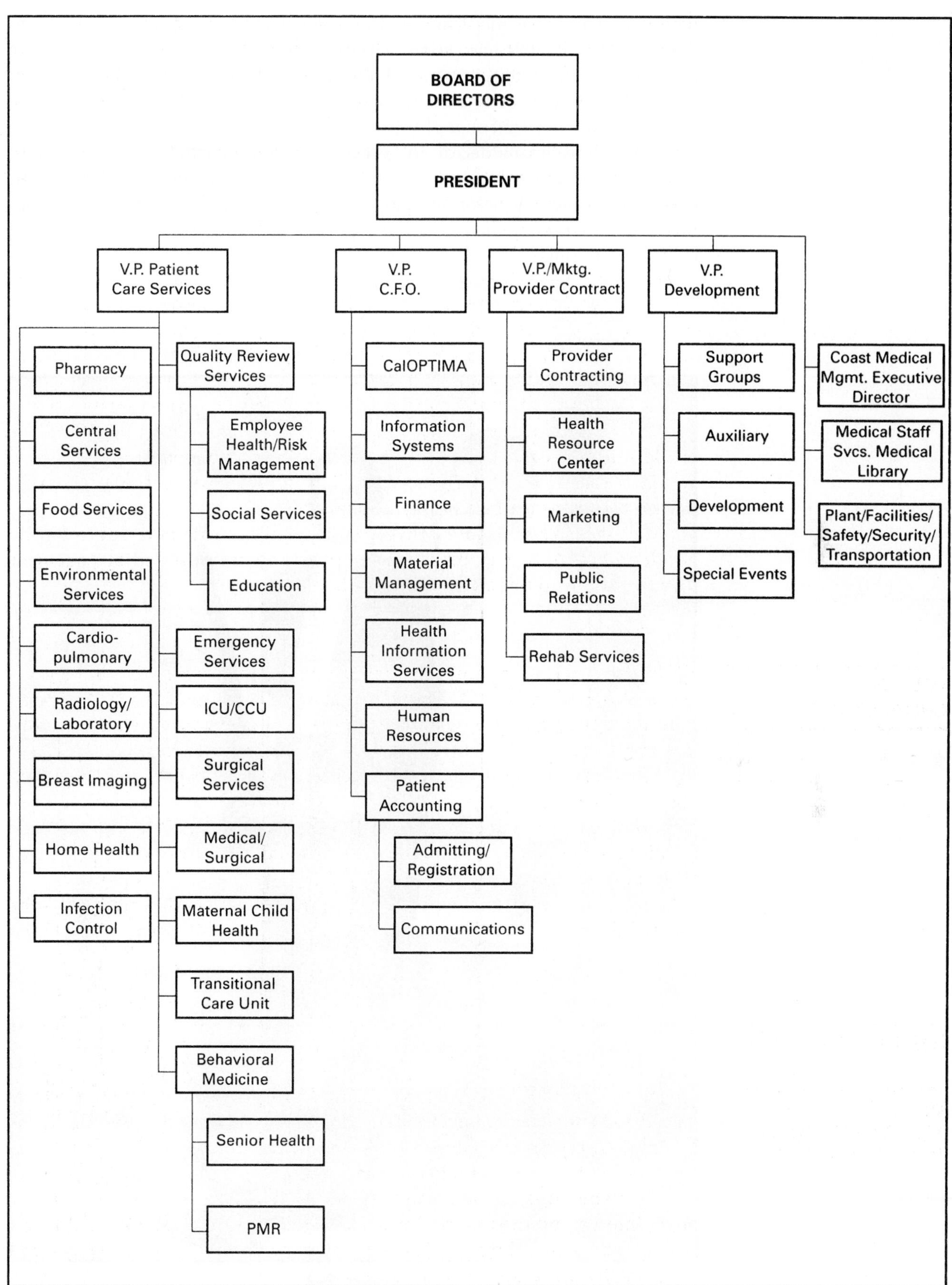

Figure 2–1 Hospital organizational chart.

KEY IDEA: EDUCATION

In order to practice medicine, a doctor must meet rigid educational standards. Although there are some variations, commonly a doctor must have graduated from college, completed a four-year course in medical school, and served for one year as a resident gaining hospital experience. After this, the doctor may be licensed as a physician by passing a state board examination.

Many physicians decide to specialize in some particular field of medicine. To do so the doctor must devote several years gaining further experience in the specialty he or she has chosen. Then the doctor becomes recognized to practice medicine in that specialty by passing a national board examination. (Fig. 2–2.)

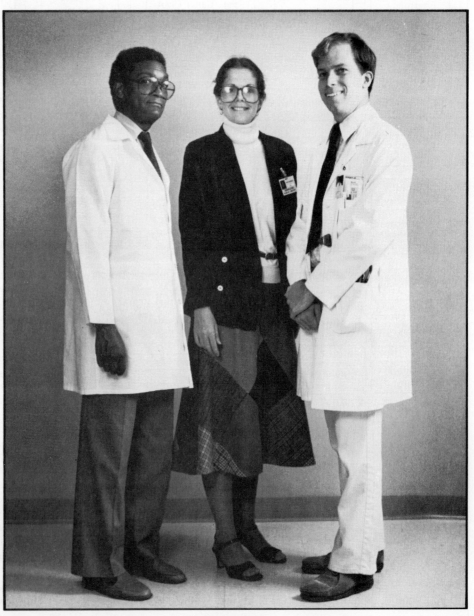

Figure 2–2

KEY IDEA: MEDICAL SPECIALTIES

A medical specialty is a branch of knowledge concerning a certain part of the body—its diseases, conditions, and treatments. A medical specialist is a physician who is devoted to a single branch of medical knowledge. You will hear medical specialties referred to in conversation by doctors and nurses. Since the health unit coordinator has a great deal of interaction with the medical staff, it will be helpful for you to know the definitions of the terms you will hear.

Table 2–1 lists definitions of most of the present-day medical specialties and the standard title of the physician practicing in those specialties.

TABLE 2–1

Medical Specialties

Specialty	*Physician's Title*	*Description*
Allergies	Allergist	A subspecialty of internal medicine dealing with diagnosis and treatment of body reactions resulting from unusual sensitivity to foods, pollens, dust, medicines, or other substances
Anesthesiology	Anesthesiologist	Administration of various forms of anesthesia in operations or procedures to cause loss of feeling or sensation
Cardiovascular diseases; Cardiology	Cardiologist	A subspecialty of internal medicine involving the diagnosis and treatment of diseases of the heart and blood vessels
Dermatology	Dermatologist	Diagnosis and treatment of diseases of the skin
Emergencies	Emergency physician	Deals with immediate-urgent care of patient in emergency rooms and emergency clinics
Endocrinology	Endocrinologist	Diagnosis and treatment of diseases of the hormone-secreting ductless glands
Family practice	Family practitioner	Diagnosis and treatment of disease by medical and surgical methods for all members of the family regardless of age
Gastroenterology	Gastroenterologist	A subspecialty of internal medicine concerned with diagnosis and treatment of disorders of the digestive tract
General surgery	Surgeon	The diagnosis and treatment of disease by surgical means without limitation to special systems or body regions
Gynecology	Gynecologist	Diagnosis and treatment of diseases of the female reproductive organs
Hematology	Hematologist	Diagnosis and treatment of diseases of the blood and blood-forming tissues
Internal medicine	Internist	The diagnosis and nonsurgical treatment of adults
Nephrology	Nephrologist	The diagnosis and treatment of diseases of the kidney

(*continued*)

TABLE 2-1 (*Continued*)

Specialty	*Physician's Title*	*Description*
Neurological surgery	Neurosurgeon	Diagnosis and surgical treatment of brain, spinal cord, and nerve disorders
Neurology	Neurologist	Diagnosis and treatment of diseases of brain, spinal cord, and nerves
Obstetrics	Obstetrician	The care of women during pregnancy, childbirth, and the interval immediately following
Oncology	Oncologist	Diagnosis and treatment of cancer
Ophthalmology	Ophthalmologist	Diagnosis and treatment of diseases of the eye, including prescribing glasses
Orthopedics	Orthopedist	Diagnosis and treatment of disorders and diseases of the muscular and skeletal systems
Otolaryngology	Otolaryngologist	Diagnosis and treatment of diseases of the ear, nose, and throat
Pathology	Pathologist	Study and interpretation of changes in organs, tissues, cells, and alterations in body chemistry to aid in diagnosing disease and determining treatment
Pediatrics	Pediatrician	Prevention, diagnosis, and treatment of children's diseases
Physical medicine and rehabilitation	Physiatrist	Diagnosis of disease or injury in the various systems and areas of the body and treatment by means of physical procedures as well as treatment and restoration of the convalescent and physically handicapped patient
Plastic surgery	Plastic surgeon	Corrective or reparative surgery to restore deformed or mutilated parts of the body or to improve the appearance of a part of the body (cosmetic surgery)
Proctology	Proctologist	Diagnosis and treatment of diseases of the rectum
Psychiatry	Psychiatrist	Diagnosis and treatment of mental disorders
Radiology	Radiologist	Use of radiant energy including x-rays, radium, cobalt, etc., in the diagnosis of disease
Rheumatology	Rheumatologist	Diagnosis and treatment of rheumatic disorders such as arthritis, gout, bursitis, and other conditions
Therapeutic radiology	Radiologist	The use of radiant energy, including x-rays, radium, and other radioactive substances in the treatment of diseases
Thoracic surgery	Thoracic surgeon	Operative treatment of the lungs, heart, or the large blood vessels within the chest cavity
Urology	Urologist	Diagnosis and treatment of diseases or disorders of the kidneys, bladder, ureters, urethra, and of the male reproductive organs

KEY IDEA: OTHER HEALTH PROFESSIONALS

Not all doctors with whom the health unit coordinator will come in contact are M.D.'s (medical doctors). Table 2–2 lists other specialties. Your hospital will have strict policies regarding the scope of practice for these individuals.

THE NURSING STAFF

KEY IDEA: NURSING STAFF RESPONSIBILITIES

Nursing personnel are responsible for carrying out the doctors' orders and giving nursing care to the patient. Nursing service plans and implements nursing care, observes the patient and records these observations, coordinates care and activities performed by other departments, conducts family and patient teaching, and works closely with the doctor in the care and rehabilitation of the hospitalized patient.

Recent revisions to nurse practice acts have expanded the role of the registered nurse, and broader definitions of nursing interpret the nurse as a colleague of the physician rather than as an assistant.

As a health unit coordinator, you are usually part of the nursing department. It is important that you understand the structure and function of nursing service and the roles of nursing service personnel. (Figs. 2–3 and 2–4.)

TABLE 2–2

Other Health Professionals

Doctor of Osteopathy (DO)	A health professional who has earned a degree by satisfactorily completing a course of education in an approved college of osteopathy. Osteopathic physicians follow almost identical courses of training and practice as medical physicians but emphasize treatment that involves manipulation of structures and the study of mechanic derangement of tissues as a cause of disease.
Doctor of Chiropractic (DC)	Provides treatment through the mechanical manipulation of the spinal column, physiotherapy, and diet. May diagnose through the use of radiology but does not employ surgery or drugs. Completes at least two years of premedical school followed by four years of education in an approved chiropractic school.
Podiatrist (DPM)	A health professional licensed to diagnose and treat diseases of the feet. Performs surgery, prescribes drugs and physical therapy. Completes at least two years of premedical courses and four years of study in an accredited college of podiatry and is awarded a DPM (Doctor of Podiatric Medicine).
Psychologist	A professional who specializes in the study of behavior and the processes of the mind especially in regard to the environment, both social and physical. A clinical psychologist has earned a graduate degree in psychology and training in clinical psychology and is qualified to provide testing and counseling services.
Optometrist	Holds a degree of Doctor of Optometry (OD) and is licensed after at least two years of college and four years in an approved college of optometry to test the eyes for visual acuity and prescribe corrective lenses.
Dentist	Practices the prevention and treatment of diseases and disorders of the teeth and oral cavity. Can prescribe pain medications, antibiotics, and some other medications that require prescriptions. Completes at least two years of undergraduate study and three to four years at an approved dental college and then may be awarded a DDS (Doctor of Dental Surgery). There are eight recognized specialties which require advanced training.

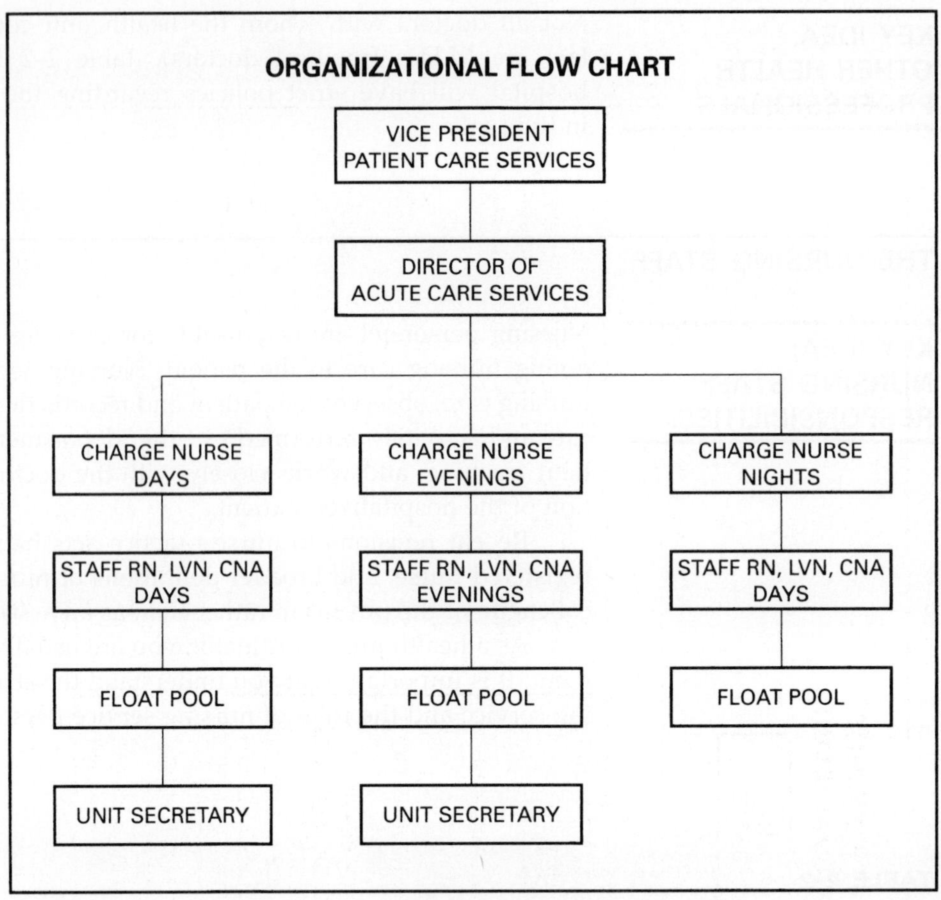

Figure 2–3

KEY IDEA: NURSING SERVICE ADMINISTRATIVE PERSONNEL

Administrative nursing personnel are registered nurses who usually have obtained advanced degrees such as BSN (Bachelor of Science in Nursing), MSN (Master of Science in Nursing), or doctorate degrees.

It is not uncommon for there to be changes in terminology to denote certain responsibilities within a hospital. For example, some hospitals refer to the head of the nursing department as the **Director of Nursing (DON)** while others call that position the **Vice President of Patient Services.** Figures 2–3 and 2–4 show two examples of organizational charts for nursing.

The Vice President of Patient Services (or Director of Nursing) is responsible for the administration of Nursing Service and is accountable to the hospital's President or Chief Administrator. An Assistant Vice President of Patient Services (or Assistant Director of Nursing) assists the Director of Nursing and assumes those duties when the Director is absent.

A **nursing supervisor** assists the Director of Nursing in carrying out administrative responsibilities and is responsible to the Director of Nursing. A hospital, depending upon its size, will employ several nursing supervisors to work on each shift so that nursing administration is represented at all times.

The **Director of Education** is responsible for the continuing education and staff development of nursing service personnel, the orientation of new nursing service personnel, and may be responsible for all hospital staff inservice. The Director of Education is responsible to the Director of Nursing.

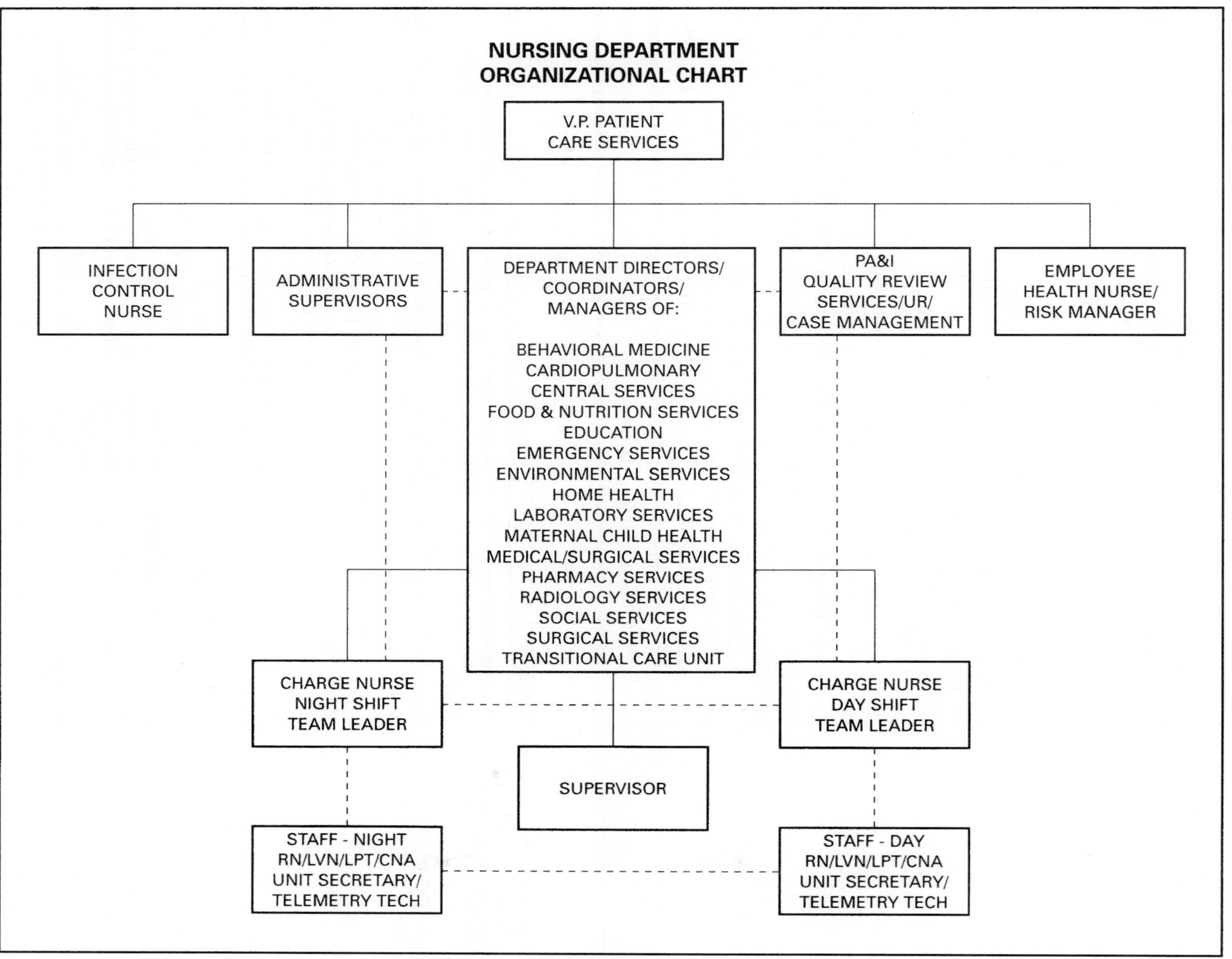
NURSING DEPARTMENT
ORGANIZATIONAL CHART
V.P. PATIENT CARE SERVICES
INFECTION CONTROL NURSE
ADMINISTRATIVE SUPERVISORS
DEPARTMENT DIRECTORS/ COORDINATORS/ MANAGERS OF:
BEHAVIORAL MEDICINE
CARDIOPULMONARY
CENTRAL SERVICES
FOOD & NUTRITION SERVICES
EDUCATION
EMERGENCY SERVICES
ENVIRONMENTAL SERVICES
HOME HEALTH
LABORATORY SERVICES
MATERNAL CHILD HEALTH
MEDICAL/SURGICAL SERVICES
PHARMACY SERVICES
RADIOLOGY SERVICES
SOCIAL SERVICES
SURGICAL SERVICES
TRANSITIONAL CARE UNIT
PA&I QUALITY REVIEW SERVICES/UR/ CASE MANAGEMENT
EMPLOYEE HEALTH NURSE/ RISK MANAGER
CHARGE NURSE NIGHT SHIFT TEAM LEADER
CHARGE NURSE DAY SHIFT TEAM LEADER
SUPERVISOR
STAFF - NIGHT RN/LVN/LPT/CNA UNIT SECRETARY/ TELEMETRY TECH
STAFF - DAY RN/LVN/LPT/CNA UNIT SECRETARY/ TELEMETRY TECH

Figure 2–4

KEY IDEA: NURSING UNIT PERSONNEL

A **registered nurse (RN)** is a graduate of a two- to four-year school of nursing, has passed a state board examination, and is licensed by the state in which he or she is practicing nursing. Many registered nurses are college graduates who have obtained the BSN, MSN, or other advanced degrees. Many nursing specialties require certification. An ACLS means that the nurse is qualified in Advanced Cardiac Life Support. A CCRN is a registered nurse who is certified by the American Association of Critical Care Nurses Certification Corporation.

Licensed Nurses

A **head nurse** (nurse manager or coordinator) is a registered nurse who has managerial responsibilities for a particular nursing unit throughout the 24-hour day. The head nurse usually works the day shift and is responsible to nursing administration.

A **charge nurse** assumes managerial responsibility for a particular unit on the evening or night shift or on the day shift in the absence of the head nurse. The charge nurse is directly responsible to the head nurse.

A **staff nurse** is a registered nurse who is able to do complete patient care and all nursing diagnosis, treatments, and other procedures, and often functions as a team leader.

A **graduate nurse (GN)** is one who is working while waiting for the results of the state board examination to become a registered nurse.

A **licensed vocational nurse (LVN)** or **licensed practical nurse (LPN)** is a graduate of a one-year nursing program, has passed a state board examination for vocational nurses, and is licensed in the state in which he or she practices. This level of nurse works under the supervision of a registered nurse and

Professional Nursing Specialties

Certified Registered Nurse Anesthetist (CRNA)	**A registered nurse who has been specially trained through postgraduate training and can administer various types of anesthetics.**
Nurse Practitioner	**Has acquired advanced skills through education and training. If specialization is in family health, may be called Family Nurse Practitioner (FNP); if in pediatrics, Pediatric Nurse Practitioner (PNP).**
Nurse-midwife	**Specializes in care of the pregnant woman from conception through the postpartum period. A registered nurse who has completed an approved nurse-midwifery program may be called a Certified Nurse Midwife (CNM). Certification denotes the passing of an examination.**
Community Health Nurse	**Public Health Nurse who works in the community to promote and provide health care.**
Clinical Nurse Specialist	**A registered nurse with advanced training and knowledge with a master's degree in nursing and a high degree of competence in a specialized area of nursing.**
Clinician	**A registered nurse with demonstrated expertise in nursing practice and a baccalaureate degree in nursing.**
Nurse Epidemiologist or Infection Control Nurse	**A registered nurse trained in the tracking and prevention of nosocomial (hospital-acquired) infections.**

provides patient care including treatment and administration of medications prescribed by the physician. Many states have career ladder programs which offer the LVN or LPN the opportunity, with further education, to take the RN state board examination and advance to the status of registered nurse.

Nonlicensed Nursing Personnel

Nursing assistants perform basic patient care and bedside tasks for the patient under the supervision of a registered nurse.

An **orderly** is a male nursing assistant who usually performs the same tasks as a nursing assistant but may have expanded duties such as responsibility for orthopedic equipment and certain male surgical preps (shaves) and catheterizations.

Nursing assistants and orderlies are trained on the job, through a vocational school, or at the beginning level of a career ladder program at a community college.

Certified Nursing Assistants (CNAs) have graduated from a training program with prescribed hours and have met certain other standards. (Fig. 2–5.)

THE NURSING HEALTH CARE TEAM

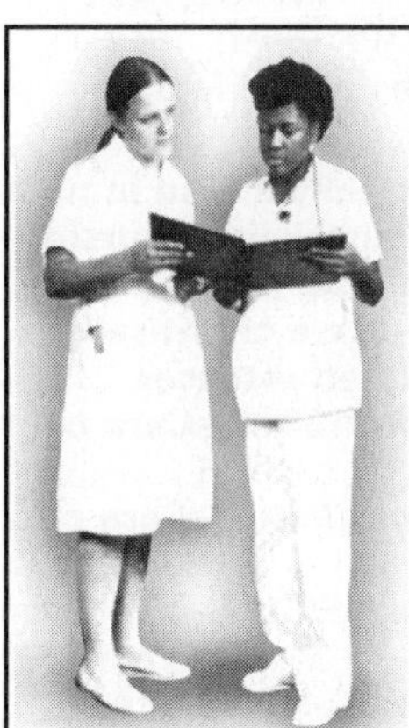

PROFESSIONAL REGISTERED NURSE

Four-year university education with a bachelor's degree
or
Two-year junior or community college education with an associate degree
or
Three-year diploma from a hospital nursing school
and
Passed state board examinations

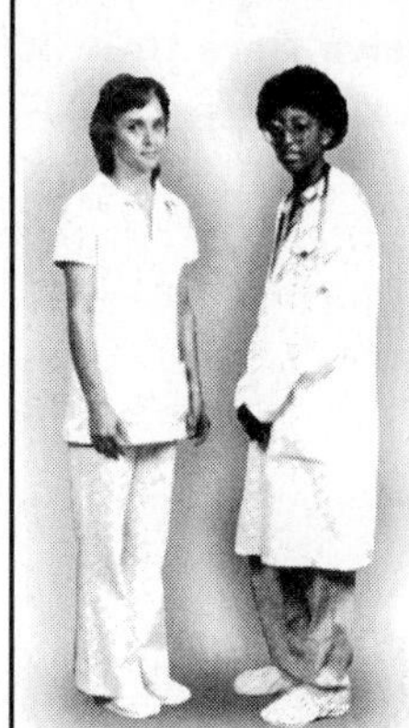

LICENSED PRACTICAL NURSE (LPN)
or
LICENSED VOCATIONAL NURSE (LVN)

One-year training program

Passed state board examinations

PLPN–Pharmaceutical Licensed Practical Nurse is one who administers drugs or medications after taking a special course and passing a special examination

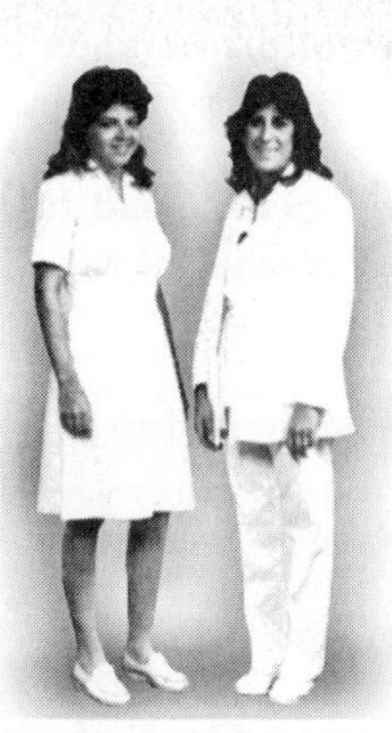

CERTIFIED NURSING ASSISTANT
NURSING ASSISTANT
NURSE'S AIDE
HOME HEALTH AIDE
GERIATRIC AIDE
ORDERLY
PATIENT CARE TECHNICIAN

All are names used for the nonprofessional worker who, under the direction and supervision of the registered nurses, carries out basic bedside nursing functions

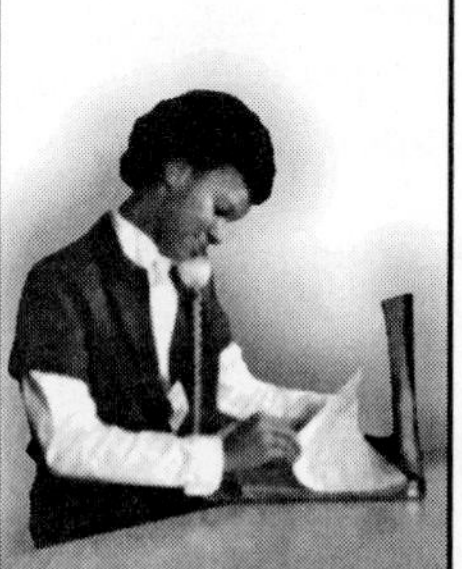

HEALTH UNIT COORDINATOR

Works at the desk of the nurses' station
- Does clerical work
- Answers the telephone at the nurses' station
- Helps to direct traffic on the floor
- Processes doctor's orders

Figure 2–5

Patient Care Technician (PCT) may be referred to as an advanced nursing assistant. The PCT provides basic care to the patient as well as being able to perform other procedures such as electrocardiograms, drawing blood (phlebotomy), and performing simple testing of specimens at the bedside. Additional tasks of the PCT may include certain procedures requiring the use of sterile technique such as simple dressing changes. The PCT may obtain skills that allow him or her to perform certain HUC functions in the absence of the health unit coordinator.

KEY IDEA: NURSING UNITS

Hospitals are divided into various nursing units according to the type of service provided to the patient (Tables 2–3 and 2–4). As a health unit coordinator, you will be assigned to a nursing unit and during the course of your em-

TABLE 2–3

Nursing Units

Unit	*Function*
Alcoholic Rehabilitation	**Care of patients receiving treatment for alcoholic abuse**
Eyes, Ears, Nose, and Throat (EENT)	**Care of patients with medical and surgical conditions in these parts of the body**
Gynecology (GYN)	**Care of women with diseases of the female reproductive system**
Intensive Care Unit (ICU)	**Care of patients who are critically ill and in need of constant supervision and specialized nursing care. May be further divided into:** • ***Coronary Care Unit (CCU)*—Care of critically ill patients with heart and related diseases** • ***Medical Intensive Care Unit (MICU)*—Care of critically ill medical patients** • ***Pediatric Intensive Care Unit (PICU)*—Care of critically ill children** • ***Surgical Intensive Care Unit (SICU)*—Care of critically ill surgical patients** • ***Neonatal ICU*—Intensive care of newborn**
Medical (Med)	**Care of patients with medical (nonsurgical) conditions**
Neurology (Neuro)	**Care of patients with diseases of the nervous system**
Nursery	**Care of newborn infants**
Obstetrics (OB)	**Care of women who are having, or have had, babies**
Orthopedics (Ortho)	**Care of patients with injury or disease of the musculoskeletal system**
Pediatrics (Peds)	**Care of children**
Psychiatry (Psych)	**Care of patients with mental and emotional disorders**
Rehabilitation (Rehab)	**Care of patients receiving treatment for physical handicaps**
Surgical (Surg)	**Care of patients who will undergo or have undergone surgery**
Transitional Care Unit (TCU)	**Care of patients requiring a reduced level of care**
Urology	**Care of patients with diseases of the urinary system and males with diseases of the reproductive tract**

ployment, you may work on several different ones. Some health unit coordinators are not assigned to a single unit but move throughout the hospital as the need arises. The term for this is "floating," and the unit coordinator who is given the opportunity to float will learn many new and interesting things about the medical field.

A large hospital may include even more divisions than those that have been listed. In all of the units thus described, the hospitalized patient is an inpatient and will receive 24-hour nursing care. There are other specialized units within a hospital in which a health unit coordinator may be employed where a patient will receive care before being either transferred to one of the units listed or in some cases discharged.

KEY IDEA: PATIENT CARE ASSIGNMENTS

Since health unit coordinators frequently need to communicate information to the nurse caring for a patient, they need to be aware of the type of patient care assignment used by the nursing unit. The nursing health care team in your hospital may be organized in one of the following ways:

Primary Nursing or Total Patient Care. Primary nursing is a method of patient care delivery in which the professional nurse is responsible and accountable for the entire nursing care of the patient. This is a patient-oriented system, and the purpose is to ensure that the professional nurse works directly with the patient—planning, implementing, and evaluating the patient's nursing care. Primary nursing is usually the type of patient care assignment employed in the critical care units and is used throughout hospitals in many parts of the country.

TABLE 2–4

Specialized Units

Unit	*Function*
Emergency Room (ER)	**Care of patients needing emergency treatment for diseases or injuries that have occurred outside of the hospital.**
Labor and Delivery (L&D)	**Care of women who are in labor or are delivering babies.**
Medical Short Stay Unit (MSSU)	**Care of medical patients requiring care and stabilization for less than 24 hours.**
Outpatient Department (OPD)	**Care of patients seen in a clinic setting for disorders not requiring hospitalization.**
Outpatient Surgery	**Care of patients having minor surgery that does not require overnight hospitalization.**
Operating Room (OR)	**Care of patients undergoing surgery.**
Postanesthetic Care Unit (PACU)	**Also called the Recovery Room. Provides care of patients immediately after surgery until condition stabilizes and they can return to nursing unit.**
Renal Dialysis	**Care of patients with kidney disorders who require artificial devices to maintain kidney function and sustain life.**
Trauma Unit	**Immediate surgical care of injured patients by special team of physicians and nurses.**

Team Nursing. The head nurse or charge nurse divides the staff into teams. Each team has a leader. The head nurse or charge nurse assigns a group of patients to each team. The team leader (usually an RN) then assigns patients for each team member to care for during the shift. Team members may be RNs, LPNs or LVNs, NAs, orderlies, or students. The team leader is teacher, adviser, and helper to all team members.

Whatever the method of patient care assignment, as a health unit coordinator you must know *which nurse is caring for which patient.* To determine this, you will refer to a patient care assignment sheet which is made out each day for each shift indicating the member of the nursing team that is assigned to each patient. These assignment sheets are posted at the nurse's station for your easy reference. (Fig. 2–6.)

Unless your hospital utilizes primary nursing or total patient care assignments and employs only RNs, you must take this process one step further. You must be able to determine which information and requests to communicate to the RN, which to the LVN or LPN, and which to the NA.

To help you in these decisions you must know what these individuals with various levels of education in nursing may do. Remember:

- **Registered nurses** perform all nursing care procedures and treatments, give medications, start and monitor IVs (intravenous administration),

PATIENT CARE ASSIGNMENT SHEET

Head Nurse — Date

Health Unit Coordinator — Shift

TEAM 1		TEAM 2	
Team Leader	J. Jones, R.N.	Team Leader	P. Pearl, R.N.
Rm. 130, 131, 132, 133	T. Smith N.A.	Rm. 139A, B, C, 140, 141	D. Stevens N.A.
134A, B, C, 135	L. Grace N.A	142, 143, 144, 145	G. Bullock N.A.
136, 137, 138	T. Johnson L.P.N.	146, 147, 148	S. Tall N.A.

(NOTE: Patient names are often included on the assignment sheet as well as room numbers.)

Figure 2–6

and take and implement doctors' orders verbally, in writing, and by telephone. Registered nurses supervise other nursing personnel.

- **LVNs and LPNs** perform most of the procedures that RNs perform. In acute care hospitals, LVNs and LPNs are usually not in supervisory positions; however, in extended care facilities in some states, LPNs/LVNs may function in that capacity. You must learn the policies of your hospital and determine the policy of your unit so that you will know which information to communicate to the LVN/LPN and which to the RN.
- **Nursing assistants** perform basic patient care. They *do not* give medication, *do not* take doctors' orders, *do not* perform sterile techniques, and *do not* start IVs. Also, they do not function in supervisory roles.
- **Volunteers** give their services without pay. Although they do not actually care for the patients, they contribute to the patients' comfort and well-being in many ways such as arranging flowers, reading to patients, and writing letters. "Candy-stripers," and other high school students, give their time after school and on weekends. Adult volunteers may escort patients, deliver messages, or run library and gift carts. They also raise money for the hospital through gift shops and hospital benefits.

LEARNING ACTIVITIES

Complete the following:

1. The five functions and purposes of the hospital are
   (a) ______________________
   (b) ______________________
   (c) ______________________
   (d) ______________________
   (e) ______________________
2. List the two ways hospitals are most commonly classified.
   (a) ______________________
   (b) ______________________
3. The meeting of an official standard by a hospital is called ______________________.

Match the following medical specialists in column A with the description of the specialty in column B.

Column A	*Column B*
(a) Allergist	____ The care of women during pregnancy, childbirth, and the interval immediately following
(b) Anesthesiologist	
(c) Cardiologist	____ Diagnosis and treatment of mental disorders
(d) Oncologist	____ A subspecialty of internal medicine dealing with diagnosis and treatment of body reactions resulting from unusual sensitivity to foods, pollens, dust, medicines, or other substances
(e) Dermatologist	
(f) Internist	
(g) Orthopedist	

Column A	*Column B*
(h) Neurologist	____ Diagnosis and treatment of diseases of the kidneys, bladder, ureters, urethra, and of the male reproductive organs
(i) Obstetrician	____ Diagnosis and treatment of diseases of the eye, including prescribing glasses
(j) Gynecologist	____ A subspecialty of internal medicine involving the diagnosis and treatment of disease of the heart and blood vessels
(k) Ophthalmologist	____ Use of radiant energy including x-rays, radium, cobalt, etc. in the diagnosis of disease
(l) Pathologist	____ Administration of various forms of anesthesia in operations or diagnosis to cause loss of feeling or sensation
(m) Pediatrician	____ The diagnosis and nonsurgical treatment of illnesses of adults
(n) Psychiatrist	____ Diagnosis and treatment of cancer
(o) Plastic surgeon	____ Diagnosis and treatment of disorders and diseases of the muscular and skeletal systems
(p) Radiologist	____ Prevention, diagnosis, and treatment of children's diseases
(q) Urologist	____ Diagnosis and treatment of diseases of brain, spinal cord, and nerve disorders
	____ Diagnosis and treatment of diseases of the female reproductive organs
	____ Corrective or reparative surgery to restore deformed or mutilated parts of the body
	____ Study and interpretation of changes in organs, tissues, cells, and alterations in body chemistry to aid in diagnosing disease and determining treatment
	____ Diagnosis and treatment of diseases of the skin

Complete the following statements regarding nursing personnel:

1. The ____________________ is responsible for the overall administration of nursing service.
2. The ____________________ is responsible for the continuing education and staff development of nursing service personnel and the orientation of new nursing service personnel.
3. The ____________________ has managerial responsibilities for a particular nursing unit throughout the 24-hour day.
4. The ____________________ has graduated from a one-year program and is licensed by the state to give direct patient care and perform less technical skills than the RN.
5. The ____________________ is not licensed and performs basic treatments and bedside tasks for the patient.

Write the correct abbreviation for each of the following nursing units in the space provided.

1. Medical ______
2. Surgical ______
3. Obstetrics ______
4. Gynecology ______
5. Orthopedics ______
6. Pediatrics ______
7. Neurology ______
8. Psychiatry ______
9. Intensive care ______
10. Coronary care ______
11. Operating room ______
12. Emergency room ______
13. Transitional care unit ______

Complete the following:

1. The nursing health care team in your institution may be organized in which of the following ways?
   (a) ______
   (b) ______
2. To determine which nurse is caring for which patient, the health unit coordinator will refer to the ______.
3. List six practices for good staff relationships:
   (a) ______
   (b) ______
   (c) ______
   (d) ______
   (e) ______
   (f) ______

True or False. Circle T if the statement is true and F if it is false.

(a) T F RNs act in supervisory positions.
(b) T F Requests for pain medications should be referred to the nursing assistant.
(c) T F Calls from doctors should be referred to the RN.
(d) T F The registered nurse may start IVs.
(e) T F LVNs and LPNs perform many of the procedures performed by RNs.
(f) T F Nursing assistants do not take doctors' orders.
(g) T F Patient care technicians are usually nursing assistants with advanced training.

In the space to the left, check the health professionals who hold the degree of M.D.

____ Rheumatologist
____ Hematologist
____ Osteopath
____ Nephrologist
____ Psychologist
____ Podiatrist
____ Chiropractor
____ CRNA

CHAPTER 3

The Hospital Departments

OBJECTIVES

When you have completed this chapter, you will be able to:

- Describe the primary functions of the various hospital departments.
- Describe the purpose of discharge planning.
- Give examples of types of "special orders" that might be placed through the dietary department.

Many departments within a hospital contribute to the care of the patient. Working in these departments are many people with various levels and types of skills. Each department is important, and the health unit coordinator in his or her coordination role must understand the functions and organization of the departments and how he or she interfaces in performing the health unit coordinator's duties.

An overview of the common departments follows. More information will be given in the chapters on Medications, and Diagnostic and Therapeutic Orders.

THE ADMINISTRATIVE AND GENERAL SERVICES

KEY IDEA: THE BUSINESS OFFICE

Departmental Organization and Services

The business office manages the hospital's business activities. This office also keeps the administration informed of the financial condition of the institution. Below is a partial list of the business office activities:

- Records all charges to be made to each patient's account, including special diagnostic tests, special treatments, and special services (e.g., telephone or television rental)

- Handles payroll records and payment of all hospital employees
- Assists in preparing budgets, taking into account the estimated needs of each department
- Secures patient valuables in a safe located in the business office
- Bills third party payers and patients, and collects payments
- Determines patient's ability to pay and verifies insurance eligibility

The business department is usually headed by a controller. The department itself has many subdivisions and may employ accountants, cashiers, bookkeepers, insurance billing specialists, clerks, a stock room manager, and stenographers to accomplish the various duties.

Execution of Forms

Because the business office issues the final bill to each patient, records of any requisitions for supplies or other items to be charged to the patient must be directed to this office. These records are computer generated and sent from the department performing the service upon completion of the test or treatment or electronically transferred via computer. Your instructor will explain whatever responsibilities you may have regarding the business office.

It is possible that you may be required to notify the business office (usually by telephone or computer) of patients about to be discharged so that their bills can be prepared.

It is obviously very important that all charges to the patient are recorded accurately and completely. (Fig. 3–1.)

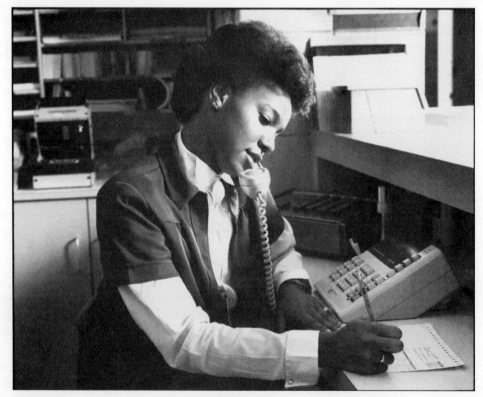

Figure 3–1

KEY IDEA: THE ADMITTING DEPARTMENT

The admitting department is responsible for admitting patients to the hospital. Admitting personnel interview patients, complete necessary forms and obtain patients' signatures, explain hospital admitting procedures to patients and notify nursing units or departments of the patients' arrival. The patient identification bracelet, addressograph plate, and face sheet for the chart usually originate in this office. Preadmissions, inpatient and outpatient admissions, emergency department registration, insurance verification, and cashiering may all be part of the duties of this department.

KEY IDEA: THE COMMUNICATIONS DEPARTMENT

Some hospitals may call this the telephone switchboard. Telephone operators handle incoming and outgoing calls and operate the doctors' paging or signal light system. In some hospitals the communications department may also act as an information station for visitors to the hospital.

KEY IDEA: THE HUMAN RESOURCES DEPARTMENT

The human resources department is responsible for interviewing and often hiring hospital employees. Human resources maintains employee records and conducts termination interviews. Information and records regarding employee benefits such as sick leave, insurance, vacations, the credit union, and retirement can be found in this department.

KEY IDEA: THE PUBLIC RELATIONS DEPARTMENT

The public relations department works to promote community relations with the hospital and provides the community with information about hospital activities. Many hospitals sponsor health fairs and offer many other community outreach programs such as seminars, CPR classes, and "Meals on Wheels"—nutritional meals prepared at the hospital and delivered each day to the homes of persons who might not otherwise enjoy a hot meal. The public relations department publicizes these activities and may also publish a newsletter for hospital employees.

KEY IDEA: THE TRANSPORTATION MESSENGER, OR ESCORT DEPARTMENT

This department may deliver mail, specimens, and reports throughout the hospital as well as pick up and deliver patients to the various departments. This service may include the transportation of patients being admitted or discharged.

KEY IDEA: THE MEDICAL RECORDS DEPARTMENT OR HEALTH INFORMATION SERVICES

Medical records is responsible for all of the charts or records of persons who have been patients in the hospital. After discharge, the patient's records are sent to this department where they are carefully reviewed by specialists to make sure that each chart is complete, accurate, and signed by all appropriate personnel. If the records are not complete, the medical records department will contact staff members and require that additional charting or signatures be added. After a certain period of time, the patient's chart is put on film called microfiche and may be viewed by the physician on a special machine in the medical records department.

One of the most important functions of health information services (formally called the medical records department) is the assigning of diagnostic and procedural codes. This is done to gather statistics and especially to obtain reimbursement for the hospital. Since 1983, the Health Care Financing Administration (HCFA) has required the use of Diagnosis Related Groups (DRGs) for Medicare patients. If a coder does not select the correct code, reimbursement to the hospital may be reduced. Another function performed by health information services is abstracting. This is the process of collecting information from the medical record for the purpose of gathering statistics. The hospital then uses this information to determine, among other things, how different physicians utilize the hospital, to analyze staffing needs, and to report required data to government agencies.

When a patient is admitted and the doctor requests the "old charts," those charts will be obtained from this department.

Medical transcription (the word processing of dictated records by the physician) is done in medical records. The health unit coordinator then files these typewritten reports (such as histories, physical examinations, consultations, surgical and pathology reports) on the patient's chart.

KEY IDEA: INFORMATION SYSTEMS

This department is responsible for the computers within a hospital. Information systems provides and works to improve computer hardware and software, provides support for systems operations, and assists hospital personnel with computer education. Working within this department are clinical data systems (CDS) analysts.

KEY IDEA: THE CENTRAL SUPPLY DEPARTMENT

Most medical and nursing equipment and supplies—probably the most frequently used items in the hospital—are stored in the central supply section. This department is also responsible for preparing and issuing the equipment and supplies. The central supply room stocks commonly used items such as cotton, bandages, dressings, and a variety of trays needed for different procedures. It may also supply more specialized appliances such as air mattresses, bed cradles, orthopedic frames, and soak machines. Central supply is also the center of sterilization; such items as surgical instruments and a variety of trays and equipment are wrapped and sterilized there. (Fig. 3–2.)

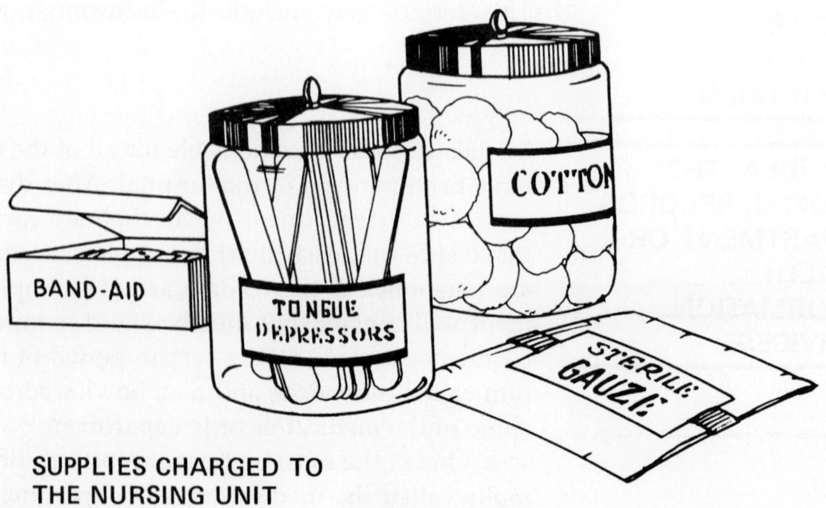

Figure 3–2

Requisitions

There are generally two types of requests when ordering from central supply, which is often done by computers.

1. Requisitions for equipment and supplies to be charged to the unit include standard equipment used in routine nursing care (e.g., tongue blades, bandages, sterile pads, and cotton). In some hospitals, stock is replenished routinely by the central supply room, through scheduled checking and delivery.
2. Requisitions for equipment or supplies to be charged to the patient include special items needed by the individual patient, who must be charged for them or their use. Suction apparatus and special trays for non-routine patient care are examples of nursing supplies that would be charged to the patient.

Most nursing supplies and equipment are charged to the patient and the health unit coordinator must be sure that all charges are made accurately.

Many central supply departments stock disposable, chargeable patient supplies on the nursing unit and attach a CS requisition stating the type of supply to each article. When nursing uses a supply, they will bring the requisition to you. You should stamp the patient's addressograph plate and then route it to CS.

Another system Central Supply may use is to keep a CS Kardex in the supply or clean utility room on the nursing unit with a CS card for each patient. Each CS item has a sticker. Nursing affixes the sticker to the patient's individual central supply Kardex when the supply is used. Central Supply tabulates the charges from each Central Supply Kardex daily for each unit. Other hospitals are using computers to accomplish this purpose. You will learn the procedure utilized in your health care institution.

Figure 3–3 illustrates a partial list used for stocking the supply cart on a medical/surgical floor.

Nondisposable equipment and supplies are also requisitioned from central supply. (Figure 3–4.)

All equipment used for patient treatment must be charged for as well. After the initial order has been placed, central supply staff may be responsible for daily tracking of use so that accurate charges may be made.

It is exceedingly important to a hospital's financial health that it be reimbursed for care that is rendered. Every hospital employee must assist in this process.

Nursing Procedure Orders are discussed in Chapter 15.

KEY IDEA: PURCHASING DEPARTMENT

As you can imagine, buying and storing huge quantities of equipment and supplies needed by the hospital is an enormous job, requiring a great deal of planning and thought. The hospital must always have a sufficient quantity of all the things it needs, and it must obtain new and better equipment as it is developed. The hospital must never run out of essential items; nor can such items be so overstocked that space and funds are not available for new purchases.

Medical Surgical Floor

Upper Cabinet

	Qty	Item
	2	Bx small latex gloves
	2	Bx medium latex gloves
	2	Bx large latex gloves
	2	Bx limb holders
	2	Arterial hand aids
	6	Posey soft belts
	10	Urinals

Drawer

	Qty	Item
	2	Bx IVAC covers
	6	Oral thermometer
	6	Rectal thermometer

Lower Cabinet

	Qty	Item
	10	Bedpans
	10	Sanpans
	20	Emesis basins
	5	Urine strainers
	5	Wash basins
	8	Fracture pans
	8	Graduates

Cart

	Qty	Item
	15	Admit kits
	10	Suction canisters
	4	Kangaroo bags
	15	Suction kits
	10	Suction tubing
	10	Wall tubing
	10	Yankauer suction tip

Medicine Room

	Qty	Item
	4	1/2" steri-strips
	2	Bx alcohol preps
	1	Bx Betadine preps
	4	Suture removal kits
	2	Staple removal kits
	4	Disposable scissors
	4	Sterile kelly's
	2	Needle holders
	1	Bx 19ga. × 1" needles
	1	Bx 19ga. × 1 1/2" needles
	1	Bx 20ga needles
	1	Bx 23ga needles
	1	Bx 25ga needles
	1	Bx 20ga syringe
	1	Bx 22ga syringe
	1	Bx 23ga syringe
	1	Bx 25ga syringe
	1	Bx 10cc syringe
	1	Bx 5cc syringe
	1	Bx insulin syringe
	1	Bx TB syringe
	20	IV start kits

In Kitchen

	Qty	Item
	10	Water pitchers

* * 5 IV pumps standby * *

Fourth Floor Circle Cart

Top Shelf

	Qty	Item
	2	Eggcrate mattress
	4	Sterile water
	4	Sterile saline
	1	Suction canister
	1	Box isolation mask

Second Shelf

	Qty	Item
	4	Baby powder
	4	Lotion
	4	Shampoo
	4	Mouthwash
	4	Dental kits
	4	Tissue
	4	Ivory soap w/ dish
	4	Razors
	4	Shave cream
	4	Odor eliminators
	6	Oral swabs
	4	Specimen cups
	2	U-bags
	2	Urine strainers

Third Shelf

	Qty	Item
	1	Sitz bath
	1	Ring cushion
	5	Chux
	5	Bedpads
	10	Adult pampers

Bottom Shelf

	Qty	Item
	1	Urinemeter w/foley
	1	Urinemeter
	1	16fr foley cath tray

Figure 3–3 Nursing care items are restocked by Central Supply as they are used.

Fourth Floor Circle Cart

	Qty	Item
	1	18fr foley cath tray
	1	Irrigation tray
	1	Drainage tray
	1	Urethral cath tray
	1	Trach care kit
	1	Bx latex gloves small
	1	Bx latex gloves medium
	1	Bx latex gloves large
	1	Box limb holders

Drawer #1

	Qty	Item
	2	Large slippers
	2	Medium slippers
	5	Combs
	1	Enema fleet
	1	Enema oil
	1	Enema bucket
	4	Lemon swabs

Drawer #2

	Qty	Item
	2	1/8" steri-strips
	2	1/4" steri-strips
	2	1/2" steri-strips
	2	1" steri-strips
	2	Kerlix rolls
	2	2" kling
	2	3" kling
	2	4" kling
	2	6" kling
	2	Small opsite
	2	Medium opsite
	2	Large opsite
	2	Vaseline gauze
	1	Bx spot band-aid
	1	Bx 1" band-aid
	1	Bx 2" band-aid

Drawer #3

	Qty	Item
	1	Bx IVAC covers
	1	Shroud
	2	Denture cups
	2	Lab cups
	5	Skin wipes
	2	1" micropore tape
	2	2" micropore tape
	2	1" transpore tape
	2	2" transpore tape

Drawer #4

	Qty	Item
	1	Bx sterile 2 × 2 dressing
	1	Bx sterile 4 × 4 dressing
	2	4 × 4 tubs

Drawer #5

	Qty	Item
	2	Suction tubing
	2	Wall tubing
	2	Yankauer suction tips
	2	60cc cath tip syringe
	2	ABG kits
	2	Culturettes
	1	Small condom cath
	1	Medium condom cath
	1	Large condom cath
	2	Cath adapters

Drawer #6

	Qty	Item
	2	Ea. Sterile gloves

	6.0		6.5		7.0
	7.5		8.0		8.5

	Qty	Item
	10	White towels
	1	Shave prep
	1	Sterile basin
	1	Peri-bottle
	5	Sterile Q-tips
	5	Sterile tongue blades
	5	Safety pins
	5	K-Y
	5	Belonging bags

In Cabinet

	Qty	Item
	4	Urinals
	4	Wash basins
	4	San pans
	4	Graduates
	4	Bedpans
	4	Fracture pans
	4	Water pitchers
	4	Admit kits

Figure 3–3 ***(Continued)***

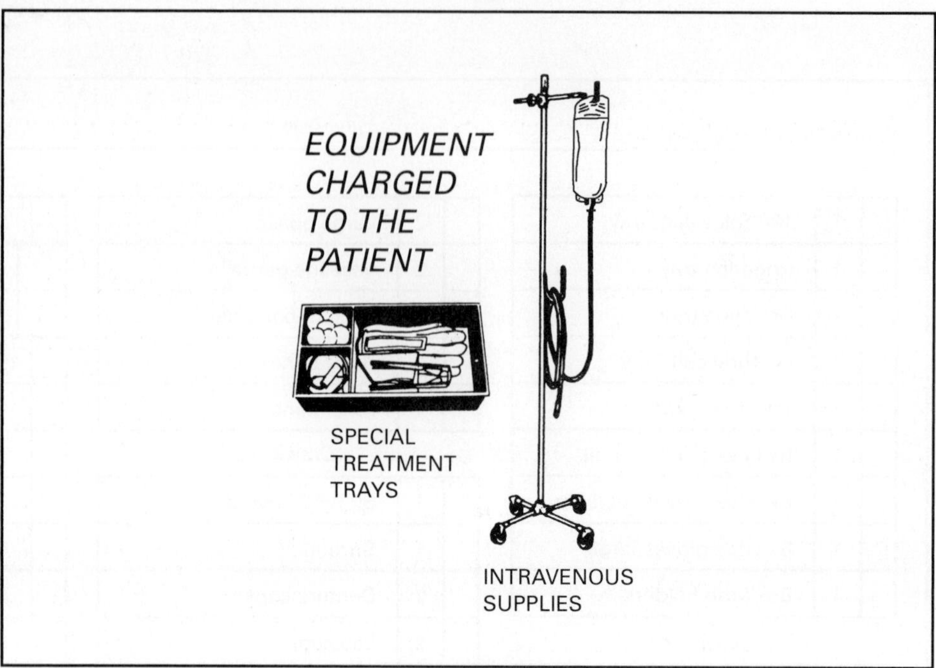

Figure 3–4

In most hospitals, all supplies, equipment, and materials used in the hospital, from pencils to the most complicated heart-lung machine, are bought by the purchasing department in cooperation with the business department. Each hospital department regularly submits a list of the supplies it needs. These supplies are then delivered on scheduled dates. Emergency requests, of course, are handled in a different manner and are delivered as soon as possible.

Forms and Requisitions

The purchasing department usually has a variety of forms to be used in requisitioning supplies. A sample form used in requesting stationery supplies is shown in Fig. 3–5.

KEY IDEA: THE ENVIRONMENTAL SERVICES OR HOUSEKEEPING DEPARTMENT

Functions

The environmental services department is responsible for maintaining the clean, sanitary, and pleasant environment that is so important to the medical and nursing care of the patient and to the entire hospital staff as well. An environment housing ill and infected people must be kept as clean as possible to aid in restoring them to good health and to prevent the spread of disease.

- Members of the environmental services staff perform the daily routine tasks that keep the various areas of the hospital (i.e., the wards, halls, restrooms, dayrooms, etc.) clean and orderly at all times.
- They also do special cleaning chores such as window washing, floor waxing, and cleaning light fixtures, on a regular basis.
- In many hospitals, environmental services aides dispense clean linen and make necessary mending repairs.

OFFICE SUPPLY REQUISITION
•STOREROOM STATIONARY ONLY

DATE	COST CENTER NO.	DEPT. NAME	DIRECTOR'S SIGNATURE X

QTY. ORDERED	UNIT	STOCK NO. NAME	QTY. ORDERED	UNIT	STOCK NO. NAME
	EA	0448 BATTERY, AA		EA	5150 OUTLET 6 PLUG
	EA	0465 BATTERY, AAA		PD	5640 PAD, POST-IT NOTE 1 1/2 × 2
	EA	0455 BATTERY, C		PD	5642 PAD, POST-IT NOTE 3 × 3
	EA	0460 BATTERY, D		PD	5585 PAD, SCRATCH 3 × 5
	EA	0472 BATTERY, 6v, J		PD	5595 PAD, SCRATCH 5 × 8
	EA	0471 BATTERY, 8.4v		PD	5600 PAD, STENO 6 × 9 GREGG 60
	EA	0474 BATTERY, 9v		PD	5580 PAD, YEL. RULED 8 1/2 × 11
	EA	6055 BINDER DATA 14 7/8 × 11 #LbC1411NJ		PD	5565 PAD, WIRE BOUND 8 1/2 × 11
	EA	5555 BINDER, 3/RG, BE, 8 1/2 × 11, 1"		RM	5662 PAPER, COPY MACHINE 8 1/2 × 11
	EA	5560 BINDER, 3/RG, BE, 8 1/2 × 11, 2"		RL	5646 PAPER, FAX F/SHARPE
	BX	5745 CARD, PATIENT, BLU., PLASTIC		DZ	5675 PEN, BALL BK, F
	BX	5120 CLIP, PAPER, JUMBO		DZ	5680 PEN, BALL BK, M BIC ROUND
	BX	5115 CLIP, PAPER, REGULAR		DZ	5690 PEN, BALL RD, M
	EA	5110 CLIPBOARD. LTR, BN, 9 × 12 1/2		DZ	5700 PENCIL, BK #2 #600
	EA	5370 CORRECT FLUID, WE 1/2 OZ.		EA	5765 PROTECTOR, SHEET 8 1/2 × 11
	EA	5374 CORRECT FLUID, COPIER		EA	5845 RIBBON, COR., SEL III
	BX	5125 DISKETTE, 3.5, DS, DD, 10/BX		EA	5846 RIBBON, COR., SEL II
	BX	5126 DISKETTE, 3.5, DS, HD, 10/BX		EA	5775 RIBBON, DIGITAL #LA75
	BX	5129 DISKETTE, 5 1/4, DS, DD, 10/BX		EA	5770 RIBBON, DIGITAL #LA424
	BX	5128 DISKETTE, 5 1/4, DS, HD, 10/BX		EA	5786 RIBBON, F/OKIDATA ML390/931 BK
	BX	5185 ENVELOPE, CLASP, 6 1/2 × 9 1/2		EA	5785 RIBBON, F/OKIDATA ML84
	BX	5190 ENVELOPE, CLASP, 9 × 12		BX	5890 RUBBER BANDS, 1/4#, REVERE 18, SMALL
	BX	5195 ENVELOPE, CLASP, 10 × 13		BX	5895 RUBBER BANDS, 1/4#, REVERE 64, LARGE
	EA	5177 ENVELOPE, INTER-DEPT., 5 × 11 1/2		EA	5915 RULER, OFFICE 12"
	EA	5178 ENVELOPE, INTER-DEPT., 10 × 13		EA	5926 SHEARS, BLACK, HANDLE 7"
	BX	5200 ENVELOPE, NO CLASP, 9 × 12		EA	6010 STAPLE REMOVER
	EA	5215 ENVELOPE, PADDED, 9 1/2 × 12		EA	6015 STAPLER, FULL BK
	EA	5220 ENVELOPE, PATIENT VALUABLES		BX	6025 STAPLES, STD FULL 5M/BX
	EA	5245 ERASER, PENCIL TIP		RL	6038 TAPE, ADDING MACHINE 2 1/4
	BX	5252 FASTENER, BASE #22		EA	6057 TAPE, CASSETTE 60 MIN.
	BX	5268 FILM, Sx70		RL	6125 TAPE, DBL STICK .75 × 1296
	BX	5261 FILM, 779BC		EA	5847 TAPE, LIFTOFF, SEL II
	PK	5270 FILM, SPECTRA		RL	4374 TAPE, MASK 1"
	BX	5295 FOLDER, FILE 1/3 ASSORT.		RL	4375 TAPE, MASK 2"
	BX	5294 FOLDER, FILE 1/3 1st POS		RL	6105 TAPE, MENDING 1/2
	BX	5296 FOLDER, FILE, PENDAFLEX, LTR		RL	6110 TAPE, MENDING 3/4
	BX	5297 FOLDER, TABS, PENDAFLEX		EA	6135 TAPE, VIDEO 120
	ST	5320 INDEX, RG/BK 8CR 8 1/2 × 11		BTL	5649 TONER CARTRIDGE, COPIER #SF830NTI
	PK	5050 INDEX CARD, WE 3 × 5, RULED		EA	5651 TONER CARTRIDGE, FAX #F033NTI
	RL	5445 LABEL, ALLERGIC, RED		EA	5020 TONER CARTRIDGE F/ LASERJET IIP, IIIP, IIP PLUS
	BX	5375 LABEL, CONT. COMPUTER 3 1/2 × 1, 5M/BX		EA	5030 TONER CARTRIDGE F/ LASERJET IIISi
	BX	5380 LABEL, FILE FOLDER		EA	5035 TONER CARTRIDGE #92295A
	RL	5475 LABEL, MEDICATION, RED		EA	5650 TONER SF 7350
	RL	5400 LABEL, PRE-CUT, PLN, 2 1/2 × 1 1/2		BTL	5648 TONER, SHARP SF80TI
	RL	5500 LABEL, RM, PT, DR, WHITE		BTL	5645 TONER, TOSHIBA T50P
	EA	5535 MARKER, FELT, BLK			
	EA	5550 MARKER, FELT, RED			
	EA	5695 MARKER, HIGHLIGHTER, PINK			
	EA	5696 MARKER, HIGHLIGHTER, YELLOW			
	EA	5532 MARKER, SHARPIE, BLK			
	EA	5533 MARKER, SHARPIE, RED			

DO NOT WRITE IN THIS SPACE

This Request For Storeroom Stationary must be presented to Purchasing by 9:00 a.m. on your order day.
See Reverse Side for Numerical Listing for cross reference

Figure 3–5

- Environmental services cleans rooms of discharged patients, makes up the bed, and prepares the unit for the next patient.

You have undoubtedly seen environmental services aides at work performing these and a variety of other tasks. In all the work they do, they must show the same consideration for the patient as is shown by the entire hospital staff. Housekeeping personnel do their jobs quietly and efficiently, disturbing the patients as little as possible. The result of their work is a clean, neat, and safe hospital. (Fig. 3–6.)

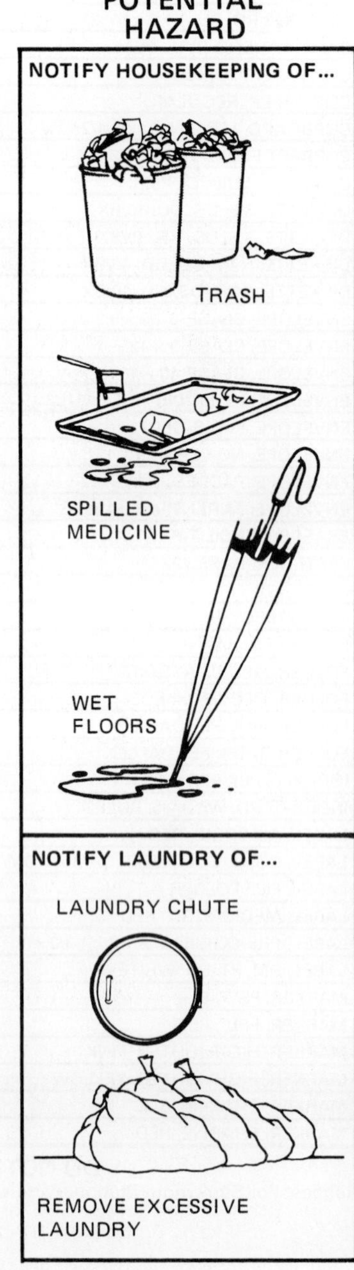

Figure 3–6

Departmental Organization

The director of environmental services directs all the activities of this department and its staff. The director of environmental services supervises the daily routine cleaning and also has an overall plan so that the larger chores are performed on a regular schedule. Other related responsibilities:

- Selection of new furnishings and recommending redecorating as the need arises
- Planning and directing an inservice training program for environmental services personnel

In large hospitals, the director of environmental services usually has an assistant. The rest of the housekeeping staff work under their direction to maintain high standards of cleanliness.

The Environmental Services Department and the Health Unit Coordinator

Although you will see environmental services aides at work on your unit every day, it is quite possible that you will have very little to do with the department as a whole. It is important, however, that you know and understand the extent of its responsibilities in your hospital so that when special situations arise, you will know the appropriate section or person to call.

Some conditions require prompt attention from environmental services personnel. You may be responsible for telephoning environmental services in the following situations:

- When medicine or something else is spilled
- When dripping umbrellas have made the halls wet and slippery
- When accumulations of trash have created a messy and potentially dangerous situation
- When patients have inadvertently hemorrhaged, vomited, urinated, or defecated on the floor

KEY IDEA: THE LAUNDRY DEPARTMENT

Functions

The laundry department collects and launders all hospital linens and maintains an adequate supply of clean, sanitary linen for all departments. Linen includes not only sheets and pillowcases but may also include patient gowns, employee uniforms, towels, and many other items.

Departmental Organization

In some hospitals, the position of laundry manager may be combined with that of executive housekeeper. In others, it is a separate department. The laundry manager supervises the laundry workers, schedules the work loads so that the entire laundering process moves efficiently, and inspects equipment frequently making any necessary minor repairs. The rest of the staff is made up of washers, marker-sorters, ironers, and tumbler (dryer) operators. The laundered items are inspected to be sure that they are clean and well ironed before they are distributed to the various hospital departments. In many hospitals, the laundry is sent out to a commercial laundry and the laundry department will coordinate this activity.

Health Unit Coordinator Responsibilities

It is unlikely that you will have frequent association with this department. Should an unusual amount of laundry accumulate on your unit between scheduled pickups, however, you might be asked to request that a member of the laundry staff come to collect it.

KEY IDEA: THE ENGINEERING AND MAINTENANCE DEPARTMENT

Function

The maintenance department provides continuous upkeep of the hospital's buildings and grounds and the safe, efficient operation of all its utilities. Among the many responsibilities of this department are:

- To service and maintain all the lighting and heating equipment in the hospital
- To make any necessary carpentry, plastering, painting, and plumbing repairs
- To repair all sorts of equipment, from boilers to furniture
- To keep electrically operated equipment, (e.g., elevators) in good running order
- To landscape and care for the hospital grounds
- To transport medical supplies and equipment, building materials, furniture and fixtures, and trash, and to service the trucks used for this purpose
- To train new employees in these tasks

Departmental Organization

The maintenance department is usually under the direction of a superintendent of buildings and grounds. In large hospitals, he/she may delegate some of his/her duties to a chief engineer and a maintenance supervisor.

The number of personnel in this department depends on the size and needs of the hospital but will generally include carpenters, painters, masons, plumbers, electricians, mechanics, repair persons, gardeners, and truck drivers. These people work together to provide and maintain safe and efficient conditions, as well as an attractive, pleasant environment for patients, staff, and visitors.

Health Unit Coordinator

In Chapter 9 you will learn about some of the hazards that may occur in the hospital. Some examples include nonfunctioning lights, faulty electrical equipment, jammed windows, etc. All these and many other situations are ordinarily corrected by the maintenance department staff. A typical form used to request repairs that may be needed in your unit is shown in Fig. 3–7. In many hospitals all ordering for maintenance is computerized.

KEY IDEA: AUXILIARY SERVICES

For some patients, illness causes problems that cannot be solved by medical and nursing care alone. Many hospitals employ nurses who have the responsibility of Discharge Planning with the doctor's consent. These nurses interview certain patients in need of auxiliary services following discharge and help arrange for these services. Auxiliary services offer assistance to alleviate the anxieties and difficulties that frequently accompany a hospitalization. Referral forms and other forms that may be issued for auxiliary services contain information regarding the patient's illness, medications provided or prescribed and instructions for follow-up care. These forms must be completed by a nurse or physician. Your hospital's routine for filling out and validating the forms will be explained by your instructor.

Home Health Services

Home health services are responsible for assisting the patient with discharge planning. Postdischarge plans are made by assessing the patient's needs before discharge from the hospital. Home health services include assisting the patient in obtaining needed supplies and equipment as well as providing nursing care and assisted care through the use of home health nurses and home health aides (HHA).

Home health care has grown and today a great deal of care is provided to patients in their homes by nurses and home health aides. (Fig. 3–8.)

REPAIR REQUISITION FOR MAINTENANCE
STAFF REPAIRS ONLY
NOT FOR NEW ARTICLES

The following repairs are required in __________

Location __________

Description __________

Date __________

Supervisor __________

Mark "URGENT" in red ink if repair is so indicated.

Job completed __________

Name __________

Date __________

SEND BOTH COPIES TO FRONT OFFICE WHEN REPAIRS ARE NEEDED.

Example of requisition for repairs.

Figure 3–7

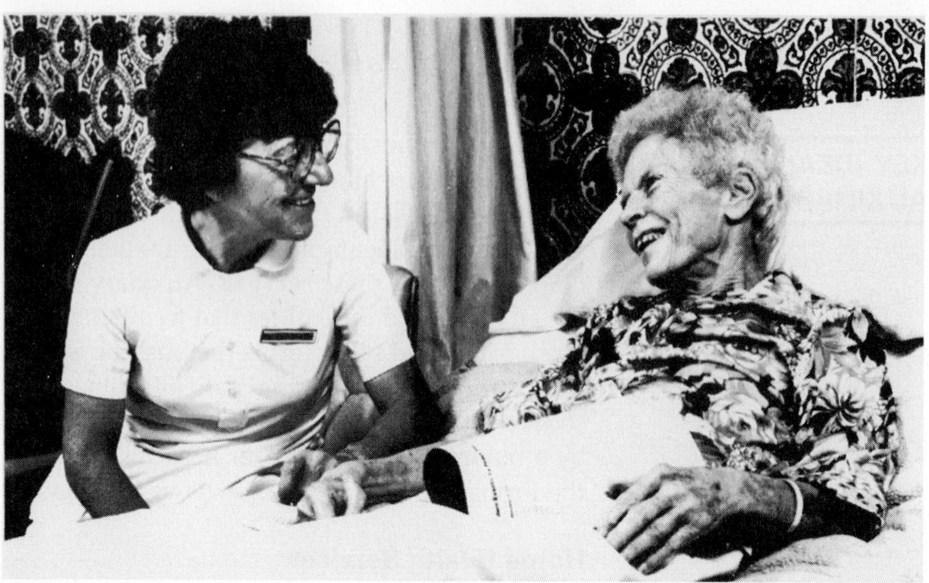

Figure 3–8

Social Services

The financial problems that often accompany a hospitalization can cause more suffering than the pain of illness. Worrying about money, a disrupted family life, or unemployment can easily delay a patient's recovery. The social service agency gives assistance to patients beset by these and other difficulties.

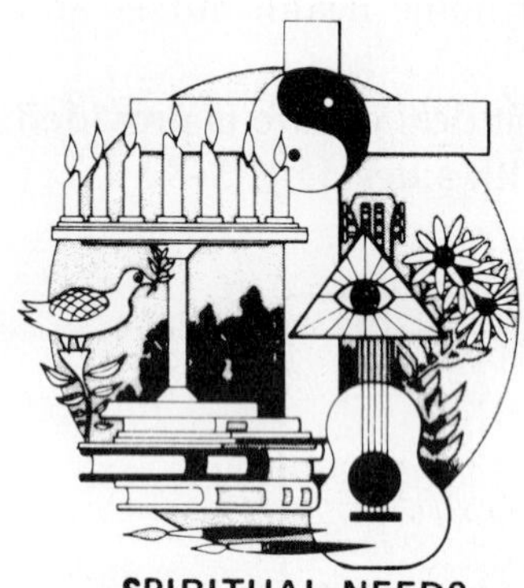

Figure 3–9

Some health care institutions have their own medical social service departments which perform patient services. These services include those for outpatients with financial problems. A social service department assists them in finding new jobs if illness has rendered them no longer suitable for their previous employment, secures the aid of specialized resources such as Home Health Agencies, and generally makes available the many community resources (such as vocational rehabilitation counseling) that may be helpful in recovery from illness and adjustment to life's circumstances. (Fig. 3–9.)

KEY IDEA: PASTORAL CARE

This department provides spiritual support to the patient and family members during their time of need. Some hospitals maintain a program for members of the clergy who wish to become hospital chaplains.

THE PROFESSIONAL SERVICES

KEY IDEA: THE HOSPITAL PHARMACY

The hospital pharmacy is operated under the direction of the chief pharmacist, a person who has graduated from a school of pharmacy and is fully trained and licensed in compounding and dispensing medicines and preparations according to prescriptions written by physicians. The pharmacist must be licensed by the state in which he or she works. Figure 3–10 shows a pharmacy organizational chart.

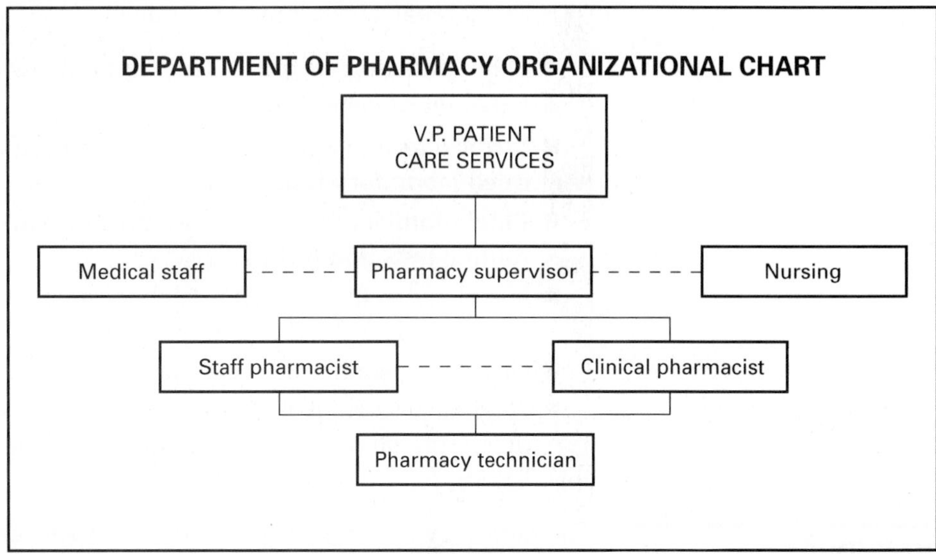

Figure 3–10

Working with the pharmacist are pharmacy technicians who, under the direct supervision and control of a registered pharmacist, perform a variety of tasks related to the processing of a prescription in a licensed pharmacy, but do not perform duties restricted to a registered pharmacist.

The pharmacy provides a variety of services to the hospital and its patients. Some of these are:

- Compounds prescriptions and dispenses medications needed for individual patient care.
- Maintains supply of stock medications which are administered to the patients as needed.
- Dispenses controlled drugs and keeps records for inspection.
- Dispenses IV solutions and often the various IV tubings.
- Adds medications to IV solutions.
- Distributes information about new drugs and often provides other educational materials.
- The pharmacy also usually stocks emergency supply cabinets or carts in specified areas of the hospital.

Medication orders are discussed in Chapter 14.

KEY IDEA: THE LABORATORY

The director of laboratories, in most hospitals, is a physician with special training in pathology. **Pathology** is a branch of medical science dealing with the nature of disease. The director is responsible for the total operation of the laboratory service, which includes testing of body specimens such as blood, urine, wound drainage, sputum, stool, and samples of tissues taken from the body. Autopsies are also a function of this department. He or she may also direct teaching and research activities in which the department is engaged.

The laboratory staff may include:

- Other pathologists or residents in pathology who assist the director
- Laboratory technicians
- Medical technologists trained and licensed to perform the more complicated laboratory tests
- **Phlebotomists** who draw blood from patients and commonly perform routine tests and duties.
- Histology technician who sections, stains, and mounts tissue for microscopic study.
- Clerical personnel who maintain records and reports
- Auxiliary personnel who perform such tasks as transporting patients, delivering laboratory results, and collecting requisitions (Fig. 3–11.)

KEY IDEA: RADIOLOGY

The radiology department provides diagnostic and therapeutic services to in-hospital patients and to patients on an outpatient basis. The department is under the direction of a **radiologist,** a doctor who specializes in the diagnosis and treatment of diseases by the use of x-rays, radioactive isotopes, and ionizing radiation. The radiologist is responsible for all radiological examinations and treatments and also interprets radiographs.

Radiologic technologists and technicians work with the doctor and operate equipment, perform many of the x-ray procedures, develop the film, and assist in other related duties. Frequently the staff also includes a group of personnel who transport the patients to and from the radiology department.

There are several major divisions of the radiology department:

- X-rays—with or without the use of contrast media and with or without special preparation
- Nuclear medicine
- Radiation therapy
- Ultrasonography

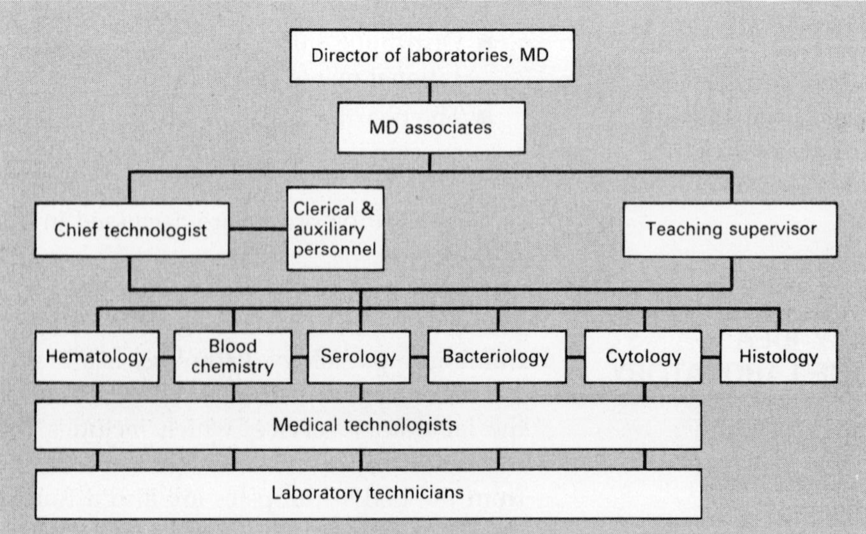

Figure 3–11

- Computerized tomography—CT Scan
- MRI—Magnetic Resonance Imaging

KEY IDEA: CARDIOLOGY

This department is responsible for both noninvasive and invasive diagnostic studies of the heart. Noninvasive tests of the heart include the electrocardiogram (ECG), the treadmill stress test, echocardiograms, and testing using the Holter monitor. Cardiac catheterization is an invasive examination done through this department in some hospitals. ECG technicians and cardiovascular technologists work under the supervision of a cardiologist, a physician specializing in the diagnoses and treatment of diseases of the heart.

Cardiac rehabilitation, consisting of prescribed exercises and other therapy for patients who have had heart attacks or have other heart disorders, is often a division of cardiology.

KEY IDEA: RESPIRATORY OR INHALATION THERAPY

Oxygen and other gases are used in inhalation therapy as a treatment for pulmonary (lung) difficulties. These gases may be administered by face mask, cannula, or tent. Respiratory therapists manage respirators, draw and analyze arterial blood gases, perform pulmonary function tests, and supervise pulmonary treatment.

KEY IDEA: PHYSICAL THERAPY

Physical therapy includes the use of exercises and massage, as well as light, heat, cold, water, and electricity in the treatment of disease and injury. The physical therapy department will ordinarily have equipment such as whirlpools, parallel bars, ramps, crutches, wheelchairs, braces, and prostheses (artificial limbs, etc.). Trained physical therapists help patients to overcome or adjust to their disabilities through instruction and supervised practice.

KEY IDEA: OCCUPATIONAL THERAPY

Occupational therapy consists of directed activities, such as games and work projects. These activities aid in the treatment and rehabilitation of patients confined to the hospital. The program is adapted to suit the particular needs of each patient to provide him with the sort of diversion and skills that will best contribute to his physical and emotional progress. In this department, partially disabled patients learn to develop and explore new vocational possibilities. In many instances, the activities of the occupational therapy department are coordinated with those of the physical therapy department, so that each patient may develop his skills both at work and in recreation.

KEY IDEA: ELECTRO-ENCEPHALOGRAPHY SECTION (EEG)

An electroencephalogram is a mechanical tracing of brain waves, used to help determine the presence and location of tumors or other brain disorders.

If the hospital is not large enough to require the services of a full-time neurologist—a doctor specializing in diseases of the nervous system—and an electroencephalograph technician, another technician may be trained to make the tests and submit the results to the appropriate member of the medical staff assigned to interpret these tracings. It is also possible that the results would be sent to a medical center for interpretation.

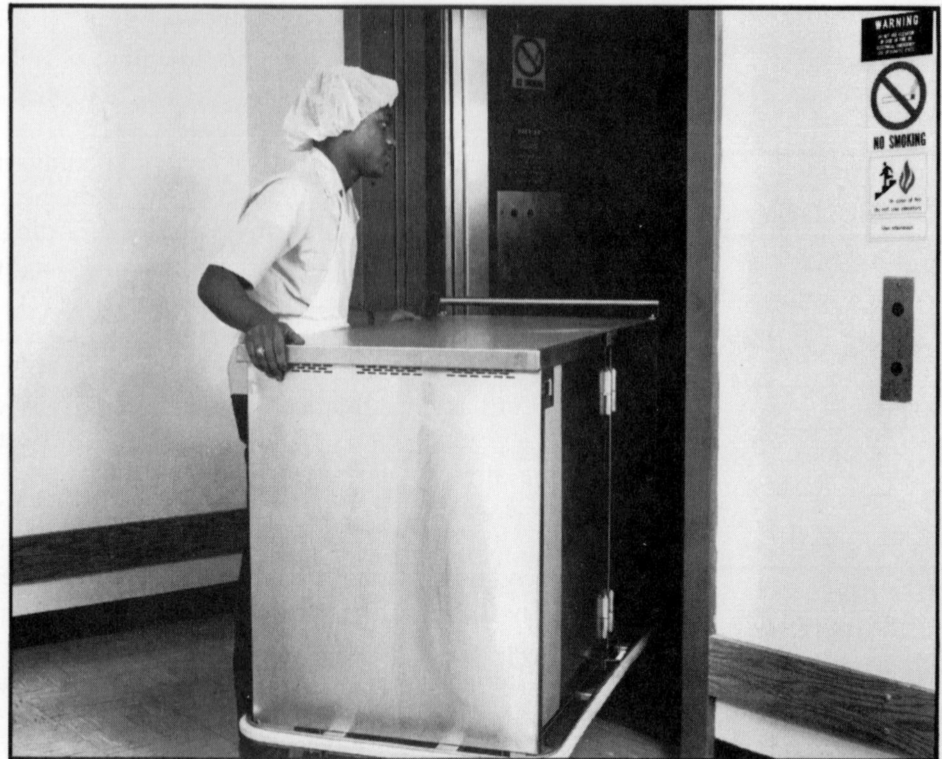

Figure 3–12

KEY IDEA: ENDOSCOPIES

An endoscopy is an examination of the body with the use of an instrument. *Endo* means inside; *scopy* means to examine or visualize. This is a diagnostic procedure done by the doctor. In large hospitals endoscopies may be done in the Endoscopy Department. In smaller hospitals (depending upon the type of endoscopy) it may be done in an examination room on the nursing unit.

KEY IDEA: THE DIETARY DEPARTMENT

Department Organization

Registered dietitians are professionals who are accredited by the Commission of Dietetic Registration, the credentialing agency of the American Dietetic Association. Their training and education is at the Bachelor's and often Master's degree level. Dietitians are an integral part of the health care team. They perform nutrition assessments, educate patients on therapeutic diet needs, and consult on enteral (by mouth or tube) and parenteral therapies.

The chief dietitian supervises all personnel concerned with the preparation and serving of food and those concerned with training in the department. (Fig. 3–12.)

Some hospitals have a large central kitchen where all the food is prepared. In other hospitals, there are smaller kitchens on each floor where the meals for the patients on that floor are prepared. There may be cooking facilities on each floor even if complete meals are not prepared; this permits nursing personnel to serve supplemental nourishments to the patients.

Functions of the Dietary Department

The responsibilities of the dietary department include:

- Planning general diets for patients and employees
- Planning menus for patients on special diets
- Preparing and serving food to patients and employees
- Training students and employees
- Preparation of a diet manual
- Preparing and distributing infant formulas

The dietary department also ordinarily provides the following services for the patients:

- Members of the dietary staff often visit patients in their rooms to determine their food preferences. In this way, the patient whose diet has been restricted to certain types of foods has the opportunity to select those most appealing to him.
- Dietary personnel also give advice and instruction to patients with special dietary problems at the time the patients are ready to be discharged from the hospital. With this help, the patients can continue the proper diet after they return home.
- The dietary staff also cooperates with the medical staff in planning, preparing, and serving experimental diets in a continuing effort to improve the entire dietary program.

Special Orders

In addition to the regular meals served to patients, the dietary department handles certain special orders. These generally include:

- Extra meals for visitors, so that a friend or family member may eat with the patient on occasion
- Supplemental nourishments for the patients, such as crackers, milk, and juices, served midmorning, midafternoon, and evening
- Stock nourishments, such as tea, coffee, milk, and crackers, served as required or desired by the patient (Fig. 3–13.)

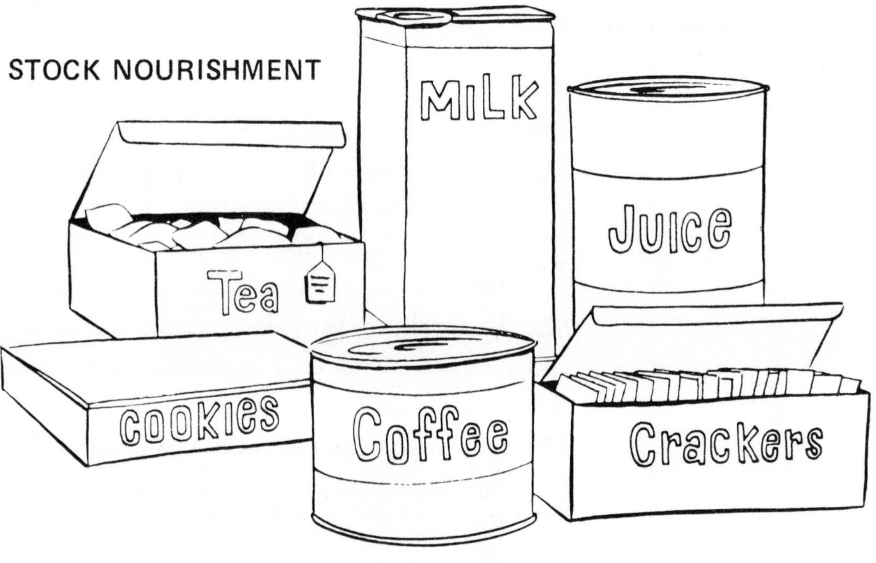

Figure 3–13

- Hold diets, for patients who must have tests or treatments that either conflict with mealtime hour or that must be completed before the patient is allowed to eat.

Diagnostic and therapeutic orders are discussed in Chapter 16.

LEARNING ACTIVITIES

Match the department in column A with the brief description of its services in column B.

Column A	*Column B*
(a) Health information services	____ Handles patients' accounts
(b) Environmental services	____ Dispenses drugs and IV solutions
(c) Radiology	____ Community outreach
(d) Pharmacy	____ Incoming and outgoing calls
(e) Purchasing	____ X-rays, radiation therapy, nuclear medicine
(f) Human resources	____ Prepares, stocks, and issues nursing supplies
(g) Business office	____ Performs tests on blood and other body specimens
(h) Engineering and maintenance	____ Reviews and maintains patients' charts after discharge
(i) Laboratory	____ Buys hospital supplies and equipment
(j) Cardiology	____ Provides clean, neat, safe hospital environment
(k) Central supply	____ Maintains buildings and grounds
(l) Physical therapy	____ Interviews, facilitates hiring, employee benefits
(m) Communications	____ Rehabilitation
(n) Public relations	____ Electrocardiograms

Complete the following:

1. List two examples of auxiliary services which may be available to help the patient after discharge.
   (a) ____________________
   (b) ____________________
2. Pastoral care provides ____________________
   ____
   ____
3. List three responsibilities of the clinical dietitian.
   (a) ____________________
   (b) ____________________
   (c) ____________________

CHAPTER 4

Medical Terminology

OBJECTIVES

When you complete this chapter, you will be able to:

- Correctly spell, pronounce, and define the medical terms in this chapter.
- Recognize word elements, abbreviations, and their meanings.
- State the rules for formulating medical terms.

Correct spelling, pronunciation, and definition of words are vitally important in a hospital. The medical staff will depend on you to transcribe doctors' orders and fill out charts, records, and reports with accuracy. It is essential for you to have a good working knowledge of terms describing diseases and medical and surgical treatments. Understanding medical terminology will also make your work more meaningful and the performance of your duties more efficient.

In this chapter, you will learn the important rules for formulating many medical terms and you will be introduced to many of the terms in common usage in modern hospitals.

Word formulation is not an exact science; there are bound to be exceptions to every rule. Learning medical terminology is comparable to learning another language. The rules of everyday English do not always apply.

The following material is designed for the primary purpose of helping you to recognize word elements and their meanings. Time, thought, and practice are required before you can become really proficient in the language of medicine. Your efforts will help you attain the goal of all hospital workers: better patient care.

KEY IDEA: GUIDE TO PRONUNCIATION

New medical terms included in this chapter will be followed by simple guides to their pronunciation. Only long vowels are marked in the pronunciation guides. Pronunciation of other vowel sounds is indicated only on words that are especially difficult to pronounce correctly. As an exercise and using the rules given below, pronounce each new word aloud.

Accents: The principal accent is written in capital letters. Example: DOC tor.

Syllables: Division between syllables is indicated by a slash (/). Example: gas/TRI/tis.

Vowels: (see following table)

Symbol	*Example*	*Name*
ā	āle	long a
ă	ădd	short a
ē	ēve	long e
ĕ	ĕnd	short e
ī	īce	long i
ĭ	ĭll	short i
ō	ōld	long o
ŏ	ŏdd	short o
ū	cūbe	long u
ŭ	ŭp	short u

KEY IDEA: WORD ELEMENTS

Many medical terms are composed of several smaller, simpler words or word elements. The three main word elements which are frequently combined to form medical terms are the *prefix*, the *suffix*, and the *root*. (Fig. 4–1.)

The *root* is the body or main part of the word and denotes the meaning of the word as a whole.

The *prefix* is a word element combined with the root, which changes or adds to its meaning. A prefix is always added to the beginning of a root.

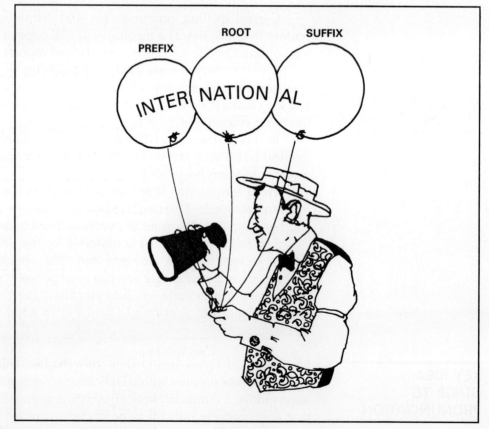

Figure 4–1

The *suffix* is also a word element used to change or add to the meaning of the root. It is always added to the end of the root.

Examples of prefixes are followed by a hyphen (e.g., pre-).

Examples of suffixes are preceded by a hyphen (e.g., -ectomy).

In addition, a *combining* vowel (usually an o) is frequently added to link a root to another root or a root to a suffix for ease in pronunciation. The combining vowel is not used if a suffix begins with a vowel (enteritis not enteroitis), but, as previously stated, it is used between two roots.

The combining form is the root plus the combining vowel (arthr + o = arthro), the combining form meaning joint.

Prefix	*Combining Vowel*	*Root*	*Suffix*	*Combining Form or Word*
dis		agree	able	disagreeable
		war	like	warlike
un		pardon	able	unpardonable
inter		nation	al	international
speed	o	meter		speedometer
		beauty	full	beautiful

The word elements of medical terms work very much like the examples shown above. The main difference is that most medical word elements are derived from foreign languages, chiefly Latin and Greek. So before you will be able to recognize easily the definitions of medical terms, you will need to learn the English meanings of the word elements in those terms. An alphabetical list of common word elements in medical terminology with their meanings and guides to pronunciation is given in this chapter.

KEY IDEA: COMBINING WORD ELEMENTS

Medical terms (like many English words) do not necessarily contain all word elements. (Figs. 4–2 and 4–3.)

- The medical term may be a combination of a prefix and a root:

Medical Term		*Prefix*	*Root*
ectoderm	EC/to/derm	ecto	derm
retropubic	RE/tro/pū/bic	retro	pubic*
endoskeleton	EN/do/skel/e/ton	endo	skeleton
hemiplegic	hem/i/PLĒ/gic	hemi	plegic*
hypertension	hy/per/TEN/sion	hyper	tension

*-ic is a suffix that means "pertaining to"

- In other medical terms, the root may be combined with only a suffix:

Medical Term		*Root*	*Suffix*
colostomy	co/LOS/to/my	col (o)	stomy
gastrectomy	gas/TREC/to/my	gastr	ectomy
myasthenia	my/as/THĒ/ni/a	my	asthenia
osteoma	os/te/O/ma	oste	oma

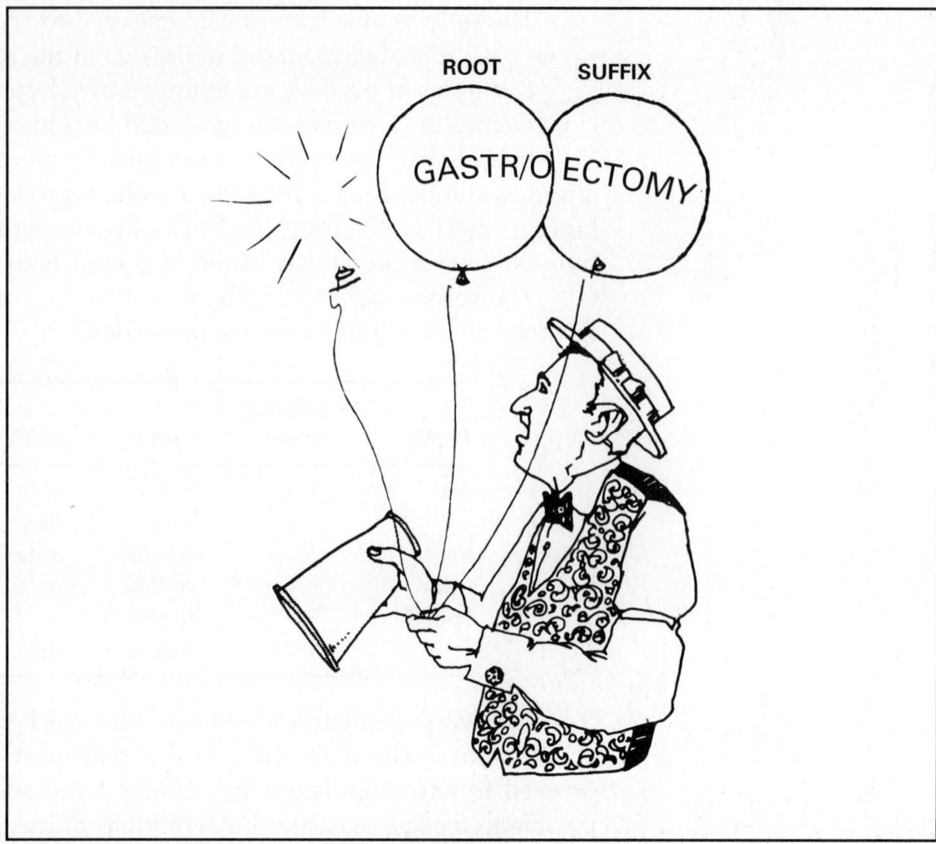

Figure 4–2

- Some medical terms may be formed by using prefixes and suffixes alone:

Medical Term		Prefix	Suffix
diarrhea	di/a/RRHĒ/a	dia	rrhea
endoscopy	en/DOS/co/py	endo	scopy
excise	ex/CISE	ex	cise
epilepsy	EP/i/lep/sy	epi	lepsy
polyuria	pol/y/U/ri/a	poly	uria

- Some medical terms are formed by combining two roots. The resulting word describes the disease or treatment more accurately:

Medical Term		1st Root	Comb. Vowel	2nd Root
bronchopneumonia	bron/cho/pneu/MO/ni/a	bronch	(o)	pneum (o)
gastroenteritis	gas/tro/en/ter/I/tis	gastr	(o)	enter
osteoarthritis	os/te/o/ar/THRI/tis	oste	(o)	arthr
pyelonephritis	py/e/lo/neph/RI/tis	pyel	(o)	nephr

KEY IDEA: WORD VARIATIONS

There are a few special problems you may encounter as you begin your study of medical terminology.

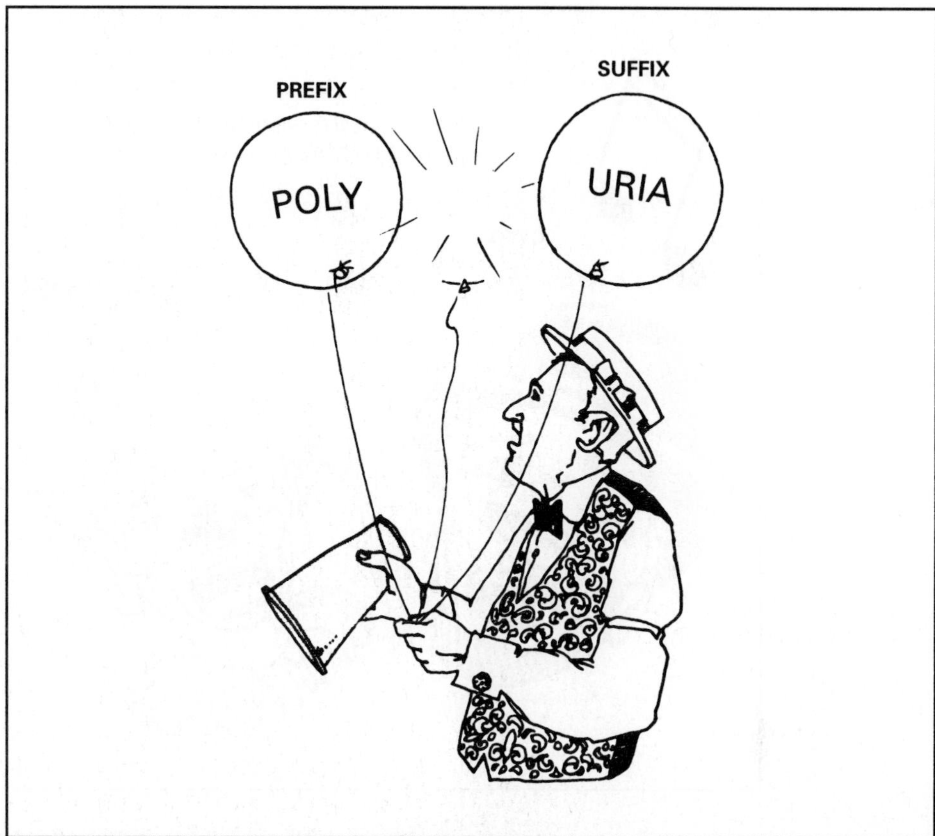

Figure 4–3

- First, a word which has been formulated from several different word elements may *omit, change,* or *add* certain letters so that it conforms to rules of spelling and pronunciation:

Prefix	*Root*	*Comb. Vowel*	*Suffix*	*Word*	
em	py		ema	empyema	em/py/Ē/ma
endo	arteri		itis	endarteritis	end/ar/ter/I/tis
	neur	(o)	logy	neurology	neu/ROL/o/gy
supra	renal			suprarenal	su/pr/RĒ/nal
	stomat		itis	stomatitis	sto/mat/I/tis

- Second, some suffixes are used to create nouns; others are used to create adjectives.

Noun Suffixes	*Adjective Suffixes*
-ax	-al
-ium, um	-ic
-on, ion	-ac
-y, -ity	-ar
-us	-ous

All of the adjective suffixes above mean "pertaining to." (Fig. 4–4.)

- Third, many of the word elements with which you must be familiar are similar in spelling but quite different in meaning. The following is a list

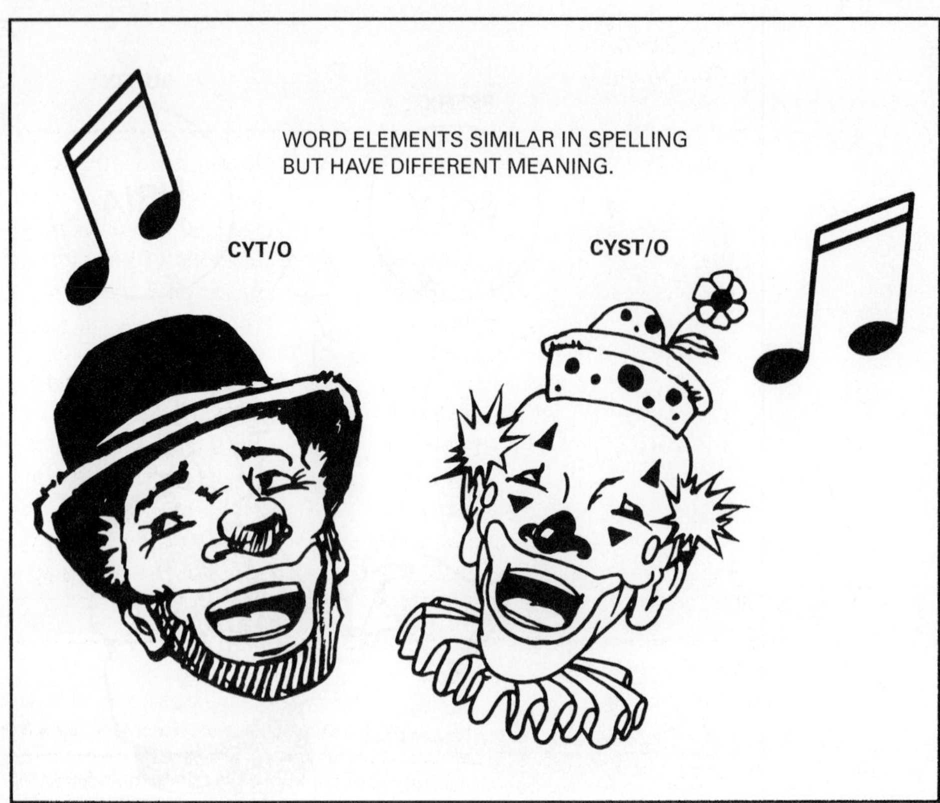
WORD ELEMENTS SIMILAR IN SPELLING
BUT HAVE DIFFERENT MEANING.
CYT/O
CYST/O

Figure 4–4

of word elements that often present difficulties. Examine this list carefully.

Prefix, Suffix, or Combining Form	*Example*	*Meaning*
ante-	antefebrile	before onset of fever
anti-	antifebrile	used against fever
a-	adipsia	absence of thirst
ad-	adrenal	near the kidney
a-, an-	anuria	absence of urine
ano-	anorectal	pertaining to anus and rectum

Prefix, Suffix, or Combining Form	*Example*	*Meaning*
ad-	adoral	near the mouth
aden	adenitis	glandular inflammation
cyt/o	cytogenesis	production (origin) of the cell
cyst/o	cystogram	x-ray record of the bladder
di-	diatomic	containing two atoms
dia-	diagnosis	to know through (recognize) a disease
dis-	dissect	to cut apart
dys-	dysmenorrhea	difficult or painful menstruation
en-	encephalitis	inflammation of the brain
enter/o	enteroplasty	operative revision of intestines

Prefix, Suffix, or Combining Form	Example	Meaning
hem-	hemangioma	tumor consisting of blood vessels
hemi-	hemianalgesia	pain relief in half of body
hem/o	hemotoxin	a blood cell poison
hyper-	hypertension	high blood pressure
hypo-	hypotension	low blood pressure
ile/o	ileocecum	ileum (section of small intestine)
ili/o	iliosacrum	ilium (part of hip bone)
inter-	interstitial	lying between spaces
intra-	intracranial	within the skull
macro-	macroscopy	seen large, as with the naked eye
micro-	microscopy	seen small, as by microscope
my/o	myology	study of muscle
myel	myeloma	tumor of the bone marrow
necr	necrosis	state of tissue death

Prefix, Suffix, or Combining Form	Example	Meaning
nephr	nephrosis	condition of the kidneys
neur	neurosis	nervous condition
oste	osteology	study of bone
ot/o	otology	study of the ear
per-	percussion	a striking through the body
peri-	pericardial	around the heart
pre-	preclinical	before the onset of disease
py/o	pyogenic	pus producing
pyr/o	pyrogenic	fever producing

- Finally, two groups of suffixes contain quite similar word elements, each of which has a specific meaning.

Suffix	Word	Definition
-gram	electrocardiogram	record of heart action
-graph	electrocardiograph	machine that makes record
-graphy	electrocardiography	process of making record

Electrocardiography is performed by a technician who connects parts of the patient's body to an **electrocardiograph,** which produces a record of the patient's heart action called an **electrocardiogram.**

Suffix	Word	Definition
-ectomy	gastrectomy	surgical removal of the stomach
-stomy	gastrostomy	surgical opening into the stomach
-tomy	gastrotomy	surgical incision into the stomach

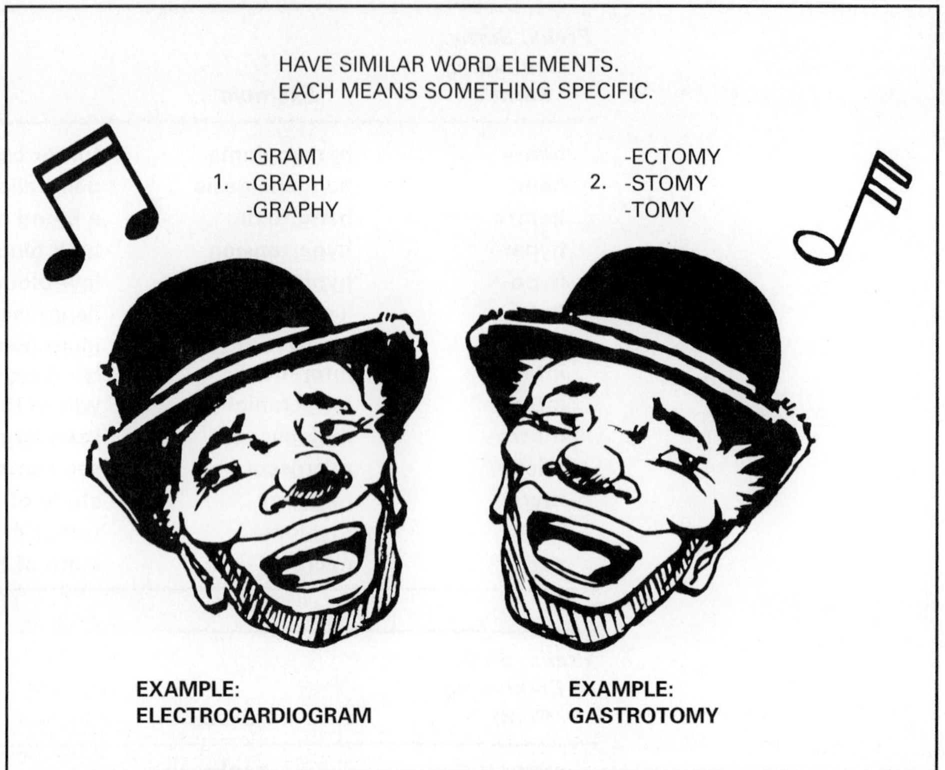

Figure 4–5

An infant who swallowed a pin requires a **gastrotomy** to remove the pin from the stomach; a patient unable to take food by mouth has a **gastrostomy** and is fed by tube directly into the stomach; the doctor performs a **gastrectomy** on a patient with bleeding ulcers. (Fig. 4–5.)

KEY IDEA: LIST OF WORD ELEMENTS

The following list of word elements is arranged alphabetically. Word elements that are most often used as prefixes are followed by a hyphen (ambi-); suffixes are preceded by a hyphen (-algia). Remember that sometimes a term changes its function (a prefix is used as a root, for example) when it is used in a different word.

- Repeat aloud each of the word elements and its meaning.
- Pronounce the words given as examples.
- Try to figure out the meaning of the sample word with the help of information given in the list. For example, the third word on the list is "adrenal." "Ad" means "near," "toward." Now look up "renal." You will find that it means "kidney." Therefore, adrenal means "near the kidney."

Prefix, Suffix, or Combining Form	*Refers to or Means*	*Example*	
A-, AN-,	**without, lack of, absent, deficient**	**asepsis** **anemia**	**a/SEP/sis** **an/Ē/mi/a**
AB-, ABS-	**from, away**	**abnormal** **abscess**	**ab/NORM/al** **ABS/cess**
AD-	**near, toward**	**adrenal**	**ad/RĒN/al**

Prefix, Suffix, or Combining Form	*Refers to or Means*	*Example*	
ADEN/O	gland	adenopathy	ad/en/OP/a/thy
AER/O	air	anaerobe	an/Ā/er/obe
ALB	white	albuminuria	al/BŪ/min/uri/a
-ALGIA, -ALGESIA	pain	analgesia	an/al/GĒ/si/a
AMBI-	both	ambidextrous	am/bi/DEX/trous
ANGI/O	vessel (blood or lymph)	angioma	an/gi/O/ma
ANTE-	before	antenatal	an/te/NĀT/al
ANTI-	against	antiseptic	an/ti/SEP/tic
ARTERI/O	artery	arteriosclerosis	ar/ter/i/o/scler/O/sis
ARTHR/O	joint	arthroplasty	AR/thro/plas/ty
-ASTHENIA	weakness	myasthenia	my/as/THĒ/ni/a
AUTO-	self	autopathy	au/to/PATH/y
BI-	two, twice	bicellular	bi/CELL/u/lar
BLEPHAR/O	eyelid	blepharoplasty	ble/PHAR/o/plasty
BRADY-	slow	bradycardia	brad/y/CAR/di/a
BRONCH/O	bronchus	bronchitis	bron/CHĪ/tis
CARCIN/O	cancer of epithelial tissue	carcinogen	car/CIN/o/gen
CARDI/O	heart	myocardium	my/o/CAR/di/um
-CELE	tumor, swelling, hernia, sac	enterocele	EN/ter/o/cēle
-CENTESIS	puncture	thoracentesis	tho/ra/cen/TĒ/sis
CEPHAL/O	head	hydrocephaly	hy/dro/CEPH/a/ly
CHOL/E	gall	cholelithiasis	chol/e/lith/I/a/sis
CHOLECYST/O	gallbladder	cholecystectomy	cho/le/cys/tect/o/my
CHOLEDOCH/O	common bile duct	choledochostomy	cho/le/do/CHOS/to/my
CHONDR/O	cartilage	chondroma	chon/DRŌ/ma
-CIDE	kill	germicide	GERM/i/cide
CIRCUM-	around	circumcision	cir/cum/CI/sion
-CISE	cut	excise	ex/CISE
COL/O	colon	colitis	co/LĪ/tis
COLP/O	vagina	colporrhaphy	col/POR/rha/phy
CONTRA-	against	contraception	con/tra/CEP/tion
COST/O	rib	intercostal	in/ter/COS/tal
CRANI/O	skull	craniotomy	cra/ni/OT/o/my
CYAN/O	blue	cyanotic	cy/an/OT/ic
CYST/O	urinary bladder	cystogram	CYS/to/gram
CYT/O	cell	monocyte	MON/o/cyte
DE-	down, from	decubitus	de/CŪ/bi/tus
DENT/I	tooth	dentistry	DEN/tis/try
DERM/O, DERMAT/O	skin	dermatology	derm/a/TOL/o/gy
DEXTR/O	right	dextrocardia	dex/tro/CARDI/a
DI-	two	diplopia	dip/LŌP/i/a
DIA-	through, between, across, apart	diarrhea	di/a/RRHE/a

Prefix, Suffix, or Combining Form	*Refers to or Means*	*Example*	
DIS-	apart	dissect	dis/SECT
DYS-	painful, difficult, disordered	dysmenorrhea	dys/men/o/RRHĒ/a
ECTO-	outer, on the outside	ectocytic	ect/o/SY/tic
-ECTOMY	surgical removal	prostatectomy	pros/ta/TEC/to/my
-EMESIS	vomiting	hematemesis	hem/at/EM/e/sis
-EMIA	blood	leukemia	leu/KĒ/mi/a
EN-	in, inside	encapsulated	en/CAP/su/la/ted
ENCEPHAL/O	brain	encephalitis	en/ceph/a/LĪ/tis
ENDO-	within, inner, on the inside	endometrium	en/do/MĒ/tri/um
ENTER/O	intestine	enteritis	en/ter/Ī/tis
EPI-	above, over	epigastric	ep/i/GAS/tric
ERYTHR/O	red	erythrocyte	er/yth/RŌ/cyte
-ESTHESIA	sensation	anesthesia	an/es/THĒ/si/a
EX- EXTRA-	out	extrahepatic	ex/tra/HEP/a/tic
FEBR/I	fever	afebrile	a/FĒB/rile
FIBR/O	connective tissue	fibroma	FĪ/bro/ma
GASTR/O	stomach	gastrocele	GAS/tro/cele
-GENE, -GENIC	production, origin	neurogenic	neu/ro/GEN/ic
GLOSS/O	tongue	glossalgia	glos/SAL/gi/a
GLUC/O, GLYC/O	sugar, sweet	glycosuria	gly/co/SUR/i/a
-GRAM	record	myelogram	MY/e/lo/gram
-GRAPH	machine	electroence-phalograph	e/lec/tro/en/CEPH/al/o/graph
-GRAPHY	practice, process	ventriculography	ven/tri/cu/LOG/ra/phy
GYNE	woman	gynecology	gy/ne/COL/o/gy
HEMAT/O, HEM/O	blood	hematology	hem/at/OL/o/gy
HEMI-	half	hemiplegia	hem/i/PLĒ/gi/a
HEPA, HEPAT/O	liver	hepatitis	hep/a/TĪ/tis
HERNI/O	rupture	hernioplasty	HER/ni/o/plas/ty
HIST/O	tissue	histology	his/TOL/o/gy
HYDR/O	water	hydronephrosis	hy/dro/neph/RŌ/sis
HYPER-	over, above, increased, excessive	hypertension	hy/per/TEN/sion
HYPO-	under, beneath, decreased	hypotension	hy/po/TEN/sion
HYSTER/O	uterus	hysterectomy	hys/ter/ECT/o/my
-IASIS	abnormal condition of	urolithiasis	u/ro/lith/Ī/a/sis
IATR/O	treatment	iatrogenic	i/A/tro/genic
ICTER/O	jaundice	icterogenic	IC/ter/o/gen/ic
ILE/O	ileum (part of small intestine)	ileitis	il/ē/I/tis
ILI/O	ilium (part of hip)	iliosacrum	il/i/o/SĀ/crum

Prefix, Suffix, or Combining Form	*Refers to or Means*	*Example*	
INTER-	between	intercellular	inter/CELL/u/lar
INTRA-	within	intramuscular	in/tra/MUS/cu/lar
-ITIS	inflammation of	appendicitis	ap/pen/di/CĪ/tis
LAPAR/O	abdomen	laparotomy	la/par/OT/o/my
-LEPSY	seizure, convulse	narcolepsy	NAR/co/lep/sy
LEUK/O	white	leukorrhea	leu/ko/RRHĒ/a
LIP/O	fat	lipoma	lip/O/ma
LITH/O	stone, calculus	lithocystotomy	lith/o/cys/TO/ tomy
-LOGY	study of	neurology	neur/OL/o/gy
-LYSIS	loosen, dissolve	hemolysis	hem/OL/y/sis
MACRO-	large, long	macrocyte	MAC/ro/cyte
MAL-	bad, poor, disordered	malabsorption	mal/ab/SORP/ tion
-MANIA	insanity	kleptomania	klep/to/MĀN/ia
MAST/O	breast	mastectomy	mas/TEC/to/my
MEG/A	large	splenomegaly	splen/o/MEG/a/ly
MEN/O	month	menstruation	men/stru/A/tion
MESO-	middle	mesocardia	MES/o/card/i/a
-METER	measure	thermometer	ther/MOM/e/ter
METR/O	uterus	metrorrhagia	met/ror/RHA/gia
MICRO-	small	microscope	MĪC/ro/scope
MONO-	single one	monocyte	MON/o/cyte
MUC/O	mucous membrane	mucocutaneous	mu/co/cu/TĀ/ne/ ous
MYC/O	fungus	mycosis	my/CŌ/sis
MYEL/O	spinal cord, bone marrow	myelomeningo- cele	my/el/o/men/IN/ go/cele
MY/O	muscle	myopathy	my/OP/a/thy
NARC/O	stupor	narcotic	nar/COT/ic
NAS/O	nose	nasopharynx	nas/o/PHA/rynx
NAT/I	birth	prenatal	pre/NĀ/tal
NECR/O	death	necropsy	NEC/rop/sy
NEO-	new	neoplasm	NĒ/o/plasm
NEPHR/O	kidney	nephritis	ne/PHRĪ/tis
NEUR/O	nerve	neuralgia	neu/RAL/gi/a
NON-	no, not	nontoxic	non/TOX/ic
OCUL/O	eye	oculomycosis	OC/u/lo/my/co/sis
-OMA	tumor	carcinoma	car/ci/NŌ/ma
OOPHOR/O	ovary	oophorectomy	o/opho/REC/to/my
OPHTHALM/O	eye	ophthalmoscope	oph/THAL/mo/ scope
-OPIA	vision	photopic	pho/TŌP/ic
ORCHI/O	testicle	orchipexy	ORCH/i/pex/y
ORTH/O	straight	orthopedics	orth/o/PĒD/ics
-OSIS	abnormal condition	neurosis	neu/RŌ/sis
OSTE/O	bone	osteoma	os/te/Ō/ma
OT/O	ear	otolith	OT/o/lith
-PARA	to bring forth or to bear	multipara	MUL/ti/para

Prefix, Suffix, or Combining Form	Refers to or Means	Example	
PARA-	alongside of, abnormal	paraplegia	par/a/PLĒ/gi/a
PATH/O	disease	pathology	pa/THOL/o/gy
PED/O (Latin)	foot	pedograph	PED/o/graph
PED/O (Greek)	child	pediatrics	pe/di/AT/rics
-PENIA	too few	leukopenia	leuko/PĒN/i/a
PERI-	around, covering	pericarditis	pe/ri/car/DĪ/tis
-PEXY	to sew up in position	nephropexy	NEPH/ro/pex/y
PHARYNG/O	throat	pharyngoplasty	pha/RYN/go/plas/ty
PHLEB/O	vein	phlebitis	phle/BĪ/tis
-PHOBIA	fear, dread	photophobia	pho/to/PHŌ/bi/a
PHOT/O	light	photolysis	pho/TO/ly/sis
-PLASTY	operative repair	rhinoplasty	RHĪ/no/plas/ty
-PLEGIA	paralysis	quadriplegia	qua/dri/PLĒ/gi/a
-PNEA	breathing	orthopnea	or/thop/NĒ/a
PNEUM/O	air, lungs	pneumonia	pneu/MŌ/ni/a
POLY-	much, many	polyuria	po/ly/U/ri/a
POST-	after	postpartum	post/PAR/tum
PROCT/O	rectum	proctoscopy	proc/TOS/co/py
PRE-	before	preoperative	pre/OP/er/a/tive
-PTOSIS	falling	nephroptosis	neph/rop/TŌ/sis
PYEL/O	pelvis of kidney	pyelonephritis	py/el/o/neph/RI /tis
PY/O	pus	pyogenic	py/o/GEN/ic
PYR/O	heat, temperature	pyrexia	py/REX/i/a
REN/O	kidney	suprarenal	su/pra/RĒ/nal
RETRO-	behind, backward	retrosternal	ret/ro/STER/nal
RHIN/O	nose	rhinopathy	rhi/NOP/a/thy
-RRHAGE	profuse bleeding, flow	hemorrhage	HEM/or/rhage
-RRHAPHY	to suture/to repair a defect	herniorrhaphy	her/ni/OR/raph/y
-RRHEA	flow	diarrhea	di/a/RRHĒ/a
SALPING/O	oviduct	salpingectomy	sal/pin/GEC/to/my
SCLER/O	hardening	scleroderma	scler/o/DERM/a
-SCOPE	instrument to view	cystoscope	CYS/to/scope
-SCOPY	look into, see	esophagoscopy	e/soph/a/GOS/co/py
SECT/O	to cut	transect	tran/SECT
SEMI-	half	semicircular	sem/i/CIR/cu/lar
SEPT/I	poison, infection	septicemia	sep/ti/CĒM/i/a
SPLEN/O	spleen	splenocele	SPLE/no/cele
STOMAT/O	mouth	stomatitis	sto/ma/TĪ/tis
-STOMY	surgical opening	colostomy	col/OST/o/my
SUB-	under	subacute	sub/a/CŪTE
SUPRA-, SUPER-	above	suprapubic	su/pra/PŪ/bic

Prefix, Suffix, or Combining Form	Refers to or Means	Example	
-THERAPY	treatment	hydrotherapy	hy/dro/THER/a/py
-THERMY	heat	diathermy	DĪ/a/therm/y
THORAC/O	chest	thoracotomy	thor/a/COT/o/my
THROMB/O	clot	thrombosis	throm/BŌ/sis
THYR/O	thyroid gland	thyroxin	thy/ROX/in
-TOME	instrument to cut	dermatome	derm/a/TOME
-TOMY	incision, surgical cutting	gastrotomy	gas/TROT/o/my
TRANS-	across	transfusion	trans/FŪ/sion
UR/O	urine	uremia	u/RĒ/mi/a
-URIA, -URIC	condition of, presence in urine	glycosuria	gly/co/SŪR/i/A
UNI	one	unicellular	u/ni/CELL/u/lar
VAS/O	blood vessel	vasoconstriction	vas/o/con/STRIC/tion

KEY IDEA: FORMULATING MEDICAL TERMS

Many medical terms referring to parts of the body systems and functions come from Latin or Greek root elements. These roots should not be seen as synonyms for English equivalents. Rather, they should be understood as referring to the English terms. Careful study will increase your familiarity with Latin and Greek roots and the English words that come from them. (Table 4–1; Figs. 4–6, 4–7, and 4–8.)

TABLE 4–1

Definitions of Latin and Greek Root Words by Body System

Word Element or Combining Form	Refers to
Integumentary system (skin)	
derm/o, dermat/o	skin
muc/o	mucous membrane
hist/o	tissue
Musculoskeletal system	
my/o	muscle
myocardi/o	heart muscle
myocolp/o	vaginal muscle
myometr/o	uterine muscle
oste/o	bone
chondr/o	cartilage
fibr/o	connective tissue
arthr/o	joint
cost/o	rib
crani/o	skull
ili/o	hipbone, ilium
sacr/o	tailbone, sacrum

TABLE 4–1 (*Continued*)

Word Element or Combining Form	*Refers to*
myel/o	bone marrow
rachi/o	spinal column; vertebrae
inguin/o	groin
Respiratory system	
aer/o	air
nas/o, rhin/o	nose
pharyng/o	throat
trache/o	windpipe
thorac/o	chest
bronch/o	bronchus
pneum/o	lung
Circulatory system	
cardi/o	heart
hemat/o, hem/o	blood
vas/o	blood vessel
arteri/o	artery
phleb/o	vein
lymph/o	lymphatic system
angi/o	blood and lymphatic vessels
erythr/o	red
leuk/o	white
cyan/o	blue
Digestive system	
stomat/o	mouth
dent/i	teeth
gloss/o	tongue
pharyng/o	pharynx, throat
esophag/o	esophagus, food pipe
gastr/o	stomach
enter/o	small intestine
hepat/o	liver
cholecyst/o	gallbladder
chol/e	bile, gall
lip/o	fat
choledoch/o	common bile duct
ile/o	ileum
col/o	large intestine
append/o	appendix
proct/o	rectum
an/o	anus
lapar/o	abdomen
Nervous system	
encephal/o	brain
myel/o	spinal cord
neur/o	nerve
ocul/o, ophthalm/o	eye
ot/o	ear
radicu/o	nerve root

TABLE 4–1 (*Continued*)

Word Element or Combining Form	*Refers to*
Endocrine system	
aden/o	gland
adren/o	adrenal gland
thyr/o	thyroid
glyc/o, gluc/o	sugar
hypophys/o	pituitary gland
Urinary system	
nephr/o, ren/o	kidney
pyel/o	kidney pelvis
hydr/o	water
ur/o	urine
ureter/o	ureter
cyst/o	urinary bladder
Reproductive system	
andr/o	man
gynec/o	woman
orchi/o, orchid/o	testicles
oophor/o	ovary
hyster/o, metr/o	uterus, womb
salping/o	oviduct
colp/o	vagina
mast/o	breasts
prostat/o	prostate
gravid/o	pregnancy
mamm/o	breast

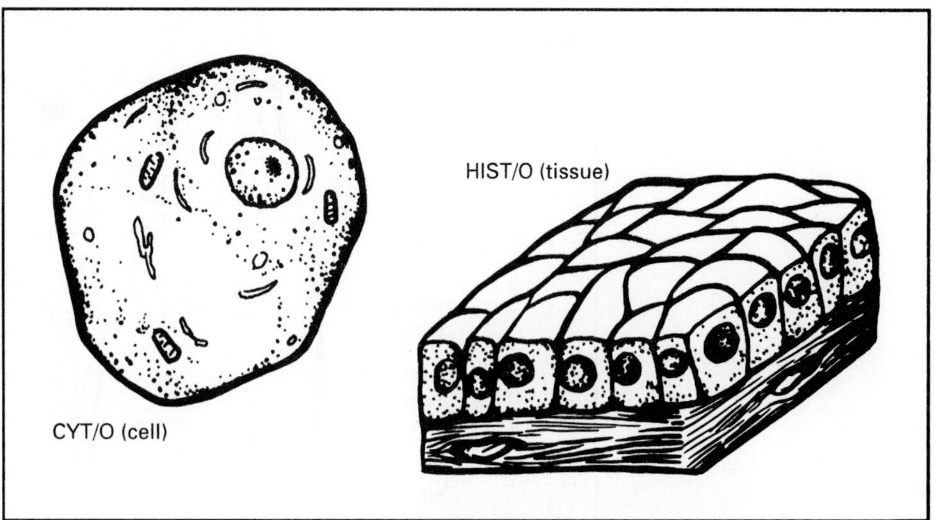

Figure 4–6

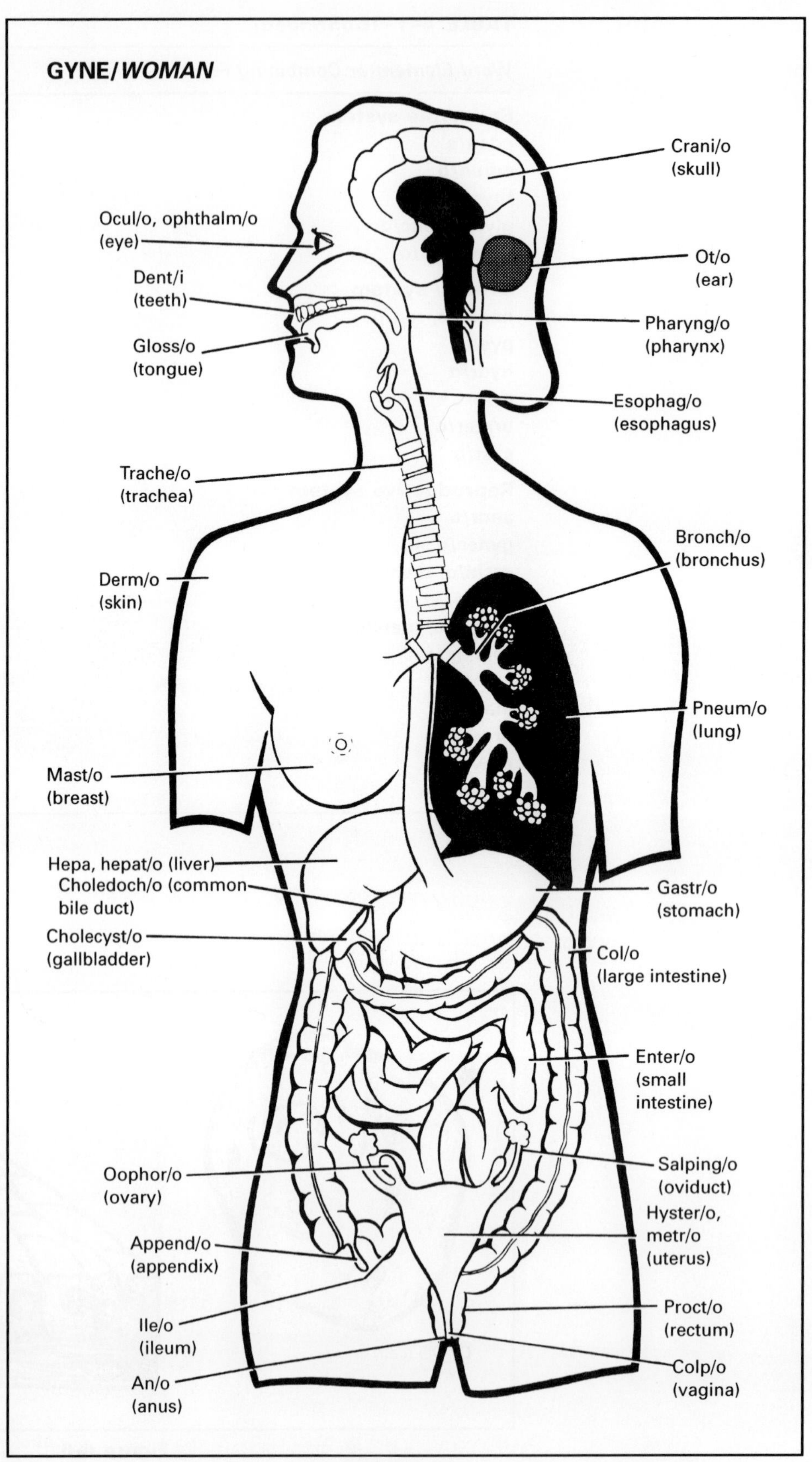
GYNE/*WOMAN*
Crani/o (skull)
Ocul/o, ophthalm/o (eye)
Ot/o (ear)
Dent/i (teeth)
Pharyng/o (pharynx)
Gloss/o (tongue)
Esophag/o (esophagus)
Trache/o (trachea)
Bronch/o (bronchus)
Derm/o (skin)
Pneum/o (lung)
Mast/o (breast)
Hepa, hepat/o (liver)
Choledoch/o (common bile duct)
Gastr/o (stomach)
Cholecyst/o (gallbladder)
Col/o (large intestine)
Enter/o (small intestine)
Oophor/o (ovary)
Salping/o (oviduct)
Hyster/o, metr/o (uterus)
Append/o (appendix)
Ile/o (ileum)
Proct/o (rectum)
An/o (anus)
Colp/o (vagina)

Figure 4–7

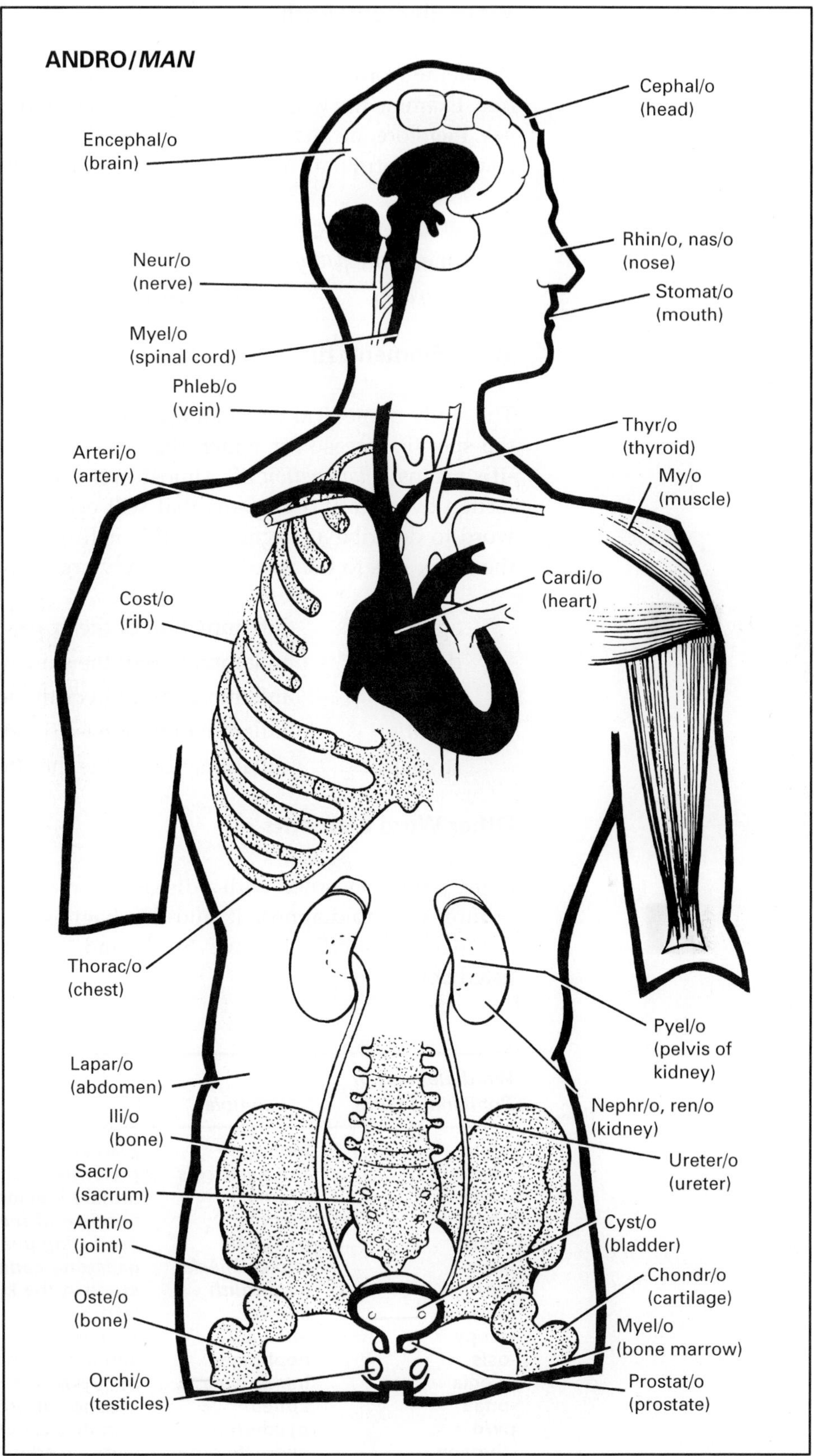
ANDRO/*MAN*
Cephal/o
(head)
Encephal/o
(brain)
Neur/o
(nerve)
Rhin/o, nas/o
(nose)
Stomat/o
(mouth)
Myel/o
(spinal cord)
Phleb/o
(vein)
Thyr/o
(thyroid)
Arteri/o
(artery)
My/o
(muscle)
Cardi/o
(heart)
Cost/o
(rib)
Thorac/o
(chest)
Pyel/o
(pelvis of
kidney)
Lapar/o
(abdomen)
Nephr/o, ren/o
(kidney)
Ili/o
(bone)
Ureter/o
(ureter)
Sacr/o
(sacrum)
Arthr/o
(joint)
Cyst/o
(bladder)
Chondr/o
(cartilage)
Oste/o
(bone)
Myel/o
(bone marrow)
Orchi/o
(testicles)
Prostat/o
(prostate)

Figure 4–8

Word Element: Path

When the word element **path** is found in a medical term, it always means *disease.* Examine the word **pathology.** The suffix **-logy** means the *study of; pathology,* therefore, means the *study* of disease. Now use the word element *path* as a suffix to formulate a whole category of medical terms.

arterio*pathy*	any disease of the arteries
pneumono*pathy*	any disease of the lungs
uro*pathy*	any disease affecting the urinary tract

Word Element: Itis

The study of medical terminology can aid you in understanding the name of the specific disease for which the patient has been hospitalized. The suffix **-itis** means *inflammation* of. Almost every organ in the body is subject to infection by disease organisms that will cause an inflammatory reaction. The word to describe a diagnosis of this nature is formulated simply by adding the suffix **-itis** to the word for the body organ so affected.

appendic*itis*	inflammation of the appendix
dermat*itis*	inflammation of the skin
hepat*itis*	inflammation of liver tissue
rhin*itis*	inflammation of nasal mucosa
stomat*itis*	inflammation of the mouth

Other Word Elements

Many terms concerned with a disease, its many symptoms, the tools and procedures used to diagnose it, and the diagnoses themselves are formulated in the manner described above. Study and learn the terms in common usage listed below.

Word Element or Combining Form	*Example*	*Definition*
-algia	neur*algia*	*pain* along the nerves
-centesis	thora*centesis*	*puncture* of chest wall to remove fluids
-emia	ur*emia*	urinary wastes in the *blood*
febr/o	a*febr*ile	absence of *fever*
-genic	pyo*genic*	*producing* pus
-iasis	cholelith*iasis*	gallstone *condition*
lith/o	nephro*lith*	*stone* in the kidney
-oma	lip*oma*	fatty *tumor*
-scopy	ano*scopy*	*visualization* of the anus
-osis	nephr*osis*	abnormal *condition* of the kidney
-plegia	hemi*plegia*	*paralysis* of one-half of the body
-pnea	a*pnea*	absence of *breathing*
py/o	*pyo*derma	skin disease caused by *pus*-forming bacteria
-therapy	hydro*therapy*	water used in *treatment* of disease
-uria	poly*uria*	excessive *urine* production and urination

KEY IDEA: SURGICAL PROCEDURES

When you are working on a surgical floor, you will encounter another large group of medical terms. These describe surgical procedures. You will need to have some idea of the type of surgery done on a patient. For this you must learn the word elements used in the names for surgical procedures.

Word Element: Ectomy

The suffix **-ectomy** means **surgical removal.** When used in combination with any word element denoting an organ or other body part, the term formed means that the organ or body part has been removed.

gastr*ectomy*	surgical removal of the stomach
thyroid*ectomy*	surgical removal of the thyroid gland
col*ectomy*	surgical removal of the large intestine

In many cases, an organ may be removed only partially. To indicate this procedure, other words are used to modify the medical term, for example:

subtotal thyroidectomy *partial* cystectomy

Other modifying words may precede the medical term. This identifies the surgery performed even more accurately.

left salpingo-oophor*ectomy*	removal of the left ovary and oviduct
vaginal hyster*ectomy*	removal of the uterus through the vagina
transurethral prostat*ectomy*	removal of the prostate through the urethra
total abdominal hyster*ectomy*	removal of the entire uterus through abdomen

Other Word Elements Used in Surgical Procedures

Word Element	*Example*	*Definition*
-rrhaphy	hernio*rrhaphy*	*suturing* of a hernia
-stomy	uretero*stomy*	*formation of an opening* for ureteral drainage
-tomy	colpo*tomy*	*surgical incision* into the vagina
-pexy	cysto*pexy*	*fixation of bladder* to the abdominal wall
-plasty	rhino*plasty*	*surgical repair* of the nose
-tripsy	litho*tripsy*	*crushing* of a stone in the kidney, bladder, or urethra

Abbreviations

Many facilities have approved lists of abbreviations, and lists can be found in many medical texts. Although used constantly, there is a lack of consistency among these sources. While some show periods or capitalization, others may not (cc, c.c. = cubic centimeter; CC, C.C. = chief complaint). One abbreviation may have several meanings (e.g., CD = carbonate dehydratase, cardiac disease, cystic duct, communicable disease, etc.). Some abbreviations are acronyms (words formed from the first letters of other words or parts of words). Some are initializations. Some are symbols and some are abbreviations of a word or words. Some are from Greek and Latin and others are from English, but all are shorter terms for longer words.

The health unit coordinator must be familiar with many abbreviations. Study the approved list from your hospital and the lists which follow. When in doubt about the meaning of any abbreviation, always remember to ask.

A list of common abbreviations and their meanings follow. Add to this list any new abbreviations commonly used in your health care institution.

	Abbreviation	*Meaning*	*Abbreviation*	*Meaning*
A	$\bar{a}$	before	AMA	against medical advice, American Medical Association
	$\overline{aa}$	of each, equal parts	Amb	ambulatory
	AA	Alcoholics Anonymous	Amp	ampule
	AAA	abdominal aortic aneurysm	Amt	amount
	@	at	ANA	antinuclear antibodies
	AB	abortion	A&P repair	anterior and posterior repair
	Abd	abdomen	Anes	anesthesia
	ABG	arterial blood gas	Ant	anterior
	ABR	absolute bed rest	AP&L	anterior, posterior, and lateral
	a.c.	before meals	Approx	approximately
	Acid phos	acid phosphatase	Appy	appendectomy
	ACL	anterior cruciate ligament	aPTT	activated partial thrombo-plastin time
	ACTH	adrenocorticotrophic hormone	Aq	aqueous
	AD	admitting diagnosis, right ear	aqua	water, H_2O
	A&D	admission and discharge	ARC	AIDS-related complex
	ADL	activities of daily living	ARDS	acute respiratory distress syndrome
	Ad lib	as desired	ARF	acute renal failure
	Adm	admission	AS	left ear
	adm spec	admission specimen	ASAP	as soon as possible
	AEO	automatic external defibrillator	ASCVD	arteriosclerotic cardiovascular disease
	AFB	acid fast bacillus	ASHD	arteriosclerotic heart disease
	AFP	alfa-feto protein	ATH	acute toxic hepatitis
	$AgNO_3$	silver nitrate	ATN	acute tubular necrosis
	A/G	albumin/globulin ratio	AU	both ears
	AIDS	acquired immune deficiency syndrome	AV	atrioventricular
	AKA	also known as, above-the-knee amputation	A&W	alive and well
	A-Line	arterial line	AWOL	away without leave
	alk phos	alkaline phosphatase	AZ test	Aschheim-Zondek test for pregnancy
	ALS	amyotrophic lateral sclerosis		
	A.M.	morning		
B	B/A	backache	BOW	bag of water
	B&B	bowel and bladder (training)	BP	blood pressure
	BBB	bundle branch block	BPH	benign prostatic hyperplasia
	Baso	basophil	BR	bedrest
	BE	barium enema	BRP	bathroom privileges
	BID	twice a day	BS	blood sugar
	bkfst	breakfast	BSC	bedside commode
	Bld	blood	BUN	blood urea nitrogen
	BM	bowel movement	BVD	bag-valve device
	BMT	bilateral myringotomy with tubes, bone marrow transplant	BW	birth weight
			Bx	biopsy
C	C	centrigrade	Ca	cancer, calcium
	$\bar{c}$	with	CABG	coronary artery bypass graft

	Abbreviation	Meaning	Abbreviation	Meaning
	CAD	coronary artery disease	COPD	chronic obstructive pulmonary disease
	Cal	caloric	CP	cocktail privileges
	Cap	capsule	CPA	carotid phonoangiography
	CAT	computerized axial tomography	CPAP	continuous positive airway pressure
	Cath	catheter or catheterize	CPK	creatinine phosphokinase
	CBC	complete blood count	CPR	cardiopulmonary resuscitation
	CBF	cerebral blood flow	CPT	chest physiotherapy
	CC	chief complaint	CRRT	continuous renal replacement therapy
	cc	cubic centimeter	CS	Central Supply or Central Service
	CCU	Coronary Care Unit, Critical Care Unit	C-S, C/S	cervical spine
	CDC	Center for Disease Control	C&S	culture and sensitivity
	C EX	cataract extraction	C-section	cesarean section
	chol	cholesterol	CSF	cerebral spinal fluid
	CHF	congestive heart failure	CSS	closed system suction
	CHO	carbohydrate	CT	computed tomography
	chr	chronic	CVA	cerebral vascular accident
	Cl	chloride	CVD	cerebral vascular disease
	Cmpd	compound	CVI	cerebral vascular insufficiency
	CMV	cytomegalovirus	CVP	central venous pressure
	CNS	central nervous system	C/W	consistent with
	C/O	complains of	CXR	chest x-ray
	CO_2	carbon dioxide	Cysto	cystoscopy
	Coag	coagulation		
	Comf	comfortable		
	Cont	continuous		
D	D 5½ NS	5% dextrose in 0.45% normal saline	DKA	diabetic ketoacidosis
	D 5¼ NS	5% dextrose in 0.25% normal saline	DM	diabete mellitus
	D5LR	5% dextrose in Lactate Ringer's	DNA	desoxyribonucleic acid, do not awaken
	D5NS	5% dextrose in normal saline	DNR	do not resuscitate
	D5W	5% dextrose in water	DOA	dead on arrival
	DAT	diet as tolerated	DOB	date of birth
	DC	discontinue	DOE	dyspnea on exertion
	D/C	discharge	DPT	diphtheria, pertussis, tetanus
	D&C	dilation and curettage	Dr.	doctor
	DDD	degenerative disc disease	dr or ʒ	dram
	Del. Rm. or DR	Delivery Room	DRG	diagnosis related group
	Dept.	department	DSD	dry sterile dressing
	Diff	differential white blood cell count	Dsg	dressing
	Dig	digoxin	D.T.'s	delirium tremens
	Dil	dilute or dissolve	DU	duodenal ulcer
			Dx	diagnosis
E	E	enema	EFM	electronic fetal monitor
	Ea	each	EGD	esophagogastroduodenoscopy
	EBL	estimated blood loss	EKG	electrocardiogram
	ECF	extended care facility	Elix	elixir
	ECG	electrocardiogram	ELOS	estimated length of stay
	ECHO	echogram	EMG	electromyogram
	ECHO virus	enterocytopathogenic human orphan virus	ENT	ears, nose, throat
	ECT	electroconvulsive therapy	EOB	edge of bed
	E.D.	emergency department	EOM	extraocular movement
	EDC	estimated date of confinement	ER	emergency room
	EDD	estimated date of delivery	ERCP	endoscopic retrograde cholangiopancreatography
	EEG	electroencephalogram	Esp	especially
	EENT	eyes, ears, nose, throat		

	Abbreviation	Meaning	Abbreviation	Meaning
	ESR	erythrocyte sedimentation rate	ETOH	alcohol
	ESS	endoscopic sinus surgery	ETT	endotracheal tube
	Etc	et cetera	EUA	examination under anesthesia
	Etiol	etiology	Eval	evaluation
			Exam	examination
F	F	Fahrenheit	FHR	fetal heart rate
	F or Fe	female	Fib	fibrillation
	FB	foreign body	FIO_2	fractional inspired oxygen
	FBS	fasting blood sugar	Fld	fluid
	Fdg	feeding	Fluro	fluroscopy
	Fe	iron	FM	fetal movement
	$FeSO_4$	ferrous sulfate	Frac	fracture
	FEF	forced expiratory flow	FS	frozen section
	FEV1	forced expiratory volume 1 second	Ft	foot or feet
	FEV3	forced expiratory volume 3 seconds	F/U	follow-up
	FF	fundus firm, force fluids	FUO	fever of undetermined origin
	FH	family history	FWB	full weight-bearing
			FWW	front wheel walker
			Fx	fracture
G	G	gravida	GER	gastroesophageal reflux
	GA	general anesthesia	GI	gastrointestinal
	Gal	gallon	Gm or g	gram
	GB	gallbladder	GP	general practitioner
	GBS	gallbladder series	gr	grain
	GC	gonorrhea	gtt	drop
	GCS	Glascow coma scale	GTT	glucose tolerance test
	GE	gastroenterology	G tube	gastric tube
	GEA	general endotracheal anesthesia	GU	genitourinary
	Gen	general	GYN	gynecology
H	H/A	heated aerosol	H_2O	water
	HA	headache	H_2O_2	hydrogen peroxide
	HAL	hyperalimentation	H/O	history of
	HAV	hepatitis A virus	HOB	head of bed
	Hg	hemoglobin	H & P	history and physical
	HBD	has been drinking	HP	hot packs
	HBP	high blood pressure	HPI	history of present illness
	HBV	hepatitis B virus	Hr	hour
	HCO_3	bicarbonate	h.s.	at bedtime
	HCG	human chorionic gonadotrophin	HSV	herpes simplex virus
	HCl	hydrochloric acid	HT	Hubbard tank
	Hct	hematocrit	Ht	height
	H & H	hemoglobin and hematocrit	HVD	hypertensive vascular disease
	HIV	human immunodeficiency virus	Hx	history
			Hyper	above or high
			Hypo	below or low
I	IBD	inflammatory bowel disease	Imp	impression
	ICD	implantable cardioverter-defibrillator	in.	inch
	ICF	intermediate care facility	Inc	incomplete
	ICP	intracranial pressure	Inc. Spiro	incentive spirometry
	ICU	intensive care unit	IND	induction of labor
	I & D	incision and drainage	Infx	infection
	IDDM	insulin-dependent diabetes mellitus	Info	information
	i.e.	that is	Int	internal
	IH	infectious hepatitis	I & O	intake and output
	IHD	ischemic heart disease	IOL	intraocular lens
	IM	intramuscular	IOP	intraocular pressure
	Immuno	immunology	IPA	independent physicians association

	Abbreviation	Meaning	Abbreviation	Meaning
	IPPB	intermittent positive pressure breathing	Isol	isolation
			IUD	intrauterine device
	IQ	intelligence quotient	IV	intravenous
	Irreg	irregular	IVC	intravenous cholangiogram
	Irrig	irrigation	IVP	intravenous pyelogram
	IS	incentive spirometer	IVPB	intravenous piggyback
J	JP	Jackson-Pratt drain	Junct	junctional
	Jt	joint	JVD	jugular vein distension
K	K	potassium	KPE	Kelman phacoemulsification
	KCl	potassium chloride	KS	Kaposi's sarcoma
	Kg	kilogram	KUB	kidneys, ureters, bladder
	KI	potassium iodide	K wire	Kirchner wire
L	L	liter, lumbar	LOC	loss of consciousness
	L&A	light and accommodation	LOS	length of stay
	Lab	laboratory	LP	lumbar puncture
	Lac	laceration	LPGD	low-profile gastrostomy device
	Lap	laparotomy		
	Lat	lateral	LPN	licensed practical nurse
	Lb	pound	L/S	lumbar spine
	LBBB	left bundle branch block	L-S	lumbosacral
	L&D	labor and delivery	LSD	lysergic acid diethylamide
	LDH	lactic dehydrogenase	Lt or L	left
	LE	lower extremity	LUQ	left upper quadrant
	LLQ	left lower quadrant	LVN	licensed vocational nurse
	LMP	last menstrual period	L & W	living and well
	LOA	leave of absence	Lymph	lymphocyte
	LOB	loss of balance		
M	m	murmur	med	medication, medium
	M	male, meter	mEq	milliequivalent
	MAA	macroaggregated albumin	mg	milligram
	MAB	management of assaultive behavior	MG	myasthenia gravis
			MHP	moist hot pack
	MAC	monitored anesthesia care	MI	myocardial infarction, mitral insufficiency
	MAE	moves all extremities		
	MAP	mean arterial pressure	Min A	minimal assist
	Mat	maternity	ml	milliliter
	Max	maximum	mm	millimeter
	Max A	maximum assist	MMPI	Minnesota Multiphasic Personality Inventory
	McB	McBurney's point		
	MCH	maternal child health	Mod	moderate
	MCHC	mean corpuscular hemoglobin count	Mono	monocyte
			MR	may repeat
	mcg	microgram	MRI	magnetic resonance imaging
	MCV	mean corpuscular volume	MRS	middle respiratory syndrome
	MD	doctor of medicine	MS	multiple sclerosis
	mec	meconium	MVP	mitral valve prolapse
N	N	nitrogen	NICU	Neonatal Intensive Care Unit
	NA	Narcotics Anonymous	NIDDM	non-insulin-dependent diabetes mellitus
	Na	sodium		
	NaCl	sodium chloride	NIL	not in labor
	NAD	no apparent distress	NKA	no known allergies
	$NaHCO_3$	sodium bicarbonate	N_2O	nitrous oxide
	NAS	no added salt	no.	number
	NB	newborn	Noc	night
	N/C	no complaints	NP	neuropsychiatric, nursing procedure
	NC	nasal cannula		
	Neg	negative	NPO	nothing by mouth
	Neuro	neurology	NS	normal saline
	N/G	nasogastric	Nsg	nursing
	NHL	non-Hodgkin's lymphoma	NSR	normal sinus rhythm

	Abbreviation	*Meaning*	*Abbreviation*	*Meaning*
	NSVD	normal spontaneous vaginal delivery	N & V	nausea and vomiting
	NTG	nitroglycerin	NWB	non-weight-bearing
O	O	none	OPG	oculoplethysmography
	O_2	oxygen	O & P	ova and parasites
	O_2 cap	oxygen capacity	OPS	Outpatient Surgery
	O_2 cont	oxygen content	OPR	Outpatient Recovery
	O_2 sat	oxygen saturation	ORIF	open reduction internal fixation
	OB	obstetrics	Ortho	orthopedics
	OBS	organic brain syndrome	os	mouth
	Occ	occasional	OS	left eye
	OCG	oral cholecystogram	OT	Occupational Therapy
	OCT	oxytocin challenge test	OTC	over the counter
	OD	right eye, overdose	OU	both eyes
	Oint	ointment	OV	office visit
	OOB	out of bed	oz or ℥	ounce
	OP	operation, outpatient		
	OPD	Outpatient Department		
P	P	pulse	PICC	peripherally inserted central catheter
	$\bar{p}$	after	PID	pelvic inflammatory disease
	PA	pulmonary artery	PIH	pregnancy induced hypertension
	P & A	percussion and auscultation	PKU	phenylketonuria
	PAC	premature atrial contraction	PLT	platelets
	P_2CO_2	partial pressure of CO_2 in arterial blood	p.m.	afternoon
	PACU	Post Anesthesia Care Unit	PMC	postmortem care
	P_2O_2	partial pressure of O_2 in arterial blood	PMH	past medical history
	Pap smear	Papanicolaou smear	PMI	point of maximal impulse
	PAT	paroxysmal atrial tachycardia	PMS	premenstrual syndrome
	Path	pathology	PND	paroxysmal nocturnal dyspnea
	PAWP	pulmonary artery wedge pressure	PNS	peripheral nerve stimulator
	PBI	protein bound iodine	P-OX	pulse oximetry
	p.c.	after meals	PO_2	partial pressure of oxygen
	PCA	patient-controlled analgesia	PO	by mouth
	PCO_2	carbon dioxide pressure	Poc	positon of comfort
	PCP	pneumocystis carinii pneumonia, primary care physician	POD	postoperative day
	PCV	packed cell volume	Polys	polymorphonuclear leukocytes
	PCXR	portable chest x-ray	Post	posterior
	PD	postural drainage	Post-op	postoperative
	PD&P	postural drainage and percussion	PPD	purified protein derivative
	PE	physical examination	PP	postpartum
	Ped	pediatric	PPBS	postprandial blood sugar
	PEEP	positive end expiratory pressure	Pre	before
	PEG	percutaneous endoscopic gastrostomy	Pre-op	before surgery
	Per	by, through	Prep	preparation
	PEFR	peak expiratory flow rate	Prev	previous
	PERL	pupils equal and reactive to light	Prog	prognosis
	PFT	pulmonary function test	PRN	when necessary
	pH	potential of hydrogen	PROM	premature rupture of membranes
	PH	past history	Prot	protein
	Phono	phonophoresis	Pro time	prothrombin time
	Phos	phosphorus	PSA	prostatic serum antigen
	PI	present illness	Pt	patient
			PT	physical therapy, prothrombin time

	Abbreviation	*Meaning*	*Abbreviation*	*Meaning*
	PTA	prior to admission	PVC	premature ventricular contraction
	PTCA	percutaneous transluminal coronary angioplasty	PVD	peripheral vascular disease
	PTL	preterm labor	PVS	persistant vegetative state
	PTT	partial thromboplastin time	PWB	partial weight-bearing
	PTX	pneumothorax	PVH	pulmonary venous hypertension
	PUD	peptic ulcer disease		
	PUW	pick up walker	Px	prognosis
Q	q	every	qhs	every night at bedtime
	qAM	every morning	q noc	every night
	QC	quad care	qid	four times a day
	qd	every day	qns	quantity not sufficient
	qh	every hour	qod	every other day
	q2h	every 2 hours	QS	quad sets
	q3h	every 3 hours	qs	quantity sufficient
	q4h	every 4 hours	Qt	quart
R	R	respiration	RR	recovery room
	RA	rheumatoid arthritis	RIA	radioimmunoassay
	Rad T	radiation therapy	RLQ	right lower quadrant
	RBBB	right bundle branch block	RN	registered nurse
	RBC	red blood cell, red blood count	R/O	rule out
			ROM	range of motion, rupture of membranes
	RDS	respiratory distress syndrome		
	Rec	recommend	ROS	review of systems
	Reg	regular	RSR	regular sinus rhythm
	REM	rapid eye movement	Rt or R	right
	Resp	respiration	RT	respiratory therapy
	RF	rheumatoid factor	RUQ	right upper quadrant
	Rh	rhesus factor	RVH	right ventricular hypertrophy
	RHD	rheumatic heart disease	Rx	prescription
S	$\bar{s}$	without	SOB	shortness of breath
	s	sacral	Sol	solution
	SA	suicide attempt	SOR	see old records
	SAB	spontaneous abortion	Spec	specimen
	SBE	subacute bacterial endocarditis	Sp gr	specific gravity
			Span	spansule
	SBS	small bowel series	SR	sedimentation rate, system review, sustained release
	Sc or Sub Q	subcutaneous		
	SCBB	stereotactic core breast biopsy	$\overline{ss}$	one half
			SSE	soap suds enema
	SCN	Special Care Nursery	SSKI	saturated solution of potassium iodide
	SDS	Same Day Surgery		
	Sed rate	sedimentation rate	stab	stabnuclear neutrophil
	SGOT	serum glutamic oxaloacetic transaminase	Staph	staphylococcus
			STAT	at once
	SGPT	serum glutamic pyruvic transaminase	Stbn	stillborn
			STD	sexually transmitted disease
	SH	social history	STK	streptokinase
	SIDS	sudden infant death	Strep	streptococcus
	SLE	systemic lupus erythematosus	STSG	split thickness skin graft
			Subling	sublingual
	SMR	submucous resection	Supp	suppository
	SNF	skilled nursing facility	Surg	surgery
	S/O	significant other	SV	stroke volume
	SO_2	oxygen saturation	Syr	syrup
	SOAP	subjective, objective, assessment, plan		
T	T	temperature, thoracic	Tab	tablet
	T & A	tonsillectomy and adenoidectomy	TAB	therapeutic abortion
			TAH	total abdominal hysterectomy

	Abbreviation	*Meaning*	*Abbreviation*	*Meaning*
	Talc	talcum	TNM	T—primary tumor, N—nodal involvement, M—distant metastasis
	TB	tuberculosis	TOB	time of birth
	Tbsp	tablespoon	Tol	tolerance
	TCDB	turn, cough, and deep breathe	TO	telephone order
	T & C	type and cross-match	TPA	tissue plasminogen activator
	TCP	transcutaneous pacing	TPN	total parenteral nutrition
	TCU	Transitional Care Unit	TPR	temperature, pulse, respiration
	Temp	temperature	Trach	tracheostomy
	TENS	transcutaneous electrical nerve stimulation	t-s, t/s	thoracic spine
	TF	to follow	Tsp	teaspoon
	THR	total hip replacement	TT	tetanus toxoid
	TIA	transient ischemic attack	TURP	transurethral resection of prostate
	tid	three times a day	TURV	transurethral vaporization of prostate
	Tinc	tincture	TV	tidal volume
	TKO	to keep open	TVH	total vaginal hysterectomy
	TKR	total knee replacement	TWE	tap water enema
	TLC	total lung capacity, tender loving care	Tx	treatment, traction
	TMJ	temporomandibular joint		
	TM	tympanic membrane		
U	U	unit	UPC	unit packed cells
	UA	urinalysis	URI	upper respiratory infection
	UCD	usual childhood diseases	US	ultrasound
	UGI	upper gastrointestinal	USN	ultrasonic nebulizer
	UOQ	upper outer quadrant	UTI	urinary tract infection
	Ung	ointment	UWB	unit whole blood
	UNOS	United Network for Organ Sharing		
V	V	vein	Vit	vitamin
	Vag	vagina, vaginal	VO	verbal order
	VC	vital capacity	Vol	volume
	VD	venereal disease	V & P	vagotomy and pyloroplasty
	VDRL	Venereal Disease Research Laboratory	VS	vital signs
	VE	vaginal examination	VSS	vital signs stable
	VF or V fib	ventricular fibrillation	VT or V tach	ventricular tachycardia
W	W/A	while awake	WNL	within normal limits
	WB	whole blood	WP	whirlpool
	WBAT	weight bearing as tolerated	WPW	Wolfe-Parkinson-White syndrome
	WBC	white blood cell, white blood count	Wt	weight
	W/C	wheelchair		
	WD/WN	well developed, well nourished		
X	x	times	XRT	x-ray therapy
Y	Yd	yard	YO	year old
	Yr	year		
Symbols				
	&	and	+	plus
	@	at	–	minus
	> or ↑	greater than	±	plus or minus
	↑	increase	–	negative
	< or ↓	less than	◯ or +	positive
	↓	decrease	×	times
	⇄	equal to	♀	female
	○	hour	♂	male

LEARNING ACTIVITIES

Complete the following:

1. The ______________ is a word element added at the end of a word to change or add to its meaning.
2. The ______________ is added to the beginning of a word.
3. The ______________ is the body or main part of the word, and denotes the primary meaning of the word as a whole.
4. The ______________ is added sometimes for ease of pronunciation.
5. The ______________ is a combination of the word elements which together make up a word.
6. Define the following word elements:
   - **(a)** gram ______________
   - **(b)** graph ______________
   - **(c)** graphy ______________
   - **(d)** ectomy ______________
   - **(e)** tomy ______________
   - **(f)** stomy ______________

Study the word elements on pages 60 to 65 and give the meaning of the following word elements/combining forms

1. ab- ______________
2. ad- ______________
3. aden/o ______________
4. angi/o ______________
5. arthr/o ______________
6. brady ______________
7. cardi/o ______________
8. -centesis ______________
9. cholecyst/o ______________
10. chondr/o ______________
11. crani/o ______________
12. cyan/o ______________
13. cyst/o ______________
14. cyt/o ______________
15. -emesis ______________
16. encephal/o ______________
17. enter/o ______________
18. erythr/o ______________
19. -esthesia ______________
20. gastr/o ______________
21. hem/o ______________
22. hepa ______________

23. hist/o ______________________
24. hyper ______________________
25. hyp/o ______________________
26. icter/o ______________________
27. lapar/o ______________________
28. -lepsy ______________________
29. leuk/o ______________________
30. metr/o ______________________
31. myel/o ______________________
32. -oma ______________________
33. ophthalm/o ______________________
34. -scopy ______________________
35. -osis ______________________
36. ot/o ______________________
37. path/o ______________________
38. phleb/o ______________________
39. -plasty ______________________
40. plegia ______________________
41. pneum/o ______________________
42. poly ______________________
43. post ______________________
44. proct/o ______________________
45. py/o ______________________
46. ren/o ______________________
47. rrhage ______________________
48. stomat/o ______________________
49. thromb/o ______________________
50. -uria ______________________

Give the meaning of the following combining terms. You have studied all of the word elements.

1. chrondroma ______________________
2. cardiology ______________________
3. arthroplasty ______________________
4. angioma ______________________
5. cholecystitis ______________________
6. erythrocyte ______________________
7. hematemesis ______________________
8. cystogram ______________________
9. craniotomy ______________________
10. anesthesia ______________________
11. leukorrhea ______________________
12. metrorrhagia ______________________
13. bronchoscopy ______________________

14. orchiectomy ______________________
15. myelogram ______________________
16. polyuria ______________________
17. apnea ______________________
18. rhinopathy ______________________
19. hydrotherapy ______________________
20. diathermy ______________________

Match the abbreviation in column A with the definition in column B.

Column A	Column B
1. $FeSO_4$	____ Anterior, posterior, and lateral
2. NTG	____ Carbohydrate
3. MI	____ Central venous pressure
4. DRG	____ Silver nitrate
5. NKA	____ Chest x-ray
6. Etiol	____ Outpatient department
7. AP&L	____ Cerebrovascular accident
8. Irrig	____ Electromyogram
9. $NaHCO_3$	____ No added salt
10. CHO	____ Incision and drainage
11. CVP	____ Central nervous system
12. CNS	____ No known allergies
13. $AgNO_3$	____ Transurethral resection prostate
14. OPD	____ As soon as possible
15. EMG	____ Shortness of breath
16. NAS	____ Complains of
17. I&D	____ Diagnosis
18. TURP	____ Ferrous sulfate
19. ASAP	____ Sodium bicarbonate
20. SOB	____ Recovery room
21. CXR	____ Magnetic resonance imaging
22. Dx	____ At once
23. CVA	____ Nitroglycerine
24. C/O	____ Etiology
25. RR	____ Tender loving care
26. ARC	____ Position of comfort
27. STAT	____ Turn, cough, deep breathe
28. TLC	____ Chronic obstructive pulmonary disease
29. POC	____ Myocardial infarction
30. TCDB	____ AIDS-related complex
31. MRI	____ Diagnosis-related group
32. COPD	____ Irrigation

CHAPTER 5

Introduction to Body Structure and Function

OBJECTIVES

When you have completed this chapter, you will be able to:

- Describe the structure and function of cells, tissues, organs, and systems.
- Explain how the body systems work together.
- Better understand orders and instructions which relate to particular parts of the anatomy.

HUMAN ANATOMY AND PHYSIOLOGY

In order to work intelligently as a health unit coordinator, you must acquire a basic knowledge of the human body. By understanding the structure and function of the body you can better grasp the meaning of medical terminology, physician's orders, treatments, diagnosis, prognosis, surgical procedures, and instructions that you receive. Knowledge of these subjects will help you perform your duties more effectively and will make your job more interesting.

In this chapter you will be introduced to ANATOMY—the study of the body's structure, and PHYSIOLOGY—the study of its function. You will learn that the living body is organized from the simple to the complex. The most basic living form is the cell. Specialized cells become tissues. Tissues group together to form organs, and these organs form systems. (Fig. 5–1.)

KEY IDEA: THE CELL

The cell is the fundamental building block of all living matter. Cells are microscopic in size. They are the living parts of organisms. The human body is made up of millions of cells. There are many kinds of cells. Each one has a special task within the body. Living cells have many things in common:

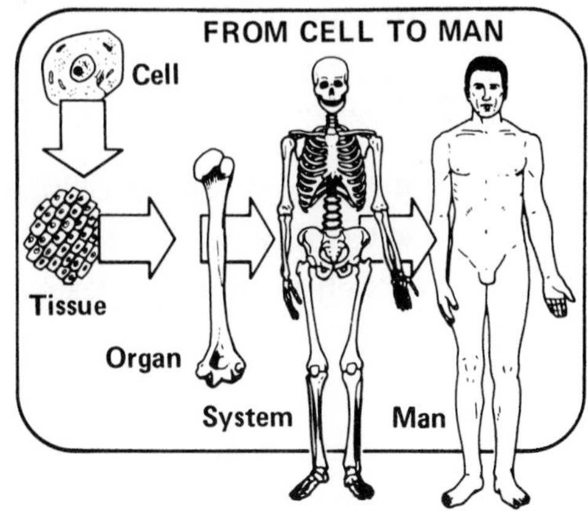

Figure 5-1

- They come from preexisting cells.
- They use food for energy.
- They use oxygen to break down the food.
- They use water to transport water-soluble substances such as sodium.
- They grow and repair themselves.
- They reproduce themselves. (Fig. 5–2.)

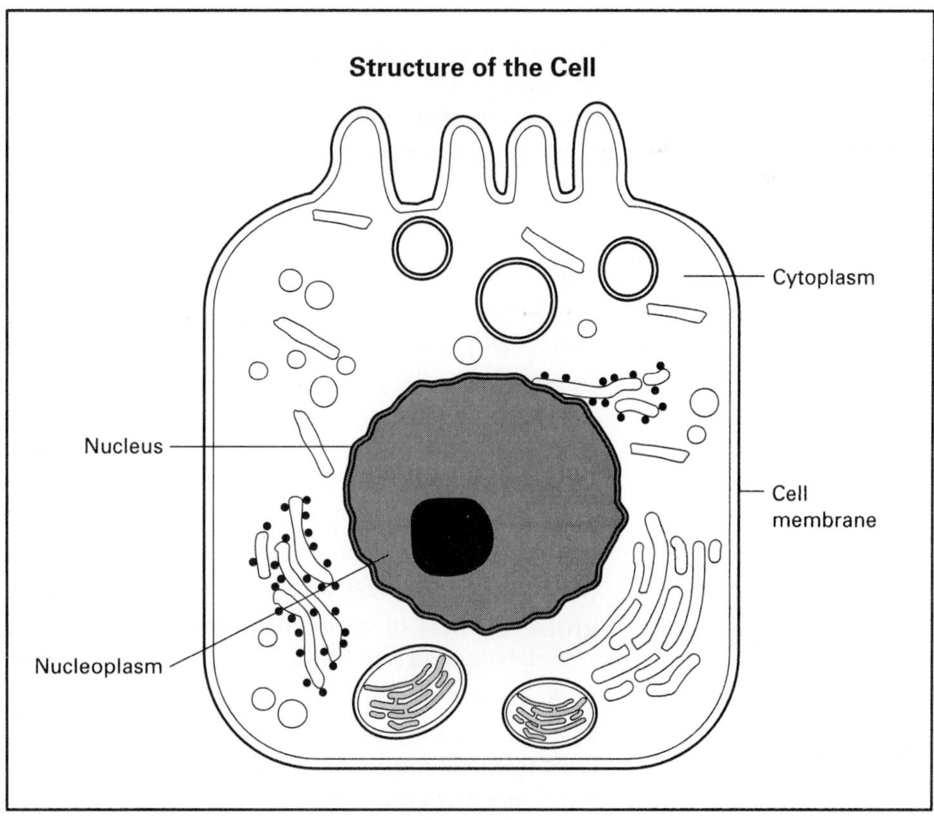

Figure 5-2

Structure of the Cell

Cells consist of three main parts:

- **Nucleus**—directs cellular activities.
- **Cytoplasm**—where the activities of the cell take place.
- **Cell membrane**—keeps the living substance of the cell, called the protoplasm, within bounds and allows certain materials to pass in and out of the cell.

Cells are made up of two main compartments: a nucleus which contains the chromosomes (the hereditary material) and a surrounding mass of cytoplasm. The nucleus is important to the process of heredity, growth, and cell division. The **chromosomes** are threadlike structures which contain deoxyribonucleic acid **(DNA)** and therefore control inheritance. There are 23 pairs of chromosomes.

DNA molecules produce messenger **RNA** molecules which are partial copies of the DNA. Each RNA passes into the cytoplasm and directs the formation of protein molecules necessary to maintain life. Through the RNA the nucleus controls the kinds of chemical reactions carried out by the cell.

Cells reproduce by division. In any cell preparing for division, the nucleus exactly duplicates its chromosomes. As the cell divides, the pairs of chromosomes pull apart and move to opposite sides of the nucleus. When division is complete the new cells are identical.

Although years away, cellular research is laying the foundation for the science of molecular pathology that will include all living things at the level of atoms, molecules, and their basic particles. It is hoped that from this research scientists will some day discover how to prevent and cure all or at least most disease.

KEY IDEA: TISSUES

Cells usually do not work alone. They are organized through the process of differentiation into collections of cells that perform specific functions. Groups of cells of the same type that do a particular kind of work are called tissues.

Some of the primary kinds of tissues in the human body are:

- **Epithelial tissue**—the function of this tissue is to protect (skin), control permeability (control what enters and leaves the body), secrete (hormones, milk, mucus, perspiration), and receive sensations.
- **Connective tissue**—the function of this tissue is to connect (tendons), to support (bones), and to cover, ensheath, or line (the thin and sometimes fatty layer of connective tissue under the skin, the tough sheet of fibrous tissue over the limbs) and to pad or protect (bursal sacs).
- **Muscle tissue**—the function of this tissue is movement. Striated tissue is found in voluntary muscles, those you can move consciously. Smooth tissue is found in the involuntary muscles such as those that push food and water through the gastrointestinal tract. Smooth muscle allows such action as a dilation and contracting of the pupil of the eye and of blood vessels. (Fig. 5–3.)

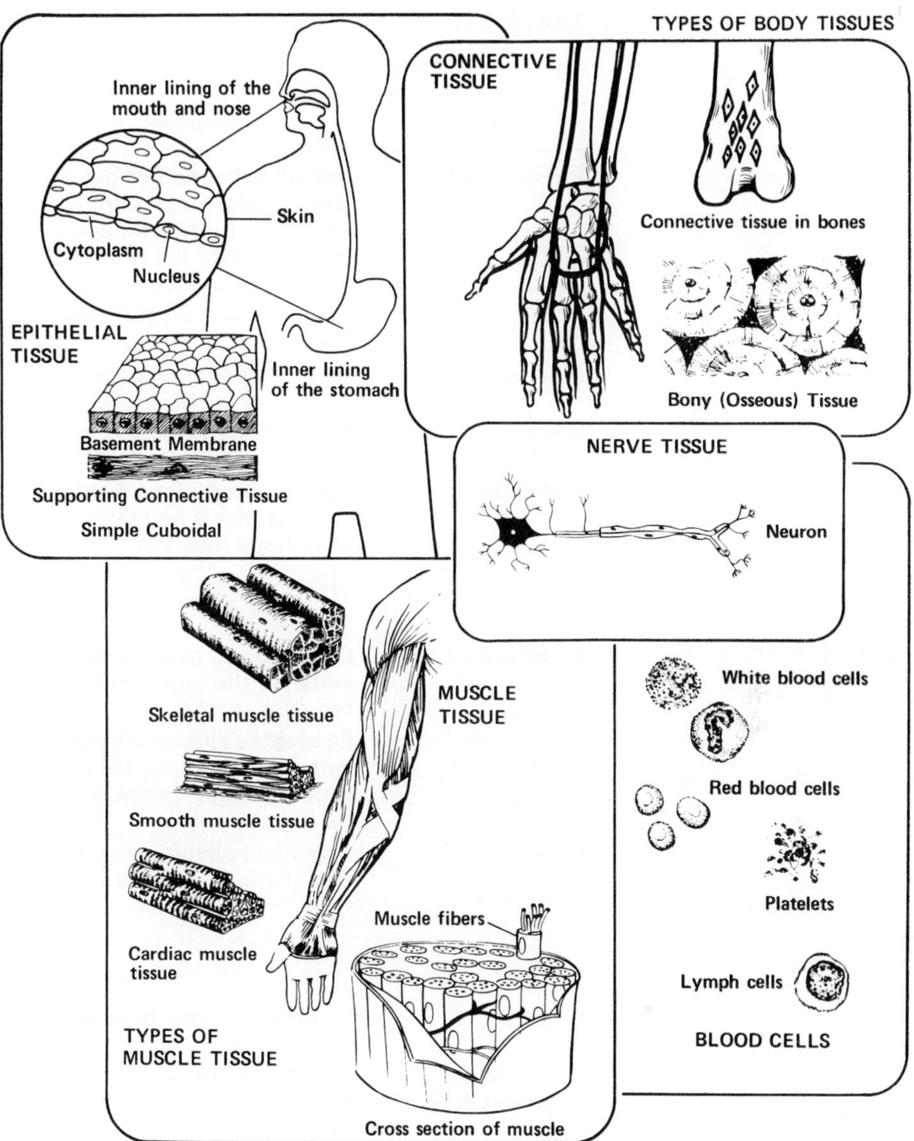

Figure 5–3

- **Nerve tissue**—the function of this tissue is to carry nervous impulses from a portion of the brain or spinal cord to all parts of the body. Generally the body cannot renew nervous tissue.
- **Blood and lymph tissue**—in this type of tissue the cells are singular and move within a fluid to every part of the body.

Cells to Systems

Tissues are grouped together to form organs, such as the heart, lungs, and liver. Each organ has a specific job. Organs that work together to perform similar tasks make up systems. It is easier to study anatomy and physiology by systems. Always remember that a system cannot work by itself. Systems are dependent, one upon the other. (Table 5–1; Fig. 5–4.)

TABLE 5–1

The Body Systems

System	*Function*	*Organs*
Integumentary	Provides first line of defense against infection, maintains body temperature, provides fluids and gets rid of wastes.	Skin; hair; nails; sweat and oil glands
Skeletal	Supports and protects the body	Bones; joints
Muscular	Gives movement to the body	Muscles; tendons; ligaments
Nervous	Controls activities of the body	Brain; spinal cord; nerves
Endocrine	Secretes hormones directly into the blood and regulates body function	Thyroid and parathyroid glands; pineal gland; adrenal glands; testes; ovaries; thymus gland; pancreatic islands of Langerhans; pituitary gland
Circulatory	Carries food, oxygen, and water to the body cells and removes wastes	Heart; blood; arteries; veins; capillaries; spleen; lymph nodes; lymph vessels
Respiratory	Eliminates carbon dioxide and gives the body air to supply oxygen to the cells through the blood	Nose; pharynx; larynx; trachea; bronchi; lungs
Digestive	Takes and absorbs nutrition and eliminates wastes	Mouth; teeth; tongue; salivary glands; esophagus; stomach; small intestine; liver; gallbladder; pancreas; large intestine; rectum; anus
Urinary	Removes wastes from the blood, produces urine, and eliminates urine	Kidneys; ureters; bladder; urethra
Reproductive	To reproduce, allows a new human being to be born	Male: testes; scrotum; penis; bulbourethral glands; epididymis; vas deferens; ejaculatory duct; seminal vesicles; prostate Female: ovaries; uterus; breasts; uterine tubes (Fallopian tubes or oviducts); vagina

KEY IDEA: THE INTEGUMENTARY SYSTEM (THE SKIN)

The skin covers and protects underlying structures from injury or bacterial invasion. Skin also contains nerve endings from the nervous system, which aid the body in awareness of its environment.

The skin helps regulate the body temperature by controlling the loss of heat from the body. To increase heat loss, the blood vessels near the skin dilate, and the increased blood flow brings more heat to the skin. Then the skin temperature rises and more heat is lost from the hot skin to the cooler environment. Even more important in heat loss is the evaporation of sweat (per-

Cells combine to form tissues, and tissues combine to form organs

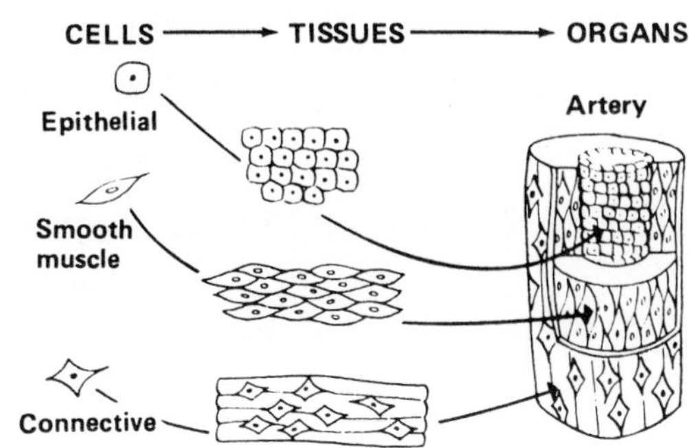

Figure 5–4

spiration). It carries heat away from the skin. When the body is conserving heat, sweating stops and blood vessels contract. This prevents the blood from carrying heat to the skin. The skin temperature falls, decreasing heat loss. In this way, the body temperature is kept almost constant.

Perspiration is released from the body through sweat glands, which are distributed over the entire skin surface. The glands open by ducts or pores. The body also rids itself of certain waste products through perspiration. Skin also secretes a thick oily substance through ducts that lead to oil glands. In this way, the skin is lubricated and kept soft and pliable. The oil also provides a protective film for the skin, which limits the absorption and evaporation of water from the surface. In elderly persons, these oil glands sometimes fail to function properly and the skin becomes quite dry, scaly, and delicate.

Appendages of the skin, in addition to the sweat and oil glands, include the hair and the nails. Each hair has a root embedded in the skin, into which the oil glands of the skin open. Fingernails and toenails grow from the nail bed at the base underneath. If the nail bed is destroyed, the nail stops growing.

The skin covers the entire body. The outer layer of the skin (the layer you can see) is called the **epidermis.** Cells are constantly flaking off or being rubbed off this outer layer of skin. Beneath the epidermis is the **dermis.** In this layer of skin are the new cells that will replace the cells that are lost from the epidermis. Pigment is found in the epidermis. This is responsible for the color of the skin. In sunlight, through a chemical reaction, the amount of pigment increases and a suntan results. (Fig. 5–5.)

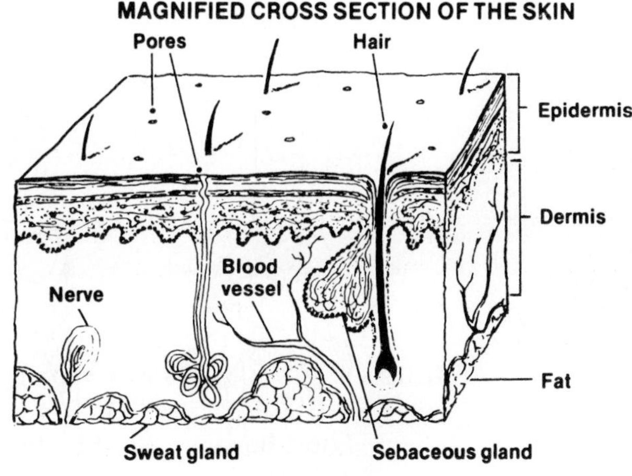

Figure 5–5

Moisture on the skin can pick up dust and dirt from the air. Moisture can also mix with the skin particles being flaked off the epidermis. This process causes a condition that promotes the growth and spread of bacteria. This is the main reason for keeping the skin clean. The skin is where the battle for asepsis (being free of disease-causing organisms) begins.

The primary functions of the skin are:

- To cover and protect underlying body structures from injury and bacterial invasion
- To help regulate body temperature by controlling loss of heat from the body
- Storage of energy in the form of fat and vitamins
- Elimination of wastes by perspiration
- Sensory perception—the sense of touch (the skin can sense heat, cold, pain, and pressure)

KEY IDEA: THE SKELETAL SYSTEM

The skeletal system is made up of 206 bones. The bones act as a framework for the body, giving it structure and support. They are also the passive organs of motion. They do not move by themselves. They must be moved by muscles, which shorten or contract. A muscle is stimulated to contract by a nerve impulse. This is an example of how systems interact. It is necessary to learn the names of the bones because they are like landmarks.

There are four types of bones (Fig. 5–6):

- **Long bones,** such as the big bone in your thigh, the femur
- **Short bones,** like the bones in your fingers, the phalanges
- **Irregular bones,** such as the vertebrae that make up the spinal column
- **Flat bones,** like the bones of the rib cage

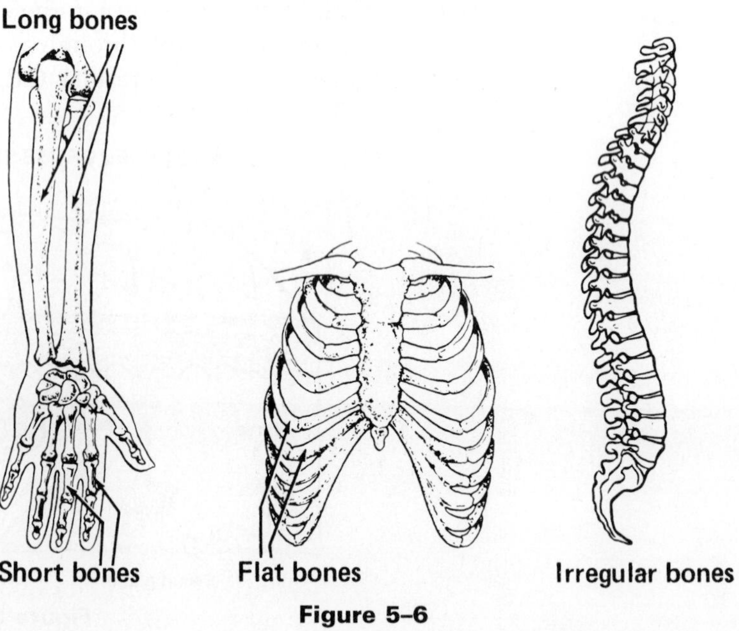

Figure 5–6

Bones are not inactive. They are dynamic and usually busy parts of the body. They store vital minerals that are necessary for many other body activities. The bones of the head are designed to protect the very delicate tissue of the brain. They are joined by sutures, similar to a zigzag embroidery pattern, and totally surround the brain and cranial nerves. Some other bones that protect vital organs include the vertebrae of the spinal column, which protects the spinal nerve cord and the rib cage, which guards the heart and lungs.

When the fetus is developing in the uterus, the entire skeleton is formed in cartilage by about two and one-half months after conception. From this cartilage, bone is formed, much as if you replaced a wooden bridge, piece by piece, with steel. The bones of the head are formed from strong membranes. They do not completely undergo **ossification** (which means development of bone) until after the child is born. This is a great aid during childbirth, when the baby's bones can overlap a little.

Broken bones can mend solidly but the process is slow and gradual. Bone cells grow and reproduce slowly. The hardening of the new bone is a gradual procedure of depositing calcium. Blood supply to bone tissue is poor, when compared with other areas of the body. Therefore, resistance to infection in the bone is relatively low.

Joints (Motion)

The systems of the body must all work together. No one system can stand alone. All the systems operate simultaneously in a healthy human body. The skeletal system, muscular system, nervous system, and circulatory system are all interacting during each body movement. Movement of the body occurs at the joints. This is a perfect example of how several systems must work together.

Joints are areas in which one bone connects with one or more bones. They are necessary levers in all motion. Joints are made up of many structures. The tough white fibrous cord, the **ligament,** connects bone to bone. The **tendons** connect muscle to bone. The meeting place of two bones—the joint—especially those in the shoulder, hip, and knee, is enclosed in a strong capsule. This capsule is lined by a membrane that secretes a fluid called **synovial fluid.** This fluid acts as a buffer, very much like a water bed, so the ends of the bones do not get worn out with a lot of motion. Other structures that protect the bone include the pad of cartilage at the end of the bone, a sac of synovial fluid (which is known as a **bursa**), and a disc of cartilage called the **meniscus.** Many such safeguards are built into the body. Injury to joints may cause a ligament or tendon to be strained in what we call a sprain. Inflammation of the bursa causes **bursitis.**

There are several kinds of joints in the human body. The hinge joint, such as in the knee, is freely movable. There are also less movable joints, such as those between the vertebrae. Some joints do not move at all. Examples are the joints between the bones of the skull, which protect the brain. (Fig. 5–7.)

KEY IDEA: THE MUSCULAR SYSTEM

The muscular system makes all motion possible, either that of the whole body or that which occurs inside the body. (Fig. 5–8.) Groups of muscles work together to perform a body motion. Other groups perform just the opposite motion. These two groups are called antagonistic groups. For example,

SYNOVIAL (MOVABLE) JOINTS

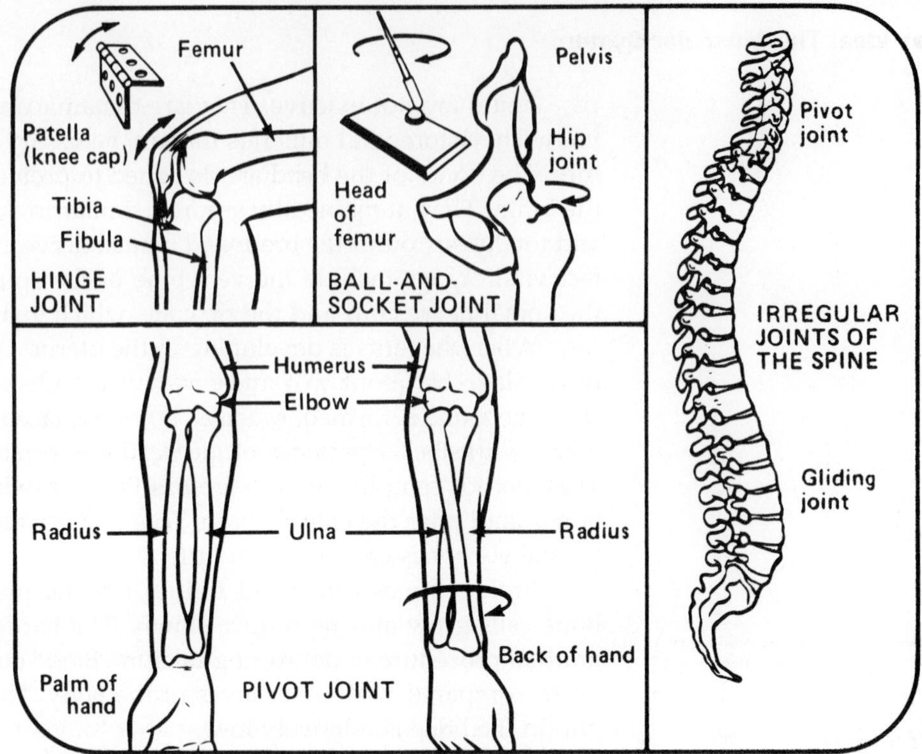

Figure 5–7

SKELETON AND SURFACE MUSCLES

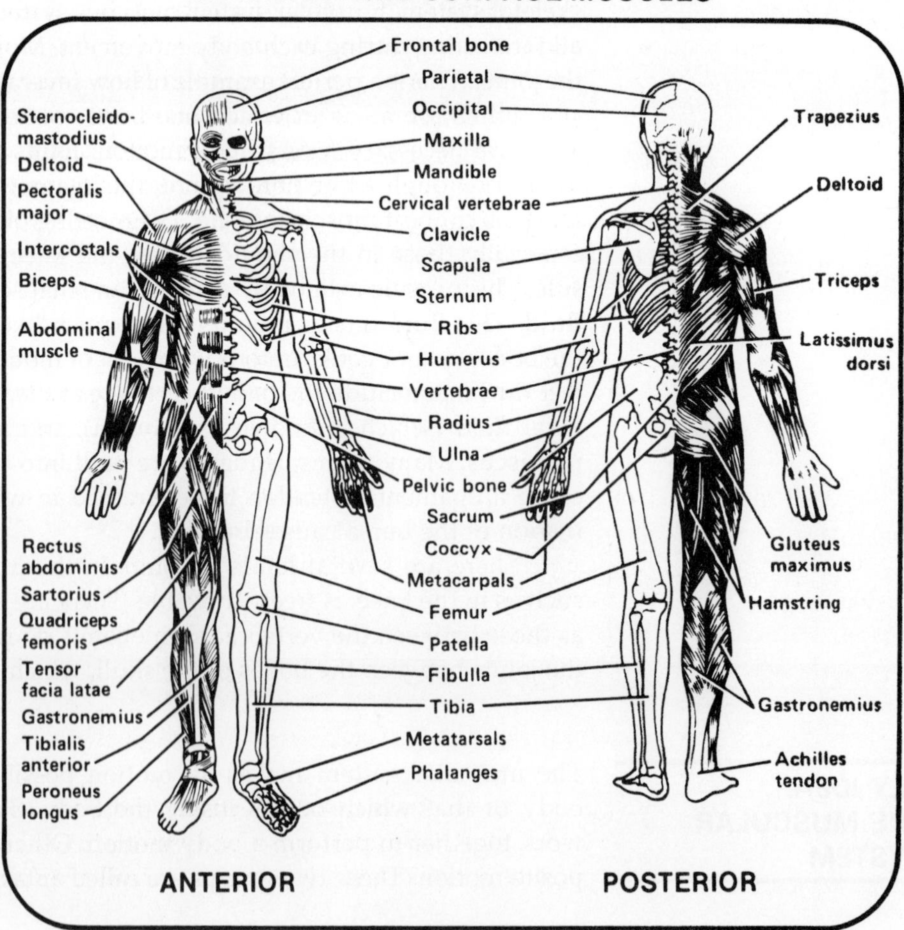

Figure 5–8

flex your arm, which means bring it toward your shoulder. Your biceps contract, and the triceps relax. Extend your arm. The biceps muscle relaxes while the triceps contracts. **Flexion** and **extension** are the two terms you should know. Two others are **abduction,** which means moving a part away from the body midline, and **adduction** which means moving it toward the body. (Figs. 5–9 and 5–10.)

Muscle is the most infection-free of all the body's basic tissues. This is largely because of its exceptionally rich blood supply. Muscles not only move the body but also help to keep the body warm, especially during activity. If a muscle is kept inactive for too long, it tends to shrink and waste away. This is called **atrophy. Contracture** is a permanent muscle shortening. This is the reason that regular exercise is so important to good health. Range of motion exercises are often given to inactive patients to prevent these problems.

KEY IDEA: THE NERVOUS SYSTEM

The nervous system controls and organizes all body activity, both voluntary and involuntary. The nervous system is made up of the brain, the spinal cord, and the nerves. The nerves are spread throughout all areas of the body in an orderly way. (Fig. 5–11.)

Nervous tissue is made up of cells called **neurons** and other supporting cells called **neuroglia.** A typical neuron is made up of a cell body with one long column called the **axon** and many small outbranchings called **dendrites.** Nerve impulses move from the dendrites through the cell body along the axon. Inside and outside our bodies, we have structures called **receptor-end organs.** Any change in our external or internal environment that is strong enough will set up a nervous impulse in these receptor-end organs. This impulse is carried by a sensory neuron to some part of the brain or spinal cord where it connects with an interneuron. The connection is called a **synapse.** This interneuron often makes hundreds of synapses (particularly in the cerebrum, the part of the brain in which we think) before a decision is made. Once that happens, the proper impulses are sent down a motor neuron to the **effector-end organs,** those organs that are going to respond to the nerve impulse.

Most nerve cells outside the brain and spinal cord have a protective covering known as the **myelin sheath.** The task of the myelin sheath is to insulate the nerve cell. The nerve cell can be compared to an electrical wire that requires insulation to keep the current in the correct pathway. This sheath helps prevent damage to the cells and often helps the nerve return to healthy function, or regenerate, if it has been injured. Nerve cells with a myelin sheath also carry an impulse faster than those without myelin. The neurons in the brain do not have this kind of protection. When they are injured, as they are by a stroke or **cerebral vascular accident** (CVA), it is necessary for another part of the brain to take over the function of the part that has been damaged. The rehabilitation department in your health care institution helps patients learn to do things again after such damage has been done.

The brain is well protected by bones, membranes, the meninges, and a cushion of fluid called **cerebral spinal fluid.** This fluid circulates outside of and within the brain as well as around the spinal cord. The brain is a very

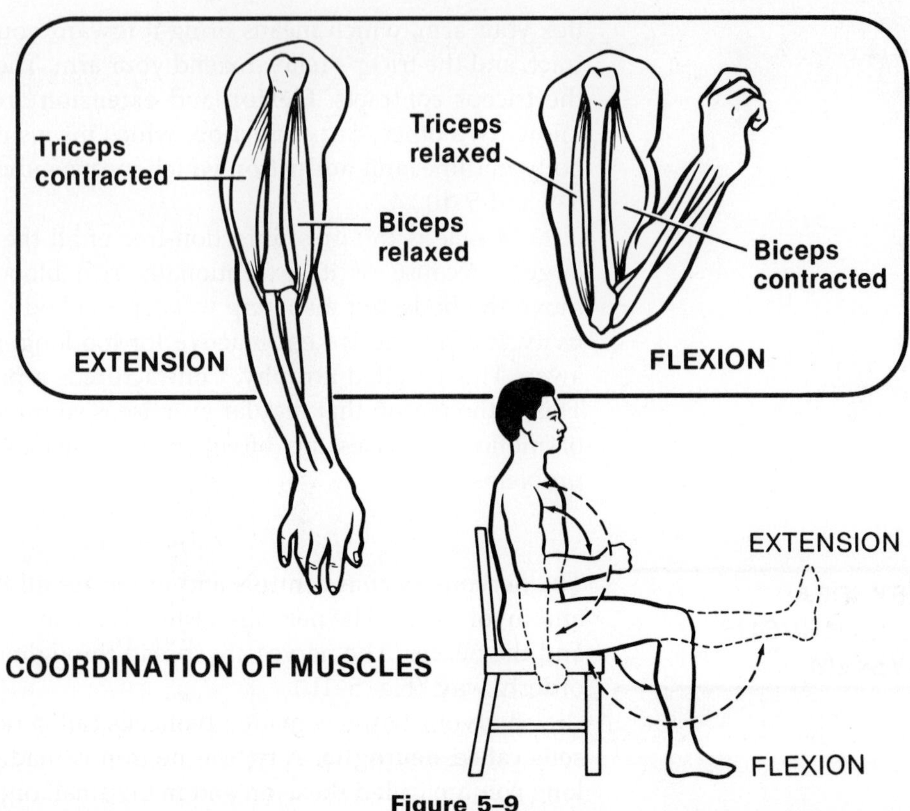

Figure 5-9

complicated organ. It is made up of five portions. The **cerebrum** is divided into two halves, called hemispheres. They are connected to one another by white material known as **corpus callosum.** The right hemisphere controls most of the activity on the left side of the body. And the left hemisphere of the cerebrum controls the activity on the right side of the body. The cerebrum has many indentations, which are known as **convolutions.** It is here that all learning, memory, and associations are stored so that thought is pos-

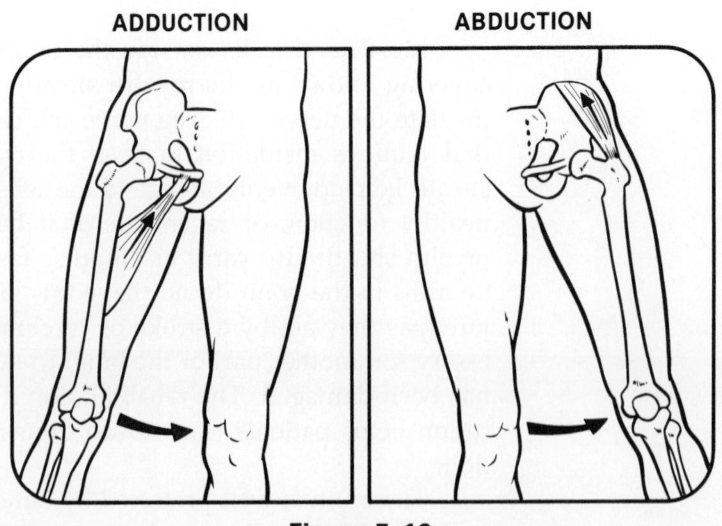

Figure 5-10

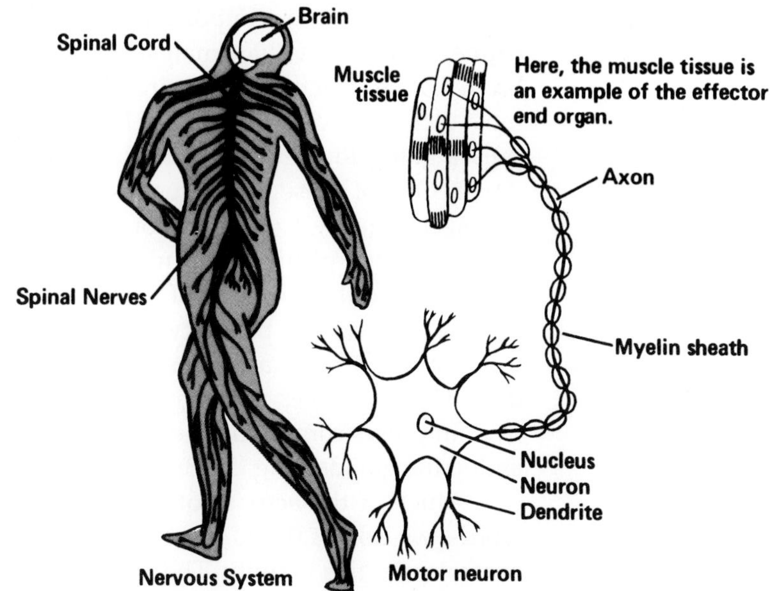

Figure 5–11

sible. Also, it is here that decisions are made for voluntary action. Certain areas of the cerebrum seem to perform special organizing activities. For example, the **occipital lobe** is the place where what you see is interpreted. The **frontal lobe** is the primary area of thought and reason. The **cerebellum** is the part of the brain that controls voluntary motion. It works with part of the inner ear, the semicircular canals, to enable us to walk and move smoothly through our world. The **midbrain, pons,** and **medulla** are primarily pathways through which nervous impulses reach the brain from the spinal cord.

Nerves throughout the body send messages into the tracts of white matter in the spinal cord, from which they rise to higher centers in the brain. There are 12 pairs of cranial nerves and 32 pairs of spinal nerves. These have many branches that go to all parts of the body. (Fig. 5–12.)

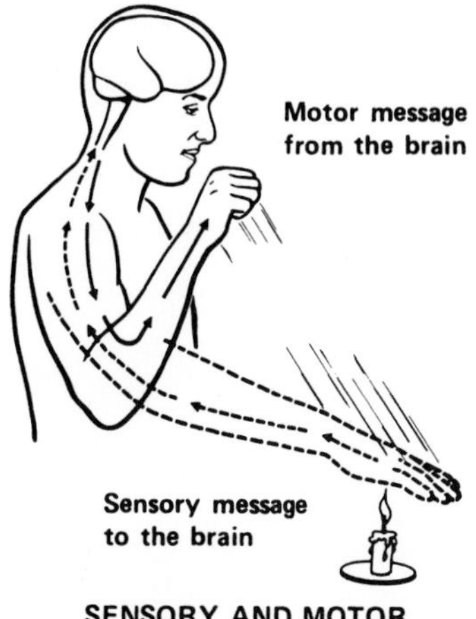

SENSORY AND MOTOR PROCESSES IN OPERATION Figure 5–12

One of the most important areas of the brain is an area called the **diencephelon.** It is here that small structures surround one of the ventricles of the brain. These structures help circulate cerebral spinal fluid and exercise an almost dictatorial control over the body's activities. They screen all nervous impulses going to the brain, either getting them there faster or slowing them down. One of these tiny structures is the **hypothalamus,** which in times of stress, emergency, excitement, or danger actually takes control of the body by controlling the **pituitary gland,** the body's master gland. Although it can be mapped, like the subways of a great city, we still know very little about the actual activity of the pituitary gland. We do know that it has tremendous control over most body activities. It seems to be the link between the mind and the body. It receives messages from the cerebrum, from the cerebellum, and from impulses coming up the spinal cord, and it has direct control over all the endocrine glands. (Fig. 5–13.)

Much of the activity of the organs of the body is involuntary. In other words, we do not think about it. Or, for the most part, we have no conscious control over this activity. The part of the nervous system that controls such things as digestion and the functions of other **visceral** (abdominal) organs is the autonomic nervous system. This is really not separate from the brain and the spinal cord. The neurons that make up the autonomic nervous system use the same pathways as those neurons that control our voluntary actions. However, the two divisions of this part of the nervous system direct and control the activity of our internal organs. Each organ is supplied with neurons from each division of the autonomic nervous system.

One division is called the **sympathetic division.** The neurons that make up this division become active during stress, danger, excitement, or illness. These neurons cause the pupils of our eyes to become larger, so we can see more clearly and can see better at a distance. These neurons also cause the heart to beat more strongly and to send more oxygen to the large muscles of the body in case it is necessary to fight or run. In today's fast paced world, we are all subject to stress and sometimes we cannot run away from it or fight it. The action of the neurons from the sympathetic system then causes changes in the shape or activity of some of our organs. This action may also cause illness.

The **parasympathetic division** of the autonomic nervous system is in control when we are relaxed. It is known to conserve our energy. Fortunately, there is a checks-and-balances system between the two divisions. When one has been in action too long, the other automatically switches on. We have all had the experience of eating a large meal after being emotionally upset and feeling as if we had lead in our stomach. This is because of the sympathetic

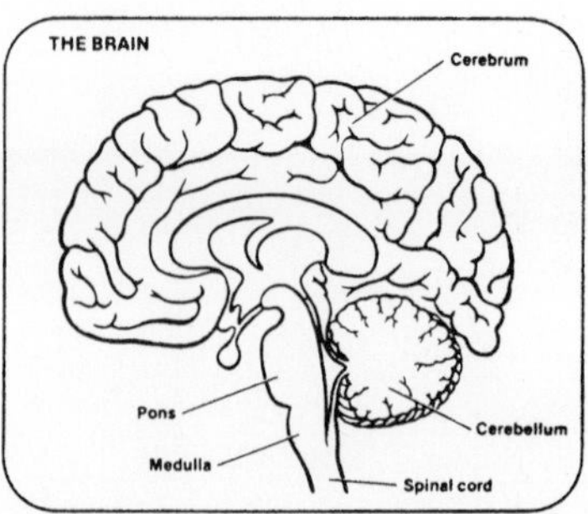

Figure 5–13

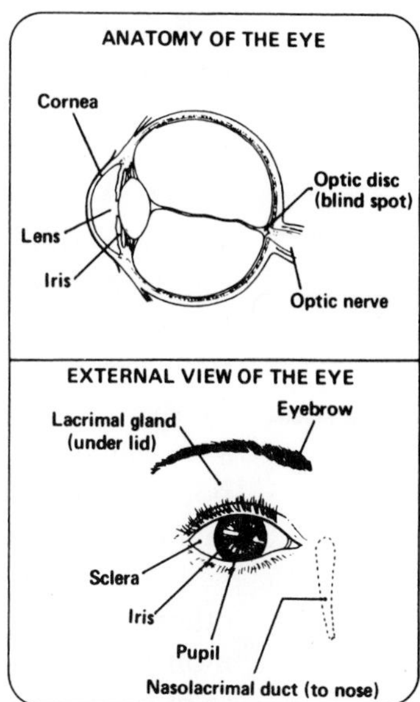

Figure 5–14

division of the autonomic nervous system. **Peristalsis** (which is movement of the gut) lessens and digestion does not go on.

The Sense Organs

The sense organs contain specialized endings of the sensory neurons. These are excited by sudden changes in the outside environment called **stimuli.**

- Eyes respond to visual stimuli (Fig. 5–14)
- Ears respond to sound stimuli (Fig. 5–15)
- Membranes of the nose respond to smells

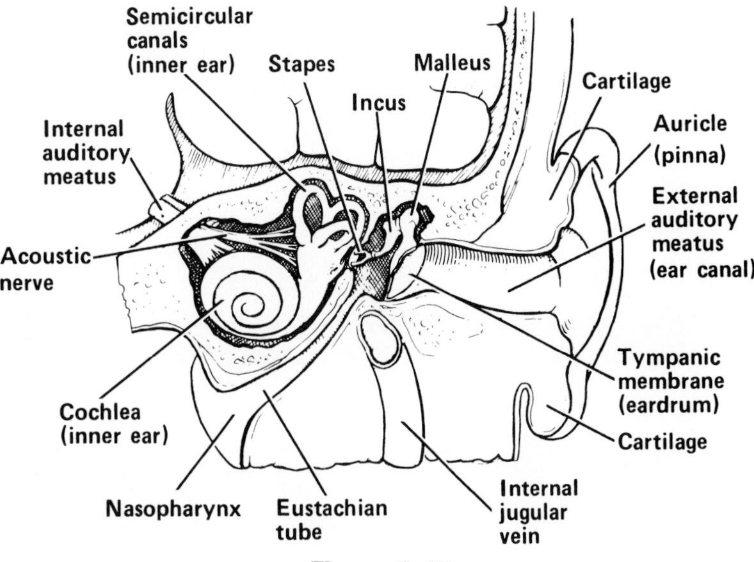

Figure 5–15

- Taste buds, located chiefly on the tongue, respond to sweet and sour and other sensations
- Skin responds to touch, pressure, heat, cold, and pain

KEY IDEA: HORMONES AND THE ENDOCRINE SYSTEMS

The endocrine glands secrete liquids called **hormones.** (Fig. 5–16.) These help the nervous system organize and direct the activities of the body. The hormones are secreted (flow) directly into the bloodstream. Exocrine glands, such as the salivary glands, deliver their products through ducts into a body cavity.

The hormones from the pituitary gland, both the anterior and posterior portions, regulate all metabolism of our billions of cells. The anterior portion manufactures and releases seven hormones.

The **pituitary gland** is the master gland. Its hormones directly affect the other endocrine glands, stimulating them to produce their hormones. Its hormones are especially important in reproduction and in all functions leading to puberty. This is the time at which a child takes on the physical characteristics of an adult man or woman. Hormones from the pituitary gland regulate the menstrual cycle in the female and sperm production in the male. Without these hormones, it would not be possible for us to reproduce.

The pituitary gland and all of these important hormones are under the direct control of the **hypothalamus,** a tiny fragment of tissue lying near the base of the brain. This structure seems to be the real link between our thinking, our emotions, and our body functions.

The **thyroid** gland produces a hormone that regulates growth and general metabolism. The **thymus** gets smaller after puberty, but it plays an important part in the body's immune system. It is this immune system that prevents us from getting many diseases.

The **parathyroids** are located within the capsule of the thyroid. They produce a hormone that regulates, along with one of the hormones in the thyroid gland, the level of calcium and potassium in the blood. Calcium is im-

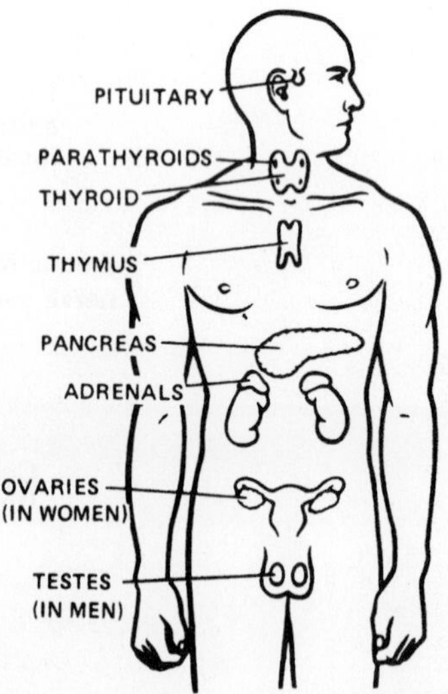

Figure 5–16

portant for many functions of our body, such as muscle contraction and conduction of nerve impulses.

The **pancreas** is both an endocrine gland and an exocrine gland, or a gland that has a duct. Its endocrine portion produces the hormone **insulin.** Insulin regulates the sugar content of the blood. If the body does not have enough insulin, the person becomes **diabetic.** He must be treated by reducing the carbohydrate or sugar intake and by regulating the balance between insulin and blood sugar.

The **adrenal glands** lie on top of the kidneys. They are very important in helping the body adapt to stress conditions, giving a lot of help to the autonomic nervous system.

The **ovaries** in the female are responsible for secreting the hormones estrogen and progesterone. The rise and fall of the levels of these hormones in the blood determine the menstrual cycle. The hormones are also important in causing an ovum, or egg, to develop and in maintaining a pregnancy.

The **testes** in the male produce testosterone, the primary sex hormone of the male, which also causes the production of sperm.

KEY IDEA: THE CIRCULATORY SYSTEM

The circulatory system is made up of the blood, the heart, and the blood vessels—**arteries, veins,** and **capillaries** and the **lymphatic system** (lymph vessels, lymph nodes, spleen, and thymus). The heart actually acts as a pump for the blood, which carries the nutrients, oxygen, and other elements needed by the cells. Important facts to know about blood include:

- The blood carries oxygen from the lungs to the cells.
- Carbon dioxide is carried by the blood from the cells to the lungs.
- Nutrients (food) are picked up (absorbed) by the blood from the duodenum (small intestine) and brought to the cells.
- Waste products from the cells are carried by the blood to the kidneys to be eliminated in urine.
- The hormones from the endocrine glands are transported by the blood.
- Dilation (enlargement) and contraction (narrowing) of the blood vessels help regulate body temperature.
- The blood helps maintain the fluid balance of the body.
- The white cells of the blood defend the body against disease.

The heart is made up of four chambers—two **atria** and two **ventricles.** The atria are the two smaller chambers. The right ventricle sends the blood only as far as the lungs. Here in the **pulmonary** circulation, the blood picks up oxygen and gets rid of carbon dioxide. This blood then returns to the heart, carrying its load of oxygen, which is pushed into **systemic** circulation by the left ventricle. (Fig. 5–17.)

The ventricles have thick walls of muscle. When they contract, the left ventricle pushes the blood through the largest blood vessel, the **aorta,** to all parts of the body. The blood vessels that carry blood having a lot of oxygen are called **arteries.** The only exception is the pulmonary artery, which carries the blood to the lungs. Arteries branch into a vast network throughout the body. As they branch, the blood vessels become smaller and smaller until fi-

THE HEART

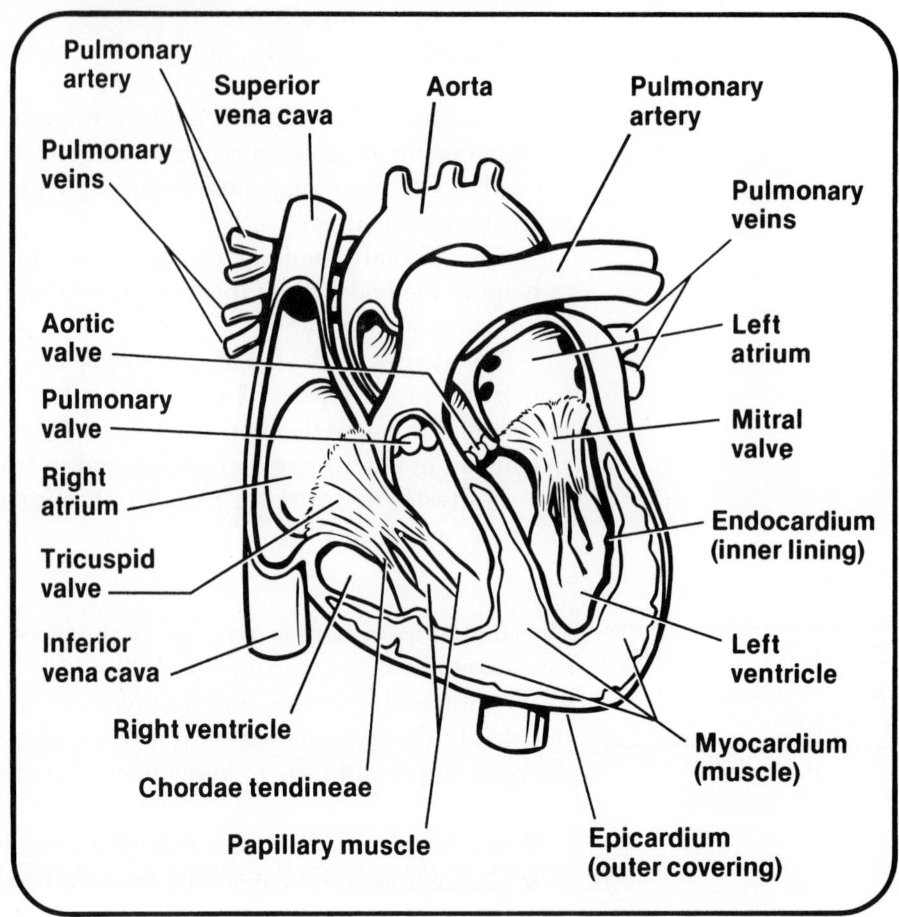

Figure 5–17

nally they are so thin they become **capillaries.** The walls of the capillaries are only one cell-layer thick. Through these walls, gases, nutrients, waste products, and other substances are exchanged among the blood in the capillaries, the tissue fluid, and the individual cell. After the blood has given up its oxygen, which is carried on the surface of the red blood cells, it is returned to the heart through the veins. Other important points are:

- All arteries carry blood away from the heart (Fig. 5–18).
- All veins carry blood back to the heart (Fig. 5–19).
- All arteries carry oxygenated blood except the pulmonary arteries.
- All veins carry deoxygenated blood except the pulmonary veins.

It is necessary that the heart muscle be supplied with blood carrying oxygen. The first branches of the aorta, which come from the heart's left ventricle, are the coronary arteries, which surround the heart. These carry needed oxygen to cardiac (heart) muscle tissue. If one of these branches of the coronary arteries is blocked by a blood clot, the patient has a heart attack (coronary thrombosis). This can result in the death of some heart tissue. The event is called a myocardial infarction (MI).

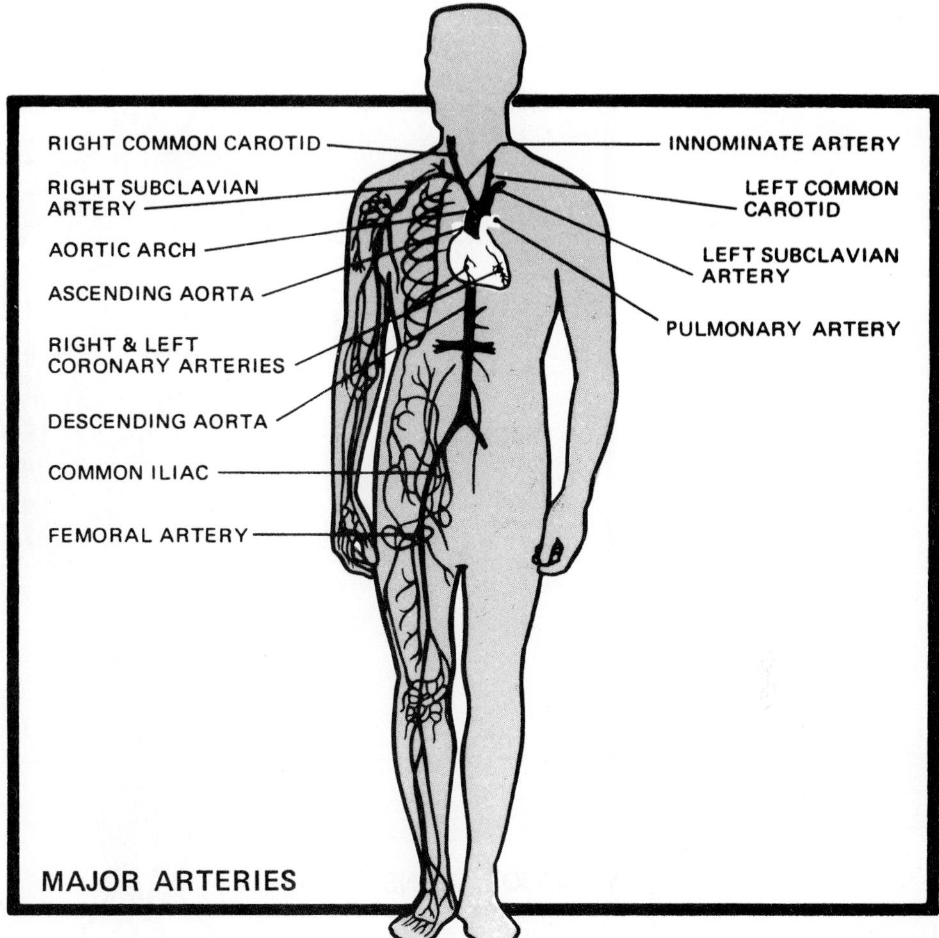

Figure 5–18

The liquid portion of the blood is called **plasma.** The cells are **red blood cells** (erythrocytes) which carry oxygen, and **white blood cells** (leukocytes) which fight infection. If a patient has an inflammation in some area of the body, a physician often prescribes warm, moist compresses. These are applied to dilate (widen) the blood vessels in the area and to bring more of those important white blood cells to the place of infection to help fight it. People who have too few red blood cells have some type of anemia. People with too few white blood cells have a lowered resistance to disease. An increase in white blood cells in the blood may mean that an infection is present somewhere in the body.

The lymphatic system has several functions. It helps defend the body against disease-causing microorganisms by producing lymphocytes and monocytes (types of white blood cells) in the spleen and thymus gland and by producing antibodies. The lymphatic system also transports proteins and fluids that have leaked into the tissue fluid and the lipids (fats) from the small intestine back into the bloodstream.

The circulatory system is responsible for getting all of the necessary ingredients to a cell for its metabolism and for carrying away its products and waste material. The circulatory system works in close harmony with the respiratory system. (Fig. 5–20.)

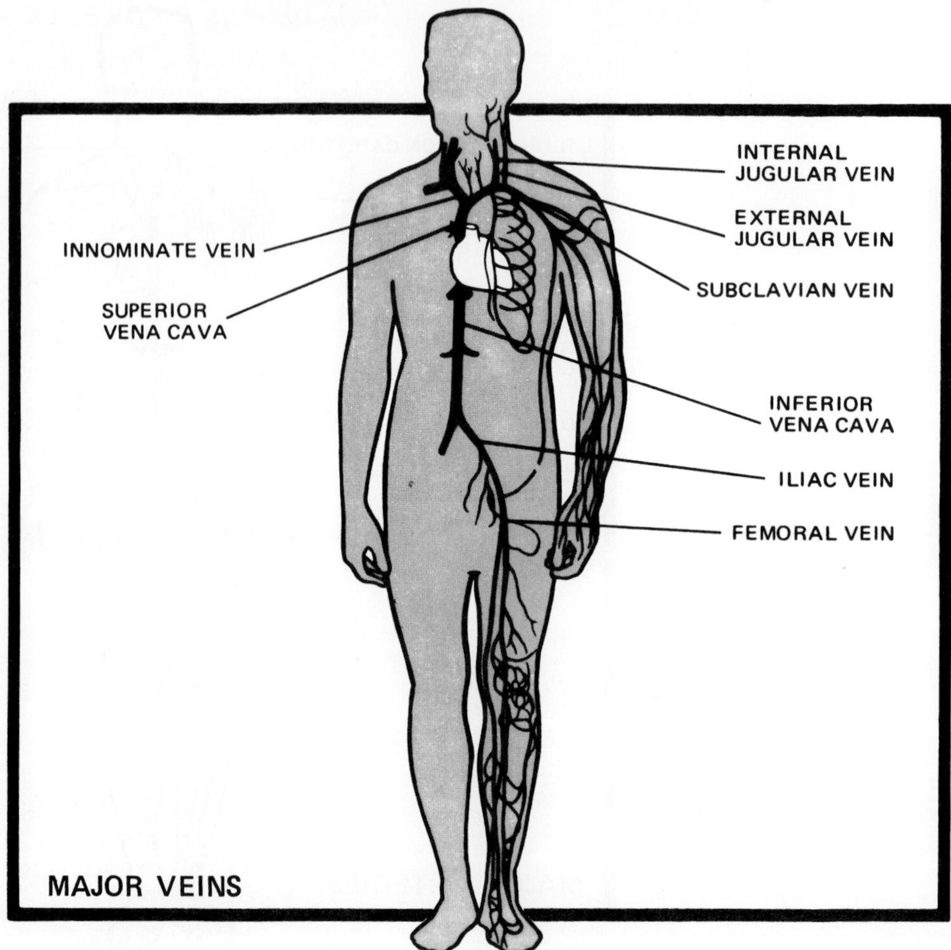

Figure 5–19

KEY IDEA: THE RESPIRATORY SYSTEM

The respiratory system provides a route or pathway for oxygen to get from the air into the lungs where it can be picked up by the blood. (Fig. 5–21.) The organs that make up this system include the **nose** and **mouth, pharynx** (throat), **trachea** (windpipe), **larynx** (voicebox), **bronchi,** and **lungs.** Because we must have oxygen to live, it is necessary to keep this pathway open. The structures themselves help to do this. The trachea and bronchi are kept open by incomplete cartilage rings.

On the top of the trachea, opening from the pharynx (the throat), is a structure known as the larynx. It is not only the opening to the trachea, it also contains the vocal cords, which make it possible for us to talk. An important piece of cartilage, the **epiglottis,** covers the opening to the trachea when food is swallowed, preventing the food from going into the lungs.

As in our other systems, the important work of the respiratory system is done at the level of the cell. The exchange of oxygen and carbon dioxide occurs in an area of the lungs that is so small you must use a microscope to see it. The last branch of the bronchus is called the **alveolar duct.** At its end is a small sac, the **alveolus.** Many oxygen molecules fill this sac after you breathe in. The blood has less oxygen and therefore is able to pick up a lot of oxygen from the alveolar sac. The blood is then returned to the heart to be sent around the body beginning in the largest artery, the aorta.

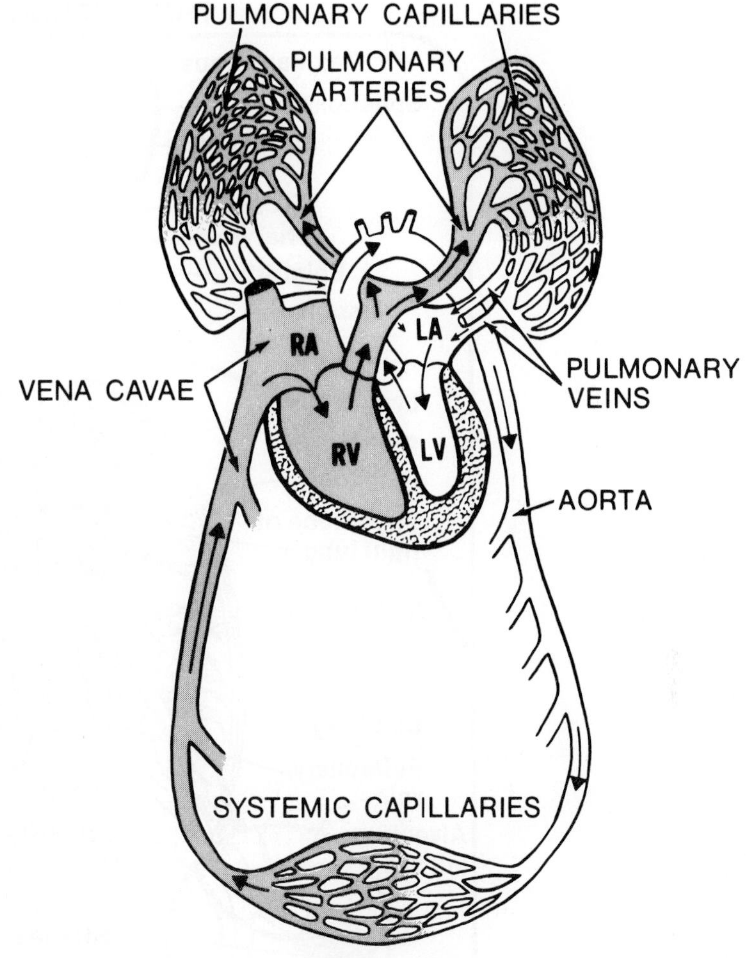

Figure 5–20

The respiratory system, then, is responsible for getting oxygen to the blood. **Internal respiration** occurs when those cells that need the oxygen receive it in exchange for carbon dioxide, which is the cells' gas waste product. Both functions are equally important.

Breathing is regulated by a center in the **medulla,** a part of the brain. Often, especially after surgery, a patient must be encouraged to breathe deeply in order to keep all the air sacs open and inflated. In many of the larger health care institutions the Pulmonary Medicine Department (Respiratory Therapy) will, by a doctor's order, institute a treatment that will force the patient to breathe deeply and cough.

KEY IDEA: THE DIGESTIVE SYSTEM (GASTROINTESTINAL SYSTEM)

The digestive system is responsible for breaking down the food that is eaten into a form that can be used by the body cells. This action is both chemical and mechanical. The digestive tract is about 30 feet long. All of it is important in reducing food to simple compounds. (Fig. 5–22.)

Digestion begins in the mouth, where food is chewed and mixed with the substance called **saliva.** During swallowing, the food moves in a moistened ball down the esophagus to the stomach. The stomach churns and mixes the food at the same time it is being broken down chemically. The most

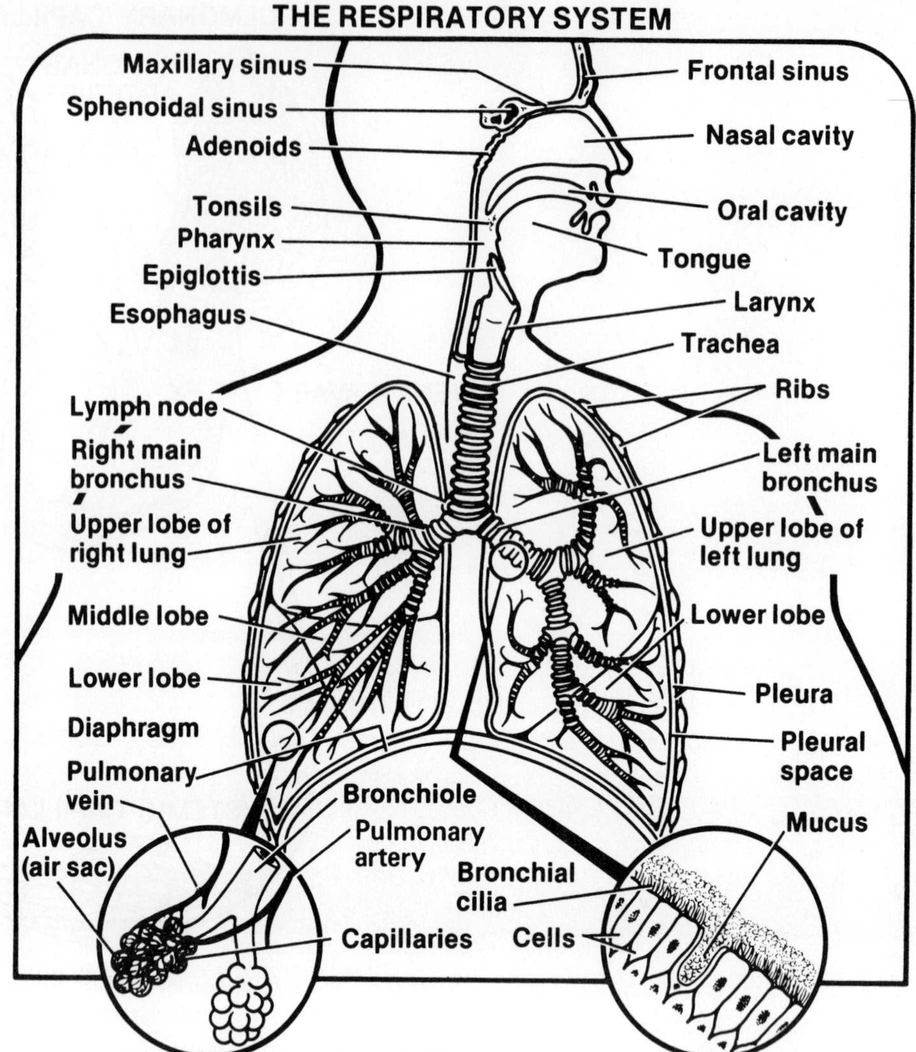

Figure 5–21

important area of digestion is the **duodenum.** This is the first loop of the **small intestine.** It is here that the digestive juices, not only from the duodenum itself but also from the pancreas, finish the job of breaking down food into usable parts. In addition, bile, which has been stored in the gallbladder after being manufactured in the liver, also enters the duodenum and helps the reduction process.

A lot of water is necessary for the chemical reduction of food into its end products. It is moved by the rhythmic contraction, called peristalsis, of the muscle walls of the organs of digestion.

Some of the final products of digestion are also absorbed in the area of the duodenum. These end products are:

- Amino acids, the building blocks for all growth and repair of body tissue, which come from dietary proteins
- Fatty acids and glycerols, from fat
- Simple sugars, such as glucose, from carbohydrates
- Water and vitamins

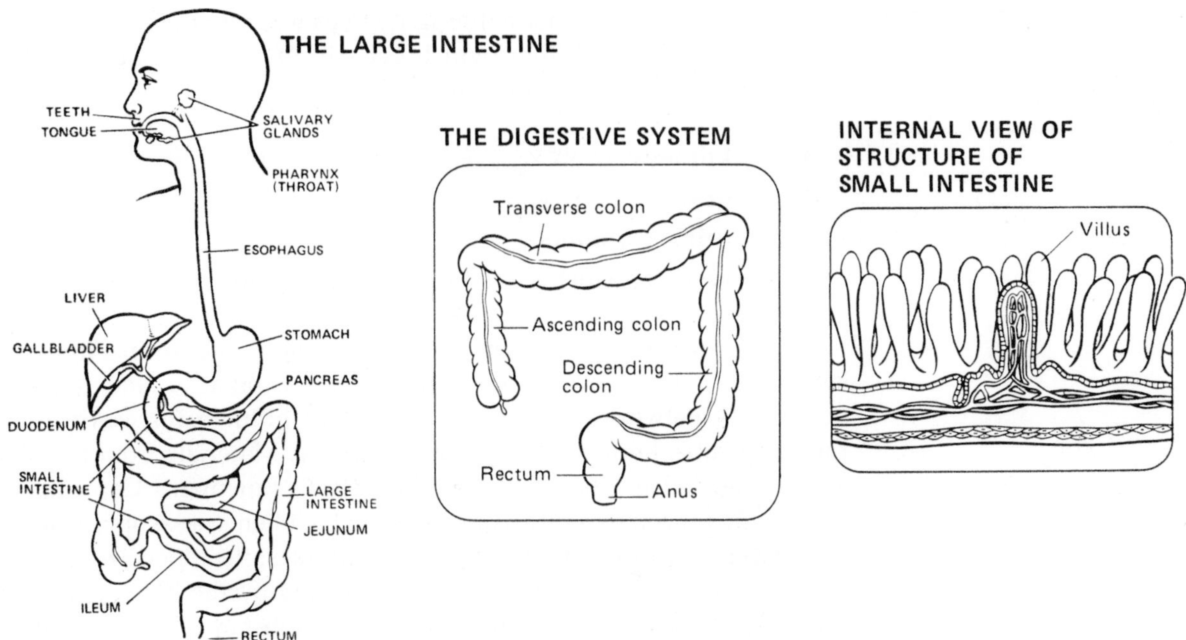

Figure 5–22

The lining of the duodenum is composed of thousands of tiny fingerlike projections called **villi.** Each villus is capable of absorbing these end products of digestion. The products are then moved into the bloodstream, where they are carried to individual cells.

Some digestion continues to take place in other parts of the small intestine. What is left of the food moves through the large intestine, where water is reabsorbed into the body. The material that cannot be used by the body is excreted from the rectum through the anus as feces.

The liver has important responsibilities aside from manufacturing bile. The liver is a storage area for glucose. This form of sugar is released in large amounts when the cells need it for energy to carry on their activities. The liver also is the place where toxins, or poisons, are removed from the blood. Damage to the liver can be caused by viruses, bacteria, drinking alcoholic substances or taking drugs that are harmful to its tissues. The liver is also responsible for production and storage of some proteins which are necessary for proper circulation of the blood and for blood clotting. Blood clots are not all bad. When a blood vessel has been injured, a clot may form that holds the blood within a closed tube (the blood vessel) until healing occurs.

On the right side of the colon, at the junction between the small intestine and the large intestine, there is a pouch with a projection of tissue called the **appendix.** Because there is very little peristalsis in this area, the appendix has a tendency to become infected, in a condition known as appendicitis. Surgery is usually performed to correct this condition.

The lowest portion of the large intestine curves in an S-shape into the **rectum.** The rectum is made of very delicate tissue. It has an internal sphincter muscle and an external sphincter muscle. Sometimes blood vessels that supply this area become enlarged and filled with blood clots, causing hemorrhoids.

KEY IDEA: THE URINARY SYSTEM

A vital body system in maintaining homeostasis (state of equilibrium or balance) is the urinary system (which gets rid of waste products). The organs that make up this system include (Fig. 5–23):

- The **kidneys**
- The **ureters** (tubes leading from the kidneys)
- The **urinary bladder**
- The **urethra** (which leads from the bladder to the outside of the body)

The functional unit of the kidneys is called a **nephron.** An exchange of substances takes place between the blood capillaries and a part of the nephron. A network of capillaries, called the **glomerulus,** lies within a cupping of a tube, known as Bowman's Capsule. Materials from the blood that are not needed by the body are filtered into Bowman's Capsule. They are then carried through a series of tubules, which help make up the nephron. As the filtered material flows through these tubules, the blood vessels surrounding them reabsorb those materials still needed by the body, particularly the water. Near the end of the winding tubules, substances from the blood, such as toxins and some drugs, pass into the urine. The filtrate that is left is collected in a larger tube. This tube joins those of all the other nephrons in a basin-like portion of the kidney. From here it drips steadily through the ureter, helped by a peristaltic motion very similar to that of the gastrointestinal tract, to the urinary bladder. There are stretch receptor-end organs in the muscular wall of the bladder. The bladder is capable of expanding greatly. When these receptors are stimulated by a full bladder, messages are sent to the brain that cause the person to urinate.

Because the urethra is open to the outside of the body, it may also provide a passageway for disease-causing organisms. These organisms may go

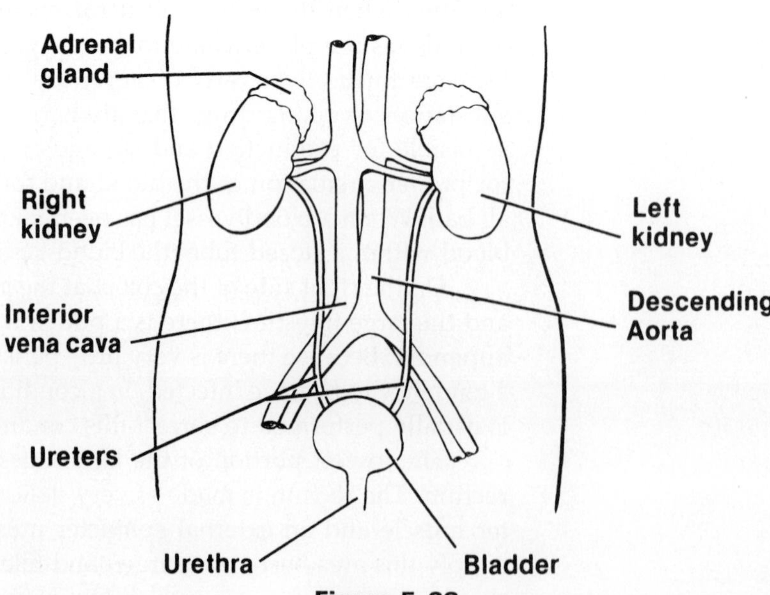

Figure 5–23

up to the bladder, infecting it and causing a disease known as cystitis. The infection may also spread through the ureters to the kidney, causing kidney damage.

The urinary system is perhaps the most important system for maintaining homeostasis. This is because the system determines the content of the blood. The blood content, in turn, determines the content of the tissue fluid, which is the immediate environment of the cells. Many changes in kidney function, some normal, can be found in urine samples. Such changes are also revealed in accurate measurement of intake and output. Sometimes in illness, especially after surgery, the patient is unable to void (urinate).

KEY IDEA: THE REPRODUCTIVE SYSTEM

In the female the primary reproductive organs are the two **ovaries.** The main task of the ovary is the production of **ova** (eggs). These are specialized cells that are able to unite with a sperm cell released from the male during intercourse and then grow over a period of forty weeks into a new human being. Developing ova lie in a lake of estrogen, a hormone that enters the blood stream during ovulation. **Ovulation** is the process whereby an ovum is released from one ovary into the opening of the oviduct (fallopian tube) and moves to the **uterus** (womb). This occurs once each month, usually 14 days before the onset of the next menstrual period. During this time, a woman is fertile (able to become pregnant). During ovulation, release of estrogen causes a buildup of the lining of the uterus (endometrium), preparing it for a possible pregnancy. (Fig. 5–24.)

Menstruation is simply the periodic (monthly) loss of some blood and a small part of the lining of the uterus, an organ that is full of blood vessels. The discharge flows out of the vagina for a period of four to seven days.

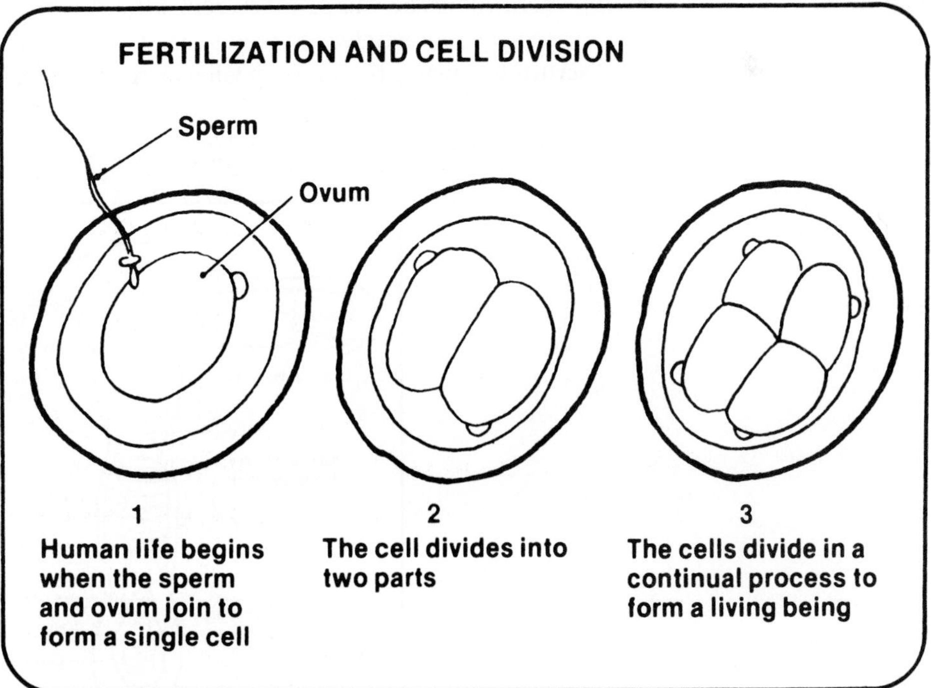
FERTILIZATION AND CELL DIVISION
Sperm
Ovum
1
Human life begins when the sperm and ovum join to form a single cell
2
The cell divides into two parts
3
The cells divide in a continual process to form a living being

Figure 5–24

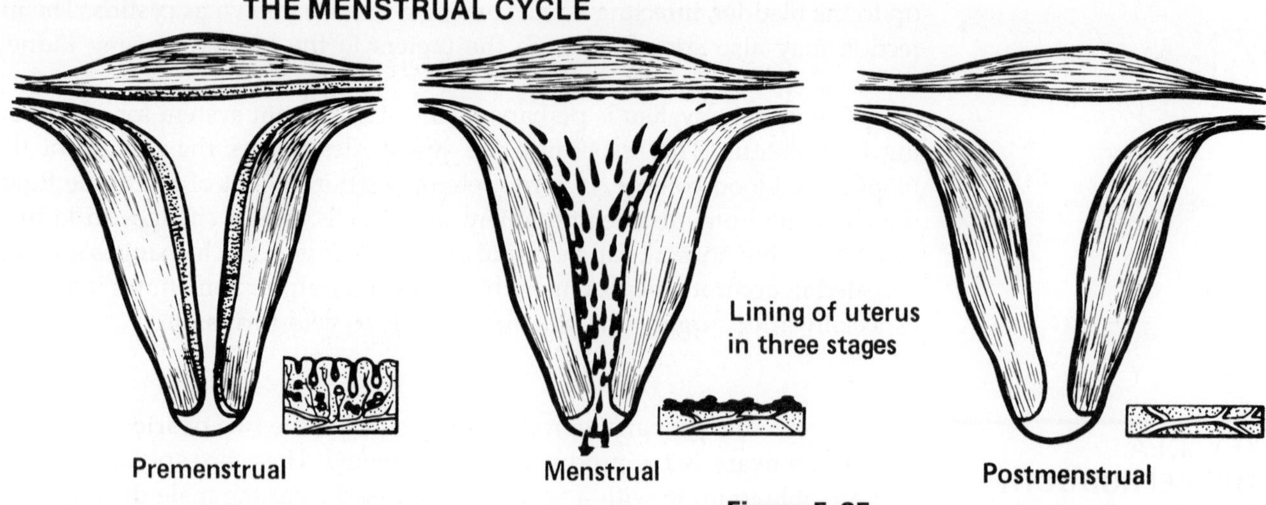

Figure 5–25

(Fig. 5–25.) The process of ovulation is controlled by hormones from the pituitary gland, under the control of the hypothalamus. The hormones from the pituitary gland are involved in the development of the ovum and in maintaining pregnancy. Menopause is the normal cessation of menstruation.

In the human female there are three openings in the perineal area. 1) The external urinary **meatus,** the end of the urethra. 2) The **vagina,** which is not only the organ for intercourse but also the birth canal. 3) The **anus,** the last portion of the gastrointestinal tract. (Fig. 5–26.)

Many women who find it necessary to have a hysterectomy, or surgical removal of the uterus, are afraid of what will happen to their bodies after surgery. Although such women will not be able to become pregnant, they usually are not affected in any other way.

In the male the primary reproductive organs are the testes, which produce sperm. **Testicles,** or **testes,** are paired glands that lie in a sac called the **scrotum** outside the body, posterior to the **penis,** which is the primary male sex organ. During intercourse, sperm travel up the **vas deferens,** or sperm duct, to a point where they enter the urethra. The entrance is made along

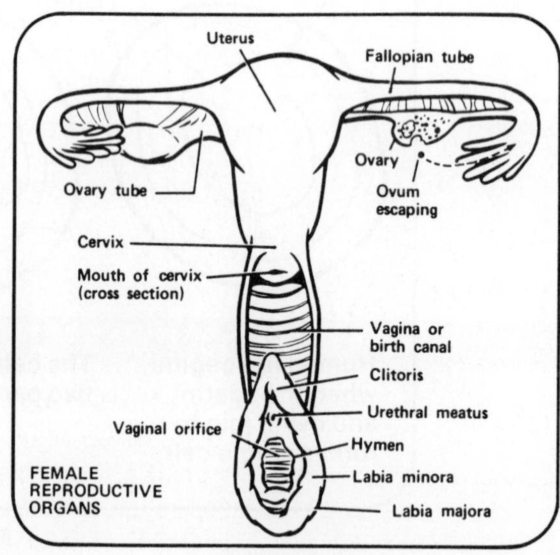

Figure 5–26

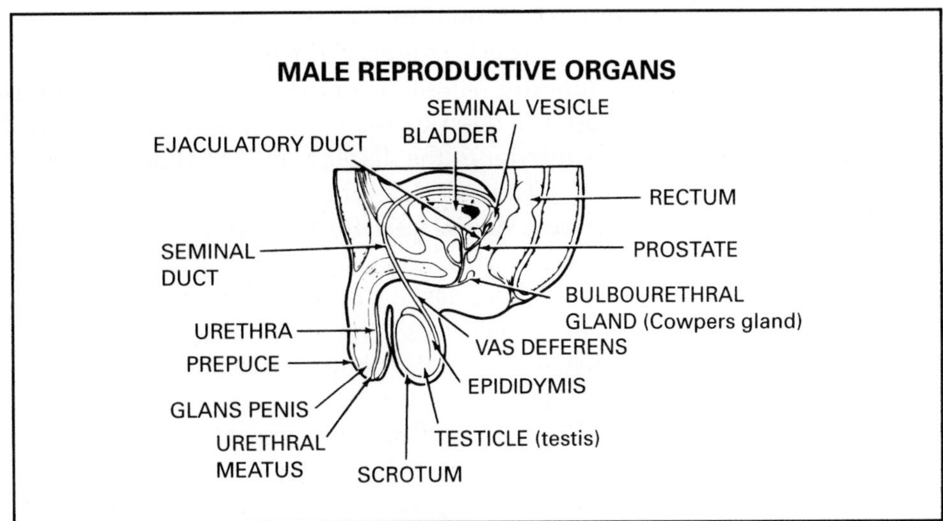

Figure 5–27

with secretions from other glands in the male reproductive system. These glands—the **seminal vesicles,** the **prostate gland,** and **bulbourethral glands** (Cowper's glands)—contribute water, nutrients, and vitamins, which, added to the sperm, make up the **semen,** a fluid that is ejaculated (expelled) at the same time the male has an orgasm. There is only one duct in the penis. It is used for the flow of urine and for the ejaculation of sperm in its carrying medium, the semen. During intercourse, the internal sphincter of the male's urinary bladder closes tightly so there is no chance for the urine to become mixed with the semen. The penis has three columns of spongy or cavernous tissue. During sexual excitement, blood rushes in through the penile artery and the veins constrict, trapping the blood so it fills these spaces. Then the penis becomes erect and turgid. All of this activity occurs under the influence of **testosterone,** the primary male sex hormone, which is also manufactured in the testes. It is secreted into the blood through the influence of the hormones from the anterior pituitary, which is under the control of the hypothalamus.

Sometimes during the aging process the **prostate gland,** which encircles the urethra like a doughnut, becomes enlarged. When the prostate expands, it squeezes the urethra, causing painful urination. Many men fear surgery on their prostate gland, because they believe it will end their sex life. The amount of semen ejaculated will be less but otherwise, men who have had a prostatectomy are almost always capable of having normal sexual relations. Vasectomy is the ligation or tying of the vas deferens to produce sterility. (Fig. 5–27.)

KEY IDEA: NAMES FOR BODY AREAS

As part of the study of each system, it would be wise to take an overall look at the body and to become familiar with the names given to body areas and cavities. In any demonstration or diagram, the body or body part shown is in the **anatomical position.** The person is standing up straight, facing you, palms out and feet together. When you look at a person in the anatomical position, remember that the left side is always on your right, as in a mirror. This is especially important in studying diagrams. The front of a person is referred to as the **anterior** (ventral) side. The back, containing the backbone, is called the **posterior** (dorsal) side. The areas of the body closer to the head are called **superior.** Those closer to the feet are called **inferior.** These terms may also be used to describe the position of an organ in the body. For example, the liver is inferior to the diaphragm. The shoulder is superior to the elbow.

The term **lateral** means pertaining to the side (the ears are lateral to the nose). **Medial** pertains to the middle (the nose is medial to the ears). **Distal** means farther from the point of attachment to the trunk and usually refers to the extremities (arms and legs). The wrist is distal to the elbow because the elbow is closer to where the arm attaches to the trunk of the body. **Proximal** means nearer the point of attachment to the trunk, so the knee is proximal to the ankle.

The body has two major cavities—the **dorsal** cavity and the **ventral** cavity. The dorsal cavity is divided into the cranial and spinal cavities. The cranial cavity is in the head. It contains the brain, its protecting membranes, large blood vessels, and nerves. The spinal cavity contains the spinal cord.

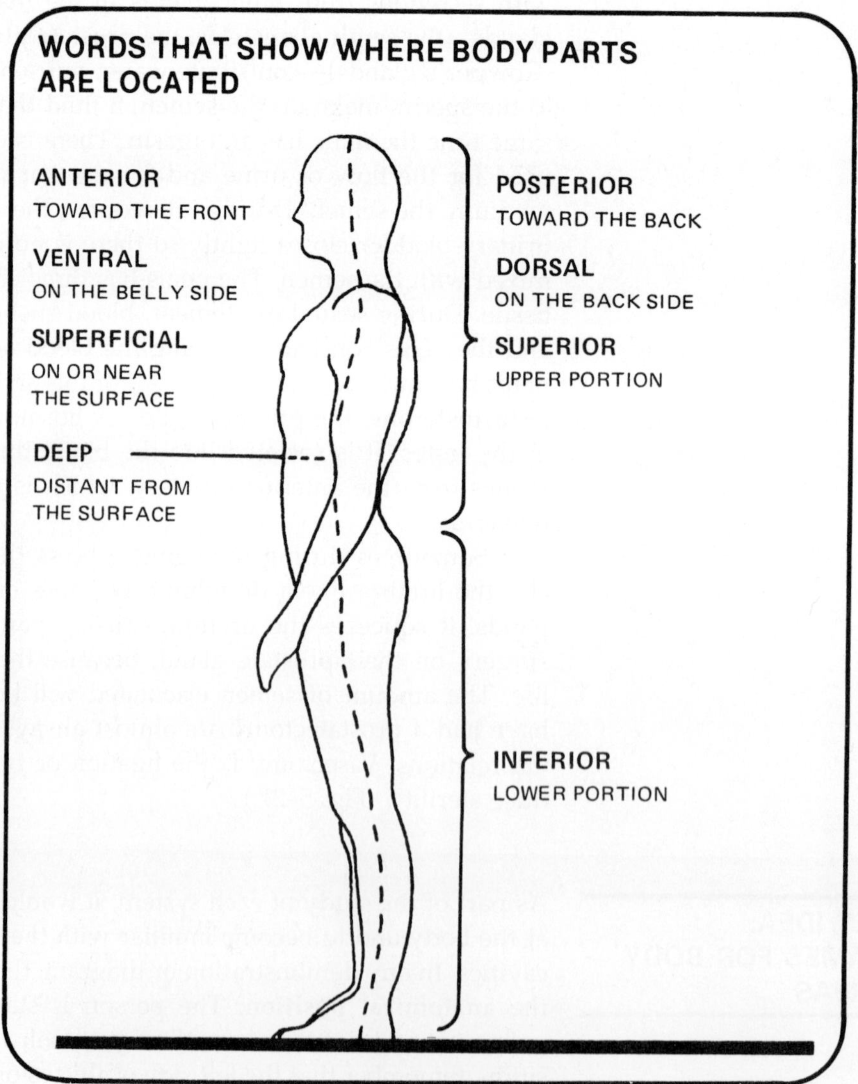

Figure 5–28

The ventral cavity is divided by a large, dome-shaped muscle—called the **diaphragm**—into the thoracic and abdominal cavities. The **thoracic** cavity is in your chest. It contains the lungs, the heart, the major blood vessels, and a portion of the esophagus. The esophagus is the food tube. It penetrates the diaphragm and enters the stomach, which is in the **abdominal** cavity.

Examples of organs in the abdominal cavity include the liver, spleen, pancreas, small and large intestines, and in the female, the ovaries and uterus.

The kidneys are located in the dorsal portion of the abdominal cavity. The kidneys are outside the large membrane that envelops all of the other organs. This membrane is known as the **peritoneum.** When this membrane becomes infected, the disease is known as **peritonitis.** The peritoneum, like all membranes in the body, is made up of both epithelial and connective tissue. It protects organs and prevents friction when they move. (Figs. 5–28 and 5–29.)

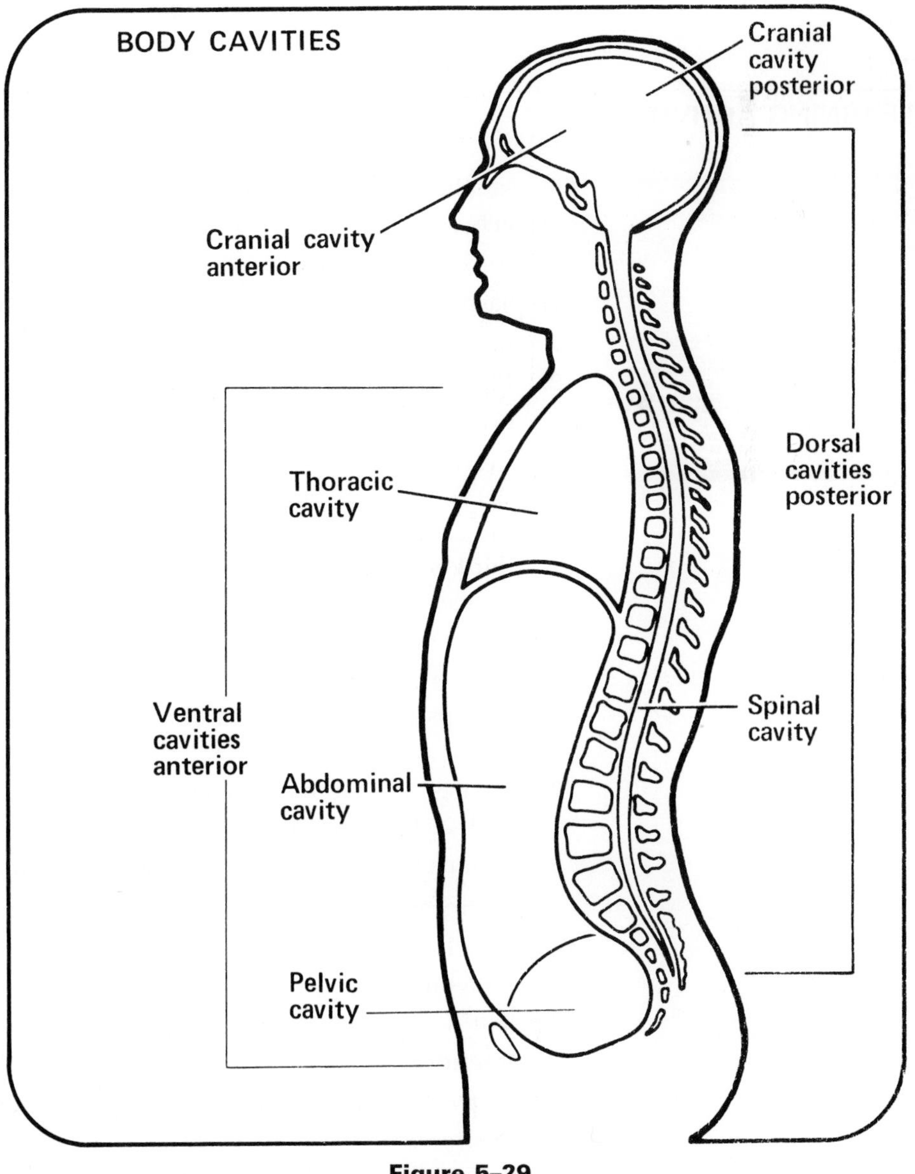

Figure 5–29

Summary

The cell is the basic unit of all living matter. The human body is made up of millions of cells. Cells reproduce by a process called cell division, which eventually produces groups of similar cells. When the cells that are similar in form and function become specialized, they are called tissues. When two or more tissues work together to perform a certain function, they form an organ, such as the heart. A system, such as the circulatory system, is formed when a group of organs act together to perform complex body functions. All cells, tissues, organs, and systems operate together to form a human being.

Good reasons for studying human anatomy are: to increase your knowledge of the science of medicine, to better communicate with the staff, and to become more efficient in the transcription of doctors' orders.

The best reason of all is that an appreciation of the design of the healthy human body and how it works will help you deliver a good quality of health care.

LEARNING ACTIVITIES

Choose the correct words from the list below to make each statement complete.

tissues	bodily	nucleus	cell membrane	structure
cytoplasm	systems	division	microscopic	organs

1. Anatomy is the study of the ______________________ of the body.
2. Physiology is the study of the ______________________ functions.
3. Cells are ______________________ in size.
4. Cells consist of three main parts. One is the ______________________, where the activities of the cell take place. The second is the ______________________, which directs cellular activities. The third is the ______________________, which keeps the living substances of a cell, called the protoplasm, within bounds and allows materials to pass in and out of the cell.
5. Cells reproduce by ______________________.
6. Groups of cells of the same type that do a particular kind of work are called ______________________.
7. Tissues are grouped together to form ______________________, such as the heart, lungs, and liver.
8. Organs that work together to perform similar tasks make up ______________________.

Write the letters of the body locations from column A in the space next to their matching description in column B.

Column A	*Column B*
(a) anterior	____ Toward the back
(b) deep	____ On or near the surface

Column A	*Column B*
(c) ventral	____ Toward the front
(d) inferior	____ Upper portion
(e) posterior	____ On the back side
(f) superficial	____ Lower portion
(g) superior	____ On the belly side
(h) dorsal	____ Distant from the surface

Fill in the blanks with the vocabulary word to remember after reading the definition carefully.

1. The region of the body between the chest and the pelvis is called the ______________________.

2. The posterior opening in the body through which feces is excreted is the ______________________.

3. A membranous sac that serves as a container within the body to hold urine is known as the ______________________.

4. The fluid circulating through the heart, arteries, veins, and capillaries that carries nourishment and oxygen to the tissues and takes away waste matter and carbon dioxide is called ______________________.

5. The ______________________ extends from the large intestine to the anus.

6. A ______________________ is a part of the body where two bones come together.

7. The total of all the physical and chemical changes that take place in living organisms and cells is called ______________________.

8. The body area between the thighs which includes the area of the anus and the external genital organs is called the ______________________.

9. ______________________ is the movement of the intestines that pushes food along to the next part of the digestive system.

10. ______________________ refers to the lungs.

11. A substance that moistens food and helps in swallowing, which also contains an enzyme (chemical) that helps digest starches, is called ______________________.

12. The ______________________ is a pouch below the penis that contains the testicles.

13. The ______________________ is the part of the digestive tract between the esophagus and the duodenum.

14. The ______________________ is a small depression on the abdomen that marks the place where the umbilical cord was originally attached to the fetus.

15. The tube leading from the urinary bladder to the outside of the body is called the ______________________.

16. Found in the female, the ______________________ is the birth canal leading from the vulva to the cervix of the uterus.

Write the letters of the body systems from Column A in the spaces next to their matching descriptions in Column B.

Column A	*Column B*
(a) Skeletal System	____ Gives movement to the body
(b) Muscular System	____ Takes in, absorbs food, converts it to energy
(c) Digestive System	____ Supports and protects the body
(d) Nervous System	____ Removes wastes
(e) Urinary System	____ Secretes hormones into the blood
(f) Integumentary System	____ Controls the activities of the body
(g) Endocrine System	____ Provides the first line of defense against infection
(h) Circulatory System	____ Carries food, oxygen, and water to body cells
(i) Respiratory System	____ Gives the body air to supply oxygen to the cells
(j) Reproductive System	____ Allows a new human being to be born

CHAPTER 6

Diseases and Diagnoses

OBJECTIVES

When you complete this chapter, you will be able to:

- Define the terms related to disease.
- List the major disease categories.
- List the seven danger signs of cancer.
- Define medical asepsis and discuss its purposes.
- Compare regular and reverse isolation and discuss the health unit coordinator responsibilities in relation to isolation.
- Define Standard Precautions, and list the three types of transmission precautions as defined by the Center for Disease Control.
- Define communicable diseases and discuss methods to prevent spread.

A doctor makes a **diagnosis,** the term denoting the name of the disease a person has or is believed to have, through careful evaluation of the patient's history, physical examination, laboratory and other tests, x-rays, and the disease process. Doctors may compare symptoms of similar diseases to determine which disease the patient may have. This is called a **differential diagnosis** (DD). They may establish a diagnosis by eliminating other possibilities. This is called diagnosis by **exclusion.** The value of establishing a diagnosis is to provide a logical basis for treatment and **prognosis**—the outcome of the disease.

The many diagnostic examinations ordered by the physician help him or her to make the correct diagnosis and to evaluate the course of the disease and the effects of the treatment prescribed. This is not a simple process, and the health unit coordinator can do a great deal to help the physician and the patient by performing the necessary duties to the best of his/her abilities.

KEY IDEA: TERMS RELATED TO DISEASE

The following list describes terms related to disease.

- **Disease**—a deviation from normal body structure or function that is harmful to the organism (person)
- **Acute disease**—a disorder of sudden onset and of short duration
- **Chronic disease**—a disorder usually having a slow onset and lasting for an extended period of time
- **Subacute disease**—a disorder not as severe as acute and of shorter duration than chronic
- **Functional disease**—a disorder of body function or performance without any observable change in the body tissues or structure
- **Organic disease**—a disorder resulting in structural change in body tissues or organs

KEY IDEA: MAJOR DISEASE CATEGORIES

There are many ways to group diseases. The following list will help the health unit coordinator understand the general categories:

- **Allergic diseases.** An allergy is an abnormal reaction to a substance that is harmless to most people and may be caused by many substances including dust, pollens, proteins, etc.
- **Congenital diseases** are disorders present at birth. These may include a wide variety such as harelip, clubfoot, or congenital heart defects. A hereditary disease is passed on in the genes. Many congenital diseases are not hereditary but are acquired **in utero** (while the baby is forming in the uterus). A mother who contracts German measles or syphilis may produce a baby with congenital disease. Hemophilia is an example of a hereditary disease passed through the genes, usually by the mother to the son, resulting in an excessive tendency to bleed.
- **Nutritional diseases**—lack of essential nutrients or inability of body to absorb and utilize them.
- **Degenerative diseases** are disorders that result from "wear and tear" on body tissues. Diseases of the heart and blood vessels rank high on the list of degenerative diseases. Lifetime habits slow down or hasten the degenerative process and all body tissues do not age at the same rate.
- **Infections or inflammatory diseases.** *Infection* is a reaction of the body to "germs" (pathogenic microorganisms) which multiply and cause symptoms. *Inflammation* is the reaction of the body to injury by pain, swelling, heat, etc. Inflammation and infection are not the same. There may be inflammation without the presence of infection.
- **Metabolic diseases** are diseases which disturb cellular activity. Diseases of the endocrine system would fall in this category.
- **Trauma** means injury. These include accidents such as falls, burns, blows, cuts, stabbings, gunshot wounds, injuries caused by heat, electricity, radiation, poisoning, snake and other bites, etc.
- **Neoplastic disease.** A *neoplasm* is a new growth or tumor. **Benign neoplasms** generally do not invade surrounding tissue, are not malignant (cancerous), and do not metastasize (spread). **Malignant neoplasms** are

cancerous tumors. They may likely invade surrounding tissue and frequently metastasize.

Cancers are classified through a process of **grading** and **staging.** Grading expresses the cancer's degree of differentiation. Benign (noncancerous) tumors are made up of well-organized and specialized (differentiated) cells which look very much like normal, mature tissue.

Staging is based on the size and spread (metastases) of the tumor. There are two main staging systems. The TNM system reports the size of the primary tumor, **T,** regional extension or nodes, **N,** and existence of metastases, **M.** Generally, the higher the number assigned to each letter, the more serious is the prognosis (forecast of outcome)—i.e., T4, N4, M4. Another method of staging uses O to IV based on the size of the tumor and the extent of its spread. Cancer is a prevalent disease in our society and there is much to learn about the subject. As a preventative health measure, the health unit coordinator should acquaint his or herself with the seven danger signs of cancer. According to the American Cancer Society they are:

Know Cancer's Seven Warning Signals

- Change in bowel or bladder habits
- A sore that does not heal
- Unusual bleeding or discharge
- Thickening or lump in breast or elsewhere
- Indigestion or difficulty in swallowing
- Obvious change in wart or mole
- Nagging cough or hoarseness

If any of these symptoms appear, a doctor should be seen at once.

KEY IDEA: PREDISPOSING CAUSES

Some conditions increase the likelihood of developing a disease. They include:

- Age—Certain age groups are more apt to contract certain diseases, for example, chicken pox in children and heart attacks in the elderly.
- Sex—Men are more likely to contract certain diseases than women, and vice versa.
- Occupation—Certain occupations predispose an individual to disease. Excessive exposure to asbestos has been linked to cancer, and coal miners are prone to lung disease.
- Genetics—Some people inherit a tendency toward certain diseases such as diabetes, heart disease, and sickle cell anemia.
- Environment—Poor, overcrowded, unhygienic living conditions can predispose to disease.
- Personal Habits—The use of drugs and alcohol, smoking, poor diet, sexual habits, stress, and overwork can lead to illness.

- Preexisting Condition—The presence of any disease can make it easier to contract others.
- Emotions—Certain diseases are linked with emotions and anxiety. Peptic ulcers and some hypertension are examples.
- Immunosuppression (e.g., in AIDS, chemotherapy, etc.)
- Chronic Illness (allergies, kidney failure, etc.)
- Drug therapy (e.g., long-term antibiotics, birth control pills, etc.)
- Pregnancy

KEY IDEA: ASEPSIS

People who work in health care institutions must learn the importance of cleanliness. Everyone tries constantly in many ways to achieve ideal sanitary conditions. You, too, take part in this team effort to keep everything absolutely clean. Why? Because cleanliness is a part of every health care institution's effort to control disease and keep communicable diseases from spreading. (Fig. 6–1.)

You will understand the importance of cleanliness in the health care institution if you know something about pathogens—the microorganisms that cause diseases. It may help to know what they are, how they spread, and how they can be destroyed. (Fig. 6–2.)

KEY IDEA: THE CAUSE OF DISEASE

People once believed that sickness was caused by evil spirits. About 500 years ago scientists began to suspect that some diseases were caused by very small living things they called *germs.*

A **germ** is a microorganism. *Micro* means very small. Microorganisms can be seen only under a microscope. *Organism* means a living thing. Different kinds of microorganisms (also called microbes) are:

Classifications of Microorganisms Which Can Cause Disease

- Viruses
- Bacteria
- Rickettsiae
- Fungi
- Protozoa

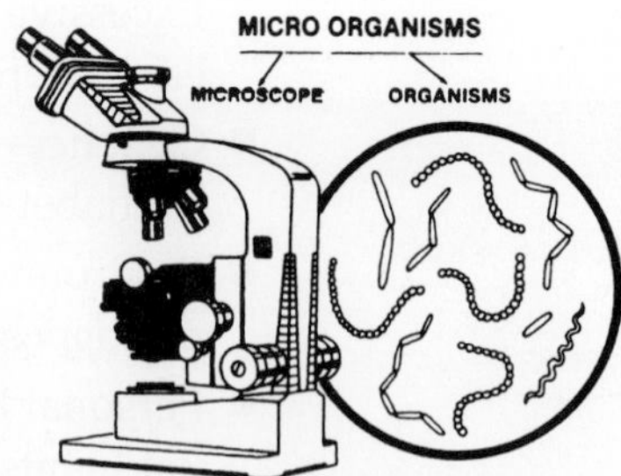

Figure 6–1

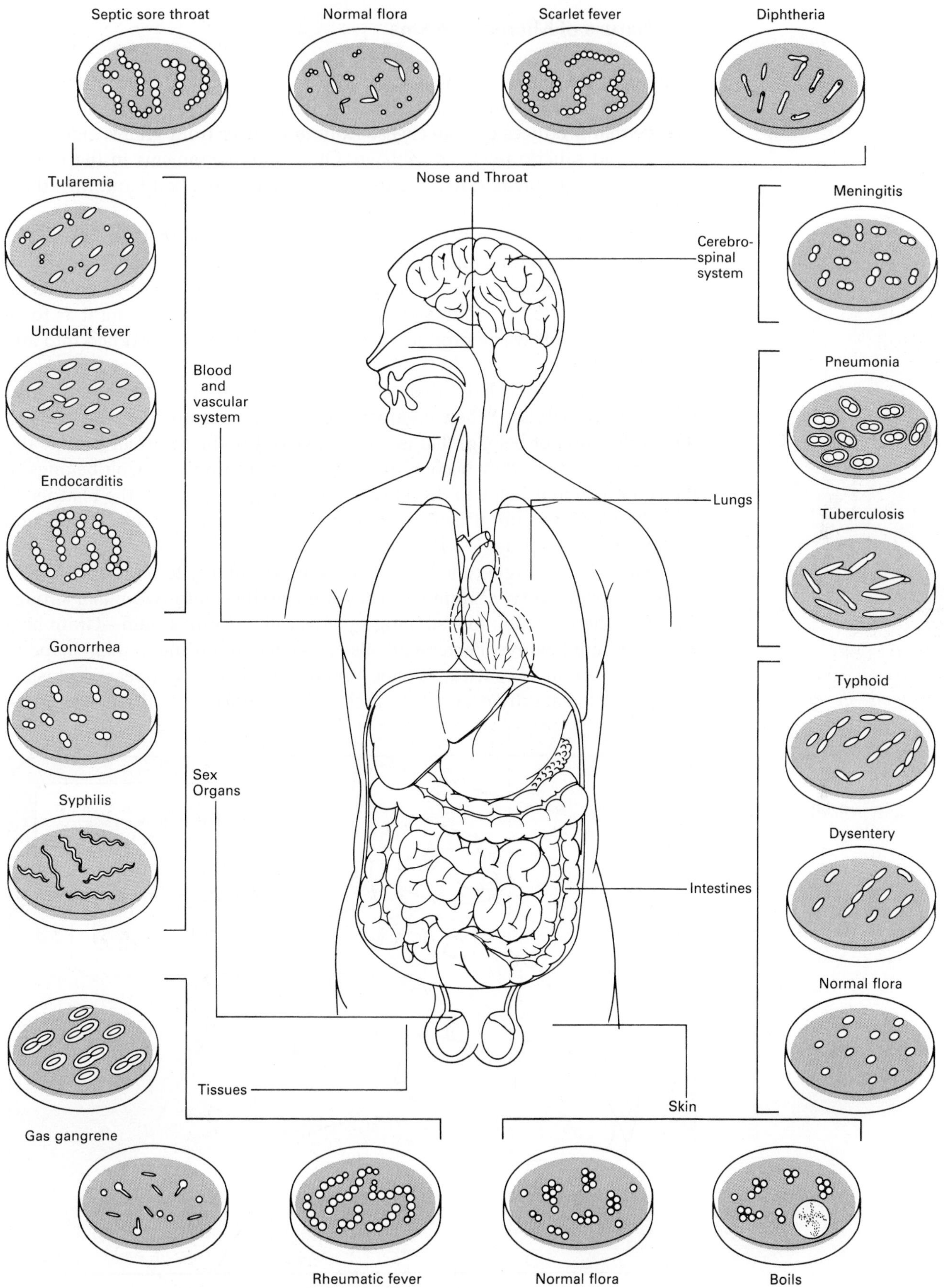
Microorganisms That Can Infect The Body And Common Portals Of Entry
Septic sore throat
Normal flora
Scarlet fever
Diphtheria
Nose and Throat
Tularemia
Undulant fever
Endocarditis
Blood and vascular system
Meningitis
Cerebro-spinal system
Pneumonia
Lungs
Tuberculosis
Gonorrhea
Syphilis
Sex Organs
Typhoid
Dysentery
Intestines
Normal flora
Tissues
Skin
Gas gangrene
Rheumatic fever
Normal flora
Boils

Figure 6–2

The Nature of Microorganisms

Some microorganisms are helpful to people. For example, certain microbes cause a chemical change in food called **fermentation.** Fermentation is the change that produces cottage cheese from milk, beer from grains, cider from apples, and sauerkraut from cabbage. Other microorganisms in the human digestive system break down the foods not used by the body and turn them into waste products (feces).

There are other kinds of microorganisms, however, that are harmful to man. These are the microbes that cause disease and infection. Disease-producing microorganisms are called **pathogens.** They grow best at body temperature, 98.6°F (37°C). Pathogens destroy human tissue by using it as food. They also give off waste products called **toxins.** These are absorbed into and poison the body.

Organisms each have their own normal environment or home called their natural habitat. When organisms gain access to areas of the body in which they do not belong, that is, they move out of their normal habitat and into a foreign area, they become pathogens. For example, E. Coli belongs in the colon where it helps to digest our food. When it gets into the bladder or into the blood stream, it can cause a urinary infection or a blood infection called **septicemia.** (Fig. 6–3.)

Bacteria are single-celled organisms with the ability to reproduce by cell division about every 20 minutes. They are classified into two major groups based on their reaction to a staining process called Gram's stain—Gram negative or Gram Positive. Bacteria are also classified according to their shape. A round bacterium is called a **coccus.** When these bacteria appear in clusters they are called **staphylocci,** when in chains, **streptococci,** and when in pairs,

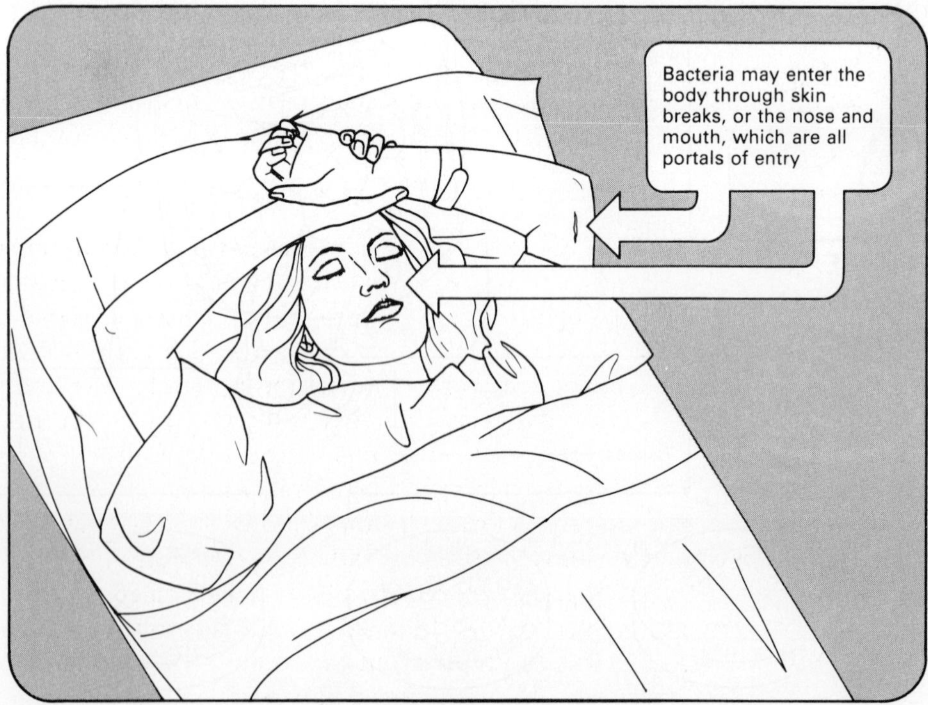
Bacteria may enter the body through skin breaks, or the nose and mouth, which are all portals of entry

Figure 6–3

diplococci. Rod-shaped bacteria are called **bacilli.** Spiral-shaped bacteria that are rigid are called **spirilla,** flexible are called **spirochetes,** and curved, **vibrios.**

In the hospital you will often hear the words staph or staphylococcus and strep or streptococcus. **Staphylococcus** and **streptococcus** are two types of bacteria that are found in all health care institutions. They are commonly found on the human skin and mucous membranes of the gastrointestinal tract **(normal flora).** They enter the body through a portal of entry. When staphylococci get inside the skin, they may produce a local infection. There may be soreness, tenderness, redness, and/or pus. Sometimes staphylococcus infections can affect the whole body. When streptococci enter the body, they may cause a septic sore throat, a local infection, or rheumatic fever, a general infection.

There are many conditions which contribute to the growth of bacteria.

- Food—bacteria grow well in the remains of food left in a patient's room
- Moisture—bacteria grow in moist places
- Temperature—High temperatures (170°F) kill most bacteria. At 50 to 110°F most disease-causing bacteria grow rapidly. The normal human body temperature of 98.6° enables bacteria to thrive easily. Low temperatures do not kill bacteria but retard their activity and growth rate.
- Oxygen—aerobic bacteria require oxygen to live; anaerobic bacteria can survive without oxygen
- Light—In darkness, bacteria become very active and multiply rapidly. Light is bacteria's worst enemy. When exposed to direct sunlight, they become sluggish and die rapidly.
- Dead and living matter—saprophytes, bacteria that live on dead matter or tissues; parasites—bacteria that live on living matter or tissue.

A **virus** is another type of microorganism. Viruses are much smaller than bacteria, and they cause many of man's diseases. Examples are measles, smallpox, influenza, and AIDS. Viruses can survive only in living cells. (Fig. 6–4.)

KEY IDEA: HISTORY OF INFECTION CONTROL

The germ theory of disease was not actually proven until a little over 100 years ago. A French scientist named Louis Pasteur made two important discoveries about bacteria. First, he discovered that many diseases are caused by bacteria. Second, he discovered that bacteria could be killed by heat.

Pasteur's name has been used to refer to this method of killing. For example, **pasteurization** is the process of heating milk to about 140°F (60°C) and keeping it at that temperature for 30 minutes. Pasteurization kills harmful bacteria and makes milk safe for us to drink. (Fig. 6–5.)

A few years after Pasteur's discoveries, a British surgeon, Joseph Lister, found that many pathogens could also be killed by carbolic acid. Lister recognized that many deaths in hospitals seemed to be connected with unclean conditions. He was the first to want surgical wounds kept clean and the air in the operating room kept pure.

Lister changed things in hospitals by introducing the principles and methods of aseptic surgery. **Aseptic** means pathogen-free, without disease-

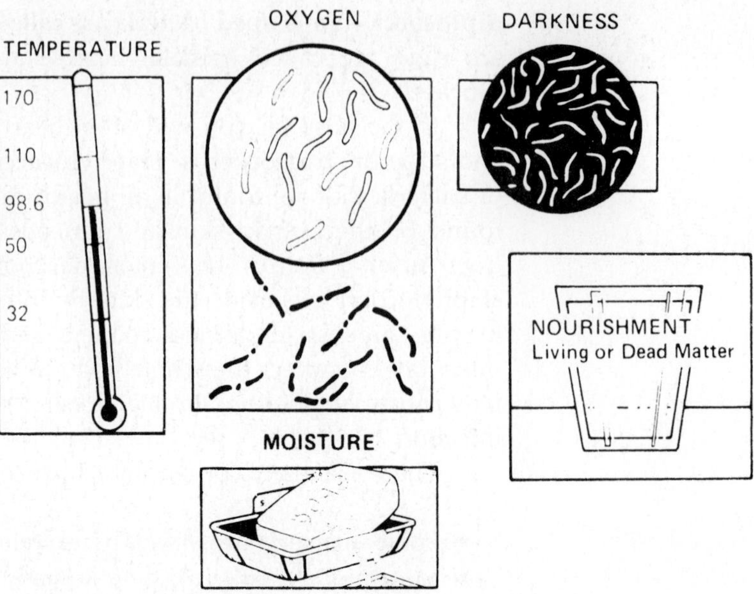

CONDITIONS THAT PROMOTE BACTERIAL GROWTH

Figure 6–4

producing organisms. Lister developed a technique to keep pathogens out of open wounds or to destroy them. His method was to spray the skin around the wound with carbolic acid. Also, surgical instruments were made aseptic by being dipped in a carbolic acid solution. This technique was a major advance in the battle against disease.

People working in hospitals began to realize that some disease-producing microorganisms are everywhere. They are in the air, on the furniture, on and inside the patients' bodies, and on all the equipment. Doctors knew that pathogens multiply very rapidly. They also know that if pathogens are not killed, they spread infection and disease from one person to another. Therefore, it was necessary to apply the principles of asepsis to the entire health care institution. (Figs. 6–6 and 6–7.)

KEY IDEA: DISINFECTION AND STERILIZATION

A continuous battle goes on in health care institutions to prevent the spread of pathogens. This battle is called **medical asepsis.** In spite of the best efforts of health care personnel, there are always some harmful microorganisms around us. They can be made harmless, however, by simple cleanliness procedures. We can keep ourselves clean by bathing and frequent handwashing.

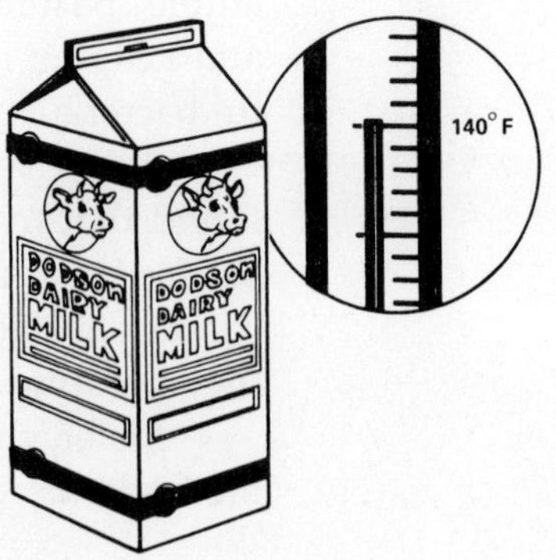

Figure 6–5

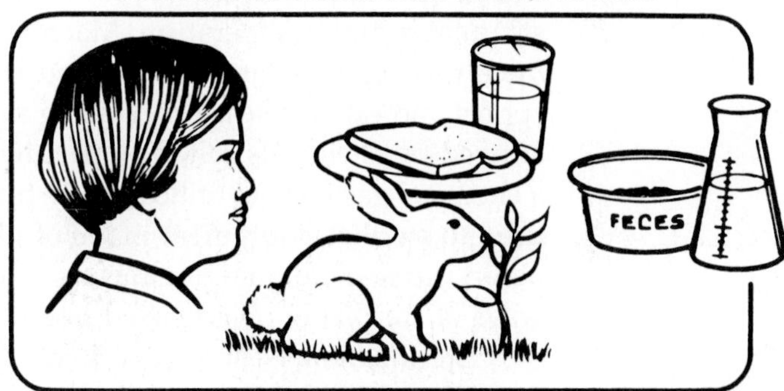

Figure 6–6

We can keep the institution and its equipment clean with soap, water, and solutions that assist in keeping down bacterial growth. Also, there are two very important methods for killing microorganisms or keeping them under control. These methods are:

- **Disinfection**—the process of destroying as many harmful organisms as possible. It also means slowing down the growth and activity of the organisms that cannot be destroyed.
- **Sterilization**—the process of killing all microorganisms, including spores, in a certain area.

Spores are dehydrated forms of some bacteria that serve as a defense for the bacteria and are very difficult to destroy. Some can even live in boiling

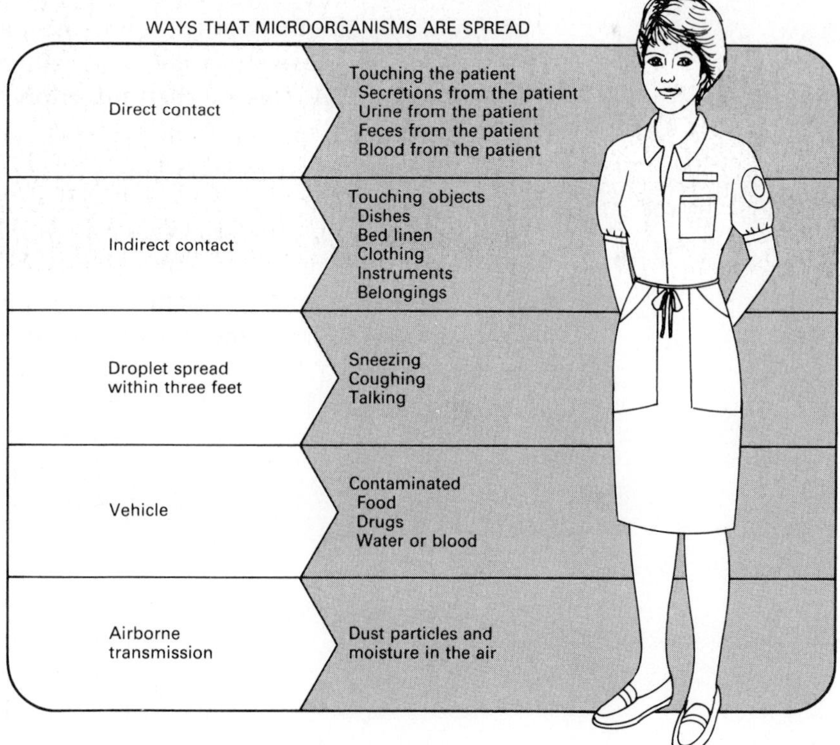

WAYS THAT MICROORGANISMS ARE SPREAD
Direct contact
Touching the patient
Secretions from the patient
Urine from the patient
Feces from the patient
Blood from the patient
Indirect contact
Touching objects
Dishes
Bed linen
Clothing
Instruments
Belongings
Droplet spread within three feet
Sneezing
Coughing
Talking
Vehicle
Contaminated
Food
Drugs
Water or blood
Airborne transmission
Dust particles and moisture in the air

Figure 6–7

water. Spores *can* be destroyed, however, by being exposed to pressurized steam at a high temperature. Machines called **autoclaves** (Fig. 6–8) can produce this high-temperature, pressurized steam. Autoclaves are used to kill spores and other disease-producing microorganisms. Spores may also be destroyed by chemicals called **sporicides.** Another method of sterilization uses a chemical gas instead of heat to destroy microorganisms. This method can be used to sterilize equipment made of plastics without melting them. When an object is free of all microorganisms, it is called **sterile.** These are both effective ways of sterilizing objects used in a health care institution.

Sterilization is necessary if the article comes in direct contact with a wound, as in the case of surgical instruments. Most supplies and equipment used in the care of patients can be disinfected to prevent them from spreading disease or infection. Disposable supplies must always be incinerated or burned.

Medical Asepsis

Medical asepsis means preventing the conditions that allow pathogens to live, multiply, and spread. As a health unit coordinator, you will share the responsibility for preventing the spread of disease and infection.

The health unit coordinator should know that the main purposes for medical asepsis are:

- Protecting the patient against becoming infected a second time by the same microorganism. This is called **reinfection.**
- Protecting the patient against becoming infected by a new or different type of microorganism from another patient or a member of the hospital staff. This is called **cross infection.**
- Protecting all other patients and hospital staff against becoming infected by microorganisms passing from patient to patient, staff to patient, or patient to staff. This is called **infection control.**
- Protecting the patient from becoming infected with his own organisms. This is called **self-inoculation.**

Handwashing. In your work you will handle supplies and equipment used in the treatment and care of patients. Pathogens will get on your hands. They will come from the patient or from the things he or she has touched. Your hands could carry these microorganisms to other persons and places.

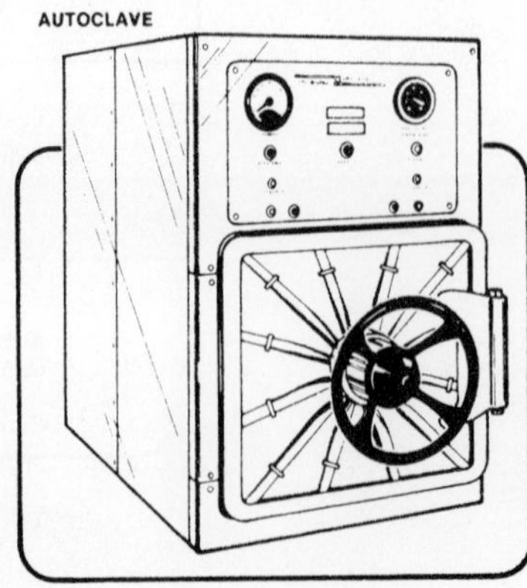

Figure 6–8

WASHING YOUR HANDS

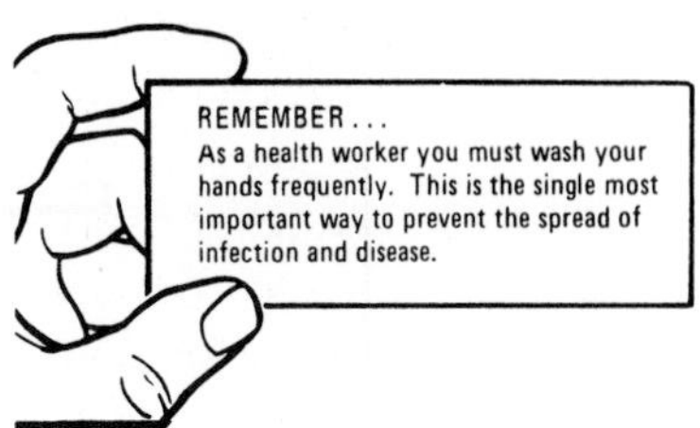

REMEMBER...
As a health worker you must wash your hands frequently. This is the single most important way to prevent the spread of infection and disease.

Figure 6–9

The pathogens could also be moved to your own face and mouth. Handwashing is the most important measure a health worker can take to prevent the spread of disease. (Fig. 6–9.)

KEY IDEA: ISOLATION

Communicable diseases spread very quickly and easily from one person to another. **Nosocomial infections** are hospital-acquired. To prevent the spread of communicable disease, hospitals employ two types of procedures:

1. **Aseptic procedures** such as handwashing and other clean techniques, as well as sterile practices which are used on certain patients as indicated.
2. **Special isolation procedures** which are used on patients who are diagnosed or suspected of having communicable diseases.

The purpose of isolation techniques is to keep the pathogens that cause the disease inside the isolated patient's unit. As you know, these pathogens are everywhere in the sick room. They are on the floor, furniture, bedding, articles brought to the bedside, and on the patient himself. The area, the articles, and the patient are said to be contaminated. Isolation technique, including the use of masks and gowns, keeps pathogens away from equipment and personnel. (Fig. 6–10.)

When strict techniques, such as the use of sterile sheets and gowns, are used to protect the patient from outside pathogens, this is called **reverse** or **protective isolation.** (Fig. 6–11.)

Isolation procedures involve separating infected patients from other patients and from health care workers by using a variety of *barriers* such as gloves, masks, gowns or plastic aprons, and through actual *isolation* (the separation of the patient from other patients and personnel) in special private rooms. These decisions are made based upon the patient's diagnosis or suspected diagnosis.

Protective isolation uses both Standard Precautions for all patients and Transmission-Based Precautions for specified patients who are immunocompromised and at increased risk for bacterial, fungal, parasitic, and viral infections from other patients and the environment. Immunocompromised patients have a diminished ability to fight off disease.

KEY IDEA: ISOLATION PRECAUTIONS

Early in 1996 the Centers for Disease Control and Prevention (CDC) and the Hospital Infection Control Practices Advisory Committee (HICPAC) published new guidelines for isolation precautions in hospitals.

The new guidelines contain two levels of precautions, *Standard Precautions* and *Transmission-Based Precautions.*

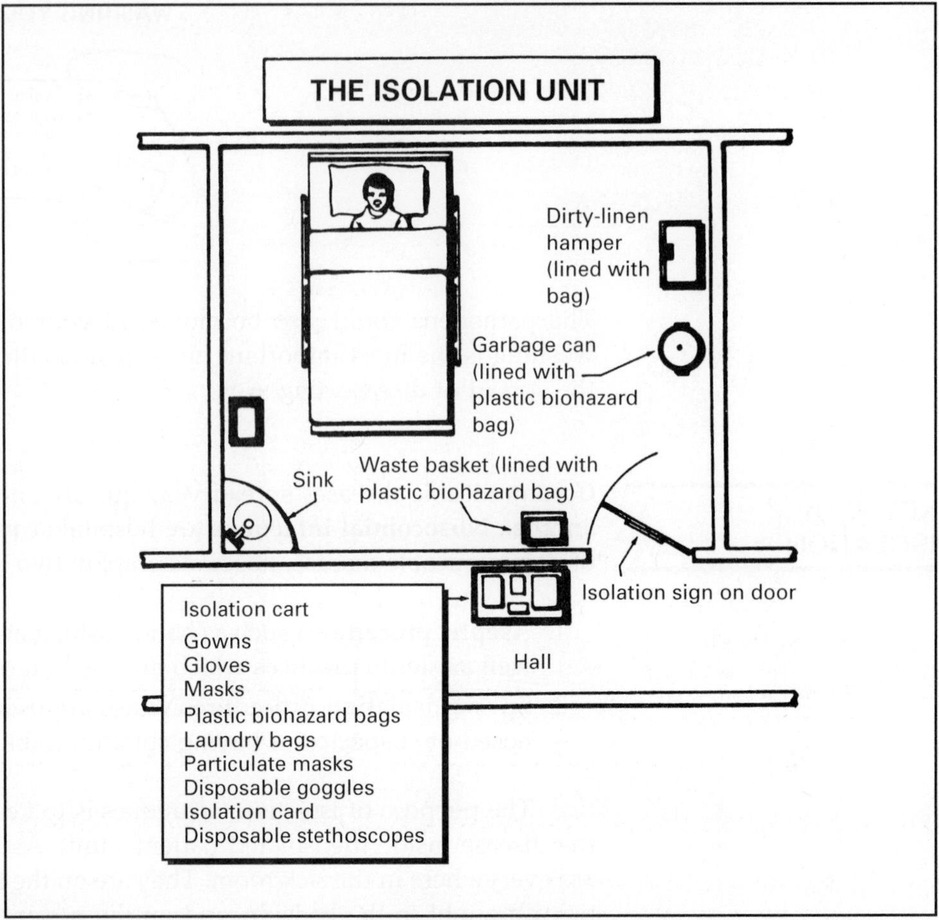

Figure 6–10

Standard Precautions are designed for the care of all patients regardless of diagnosis or infection status. They were formerly known as Universal Precautions.

Standard Precautions integrate the characteristics of Universal Blood and Body Fluid Precautions and Body Substance Isolation Precautions.

Standard Precautions are used when any procedure is performed that may cause the health care worker to come in contact with blood; body secretions (except perspiration); excretions; nonintact skin; or mucous membranes. The application of Standard Precautions includes:

- Proper handwashing technique
- Proper use of gloves
- Appropriate and correct use of personal protective equipment
- Correct handling of used needles and other sharps
- Proper handling of used patient-care equipment, environment, and linen
- Careful consideration of patient placement (i.e., private room)

Transmission-Based Precautions are used for patients who are known or suspected to be infected with pathogenic microorganisms or communica-

ISOLATION

PURPOSE OF ISOLATION

ISOLATION TECHNIQUES ARE USED WHEN PATIENTS HAVE INFECTIOUS OR COMMUNICABLE DISEASES THAT CAN BE SPREAD TO OTHERS. THE PURPOSE OF ISOLATION TECHNIQUES IS TO PREVENT THE SPREAD OF THESE DISEASES TO OTHER PATIENTS, STAFF, AND VISITORS.

REGULAR ISOLATION

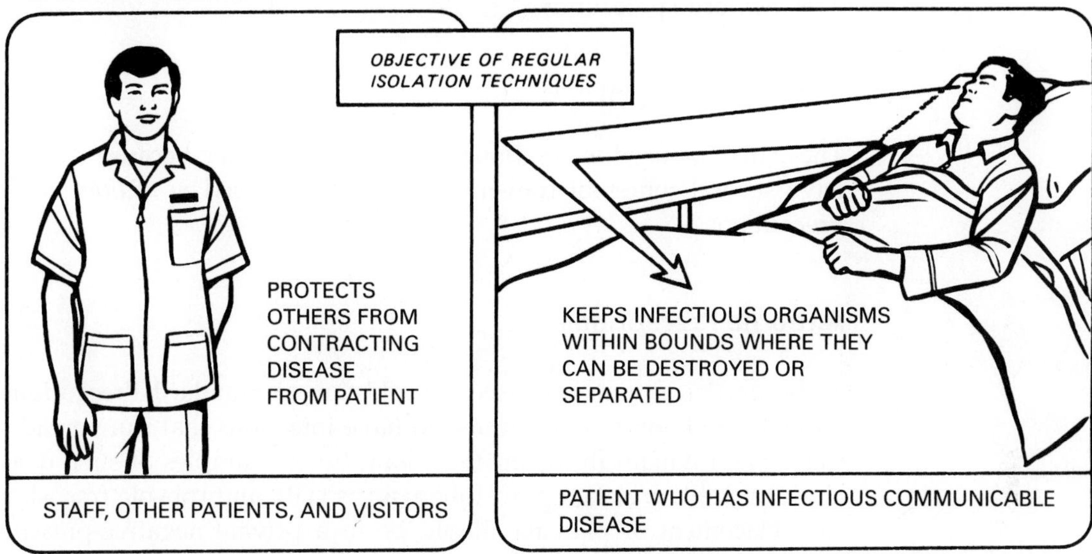
OBJECTIVE OF REGULAR ISOLATION TECHNIQUES
PROTECTS OTHERS FROM CONTRACTING DISEASE FROM PATIENT
KEEPS INFECTIOUS ORGANISMS WITHIN BOUNDS WHERE THEY CAN BE DESTROYED OR SEPARATED
STAFF, OTHER PATIENTS, AND VISITORS
PATIENT WHO HAS INFECTIOUS COMMUNICABLE DISEASE

IN REGULAR ISOLATION, CONTAMINATION IS PREVENTED FROM SPREADING FROM THE ROOM.

REVERSE OR PROTECTIVE ISOLATION

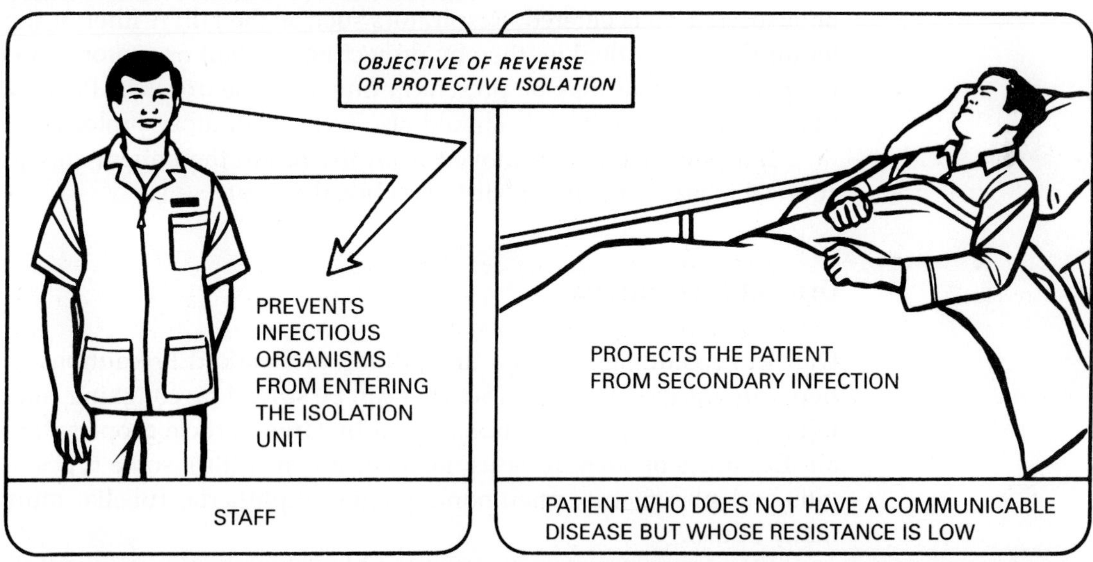
OBJECTIVE OF REVERSE OR PROTECTIVE ISOLATION
PREVENTS INFECTIOUS ORGANISMS FROM ENTERING THE ISOLATION UNIT
PROTECTS THE PATIENT FROM SECONDARY INFECTION
STAFF
PATIENT WHO DOES NOT HAVE A COMMUNICABLE DISEASE BUT WHOSE RESISTANCE IS LOW

SOMETIMES A PATIENT WHOSE RESISTANCE IS LOW AND WHO COULD EASILY CATCH A DISEASE IS ISOLATED FROM POSSIBLE INFECTIONS. THIS IS COMMONLY DONE FOR BURN PATIENTS OR FOR THOSE WHO ARE IMMUNOCOMPROMISED. IT IS CALLED *REVERSE* OR *PROTECTIVE* ISOLATION. IN PROTECTIVE ISOLATION, CONTAMINATION MUST BE PREVENTED FROM ENTERING THE ROOM.

Figure 6–11

ble disease, or **colonized** (when a positive bacterial culture shows a developing infection even in the absence of symptoms) by pathogenic microorganisms.

These guidelines combine and revise the previous category and disease-specific isolation procedures into three types of precautions:

- Airborne precautions
- Droplet precautions
- Contact precautions

These may be used in combination with one another, because many diseases have several routes of transmission. They are used *in addition to* Standard Precautions.

Airborne Precautions

Airborne Precautions are used (in addition to Standard Precautions) when patients are known or suspected to have infections that can spread through the air and remain in the air for a long time. Examples of such diseases include varicella (chicken pox), tuberculosis (TB), and rubeola (measles).

Placement of patients should be in a private negative-pressure isolation room with the door closed. If this is not possible, nursing will consult with the Epidemiology Department (department responsible for infection control).

Respiratory protection is worn when the room of a patient with known or suspected TB is entered. Respirators such as the HEPA-filter or the N95 filter air that is breathed in, thereby protecting the staff or visitor from inhaling the pathogens that may be present in tiny airborne droplets. Persons susceptible to varicella or rubeola should also wear respiratory protection.

If a patient must be moved from the room, the patient should wear a surgical mask which filters air that is breathed out.

Droplet Precautions

Droplet Precautions are used (in addition to Standard Precautions) when patients are infected with diseases that can be spread by coughing, sneezing, or talking. These diseases are transmitted by large-particle droplets through the air. Examples of such diseases include influenza (flu), some types of meningitis and pneumonia, pneumonic plague, diphtheria, rubella, mumps, and many others.

Placement of such patients should be in a private room or, if that is not available, with another patient with the same disease. Caregivers and visitors should wear a surgical mask when within 3 feet of the patient. Large-particle droplets generally travel no more than 3 feet before dropping from the air. If the patient must leave the room, he or she should wear a surgical mask.

Hospitals use special signs and symbols to let others know about the type of isolation that is being used. The accompanying chart shows the category-specific color-code labels for communication. (Fig. 6–12.)

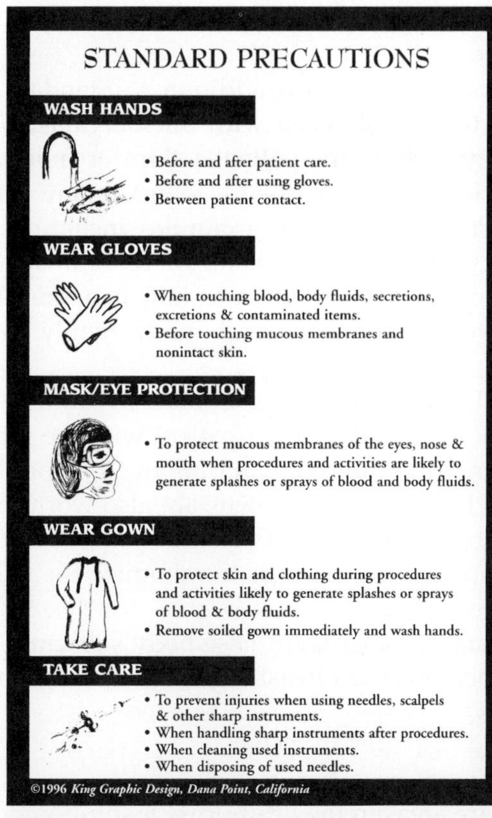
STANDARD PRECAUTIONS
WASH HANDS
• Before and after patient care.
• Before and after using gloves.
• Between patient contact.
WEAR GLOVES
• When touching blood, body fluids, secretions, excretions & contaminated items.
• Before touching mucous membranes and nonintact skin.
MASK/EYE PROTECTION
• To protect mucous membranes of the eyes, nose & mouth when procedures and activities are likely to generate splashes or sprays of blood and body fluids.
WEAR GOWN
• To protect skin and clothing during procedures and activities likely to generate splashes or sprays of blood & body fluids.
• Remove soiled gown immediately and wash hands.
TAKE CARE
• To prevent injuries when using needles, scalpels & other sharp instruments.
• When handling sharp instruments after procedures.
• When cleaning used instruments.
• When disposing of used needles.
©1996 King Graphic Design, Dana Point, California

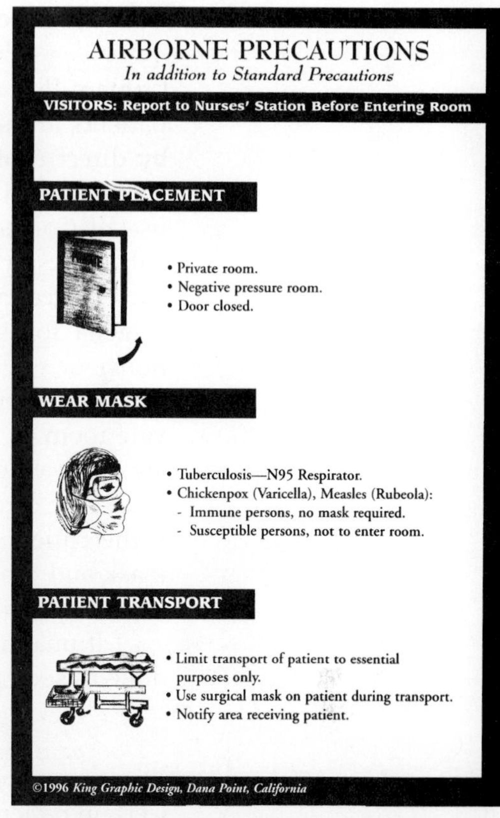

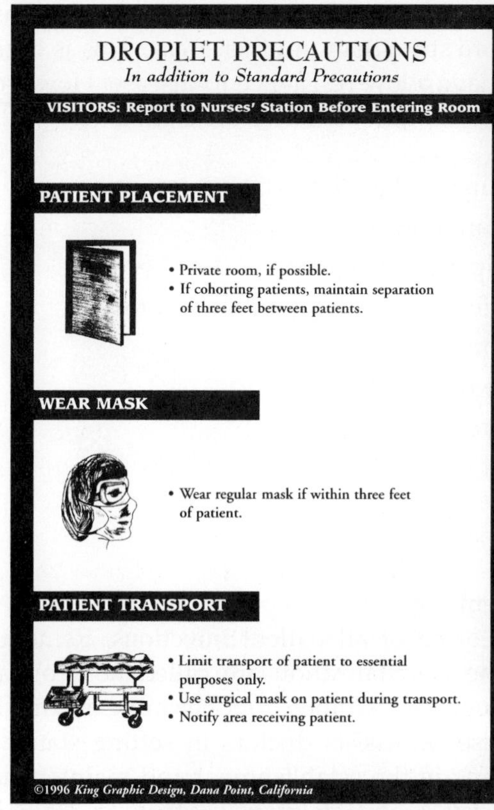

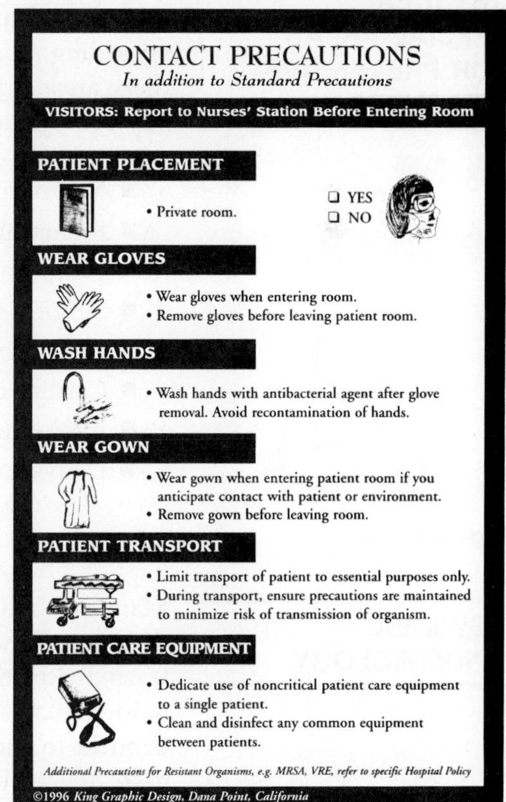

Figure 6–12 (Courtesy King Graphic Design, Dana Point, CA. To order call Etna Communications, 3023 North Clark St., Suite 744 Chicago, IL 60657-5200 1-800-347-6893.)

Contact Precautions

Contact Precautions are used (in addition to Standard Precautions) when patients are infected or colonized with microorganisms that can be spread by direct contact (touching the patient's skin) or indirect contact (touching contaminated articles in the patient's room). Many infections require the use of Contact Precautions. Some examples include wound, gastrointestinal, or respiratory infections or colonizations with multiple drug-resistant bacteria; certain enteric infections including hepatitis A, some E. coli and shigella for incontinent patients, and many highly infectious skin infections.

Placement of patients requiring Contact Precautions should be in a private room or, if not available, with a patient with the same infection. Gloves are worn when entering the room and removed before leaving, followed of course by careful handwashing. Gowns are also worn for most patient care. If the patient is transported outside of the room, the patient should wear a mask and other appropriate barriers to minimize the risk of transmission of microorganisms to others.

If unanticipated contact with these body substances occurs, washing is done as soon as possible (handwashing, face washing, showering, etc.).

KEY IDEA: SPECIAL AREAS FOR PREVENTIVE MEASURES

Certain patient care areas in the health care institution need special attention to ensure cleanliness. Precautions to prevent communicable conditions from spreading are more strict than in other areas. This is because the patients in these areas may have a low resistance to disease. However, they do not have any communicable conditions. These areas include:

- Newborn nursery (Fig. 6–13.)
- Premature care nursery
- Postpartum patient care unit
- Surgical patient care unit (operating room)
- Delivery room
- Cardiac care unit
- Intensive care unit
- Dialysis unit (Fig. 6–14.)

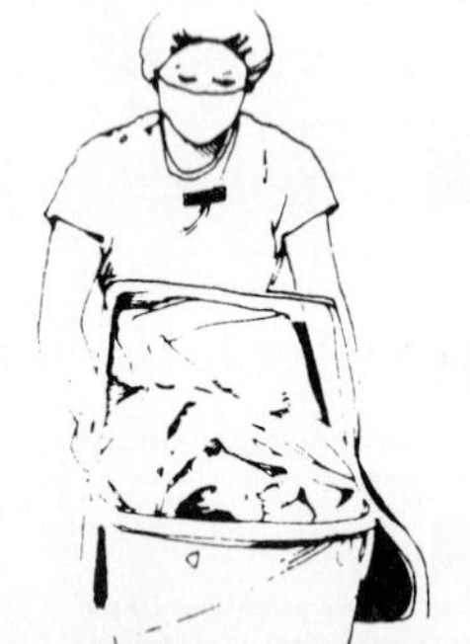

Figure 6–13

KEY IDEA: EPIDEMIOLOGY

Many hospitals employ a nurse epidemiologist. This RN is responsible for the careful monitoring of all patient infections. Remember, infections contracted during the hospitalization are called nosocomial infections. Nurse epidemiologists conduct studies to determine if the hospital itself contributes to the disease, assists doctors in setting standards to prevent disease, assists nursing in the establishment and maintenance of isolation techniques, and compiles and delivers records to state health agencies as necessary.

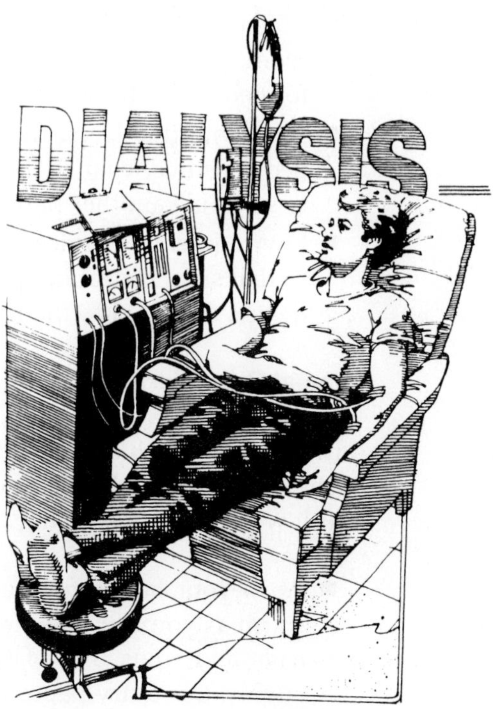

Figure 6–14

KEY IDEA: ISOLATION AND THE HEALTH UNIT COORDINATOR

It is a nursing responsibility to see that all patients are isolated properly according to the CDC guidelines.

- The appropriate isolation precaution sign (Standard Precautions, Airborne Precautions, Droplet Precautions, or Contact Precautions) is placed on the patient's door. Sometimes more than one sign will be necessary because some infections and conditions have multiple routes of transmission.
- All departments who will have contact with the patient are notified.
- Isolation supplies such as gloves, gowns, and masks are ordered for the patient's room.
- The physician is notified by nursing, and a written order for isolation is requested.
- The infection control officer or nurse epidemiologist is notified immediately.
- The word "isolation" and type of isolation will be indicated on the patient's chart, Kardex, and other forms as explained by your instructor.
- Family and other visitors will be directed to the nurse for an explanation of the isolation procedure.
- Isolation will be indicated when requisitioning from other departments. Dietary will use disposable dishes and utensils. Other departments will take special precautions.
- Whenever possible, the use of noncritical patient care equipment will be dedicated to a single patient.

- When a patient must be transported to an area outside of the patient's room, personnel in the area to which the patient is being sent are informed of the transport and of the precautions that must be used.
- The Admitting Department will be notified when isolation is discontinued (this may change the cost of the room to the patient) to allow them to schedule another patient for the room.
- Environmental Services will be notified when isolation is discontinued so that special cleaning procedures may be employed before another patient is admitted to the room.

Special Considerations

Although the health unit coordinator does not perform direct patient care, he or she must be acutely aware of the necessary precautions to be taken by all health workers in preventing the contraction of disease.

- Wash your hands frequently. Scrub with plenty of soap and water as warm as you can tolerate. Use a lot of friction and be sure to get under nails and rings. FRICTION GETS RID OF PATHOGENS. Rinse thoroughly. Use a dry paper towel to turn off the water and dry your hands well. Do not touch the sink or area around it with your clean hands.
- Protect yourself from body substances. When handling laboratory specimens destined for the lab, wear gloves. These specimens should be bagged in plastic for transportation. Always wash your hands after handling any specimen container.
- Remember that *any* health worker in danger of contamination must wear protective gear—masks, gowns, gloves, and so on.

LEARNING ACTIVITIES

1. Complete the following:

(a) Prognosis ______

(b) Disease ______

(c) Acute disease ______

(d) Chronic disease ______

(e) Functional disease ______

(f) Organic disease ______

(g) Metastasis ______

(h) Malignant ______

2. List the seven danger signs of cancer.

(a) ______

(b) ______

(c) ______

(d) ______

(e) ______

(f) ______________________________

(g) ______________________________

3. List the five types of microorganisms.
   (a) ______________________________
   (b) ______________________________
   (c) ______________________________
   (d) ______________________________
   (e) ______________________________
4. Define the following:
   (a) Aseptic ______________________________
   (b) Sterile ______________________________
   (c) Medical asepsis ______________________________
   (d) Isolation ______________________________
   (e) Nurse epidemiologist ______________________________
   (f) Nosocomial infection ______________________________
5. List five patient care areas where extra precautions are taken to prevent the spread of communicable diseases.
   (a) ______________________________
   (b) ______________________________
   (c) ______________________________
   (d) ______________________________
   (e) ______________________________
6. What are the two levels of isolation precautions?
   (a) ______________________________
   (b) ______________________________
7. What are the three types of transmission-based precautions?
   (a) ______________________________
   (b) ______________________________
   (c) ______________________________
8. When should Standard Precautions be used? ______________________________

   ____

   ____

   ____
9. The purpose of isolation is ______________________________

   ____
10. Regular isolation protects ______________________________
11. Reverse or protective isolation protects ______________________________
12. The single most important way to prevent the spread of infection and disease is to ______________________________
13. Discuss the health unit coordinator's responsibilities in regard to isolation. ______________________________

    ____

    ____

14. Match the following terms in column A with the description in column B.

Column A	*Column B*
(a) Allergic diseases	____ New growth of tissue
(b) Congenital disease	____ Abnormal reaction to generally harmless substance
(c) Degenerative disease	____ Injuries
(d) Neoplastic disease	____ "Wear and tear" disorders
(e) Trauma	____ Disorder present at birth

CHAPTER 7
Medical Law and Ethics

OBJECTIVES

When you have completed this chapter, you will be able to:

- Recognize the definitions of legal terms from the glossary.
- Discuss the purpose of licensing of medical personnel.
- Discuss the legal physician-patient relationship.
- Demonstrate your understanding of the terms duty of care and reasonable care.
- Demonstrate your knowledge of the rights of the individual under the law and how these rights might be violated.
- Discuss your knowledge of responsibility in relation to legal records.
- List several basic rules to follow for the prevention of litigation.
- List and define the forms and elements of negligence.
- Define ethics.
- Define advance directive.
- Discuss the difference between legal aspects and ethical considerations.
- State the necessity for and utilization of ethics in hospital situations.
- Apply guidelines of ethical behavior in health-related situations.

The practice of medicine is carried on within a framework of laws. It is important that those in the medical field be familiar with the basic legal ground rules of the profession. Laws concerning patients and workers in health care institutions were written to protect both the patient and the worker. As a health unit coordinator, you need to understand how the law affects you, the patients, and the health care institution. You will want to become aware of potential legal hazards and know how to avoid legal trouble as a result of your work.

KEY IDEA: GLOSSARY OF LEGAL TERMS

- **Abandonment**—the withdrawal of a physician from the care of a patient without reasonable notice of such withdrawal or without discharge from the case by the patient
- **Advance Directive (AD)**—a legal document in which an individual gives written instructions expressing his or her wishes regarding health care in the event a person can no longer make those decisions
- **Assault**—an unlawful threat or attempt to do bodily injury to another
- **Battery**—unlawful touching of another person without their consent with or without resultant injury
- **Breach**—breaking of a law, promise, or duty
- **Civil law**—a statute that enforces private rights and liabilities, as differentiated from criminal law
- **Consent**—permission granted by a person voluntarily and in his right mind
- **Contract**—an agreement between two or more parties for the doing or not doing of some definite thing
- **Defamation**—an attack on a person's reputation, called "libel" when written or "slander" when spoken
- **Defendant**—a person sued—in criminal proceedings, also called the accused
- **Do-not-resuscitate (DNR)**—an order by a physician not to administer cardiopulmonary resuscitation (CPR) if the patient goes into cardiac or respiratory arrest
- **Durable power of attorney**—a legal document that allows an individual named in the document to act on behalf of another. A durable power of attorney for health care (DPAHC) allows the patient to express his or her health care decisions and the amount of authority he or she wishes his agent to assume
- **Duty of care**—the obligation under law for a health worker to perform services for a patient which meet the common standards of practice expected for a comparable worker; the *patient* is protected by recognition of the health worker's responsibility for duty of care
- **Euthanasia**—an act by an individual to assist a person to die when that person is suffering from an incurable condition
- **Expert witness**—a person who offers testimony in court because he or she possesses special knowledge, training, or skill in an area that is important to the case
- **False imprisonment**—holding or detaining a person against his will
- **Felony**—a major crime for which greater punishment is imposed than for a misdemeanor
- **Guardian**—a court-appointed person whose duty it is to make decisions for and protect the interests of another person who can not make his or her own decisions
- **Incompetent**—want of physical or mental fitness
- **Invasion of privacy**—to make public knowledge any private or personal information without the individual's consent
- **Judgment**—the final decision of a court in an action or suit

- **Libel**—written defamation
- **Licensure**—authorization by the state to practice one's profession or vocation; involves control of educational standards, licensing examinations, means for revocation of license, and prohibitions for the unlicensed
- **Litigation**—a lawsuit
- **Malpractice**—literally, "bad practice" by a professional; care below the expected community standard that has led to injury
- **Negligence**—failure to do something a reasonable person *would do* under ordinary circumstances, or doing something a reasonable person would not do under ordinary circumstances; negligence can work in two ways, by action or by omission
- **Plaintiff**—one who institutes a lawsuit
- **Privileged communication**—information given by a patient to medical personnel which cannot be disclosed without consent of the person who gave it
- **Proximate**—in a case where negligence has been claimed, the act must be immediately related to (or the *proximate* cause of) the injury
- **Reasonable care**—the *health worker* is protected by law if it can be determined that he or she acted reasonably as compared with fellow workers
- **Respondeat superior**—responsibility of an employer for the acts of an employee
- **Slander**—oral or spoken defamation
- **Statute**—that law which has been enacted by a legislative branch of the government
- **Statute of limitations**—the time established for filing lawsuits
- **Subpoena**—a writ that commands a witness to appear at a trial or other proceeding and to give testimony
- **Tort**—a private or civil wrong
- **Will**—a document in a form prescribed by law and stating the orders of a person for the disposition of his property after his death
- **Living Will**—a written agreement between the patient and physician to withhold heroic measures if the patient's condition is such that it cannot be reversed

Note: The student should be aware that these definitions are simplified as an introductory study.

KEY IDEA: LICENSING

The principal way in which medicine is regulated by law in this country is by licensing. Every state in the nation requires that hospitals be licensed. A doctor must have a license to practice medicine; a nurse must have a license to practice nursing. Many other groups of health workers must be licensed to practice their vocation (e.g., licensed radiology technicians, licensed physical therapists, etc.).

The statutes dealing with licensing of physicians and nurses are commonly referred to as medical practice or nurse practice acts.

The laws which grant health workers licenses also have the power to take those licenses away.

KEY IDEA: THE LEGAL SIDE OF THE PHYSICIAN/PATIENT RELATIONSHIP

In the legal sense, the relationship between the doctor and the patient is contractual. That is, each of the parties agrees to do something. In the case of many hospitalized patients, this contract was begun in the doctor's office prior to hospitalization. Although this contract is rarely written, the simple sequence of a person asking for treatment and the doctor undertaking to treat is sufficient to create a contract and set up certain obligations each has to the other.

The patient's obligation is to pay for the services received. The doctor's legal responsibility is more complicated. The law requires of every doctor the duty to apply knowledge and skill with reasonable care and to use his or her best judgment. The doctor is duty-bound by law to give that patient a standard of care which is equal to that provided by similar physicians. In the eyes of the law, all patients regardless of race, religion, or financial status are entitled to the same skillful care.

The legal duty of the doctor does not require that the patient be cured or even be improved. The test of legality is whether the quality of care is up to the legal standard. If a promise of cure is made which does not indeed occur, the failure to perform could result in a suit for breach of contract. The health unit coordinator should avoid comments that would lead a patient or his family to believe that treatment will definitely be successful.

KEY IDEA: DUTY OF CARE

In a hospital, the patient must be guaranteed safe care, and the conscientious health worker must be protected from lawsuits. The patient is protected by the term **duty of care.** The patient is entitled to and expects safe care. The law requires every health worker to perform services for the patient in such a way that the health worker is meeting the common or average standards of practice expected for a comparable worker. In other words, the patient can expect that the health unit coordinator will perform his or her duties in a manner that will be at least average to those of other health unit coordinators in the community under similar circumstances.

The health worker is protected by the law if he uses what is termed **reasonable care.** Reasonable care describes the standard or level of care which is equal to the care given by a worker of comparable training and experience under similar circumstances. If the health worker does not equal this standard of reasonable care and harm comes to the patient as a result, he may be judged as negligent.

Negligence and Malpractice

Negligence is the failure to give reasonable care or the giving of unreasonable care. That is, the worker may do something wrong or may fail to do something she should have done under the circumstances, and the patient was harmed.

The Forms of Negligence

- **Malfeasance**—the performance of an unlawful or improper act
- **Misfeasance**—the performance of an act in an improper manner that results in injury to the person
- **Nonfeasance**—failure to perform an act when there is a duty to do so
- **Malpractice**—negligence performed by a professional
- **Criminal negligence**—reckless disregard for the safety of another person

The Four Elements of Negligence

In order for a plaintiff to recover for damages (usually money) for a claim of negligence, four elements of negligence must be proven. They are:

- **Duty of care.** (It is clear that a duty to the patient existed.)
- **Breach of duty.** (There was a failure to meet the duty of care.)
- **Injury.** (An injury resulted.)
- **Causation.** (The breach of duty was the proximate cause of the injury.)

The higher the educational level and requirements of the health worker the greater the possibility that he may be held responsible for his actions.

Although the health unit coordinator works under the supervision of the registered nurses, you must exercise great care in the performance of your duties and keep in mind that the terms *duty of care* and *reasonable care* apply to all health workers in the health care institution.

KEY IDEA: PATIENT'S BILL OF RIGHTS

The American Hospital Association published a document called *A Patient's Bill of Rights* with the hope that it will be posted in hospitals and given to patients upon admission. The intent of this document is to make both patients and personnel aware of what the patient has a right to expect.

The law operates to protect the patient but it also operates to protect the public. Certain diseases and conditions must be reported by physicians and hospitals. They include syphilis; trauma such as stabbings, gunshot wounds, attempted suicide; child or elder abuse; births and deaths; and requests for plastic reconstruction to change the identity.

Patient's Bill of Rights

1. **The patient has the right to considerate and respectful care.**
2. **Patients have the right to obtain from their physician complete current information concerning their diagnosis, treatment and prognosis in terms they can be reasonably expected to understand.**
3. **An informed consent should include knowledge of the proposed procedure, along with its risks and probable duration of incapacitation. In addition, the patient has a right to information regarding medically significant alternatives.**
4. **The patient has the right to refuse treatment to the extent permitted by law, and to be informed of the medical consequences of his action.**
5. **Case discussion, consultation, examination, and treatment should be conducted discretely. Those not directly involved must have the patient's permission to be present.**

(Continued)

Patient's Bill of Rights ***(Continued)***

6. **The patient has the right to expect that all communication and records pertaining to his care should be treated as confidential.**
7. **The patient has the right to expect the hospital to make a reasonable response to his request for services. The hospital must provide evaluation, service and referral as indicated by the urgency of the case.**
8. **The patient has the right to obtain information as to any relationship of his hospital to other health care and educational institutions, insofar as his care is concerned. The patient has the right to obtain information as to the existence of any professional relationships among individuals, by name, who are treating him.**
9. **The patient has the right to be advised if the hospital proposes to engage in or perform human experimentation affecting his care or treatment. The patient has the right to refuse to participate in such research projects.**
10. **The patient has the right to expect reasonable continuity of care.**
11. **The patient has the right to examine and receive an explanation of his bill regardless of the source of payment.**
12. **The patient has the right to know what hospital rules and regulations apply to his conduct as a patient.**

KEY IDEA: ADVANCE DIRECTIVES

The Patient Self-Determination Act of 1991 is a federal law that requires hospitals to inform their patients about the advance directive laws in their state. Advance directives give adult patients the opportunity to formulate decisions and give instructions about the health care they wish to receive (or not receive) should they become incompetent. Forms are made available to the patient upon admission and the completed form is placed on the medical record. If the advance directive is not completed when the patient is admitted, it can be done later, revised, or not done at all.

KEY IDEA: AIDS

AIDS—Acquired Immune Deficiency Syndrome—is an incurable but preventable disease which has reached epidemic proportions in the United States. As a result of the widespread prevalence of the disease, the fact that it is universally fatal, and the availability of blood testing for exposure to the virus, a number of laws dealing with AIDS and AIDS-related issues have been passed. These laws vary widely among the states. Keep in mind as you read the statements that follow (from California guidelines) that you must be aware of the laws that apply to your state and that these are simply representative of the areas of concern.

1. Mandatory Testing by Blood Banks and Plasma Centers:
   (a) Required testing of blood and blood components before use: Generally blood or blood components may not be used for humans unless they have been tested and found nonreactive for the probable causative agents of AIDS and to detect viral hepatitis.
   (b) Reporting for donor referral register: If donor blood tests positive, blood banks or plasma centers must provide the information to the Department of Health Services for inclusion on the Donor Referral Register.
2. Provision of Testing Sites for Free Testing to Detect Antibodies to HIV, which is the probable causative agent of AIDS.

3. Mandatory Reporting of Diagnosis of AIDS:
   (a) Duty of physicians and hospitals to report: This includes the reporting to county or state health officers of all transfusion-associated AIDS cases and all hospitalized patients with a confirmed diagnosis of AIDS.
   (b) Follow-up contact: Health officials must contact persons with confirmed AIDS diagnosis to instruct them not to donate blood and suggest treatment sources and to conduct follow-up studies.
4. Testing by Health Care Providers:
   (a) Written consent prior to testing: Before a person's blood is tested to detect antibodies to the probable cause of AIDS (HIV virus), a written consent must be obtained. Some exceptions to this may apply.
   (b) Confidentiality of test results:
      (1) Generally no disclosure of test results may occur without the written permission of the patient that includes to whom the disclosure will be made. Written authorization may be required for each separate disclosure of test results.

         NOTE: These guidelines indicate there is no mandatory reporting requirement for HIV antibody test results but a *diagnosis* of AIDS must be reported by the physician.
      (2) Penalties for unauthorized disclosure: Penalties are provided for the disclosure of the results of a blood test to detect antibodies to the probable causative agent of AIDS to anyone without the written authorization of the patient. Penalties may vary based on whether the disclosure is negligent or willful. It can result in fines and even imprisonment.
      (3) Limitations of use of test results: Much controversy exists regarding employment and insurance decisions and AIDS. The results of a blood test to detect antibodies to HIV may not be used to determine insurability or employability. However, a diagnosis of AIDS, established by other means, may not be expressly forbidden by law.

KEY IDEA: CONSENTS

The underlying relationship between the hospital and the patient is contractual and the law holds that a person has the exclusive right to determine what shall be done with his or her body. Therefore, it is essential that this contractual relationship be clearly defined and that the patient's understanding be expressed in a written agreement signed by him or his personal representative.

Consider the following information as guidelines when dealing with consents. Consult your policy manual or ask your head nurse/nurse manager for specific information relative to your hospital.

1. The patient should first read, or have read to him/her, the consent in order that he/she knows what he/she is signing. The law requires that to be legally valid the consent must be an *informed consent;* that is, the procedures and risks involved should be fully explained in terms understandable to the patient.

Patient's Name: ______________________________

I am consenting to be tested to see whether I have been infected with the Human Immunodeficiency Virus (HIV), which is the probable causative agent of Acquired Deficiency Syndrome (AIDS).

THE MEANING OF THE TEST

This test is not a test for AIDS but only for the presence of HIV. Being infected with HIV does not mean that I have AIDS or that I will have AIDS or other related illnesses. Other factors must be reviewed to determine whether I have AIDS.

Most test results are accurate, but sometimes the results are wrong or uncertain. In some cases the test results may indicate that the person is infected with HIV when the person is not (false positive). In other cases the test may fail to detect that a person is infected with HIV when the person really is (false negative). Sometimes, the test cannot tell whether or not a person is infected at all. If I have been recently infected with HIV, it may take some time before a test will show the infection. For these reasons, I may have to repeat the test.

CONFIDENTIALITY

California law limits the disclosure of my HIV test results. Under the law, no one but my doctor and other care givers are told about the test results unless I give specific written consent to let other people know. Additionally, doctors may inform my spouse, any sexual partner(s) or needle-sharing partner(s), or the county health officer if a doctor thinks that is necessary. All information relating to this test is kept in my medical record.

BENEFITS AND RISKS OF THE TEST

The test results can help me make better decisions about my health care and my personal life. The test results can help me and my doctor make decisions concerning medical treatment. If the results are positive, I know that I can infect others and I can act to prevent this.

Potential risks of the test include psychological stress while awaiting the results and distress if the results are positive. Some persons have had trouble with jobs, housing, education or insurance when their tests results have been made known.

MORE INFORMATION

I understand that before I decide to take this test I should be sure that I have had the chance to ask my doctor any questions I may have about the test, its meaning, its risks and benefits, and any alternatives to the test.

By my signature below, I acknowledge that I have read and understood the information in this form, that I have been given all of the information I desire concerning the HIV test, its meaning, expected benefits, possible risks, and any alternatives to the tests, and that I have had my questions answered. Further, I acknowledge that I have given consent for the performance of a test to detect HIV.

Signature: ______________________________ ______________

(patient / parent / conservator / guardian) *If signed by other than patient, indicate relationship Date and Time

Witness: ______________________________

*This consent may be signed by a person other than the patient only under the following circumstances:

1. The patient is under twelve (12) years of age or, as a result of his/her physical condition, is incompetent to consent to the HIV antibody blood test; and
2. The person who consents to the test on the patient's behalf is lawfully authorized to make health care decisions for the patient, e.g., an attorney-in-fact appointed by the patient under the Durable Power of Attorney for Health Care; the parent or guardian of a minor; an appropriately authorized conservator; or, under appropriate circumstances, the patient's closest available relative (see chapters 2 and 20);
3. It is necessary to obtain the patient's HIV antibody test results in order to render appropriate care to the patient or to practice preventative measures. Health and Safety Code section 199.27.

CONSENT FOR THE HIV TEST

Authorization for Disclosure of the Results of the HIV Antibody Blood Test

A. EXPLANATION
This authorization for use or disclosure of the results of a blood test to detect antibodies to the HIV virus, the probable causative agent of Acquired Immune Deficiency Syndrome (AIDS), is being requested of you to comply with the terms of the Confidentiality of Medical Information Act, Civil Code Section 56 et seq. and Health and Safety Code Section 199.21(g).

B. AUTHORIZATION
I hereby authorize ______________________________
(Name of Physician, Hospital or Health Care Provider)

to furnish to ______________________________
(Name or Title of Persons Who Is to Receive Results)
the results of the blood test for antibodies to the HIV virus.

C. USES
The requester may use the information for any purpose, subject only to the following limitations: ______________________________
____

D. DURATION
This authorization shall become effective immediately and shall remain in effect indefinitely or until __________,19 ____, whichever is shorter.

E. RESTRICTIONS
I understand that the requestor may not further use or disclose the medical information unless another authorization is obtained from me or unless such use or disclosure is specifically required or permitted by law.

F. ADDITIONAL COPY
I further understand that I have a right to receive a copy of this authorization upon my request.
Copy requested and received: _____ Yes _____No Initial _____

Date: __________, 19 ____ ______________________________
Signature

____
Printed name

2. The patient must be of sound mind and not sign under duress. The mental competency of the patient is important. Patients may not sign when they are under the influence of drugs or alcohol.
3. The signature on a consent must match the signature on the conditions of admission. The Conditions of Admission form is signed upon entering the hospital.
4. All signatures must be in black ink. Full legal names must be used. A married woman may sign Mary K. Jones or Mrs. John H. Jones.

5. All dates, times, signatures, including the signature of witnesses, must be legible and the witness must be over 21.
6. No abbreviations may be used. All words must be spelled out.
7. Witnesses, in the number indicated, must always sign in the space so allocated in the form as witness to the signature of the person signing the permit.
8. All signatures must be witnessed and dated.
9. The patient may indicate an X if unable to write and there are two witnesses.

Who May Sign: States vary on their laws regarding consents. Each state will have laws regarding special consideration for people in custody, married minors, and unmarried minors. Generally:

1. Any adult, male or female, 18 years of age and over must sign their own consents with two possible exceptions:
   (a) An actual emergency when two physicians sign a statement, incorporated in the consent. "The immediate treatment of the patient is necessary because ______________________________."
   (b) When the patient has been declared incompetent and has a guardian.
2. All persons in custody of the law must give their consent for treatment.
3. Married minors are freed from parental authority and may sign their consent, including a divorced minor.
4. Unmarried minors must have their consent signed by one parent or legally appointed guardian. Consent of both parents is recommended. A stepparent may not consent unless the child has been legally adopted.
5. Emancipated minors who through legal action have established that they are living away from home and are financially responsible may sign their own consents.
6. An executor of the patient's estate does not have the legal right to consent to treatment. Only in the case of legal guardianship determined by the court may a member of the family consent (such as a son consenting to treatment of his mother).

Consent for Operation

Purpose: Any procedure which breaks the skin may be interpreted as an operation. The patient's valid surgical consent is necessary to preclude liability for battery, unless the patient needs immediate care to save his life. (Fig. 7–1.)

Any invasive procedure requiring entrance into a body cavity such as the various endoscopies, many diagnostic procedures using injections of radiopaque substances, insertion of catheters into vessels, and procedures requiring general, local, or regional anesthesia requires consent.

Consent for Sterilization

(a) This release is to be completed in addition to the "Consent to Operation" whenever it is anticipated that a particular operation will possibly render the patient, either male or female, sterile (unable to reproduce).

AUTHORIZATION FOR AND CONSENT TO SURGERY OR SPECIAL DIAGNOSTIC OR THERAPEUTIC PROCEDURES

To____
Name of Patient

Your/the patient's attending physician is____, M.D.

Your/the patient's supervising physician or surgeon is____, M.D.

1. The hospital maintains personnel and facilities to assist your/the patient's physicians and surgeons in their performance of various surgical operations and other special diagnostic or therapeutic procedures. These operations and procedures may all involve risks of unsuccessful results, complications, injury, or even death, from both known and unforeseen causes, and no warranty or guarantee is made as to result or cure.

   You have the right to be informed of such risks as well as the nature of the operation or procedure; the expected benefits or effects of such operation or procedure; and the available alternative methods of treatment and their risks and benefits.

   You also have the right to be informed whether your physician has any independent medical research or economic interests related to the performance of the proposed operation or procedure. Except in cases of emergency, operations or procedures are not performed until you have had the opportunity to receive this information and have given your consent. You have the right to consent or to refuse any proposed operation or procedure any time prior to its performance.

2. Your/the patient's physicians and surgeons have recommended the operations or procedures set forth below. Upon your authorization and consent, the operations or procedures set forth below, together with any different or further procedures which in the opinion of the supervising physician or surgeon may be indicated due to any emergency, will be performed on you/the patient. The operations or procedures will be performed by the supervising physician or surgeon named above (or in the event of any emergency causing his or her inability to complete the procedure, a qualified substitute supervising physician or surgeon), together with associates and assistants, including anesthesiologists, pathologists and radiologists from the medical staff of   whom the supervising physician or surgeon may assign designated responsibilities. The persons in attendance for the purpose of performing specialized medical services such as anesthesia, radiology or pathology are not agents, servants or employees of the hospital or your/the patient's supervising physician or surgeon but are independent contractors, and therefore your agents, servants, or employees.

3. If your physician determines that there is a reasonable possibility that you may need a blood transfusion as a result of the surgery or procedure to which you are consenting, your physician will inform you of this and will provide you with a brochure regarding blood transfusions. This brochure contains information concerning the benefits and risks of the various options for blood transfusions including predonation by yourself or others. You also have the right to have adequate time before your procedure to arrange for predonation, but you can waive this right if you do not wish to wait. You should understand that transfusions of blood or blood products involve certain risks, including the transmission of disease such as hepatitis or Human Immunodeficiency Virus (HIV) and that you have a right to consent or refuse consent to any transfusion. You should discuss any questions that you may have about transfusions with your physician.

4. The pathologist is hereby authorized to use his or her discretion in disposing any member, organ, or other tissue removed from your/the patient's person during the operation(s) or procedure(s) set forth below.

5. To make sure that you fully understand the operation or procedure, your physician will fully explain the operation or procedure to you before you decide whether or not to give consent. If you have any questions, you are encouraged and expected to ask them.

6. Your signature below constitutes your acknowledgment (1) that you have read and agree to the foregoing; (2) that the operation or procedure set forth below has been adequately explained to you by the above-named physician or surgeon and by your/the patient's anesthesiologist and that you have received all of the information you desire concerning such operation or procedure; (3) that you have had a chance to ask questions; and (4) that you authorize and consent to the performance of the operation or procedure.

Operation or Procedure ____

____

____

________________________ Signature ________________________
Date *(Patient / Parent / Conservator / Guardian)*

________________________ If signed by other than patient, indicate relationship:
Time

________________________ ________________________
Witness

AUTHORIZATION FOR AND CONSENT TO SURGERY OR SPECIAL DIAGNOSTIC OR THERAPEUTIC PROCEDURES

Figure 7–1

(b) In most states, the signature of the spouse is desirable for married persons to avoid a charge of conspiracy between physician and the spouse, if available. If not available, the patient possesses full power to consent. (Fig. 7–2.)

Telephone Consents

May be obtained in an emergency situation in which a delay of treatment would jeopardize the life or health of the patient. Generally:

(a) Two people must listen to a consent by telephone. Both people must witness the consent noting time and date.
(b) Confirmation by written letter or telegram must follow immediately, which is to be attached to the consent and remains a part of the permanent record.

MEMORIAL HOSPITAL
STERILIZATION PERMIT

Date ______________ Hour ________.M.

I hereby authorize and direct Doctor ______________________________ and assistants of his choice to perform the following operation upon me at the above named hospital: ______________________________ and to do any other procedure that his (their) judgment may dictate during the above operation. It has been explained to me that I may (or will probably) be sterile as a result of this operation but no such result has been warranted. I understand that the word "sterility" means that I may be unable to conceive or bear children and in giving my consent to the operation have in mind the possibility (probability) of such a result. I absolve said doctor, his assistants and the hospital from all responsibility for my present condition or any condition that may result from said operation.

Signed ______________________________

Signature Witnessed:

By ______________________________ By ______________________________

I have read the foregoing matter and, as the spouse of the above named patient, do hereby join in authorizing the performance of the surgery under the terms set forth and consented to above.

Signed ______________________________

Signature Witnessed:

By ______________________________ By ______________________________

Figure 7–2

Length of Consents

Consents are considered valid for a reasonable time after signing, as long as no changes in the anticipated surgery occur as a result of further tests and study of the patient, and as long as the patient is not discharged.

KEY IDEA: TERMINATION OF PATIENT CONTRACT

The legal aspects of terminating a contract with a patient are as important as those involved in establishing the relationship. A doctor cannot lawfully abandon a case. The law says that once a doctor has entered into a contractual relationship with a patient he is obligated to continue to care for that patient until there is no need for further treatment, the patient dismisses the doctor, or the doctor withdraws from the case. If the doctor does withdraw, he legally must advise the patient of any further need for treatment and give him sufficient time to obtain the services of another physician.

KEY IDEA: DOCTOR AVAILABILITY

A doctor must be reasonably available to his or her patients. If a doctor is ill or out of town, arrangements will have been made for another qualified physician to take care of the patients. The health unit coordinator should make every effort to assist the doctor and his office staff in the communication of messages so that the doctor can be made available to his patients with a minimum of delay.

KEY IDEA: THE PATIENT'S RECORDS

The patient's chart is a legal document and is the property of the hospital. It must be accepted as evidence of truth in a court of law. The patient's chart should be used only by health workers authorized to do so. To meet the standards of the law the patient's chart must be:

- Complete
- Accurate
- Neat
- Honest
- Legible
- Signed
- In ink

Careful documentation is essential. In a court of law the usual rule is "If it wasn't charted, it didn't happen."

Corrections

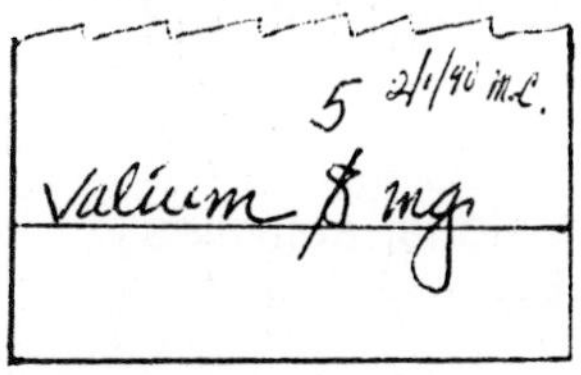

If corrections are necessary, the proper technique is to line out the original entry so that it can still be read. Then the correction should be made, initialed, and dated. **DO NOT ERASE.** Any chart with erasures will not be admitted as legal evidence. (Fig. 7–3.)

Figure 7–3

KEY IDEA: AVOIDING LITIGATION

Legal actions against health care workers are more common today than ever before. Although legal problems do arise, the health unit coordinator should be able to work with confidence after you realize legal problems can often be prevented. Remember:

- Stay within the limits of your training. Do not attempt to give nursing care when you have been trained to work as a health unit coordinator.
- Do not recommend treatment, make a diagnosis or give a prognosis.
- Consistently practice with conscientious care and with an understanding of the terms *duty of care* and *reasonable care.*
- Obtain written consents.
- Always consider human rights.
- Keep up-to-date, comprehensive, and accurate records.

KEY IDEA: ETHICS

Ethics is a code of behavior that represents ideal conduct for a particular group. Each group of health care professionals requiring a license has a code of ethics that has been adopted by its membership. Codes of ethics for different groups have many things in common. They are based upon good judgment, reason, and an understanding of the difference between right and wrong.

The National Association of Health Unit Coordinators has adopted the following code of ethics:

National Association of Health Unit Coordinators Code of Ethics

This code of ethics is to serve as a guide by which Health Unit Coordinators may evaluate their professional conduct as it relates to patients, colleagues, and other members of the health care profession. This code of ethics shall be subject to monitoring, interpretation, and periodical revision by the association's Board of Directors.

Therefore, in the practice of our profession, we the members of the National Association of Health Unit Coordinators accept the following principles:

- ***Principle One:*** Each member shall conduct themselves in such a manner as to gain the respect and confidence of the patients, health care personnel, and the community, as well as respecting the human dignity of each individual.
- ***Principle Two:*** Each member shall protect the patients' rights, including the right to privacy.
- ***Principle Three:*** Each member shall strive to acheive and maintain a high level of competency.
- ***Principle Four:*** Each member shall strive to improve their knowledge and skills by participating in educational and professional activities and sharing the benefits of their attainments with their colleagues.
- ***Principle Five:*** Unethical and illegal professional activities shall be reported to the appropriate authorities.

(Printed courtesy of NAHUC)

Ethics deal with our moral responsibility. Unethical behavior is not always illegal, but it may reflect unfavorably upon the hospital and can result in discipline or even loss of employment.

Legal requirements are set by society. Violation of these requirements can result in legal discipline. Many times the line between ethical behavior and legal requirements is not entirely clear. For example, it would be unethical if a health unit coordinator were to ask a nurse to *give* her some of the patients' medications. If she were to *take* the medications, it would be stealing, which is, of course, illegal.

If a health unit coordinator were to go to another unit, see the chart of a neighbor, and read it, this would be unethical. If she were to talk about the contents of the chart, this would be illegal.

The health worker who consistently practices ethical behavior should not have to worry about meeting the requirements of the law.

Confidentiality

Information acquired in a doctor-patient relationship is considered a confidential or privileged communication. Employees are obligated to safeguard information regarding patients and the hospital.

As a health unit coordinator, you have access to certain clinical and personal patient information. You must be thoroughly aware of the grave responsibility you have of maintaining the confidentiality of all matters relating to patients. (Fig. 7–4.)

Ethical behavior means keeping your promises and doing what you ought to do. As a health unit coordinator, you should observe the following code of ethical behavior:

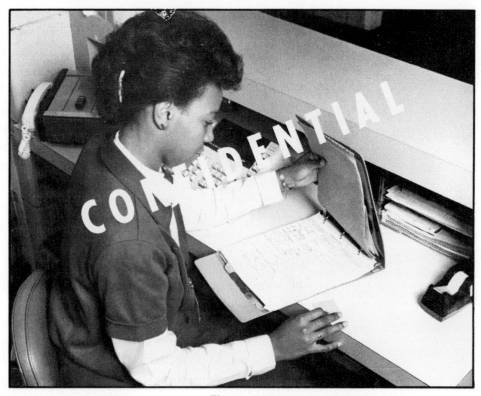

Figure 7–4

- Be conscientious in the performance of your duties. This means do the best you can.
- Be generous in helping your patients and your fellow workers.
- Carry out faithfully the instructions you are given by the nurse in charge.
- Respect the right of all patients to have beliefs and opinions that might be different from yours.
- Let the patient know that it is your pleasure, not your job, to assist him.

LEARNING ACTIVITIES

Match the legal terms in column A to the appropriate definition in column B.

Column A	*Column B*
(a) Duty of care	____ To threaten to injure another person
(b) Consent	____ "Bad practice" by a professional
(c) Invasion of privacy	____ The highest concept of right and wrong
(d) Slander	____ Information kept in trust by medical personnel
(e) Ethics	____ Meeting expected standards
(f) Assault	____ Written defamation
(g) Negligence	____ Verbal defamation
(h) Privileged communication	____ To make public knowledge any private or personal information without the individual's consent
(i) Libel	____ A lawsuit
(j) Battery	____ Permission granted by a person voluntarily and in his right mind
(k) Tort	____ Private or civil wrong
(l) Litigation	____ Unlawful touching of another person without their consent
(m) Misdemeanor	____ Failure to give reasonable care
(n) Incompetent	____ Major crime
(o) Malpractice	____ Less serious crime
(p) Felony	____ Want of physical or mental fitness

Complete the following:

1. The principle way in which medicine is regulated by law is through ____________________.
2. In a legal sense, the relationship between the doctor and the patient and the hospital and the patient is ____________________.
3. The person protected by the law by "reasonable care" is the ____________.
4. The person protected by the legal term "duty of care" is the ____________.

5. To meet the standards of the law the patient's chart must be:
   (a) ______
   (b) ______
   (c) ______
   (d) ______
   (e) ______
   (f) ______
6. The document published by the American Hospital Association with the intent of making both patients and personnel aware of what the patient should be able to expect is called ______.
7. What is an advance directive? ______
8. List five ways to prevent involvement with lawsuits:
   (a) ______
   (b) ______
   (c) ______
   (d) ______
   (e) ______
9. List the four elements of negligence.
   (a) ______
   (b) ______
   (c) ______
   (d) ______

True or False—Circle *T* if the statement is true and *F* if it is false.

T F **(a)** To be legal a consent must be an informed consent.
T F **(b)** Abbreviations may be used on a consent.
T F **(c)** All persons in the custody of the law must give their consent for treatment.
T F **(d)** Emancipated minors may give their own consent for medical or surgical treatment.
T F **(e)** Consents must be in ink.

Choose and circle the one best answer.

1. Health unit coordinators may be said to have acted with reasonable care if they:
   (a) Have been a unit manager
   (b) Have taken college classes
   (c) Have been health unit coordinators for ten years
   (d) Did what other health unit coordinators of similar background would have done under similar circumstances
2. A health unit coordinator decided that since she was not busy she would help the nurses by giving a patient a bedpan. The patient had undergone surgery that morning and was injured when the health unit coordinator turned him improperly. The unit coordinator could have

avoided this tragedy if she had:
(a) Obtained a written consent
(b) Asked another unit coordinator to help her
(c) Stayed within the limits of training
(d) Had the patient walk to the bathroom

3. A consent is not valid if the patient, when signing it, can be proven to have been:
(a) Under the influence of sleeping pills
(b) Not mentally competent
(c) Forced to sign
(d) All of these

4. A health worker read the history on a neighbor's chart and then talked about it at a party. The neighbor accused him of defamation of character. The health worker was most likely guilty of:
(a) Assault
(b) Slander
(c) Libel
(d) Abandonment

5. Your child is ill, and you ask the medication nurse to give you some of a patient's medications. This is:
(a) Malpractice
(b) Negligence
(c) Unethical
(d) Illegal

6. If a health worker were to take the medication, this would be:
(a) Assault
(b) Unethical
(c) Illegal
(d) (b) and (c)

CHAPTER 8

Communications

OBJECTIVES

When you have completed this chapter, you will be able to:

- Define the elements and the components of communication.
- Discuss the responsibilities of both the sender and the receiver in the communication process. List some barriers to communication.
- Define kinesics and the importance of body language in the process of communication.
- Describe the proper use of the telephone and intercom system.
- Discuss the importance of effective communication.
- Describe the several types of paging systems.
- Discuss written communication and accepted techniques for message taking and composition.
- Compare ways we are alike and different.
- List the possible concerns of the hospitalized patient.
- Discuss various methods of intra- and interdepartmental communication.
- Stress the importance of confidentiality.
- Discuss the importance of effective communication with the patient's family and visitors and rules for dealing with visitors.
- Contrast negative and positive personalities; assertive and aggressive responses.
- Define stress and ways to reduce stress.
- Discuss Maslow's Hierarchy of Needs.

Communications is one of the most fundamental functions you will perform. More than ever in today's busy world of information systems it is essential that you, as the human communication link of your unit, become an expert communicator.

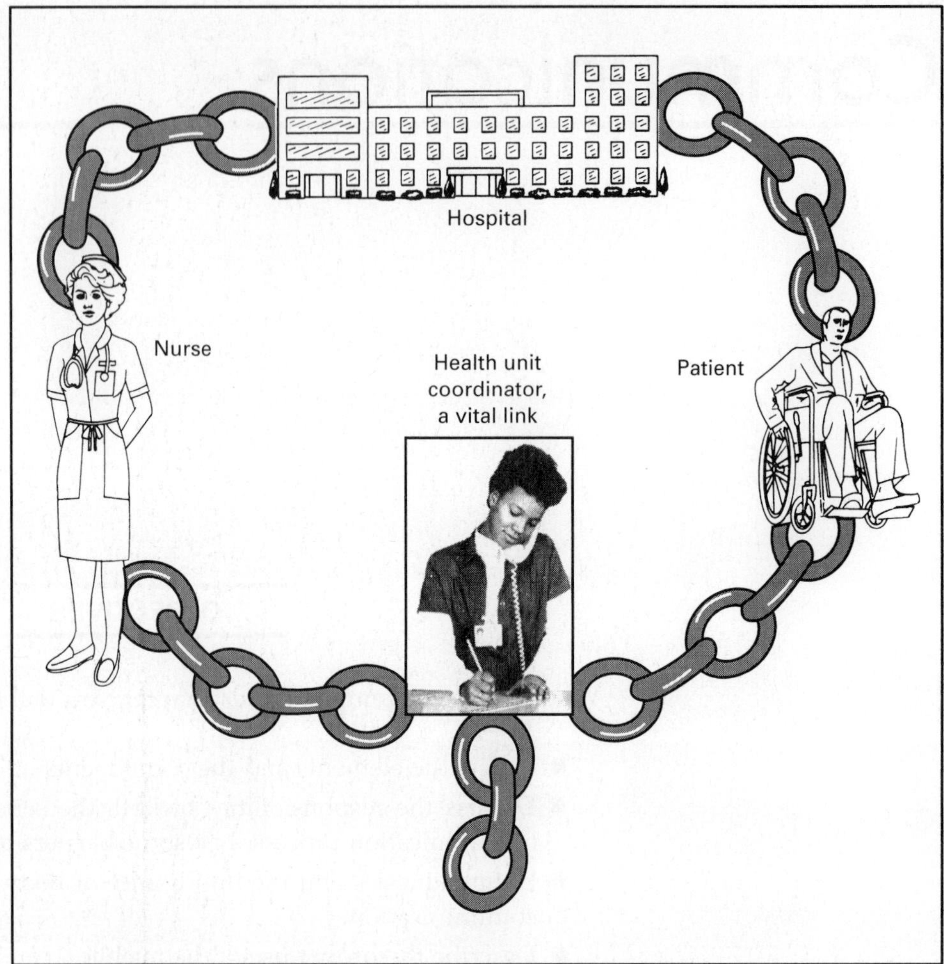

Figure 8–1 The health unit coordinator serves as a vital link between the nursing unit and the rest of the hospital, doctor's offices, the patient's family and friends, and the community.

It has been estimated that health unit coordinators communicate with someone at least once every 60 seconds and at the hectic, often heavily populated nurse's station, the health unit coordinator is often challenged to use his or her skills of communication effectively.

Not all of us possess the same level of communication skills but we can learn and practice speaking, listening, and writing. It can be both fun and satisfying to become capable of handling each situation so pleasantly and efficiently that you are recognized for your outstanding reception techniques.

The health unit coordinator is a vital link between the patients and staff of the nursing unit and between the unit, the rest of the hospital, and the outside world. (Fig. 8–1.)

Communication is simply defined as the **sending and receiving of a message.** Messages are a very important part of the health unit coordinator's job. It is essential to understand the various means of communication you will use, the type of information you will transmit, and the appropriate procedure in each case because a patient's welfare, or perhaps even his life, may depend on the health unit coordinator's ability to communicate a message.

PRINCIPLES OF COMMUNICATION

Remember the definition of communication—the sending and receiving of a message. In order for effective communication to take place, both the sender and the receiver must share the responsibility. (Fig. 8–2.)

1. **Sender**—who transmits the message
2. **Symbols**—the writing or words we use to convey a message
3. **Receiver**—who receives and interprets the message
4. **Feedback**—the receiver repeats the message to the sender (i.e., interprets) to establish accuracy

Therefore, when a message is sent, the sender turns his ideas into words (symbols) and transmits these words to the receiver. The receiver then must change his words back into ideas. If effective communication has taken place, both ideas will be the same.

KEY IDEA: THE SENDER

As the sender of a message, there are things you can do to make the communication more effective. First, an effective message must have three objectives (what it is to achieve) and three components (what it is to contain). It must also be conveyed in a manner that will make it easy for the receiver to listen and to understand.

Objectives of an Effective Message

1. **To be understood**—Construct your message in a logical manner and speak or write clearly.
2. **To result in the action that you want**—Your message was ineffective if this does not occur.

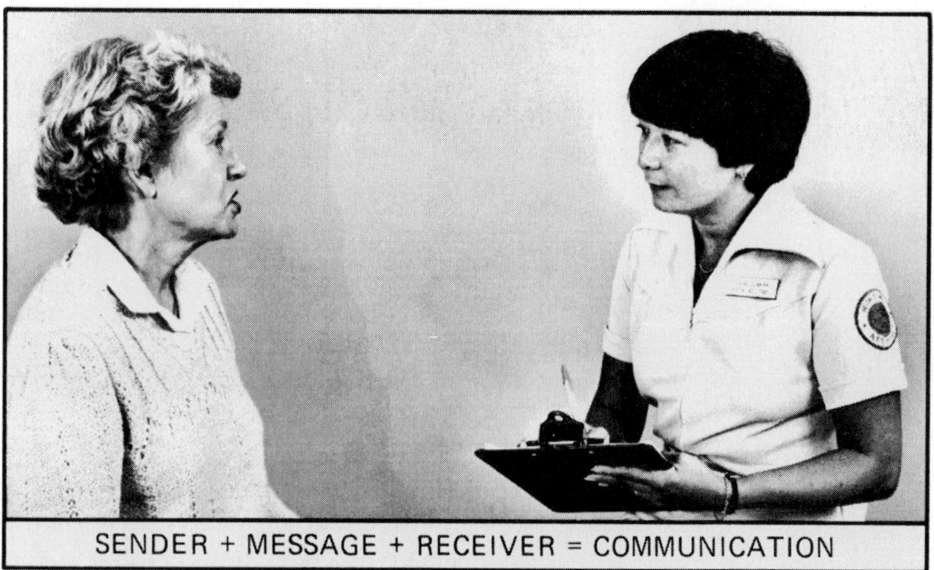

Figure 8–2

3. **To maintain good feelings**—Speak with courtesy and in a pleasant tone of voice at all times.

Components of an Effective Message

1. An effective message must contain all the necessary information.
2. The information must be meaningful to the receiver. Do not use unfamiliar "medical jargon" the receiver may not understand.
3. The message should be simple and should get to the point.

When your responsibility is the sending of verbal messages, practice your skills of communication.

1. Avoid distractions. If you are communicating face-to-face, do not fidget or use distracting hand movements.
2. Look the receiver in the eye.
3. Think about your body language. It is often effective to lean forward when talking to another.
4. Use your personality and whenever it is appropriate, smile!

KEY IDEA: THE RECEIVER

As the receiver of a message, you also have a responsibility to see that effective and satisfying communication takes place. There are many reasons why you may shut out a message:

- The message does not seem important.
- The sender is a poor communicator.
- You are preoccupied with something else.
- You feel defensive or hostile toward the sender.
- The physical environment distracts you.
- The way you feel emotionally or physically.

Since inadequate or inaccurate communication may directly affect a patient's welfare, you must learn the skills of receiving as well as of sending messages.

1. Really listen to what the sender is saying. To be an ACTIVE LISTENER you must concentrate and not think of other things at that moment.
2. Keep an open mind and don't prejudge.
3. Avoid selective listening, which means hearing just what you want to hear.
4. Think about what the message means.
5. Repeat the message as you understand it. *Always* repeat numbers such as telephone numbers, laboratory results, and so on.
6. Give feedback. Ask questions and get actively involved in the exchange.

7. If the communication is face-to-face, look at the sender. Through your body language, indicate your interest in the message and your willingness to participate in the communication.

KEY IDEA: BODY LANGUAGE

There are two main avenues of communication—*verbal and nonverbal.* Verbal is the use of words in speaking and writing. **Nonverbal communication** is unspoken and includes facial expressions, movements, posture, and gestures. This is called body language. Probably the greatest part of communication is nonverbal. Our gestures and expressions are often the truest indicator of our inner feelings no matter what the specific words we use.

Kinesics, the study of body language, can be fascinating. The health unit coordinator, as the constant communicator, must be aware of the implications of body language. A smile, a frown, or the way that you sit or stand can reflect such feelings as acceptance, hospitality, or hostility and can enhance or impede your ability to communicate effectively.

If your posture is erect when you sit at your desk, if you seem alert, and if you look at others straight in the eye when you talk with them, leaning forward and smiling, your body language is saying, "I like my job. I'm happy to be here, and I want to communicate with you." If you slouch, look away, or use other body gestures that indicate negativism, your body language is saying something else.

Integrate your understanding of kinesics with your new information on verbal communication and practice your skills to become the most effective communicator you can be.

METHODS OF COMMUNICATION

KEY IDEA: THE TELEPHONE

There will be a telephone on each health unit coordinator's desk which is an extension of the hospital's central switchboard. There are similar extensions in all other units and in all the various departments of the hospital, such as the laboratory, radiology, pharmacy, etc. The **multibutton key telephone** is the most common telephone set used in the hospital because it allows the user to handle several incoming and outgoing calls simultaneously. The buttons at the bottom of the telephone glow intermittently—a steady light indicating lines are in use, or a flashing light indicating a line is on hold. A hold button provides complete privacy by closing off all other extensions and should always be used so that the caller will not overhear conversation at the nurses' station while he is waiting. This telephone operates as follows:

1. **To place a call:**
   - Choose a line that is not in use—the button will be unlighted.
   - Push down the button (key), pick up the receiver, and dial the number. (*Note:* Your instructor will explain exactly how the telephone works in your hospital. If you are calling outside the hospital, it is often necessary to dial one or several numbers to get an outside line.)

- If you accidentally choose a line that is on hold, depress the hold key to reestablish the hold.

2. **To answer a call:**
   - Determine the line to be answered by the ring and/or by the lighting of the button at the bottom of the telephone.
   - Before removing the receiver, depress the key for the line to be answered, and speak.
3. **To hold a call:**
   - After picking up the receiver, ask the caller if he will please hold the line and wait for his reply.
   - Depress the hold key for 2–3 seconds until you are sure the line is holding. When the call is on hold, both the line and hold key will return to normal positions with the light on.
   - You may now place or answer another call on a different line.

The **Touch-A-Matic Touch Tone telephone** is a multibutton memory telephone that can be programmed to reach frequently called numbers (such as other hospital departments) automatically simply by depressing a single button.

Many hospitals use a system in which a recording is received by outside callers stating the button to press for various departments or services, when to dial their party's extension, and to otherwise stay on the line for operator assistance. (Fig. 8–3.)

Rules of Telephone Courtesy

One of your most important duties is using the telephone. You will constantly be answering and placing telephone calls and must learn to use the telephone skillfully and courteously. Make a special effort to become expert at using the

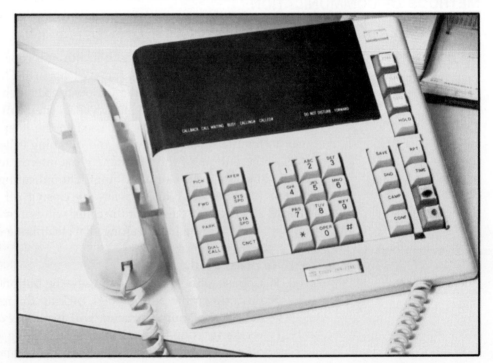

Figure 8–3

telephone. Ask yourself how you feel when someone is nice to you on the telephone—when they are helpful and efficient and when their voice is clear and pleasant.

Efficiency and courtesy go hand in hand. If you follow these simple rules and use your common sense, you will find that your work will be done more smoothly and easily.

- Answer all calls promptly.
- Keep a pencil and pad handy so that you can take down messages immediately and avoid omissions and inaccuracies.
- Always be polite. Use courteous terms such as "please" and "thank you." Avoid the use of slang such as "O.K." and "bye bye." If someone says "Thank you" say "You're welcome" rather than "No problem," which is less polite.
- Use a pleasant voice at all times. Speak distinctly but do not shout. Hold the mouthpiece about one inch from your lips.
- Never answer anger with anger. Be calm, listen, and determine what action can be taken. Smile—it will show in your voice.
- Do not leave the phone untended. If you must leave your station, arrange for someone else to take your calls. Leave word where you can be located and when you will return.

Answering Incoming Calls

- Answer the telephone by giving your location and your title, "2E, Unit Coordinator." If your hospital also wishes you to use your name, you will be so instructed.
- If the caller does not identify himself, always ask "To whom am I speaking?" Then repeat the name as soon as possible.
- If the caller asks for information which you do not immediately have, say, "Will you please hold the line while I get the information?" and wait for his reply. When you return to the phone, thank him for waiting. If it will take you some time to get the information, offer to call back.
- If the call is for someone who is not immediately available, ask the caller whether he prefers to hold the line, to call back, or to leave a message. If he chooses to wait, return to the line at frequent intervals to give him a chance to leave a message.
- Never give out information about a patient. Never divulge medical orders pertaining to a patient. This rule applies to members of the hospital staff as well as to the patient's family. It is the nurse's responsibility to observe and describe accurately a patient's condition. When information about a patient is requested, say pleasantly but firmly, "Let me get the nurse for you, Dr. Jones," or "I don't know, sir, but I will get Miss Smith, the nurse manager. Perhaps she can help you."
- If you are asked to take a message, or if the caller has some complex instructions for you, write them down promptly.
- Hospital policy usually states that personal telephone numbers of hospital staff are not given out. You should refer such calls to the nurse in charge or hospital supervisor.

Placing Outgoing Calls

- A list of the other hospital extensions and frequently called outside numbers should be kept at your desk. Do not ask information for a number unless you cannot find it yourself.
- Plan your conversation before you make a call. Know the points you want to cover. Have any records or other materials you may need in front of you.
- Give the person you are calling ample time to answer before you hang up—about ten rings. However, do not tie up the line indefinitely hoping someone will answer. If the line is busy, hang up immediately.
- When the person answers, identify yourself. "This is Miss Brown, Unit Coordinator from 2E." If you are calling outside the hospital, give the name of the hospital rather than the floor.
- If the person who answers is not the one you want or does not identify himself, ask pleasantly for that person: "May I speak to Dr. Jones, please? This is Miss Brown, Unit Coordinator on 2E."
- If you want to leave a message for someone, state your name and why you are calling: "This is Miss Brown, Unit Coordinator on 2E. I'd like to leave a message for Dr. Jones." Be sure to state the message clearly. Repeat any part of the message that is lengthy or might be confusing.

Transferring Calls

Do not transfer a call if you can handle it properly yourself. Otherwise:

- Offer to transfer the caller to someone who can handle his call: "That is handled by our admissions department. If you wish, I can have your call transferred."
- Be sure that the person knows what you are doing so that he does not think you have disconnected him.
- If your hospital's telephone system requires that you reach the switchboard operator for the transfer, say: "Will you please transfer this call to the admissions department?"

KEY IDEA: PAGING

If asked by the nurse to page a doctor who is elsewhere in the hospital, follow standard procedures for your hospital. Here is one type of paging system:

- Dial "0" to reach the switchboard operator.
- Tell the operator the name of the doctor to be paged and your location. "Please page Dr. Jones for extension 275." The operator will then page the doctor over a public address system.
- Keep the line free until the doctor has called back.

To call departments within the hospital there will be a list of extensions at your desk. To call physicians and other numbers outside of the hospital you will use a roster, Rolodex®, or other list that has been compiled for that purpose. You may need to add frequently called numbers to that list.

Another popular system utilizes **individual pocket pagers** worn by physicians and key hospital personnel. To page a person with this system, the health unit coordinator would call the hospital operator and ask that the doctor or other individual be paged for the unit extension. You may also use the hospital's internal paging system and place the page yourself.

The operator will call the person being paged by dialing a preassigned number which will cause the pocket pager to buzz or beep; your page request will follow. The person should then dial your extension to receive the message.

The **light system of paging** utilizes a light panel installed at intervals in the hallways of the hospital. Again, doctors and key personnel will have assigned numbers. When the hospital operator receives a message, he/she will light a number in the panel. The person assigned that number will respond by calling the switchboard.

KEY IDEA: MESSAGE RECORDING AND DELIVERY

An important part of correct telephone procedure is to record messages *accurately.* If possible, always relay any message directly to the person concerned. If the person is not in the nurses' station, take down the message in detail and see that it is delivered as soon as possible.

- Use the hospital message pad.
- Write the date, time, and name of the person for whom the message is intended.
- Be sure your recorded message answers the following five questions: who, what, when, where, and why.
- Listen carefully and repeat all messages to assure accuracy. Always repeat numbers (feedback) because it is common to transpose (switch) them by mistake when they are written down.
- Always ask for the spelling of names when you are in doubt.
- Sign the message with your name and title. (Fig. 8–4.)

KEY IDEA: THE INTERCOMMUNICATIONS SYSTEM (INTERCOM)

An intercom system is located at each nurses' station. This system enables the health unit coordinator to have direct communication between the patient's room and the nurses' station. When the patient has a request, he signals from his room by depressing a button by his bed. When he does this, a light flashes over the room number on the intercom at your desk, and it makes a buzzing sound.

Answering the Intercom

- Respond promptly by depressing the appropriate key (you will be shown your hospital's system) and say "Unit Coordinator, may I help you?" As in the answering of the telephone, your hospital may wish that you also state your name—"Miss Brown, Unit Coordinator, may I help you?"
- Listen to the patient's reply.
- Always be courteous. The same general rules apply to the intercom as to the telephone, but remember that this device may be unfamiliar to a

Date ______________ Time ________

To ______________________________

☐ You were called by ☐ You were visited by

____

Phone No. ________________________

☐ Please call ☐ Will call you

☐ Returning your call ☐ Waiting to see you

MESSAGE:

____

____

Call taken by J. Brown HUC

Figure 8–4

patient and he may not be accustomed to hearing a voice come out of "the wall."

- Write down the message using the technique for message recording.
- Relay the patient's request to the appropriate personnel.

The Pneumatic Tube

The pneumatic tube is a system in which air pressure sends tubes carrying messages, requisitions, or sometimes supplies from one hospital department to another. You will be instructed in the operation of the pneumatic tube if your hospital utilizes this system.

The Computer

Today computer use in hospitals is universal. The degree to which they are used varies. Vital information about the patient is entered by the Admitting Department and added to by other hospital departments during the patient's hospitalization. This information can be retrieved at any time, and hospitals have strict guidelines regarding who has access to the information.

The computer is discussed in Chapter 11.

Communication within the Nursing Unit

Within the nursing unit some of the most important forms of communication include:

- **Kardex.** The patient care record card is a consolidated record of all procedures, treatments, medications, and tests for each patient. It is a unit

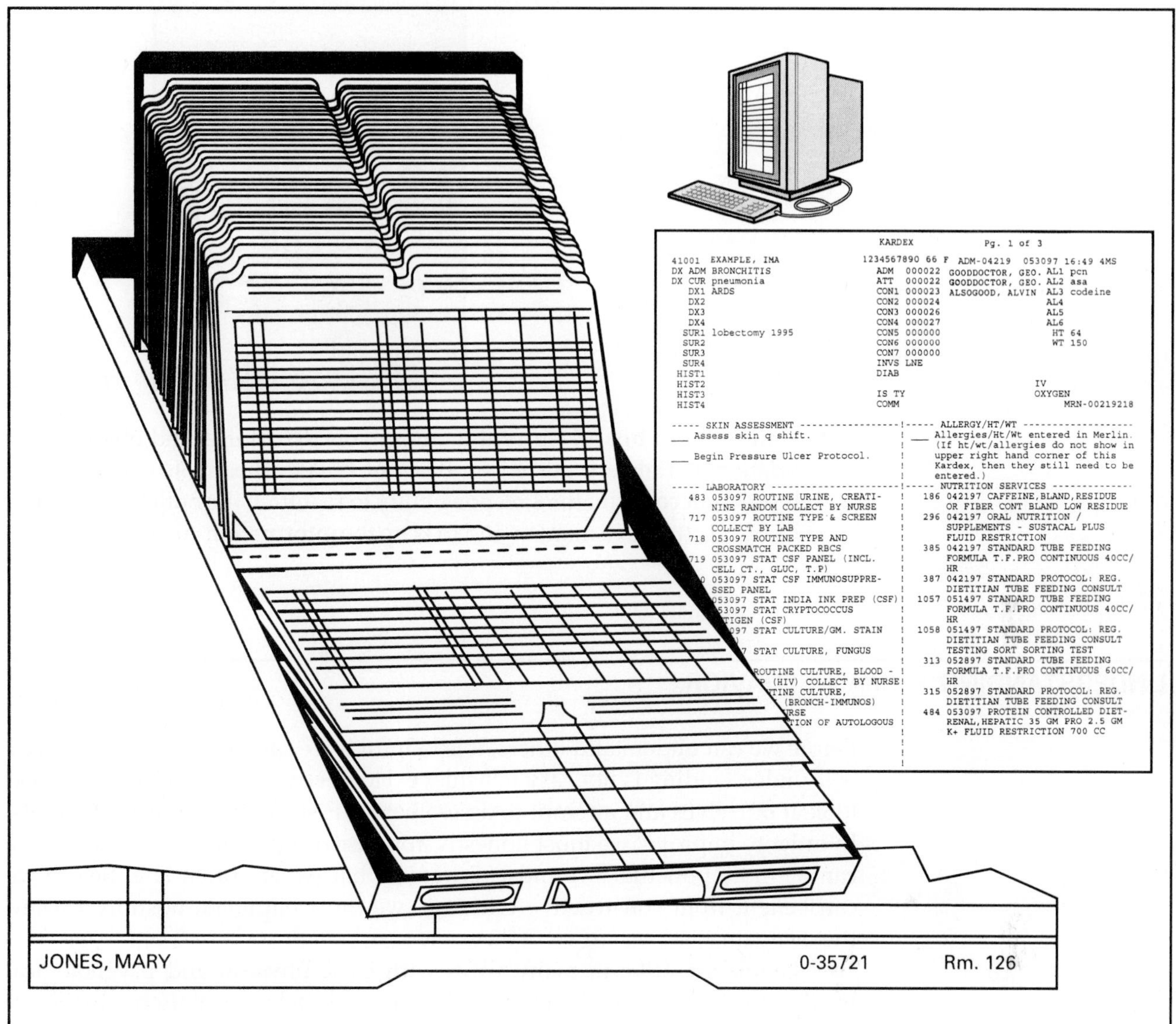

Figure 8–5

worksheet used by the nursing staff, kept during every patient's stay, and discarded upon discharge. The record card may be kept in a Kardex holder, but computerized Kardexes are widely used. A common practice is to print out patient care information on each patient at the beginning of the shift. Nurses keep this information on clipboards or in notebooks, and the old-time Kardex is fast becoming a thing of the past. (Fig. 8–5.)

- **Assignment sheet.** The use of the assignment sheet was explained in Chapter 2. The assignment sheet tells you which nurse is caring for which patient.
- **Unit chalkboard or other erasable board.** Some nursing units utilize a chalkboard as a method of intradepartmental communication. The chalkboards may either reflect patient care assignments or indicate special information regarding patient care such as patient's schedule for surgery or x-ray, or those who will receive laboratory or other tests or treatments.

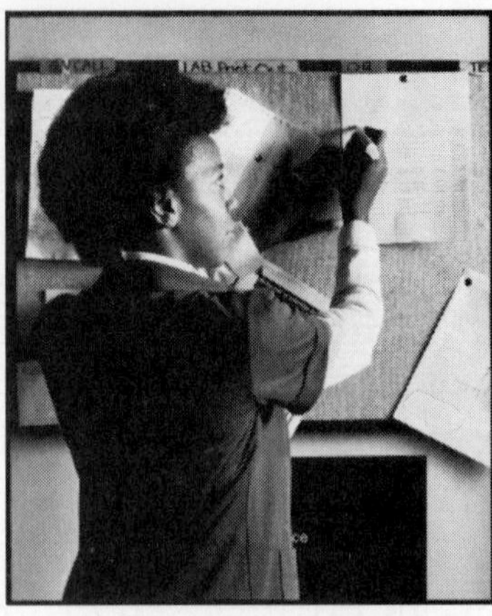

Figure 8–6

- **Unit bulletin board.** Current memos, work schedules, and other appropriate materials are posted on the unit bulletin board. It is usually the health unit coordinator's responsibility to maintain the bulletin board in a neat and attractive manner and to keep the information current. (Fig. 8–6.)

UNDERSTANDING HUMAN BEHAVIOR

Before we can understand others, it is helpful if we can understand ourselves. Self-understanding is not easy to achieve. However, it is useful to take a good look at ourselves and attempt to assess both our strong and our weak points. In order to improve, we must honestly appraise our personal traits. Before we can be more punctual, we must recognize that we are often late. Before we can benefit from constructive criticism, we must eliminate hostility toward the evaluator.

People are alike in many ways with basic physical and psychological needs, but each person develops his or her own behavior patterns for meeting these needs. Many factors influence our behavior and make us unique individuals such as: hereditary traits inherited from our parents; our rate of development; prenatal influences including the mother's general health and habits (drugs, tobacco, and alcohol can cause birth defects); our home conditions and social environment; our interests; and our value systems.

Value systems strongly influence a person's behavior and consist of character traits such as honesty and loyalty, beliefs about love, sex, religion, family, work, and so on. Along with this are our internal rules—our o.k.'s and not o.k.'s that are part of the way we view the world. Values and standards of behavior are learned early and modified throughout our lives. It is important to realize that there are vast differences among individuals as a result of these influences on behavior.

In the sense that all of us *share* certain basic needs and have inner pressures that drive us to fulfill these needs, we are alike. In the ways that we strive to *satisfy* these needs, we are all different. We also differ greatly in our expectations and ambitions.

There have been many studies of human behavior, and one of the most famous and useful was a model created by Abraham Maslow. The model by

Professor Maslow is known as "Maslow's Hierarchy of Needs" and ranks human needs in levels of priority. (Fig. 8–7.)

In this model, physical or survival needs are most basic; then the need for safety; then love, affection, and belonging; then self-esteem; and finally, self-actualization or the full development of one's potential or talents.

Dr. Maslow believed that each level of need had to be satisfied before an individual could attempt to satisfy the next. A person must be fed, clothed, and safe before they can deal successfully with goal-setting, social, and professional needs.

Emotions and Behavior

All of us have emotions—inner feelings that are responses to life situations. They are natural responses that vary in intensity according to what is happening and how we feel about what is happening. They can affect us both physically and mentally, and over a period of time emotions inadequately dealt with can actually make us ill.

Built into our bodies is a reaction to alarm called the "fight or flight" response designed to allow the body to deal with emergencies. The heart and respiration speed up, adrenalin is produced in large amounts, and muscles are prepared for extra activity. This syndrome usually disappears when the emergency passes.

There is another generalized reaction (both physical and emotional) that occurs in response to exciting, frustrating, confusing, demanding, irritating, and pressured, outside influences. These influences may be either positive or negative but the body's reaction does not go away quickly, does not serve a useful purpose, and if allowed to continue, can result in interference with our health. This reaction is called *stress.*

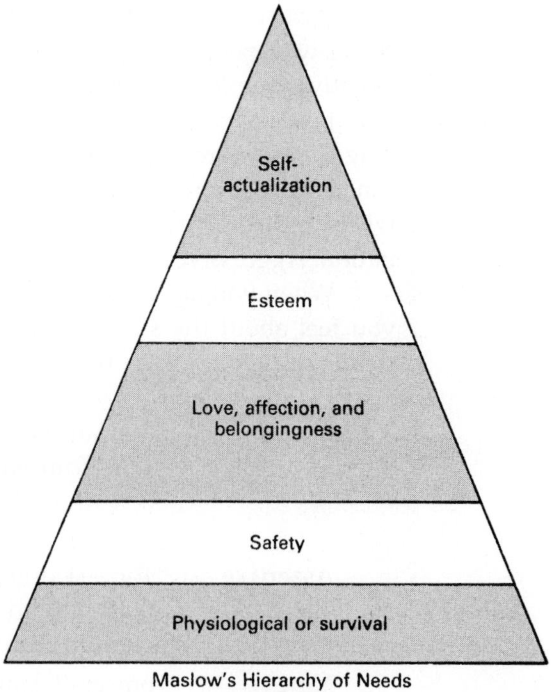

Maslow's Hierarchy of Needs

Figure 8–7

For example, improper diet, long and hectic working hours, lack of exercise and recreation and/or a personal support system, alone or in combination, can equal stress. Although some stress is good because it motivates us to accomplish and achieve, too much stress can result in serious physical and psychological problems.

Some physical reactions to stress can include hypertension, gastrointestinal problems, headaches, reduced resistance to infection, and so on. Emotional reactions can include nervousness, tearfulness, depression, anxiety, withdrawal and inability to function, anger, and alcohol and drug abuse.

Burnout is a term often used to describe a state in which a person no longer feels able to cope with their circumstances and may suffer decreased energy and productivity.

It is imperative that you learn to combat stress and burnout and use your emotional responses constructively. Eat properly, get plenty of rest and physical exercise, develop hobbies you enjoy, learn to relax, and develop techniques to reduce mental and physical pressures.

Positive vs. Negative Personality

A positive personality is one which has developed healthy methods of coping with life. All of us are faced with difficulties at one time or another in our lives—financial, family, social, health, and so on. All of us are faced with making decisions and we must constantly analyze our problems and choose paths that will hopefully lead us to successful solutions.

Positive people cultivate emotions that make them feel good. They like themselves and others. They try to see the bright side of the situation and they know that there are solutions to problems, and work to make things better.

Positive people don't let others drag them down. They surround themselves with people who are interested in growing and enjoying rather than by negative people who obstruct and complain.

Positive people are assertive. They can communicate with others in a way that declares confidence and strength without being unpleasant. They can disagree without being disagreeable but can stand up for their rights when they feel threatened. Assertive behavior is a positive approach to a situation. Aggressive behavior is negative and generally offensive.

When you are being assertive, try to use "I" statements to describe how you feel about the situation and try to avoid "you" statements which may seem accusatory to the receiver.

Example: Mary, an HUC, works the day shift and is very conscientious. Tom works 3–11:30 and for the last two weeks has been 10 to 15 minutes late, causing Mary to have to work overtime.

Assertive "Tom—I don't intend to stay late to cover for you when you're late to work. I have to be home on time to pick up my child from the babysitter and I won't be late again."

Note Tom isn't late again. You get treated the way you teach people to treat you.

Aggressive "Tom—You are always late and you are really a terrible employee," etc. etc. etc.

Example: Jim is in an HUC on ICU. A respiratory therapy technician persistently asks him to place her telephone calls to other departments rather than dialing the telephone herself.

Assertive "Janet—I would prefer not to place your telephone calls for you. I have my own work to do and I know we'll both be more efficient if you make the calls yourself."

Aggressive "No way! You are asking me to do your work! Forget that!"

Remember Be assertive and you won't be a victim. But choose your responses carefully. In general, work with a cooperative spirit.

KEY IDEA: COMMUNICATING WITH THE HOSPITAL STAFF

You have learned a great deal about the art of communications. The relations between yourself and your fellow workers depend upon your approach to them. If you have a kind, courteous, tactful, sympathetic, and open manner you will find it easier to form positive relationships.

As a health unit coordinator, you will be working with all other members of the hospital staff for one main purpose—to help care for the patients. You should perform all of your duties in a spirit of cooperation and follow orders willingly. You should always maintain a professional attitude toward the other members of the staff no matter how well you may come to know them. (Fig. 8–8.)

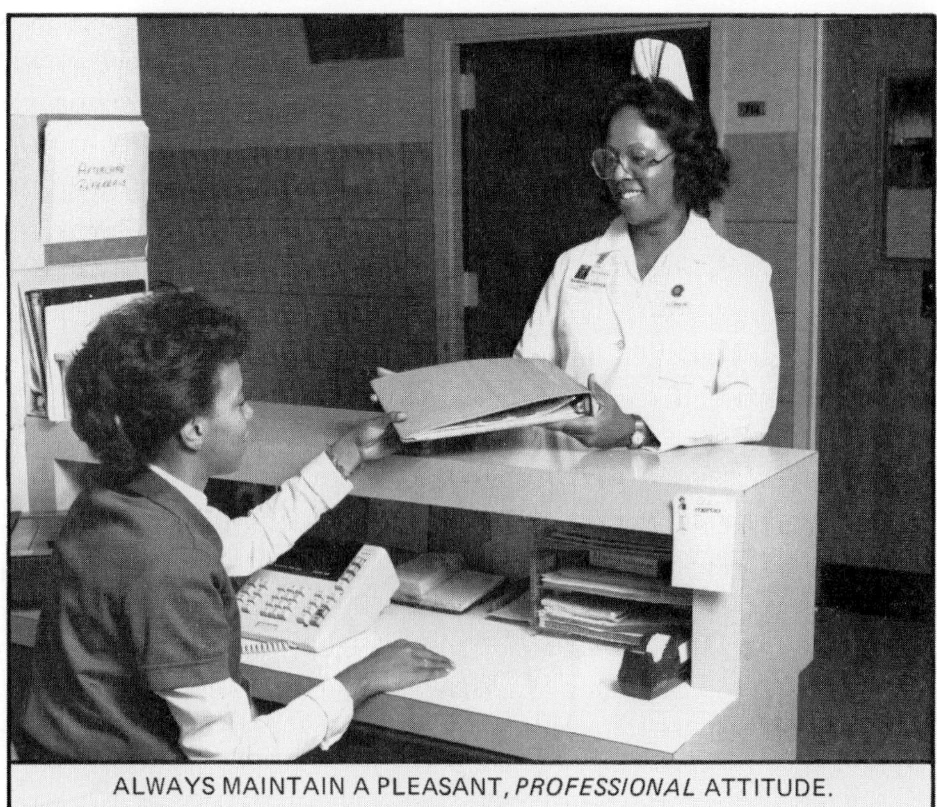

ALWAYS MAINTAIN A PLEASANT, *PROFESSIONAL* ATTITUDE.

Figure 8–8

Behaving courteously means putting the needs of another person before your own. It means cooperating, sharing, and giving. Being polite and considerate of others shows them that you care about them. Give your fellow workers support and work as a team.

Sometimes another staff member can upset you so much you get angry. You may feel like making a rude remark. *Don't* do it. Stop and think! Your fellow worker may be under stress because of a problem at work or at home. Try to be understanding and let the anger fade.

Learn to take criticism and accept suggestions without feeling you are being attacked. Try to avoid being defensive. Your supervisor may criticize you or tell you to do something. You may feel like saying "That's not my job" or "Why do you pick on me?" Stop, think, and examine your attitude. Calm down. Go ahead and do the right thing. Develop a positive, mature attitude. Don't allow yourself to be caught up in the negative attitudes of others. Enjoy your job! (Fig. 8–9.)

You will find your fellow workers and other health care personnel more agreeable and helpful if you treat them properly. Some good practices are:

- Report to the nurse manager or charge nurse whenever you leave the nurses' station or the unit for any purpose and again when you return.
- Take all questions you may have about your work to your head or charge nurse.
- Tell the head or charge nurse about personal problems that you feel might be interfering with your work.
- Do not talk about your personal problems with other staff members.
- Do not discuss your personal problems with patients or their visitors.
- Follow all instructions you receive from your head or charge nurse.

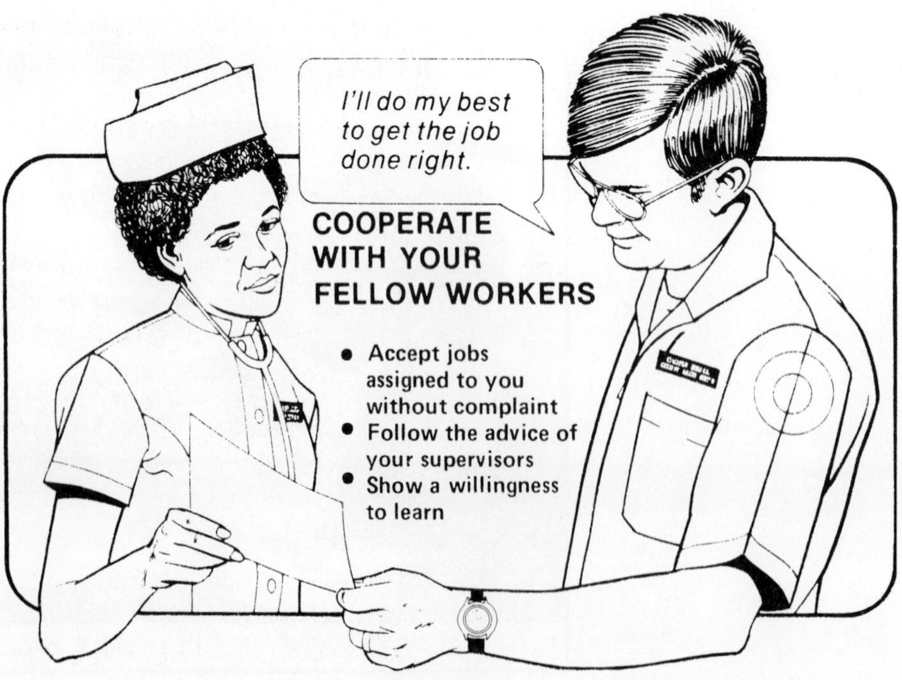

Figure 8–9

- Report all complaints from patients and visitors to the head or charge nurse. Never ignore complaints, no matter how insignificant they may seem to you.
- Perform all of your duties in the spirit of cooperation and follow orders willingly.
- Accept tasks assigned to you without complaint.
- Follow the advice of your supervisors.
- Show a willingness to learn.

KEY IDEA: COMMUNICATING WITH THE PHYSICIAN

As a health unit coordinator, you are in a position which requires frequent communication with the various physicians who visit the nursing unit.

Doctors are highly educated, dedicated, and busy individuals who come to the nursing units to visit their patients and to prescribe examinations and treatments to aid in the patient's recovery.

The health unit coordinator who learns the doctors' names, and their desire for speed and accuracy, and is willing and able to assist each doctor as efficiently and courteously as possible will do much to preserve or improve communication between the medical and nursing staffs.

PATIENT RELATIONSHIPS

Relating to people means making a connection between yourself and another human being; putting yourself in another's place—**using empathy.**

Many things make a difference in a patient's behavior and attitude during an illness. The patient may be frightened, angry, or sad. Some factors are the diagnosis, seriousness of the illness, age, culture, previous illnesses, past experience in hospitals, and the patient's mental condition. Other things that can make a difference are the patient's personality and disposition and perhaps his financial condition.

Each patient is different in his reaction to pain, treatment, annoyances, and even kindness. Always treat each patient as an individual—a person who needs your help. Practice the special kind of consideration that all patients need on an individual basis. (Fig. 8–10.)

Although you will not have as much direct contact with patients as the nursing personnel do, you will, however, greet newly admitted patients, speak with them frequently over their intercom, and perhaps enter their rooms to deliver mail or perform some other occasional nonnursing task.

You represent the entire hospital: the patient's reaction to you may influence his opinion of the whole hospital. (Fig. 8–11.)

Remember:

- Always be courteous.
- Greet patients pleasantly and address them by name. Do not use first names (except those of children) unless you are asked to do so.
- Introduce yourself to patients and explain your position and how you may be of service.

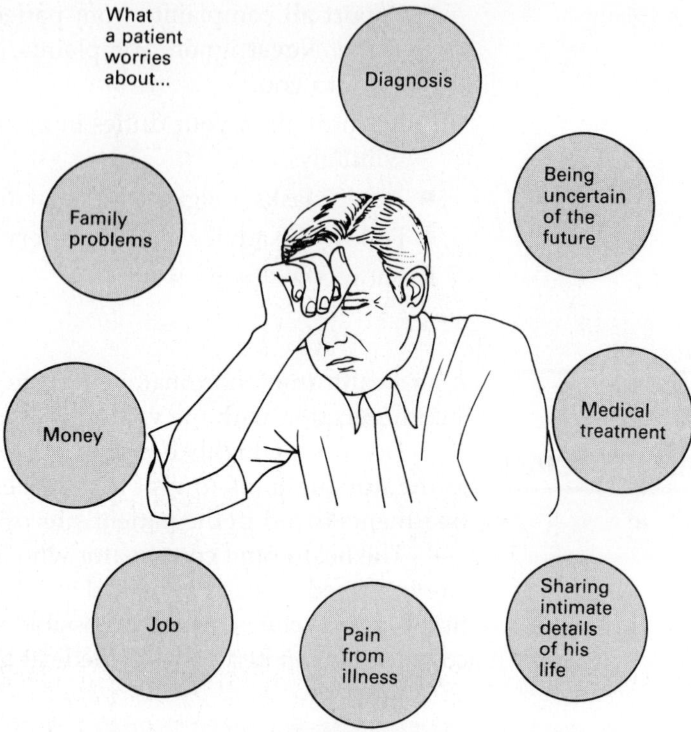

Figure 8–10

- Do not disturb patients by being noisy. Keep your voice down and avoid slamming drawers and doors.
- Be friendly but avoid becoming too familiar with the patients. This means that you do not discuss your personal life with the patients.
- Never ignore a patient who speaks to you about a problem whether it concerns his own condition or another member of the staff. All complaints must be relayed to the nurse, no matter how trivial or unreasonable they may seem to you.
- All requests from patients for equipment or care must be relayed to the nurse. You are not authorized to handle such requests yourself.
- Questions regarding hospital charges should be relayed to the business office.
- There are certain privileges and restrictions that apply to particular patients.
- All information about a patient is confidential.

KEY IDEA: PATIENT REQUESTS

In handling patient requests, you must distinguish between those which are **medical** and must be referred to the nurse, and those which are **nonmedical** which you will be able to handle yourself. If you are in any doubt, ask the nurse.

There are many things that a patient may ask for that seem to you to be totally unrelated to his treatment (e.g., raising or lowering the bed, opening or closing the window, getting a drink of water or an additional pillow). There may, however, be good medical reasons for denying these requests. Explain to the patient that you are the health unit coordinator and that you will relay his request to a nurse who will help him. **Remember that if, as a health**

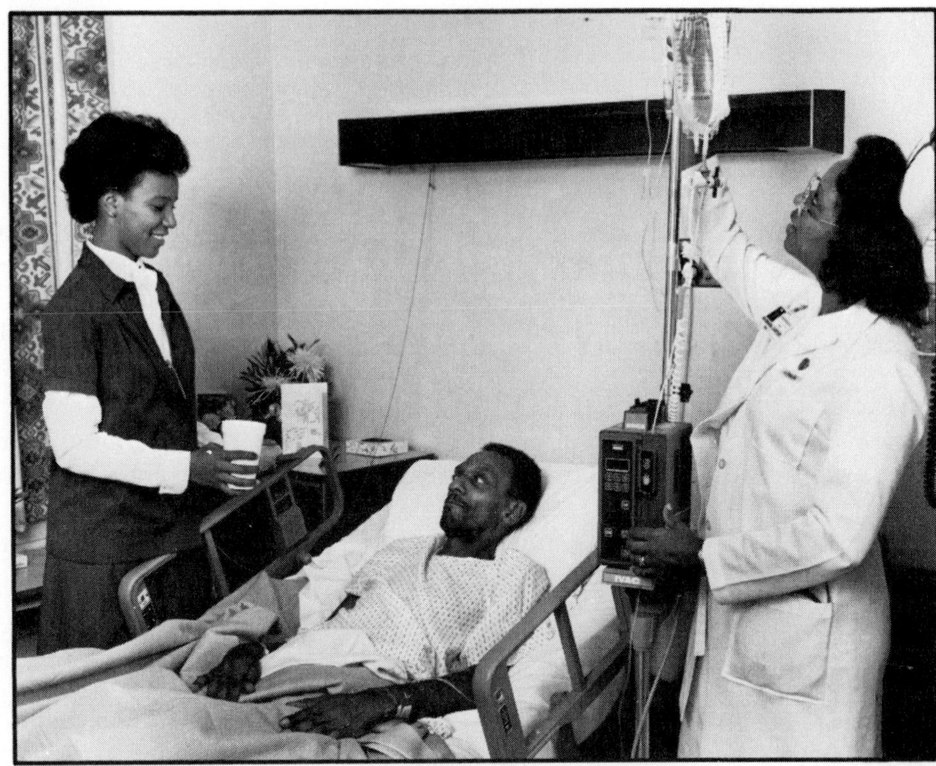

Figure 8–11

unit coordinator, you attempt to give nursing care, you are functioning outside of your scope of training.

Be sure to keep your word and deliver the message as quickly as possible to the appropriate nursing personnel.

KEY IDEA: RELATIONSHIPS WITH VISITORS

Your direct contact with not only patients but with their visitors requires complete dedication to the rules of courtesy and kindness. Remember that they are often worried and uncomfortable. The hospital environment is unfamiliar, and the staff are probably unknown to them.

Visiting hours are often the highlight of the day for patients. Knowing his family and friends are interested and concerned about him can do a lot to relax his tensions, ease his feelings of loneliness or isolation, relieve his fears, and cheer his spirit.

Visitors may be worried and upset over the illness of a member of the family. They need your kindness and patience. Pleasant comments about flowers or gifts brought by visitors for the patient may be helpful. Make all visitors feel welcome in the hospital.

If the patient is seriously ill or is an obstetrical patient, visiting hours may be different. Your instructor will tell you about the visiting hours and any rules for visitors in your health care institution. These rules, of course, must be followed. Three main rules usually apply to visitors in all health care institutions:

1. Visitors are not allowed to take institutional property away with them.
2. Visitors are not allowed to give nursing or medical care to a patient (they may help with care with the doctor's or nurse's permission).

3. Visitors cannot bring food or drink to the patient unless permission has been given by the nurse.

Actions Helpful in Visitor Contacts

- Listen to the family member. Whether it is a suggestion, a complaint, or "passing the time of day," listen to the person. Some suggestions by visitors can be very helpful. Some complaints may be valid, others not. When a complaint is first presented, you probably need to get more information. You might ask, "Where did this happen?" or "What did you do?" Say to the person, "I will tell the nurse manager about this," and then report it to the nurse in charge.
- If the visitor asks for a patient's room number, check to be sure there have been no changes. Give the visitor the room number and directions to help find it.
- Do not get involved in the family's private affairs and feelings. Never take sides in family quarrels. Never give information or opinions to someone about other family members.
- When a visitor comes to the desk, stop whatever you are doing, direct your attention to the visitor, and answer his questions. Always let the visitor know he is welcome in the hospital; do not give the impression that he has interrupted you.
- Be prepared to give information to visitors. Tell them under what circumstances family members are allowed to eat in the employee cafeteria. Mention where the coffee shop is and what hours it is open. Tell them where the public telephone is. Direct them to other places in the institution (e.g., the public restrooms, business office, gift shop, or chapel). (Fig. 8–12.)
- Avoid assuming familial relationships until you know who the visitor is. It is best to say, "Mr. Brown is in room 200" rather than "Your husband is in room 200."
- Remember that a "significant other" may be the most important member of a patient's family.

Visitor Situations

Situations will arise occasionally that you cannot handle alone. Sometimes visitors, in their concern for the patient, will be very critical and complain about the care being given, the quality of the meals, the room location, etc. If a polite answer from you does not seem to suffice, call the nurse in charge.

If you feel that a particular visitor upsets the patient in any way, report it to the head nurse. Certain visitors must sometimes be restricted from seeing the patient.

Drunken, noisy, or obstreperous visitors may disturb patients. Notify your head nurse or, when necessary, call the hospital security guard to remove the visitor.

If a visitor falls or is injured on hospital property, get a nurse immediately to help him. In such cases, there are additional procedures you must follow; these will be explained on page 186.

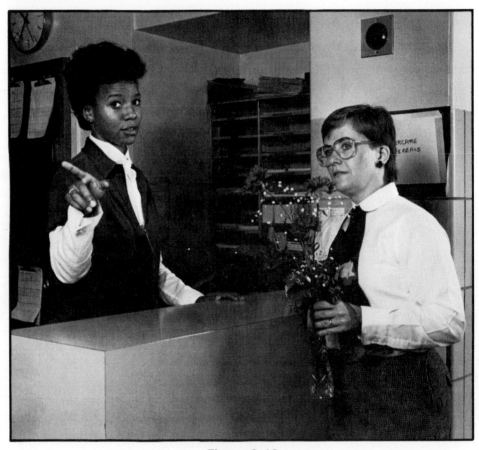

Figure 8–12

KEY IDEA: RELATIONSHIPS WITH CHILDREN AND THEIR PARENTS

Several important things need to be considered and remembered with the pediatric patient (Fig. 8–13):

- Parents need to be with their children, and children need their parents.
- Parents are normally concerned and often are worried, frightened people.
- Most children first learn about the world from their parents.
- The younger the child, the more he needs his parents.

There are several things the unit coordinator can do to help:

- Do the best possible job of caring for the child. This is usually reassuring to the parents.
- Show interest and concern about the parents' welfare. Ask, "Is there anything we can do for you?"
- Do not make judgments about the parents' attitudes or behavior, even if they seem strange to you.
- Sometimes parents seem to be worried about something concerning their child in the hospital and are afraid to talk about it. If you suspect this, tell the nurse in charge.

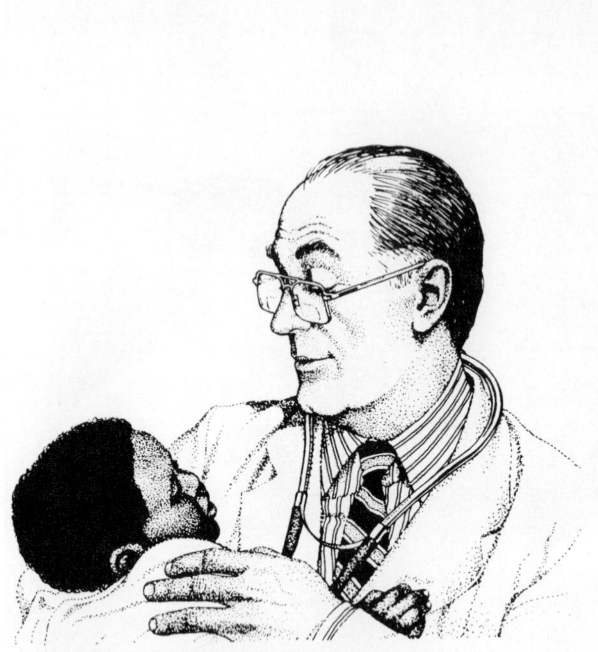

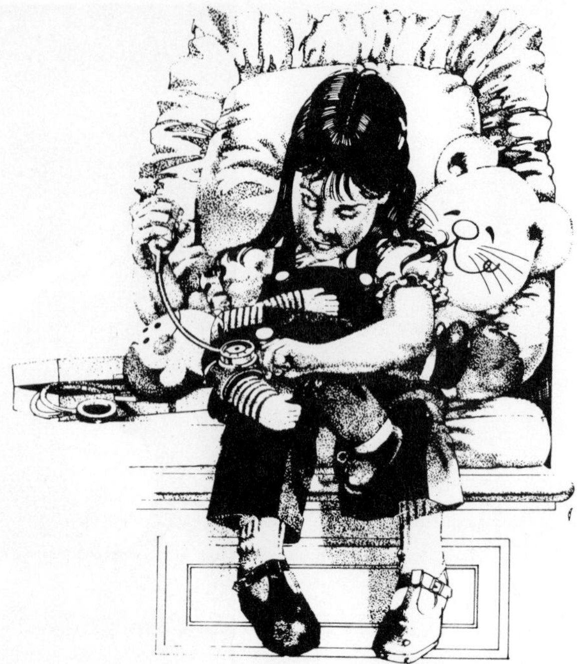

Figure 8–13

LEARNING ACTIVITIES

Complete the following:

1. Define communication ______
2. List the four elements of communication:
   (a) ______
   (b) ______
   (c) ______
   (d) ______
3. In order to be an effective listener you must first ______
   ______.
4. List the three components of an effective message:
   (a) ______
   (b) ______
   (c) ______
5. List eight general rules of telephone courtesy:
   (a) ______
   (b) ______
   (c) ______
   (d) ______
   (e) ______
   (f) ______
   (g) ______
   (h) ______

6. List three rules for answering the telephone:
   (a) ______
   (b) ______
   (c) ______
7. List three rules for placing a call:
   (a) ______
   (b) ______
   (c) ______
8. When answering the telephone or placing a call, you must always ______ yourself.
9. When placing a call outside of the hospital, you always state the ______ first.
10. The device that allows direct communication between the nurses' station and the patient's room is the ______.
11. When you take a message, you must always ______ numbers.
12. The health unit coordinator may never discuss a patient with ______.
13. The health unit coordinator may only discuss a patient with ______.
14. List the five concerns a patient may have while in the hospital.
    (a) ______
    (b) ______
    (c) ______
    (d) ______
    (e) ______
15. List two rules that apply to all visitors.
    (a) ______
    (b) ______.

DETERMINING RESPONSES TO HOSPITAL SITUATIONS

Discuss how you would handle each of the following situations.

1. You have the opportunity to go away for the weekend and are scheduled to work.
2. The doctor reprimands you because the lab results for his patient are not on the chart.
3. You call the laboratory and they swear they never received the order.
4. A patient calls on the intercom and says he has asked for pain medication three times and still hasn't received it and he is really angry!
5. The hospital supervisor asks you to "float" to another floor for the rest of your shift because the regular unit coordinator got sick and went home.
6. A nursing assistant asks you to help one of her patients to the bathroom.
7. A patient's visitor comes to the desk holding an empty water pitcher.
8. A patient's daughter asks you if you think her mother is going to die.

9. Another unit coordinator tells you that she overheard the nurses saying they were going to be cutting back on staff.
10. The hospital calls you at home and tells you not to come in to work because the census is low.
11. You can't read a doctor's writing on the chart and she is just walking down the hall.
12. A visitor asks you where the gift shop is located.
13. Friends of Joe Doyle (in room 342) walk in carrying a large pizza.
14. A patient complains to you because his roommate is playing the radio too loud.

TELEPHONE PRACTICE

Pretend that you are the health unit coordinator and handle the following telephone situations:

1. A friend of a patient calls to ask about her condition. She also wants to know what is wrong with the patient and whether or not she is going to have to have surgery.
2. Dr. Know calls to leave orders on Mrs. Pothier's chart.
3. The laboratory calls with stat results on your patient, Mr. Behncke. The doctor left instructions that his office was to be called immediately with the results.
4. Radiology calls and wants to know whether or not Mrs. Pothier's prep for the barium enema was successful.
5. The head nurse asks you to call Acme Ambulance Company. They are to transport your patient, Mr. Blackstone, to Riversweet Convalescent Hospital today.
6. Mr. O'Hearn, the husband of a patient from your floor who is in surgery, calls to find out what time she is expected back from Recovery Room.
7. Dr. Merryweather calls to find out how his patient, Mr. Gomez, is doing.
8. Mr. Goldstein calls to find out what time visiting hours are so that he can visit his wife. He asks if it is alright to bring in a hot water bottle.
9. Dr. Chino calls and starts to give you admitting orders on his new patient.
10. O.R. calls and says they are ready to pick up Mrs. Henry and they say that she should have her on-call medicine.
11. The nurse asks you to call dietary and order a low-salt 1500-calorie diet for Miss Strong in room 440.
12. Dr. Amada asks you to call Dr. Morgan at her office and arrange for a consultation. The patient is Linda Bowman, age 48, room 610, diagnosis—acute pyelonephritis. Dr. Morgan is a urologist.

CHAPTER 9

Hospital Safety and Emergencies

OBJECTIVES

When you have completed this chapter, you will be able to:

- List the general rules of hospital safety.
- State the general rules of good body mechanics.
- Explain what you can do to prevent fires.
- Explain what to do in case of fire.
- Define PASS and RACE.
- Discuss your responsibilities during a medical emergency.
- Define and discuss the International Code.

GENERAL SAFETY REGULATIONS

In hospitals, as everywhere, it is easier to take precautions against accidents than to handle them after they occur. By constantly being on the alert for potentially dangerous situations, you can do a great deal toward maintaining safe conditions for the patients, visitors, and the entire hospital staff. (Figs. 9–1 to 9–3.)

KEY IDEA: SAFE MOVEMENT WITHIN THE HOSPITAL

- Walk! Never run in the hallways. Running in the halls may cause injury to yourself or others or may create panic in the hospital.
- Walk on the right side of the hall—not more than two abreast. Be cautious of intersections. In doing this you should avoid traffic jams, collisions, and injury to yourself or others.
- Use handrails when using the stairs so that you won't fall and injure yourself.
- Watch out for swinging doors which can hit you or someone else and cause injury.

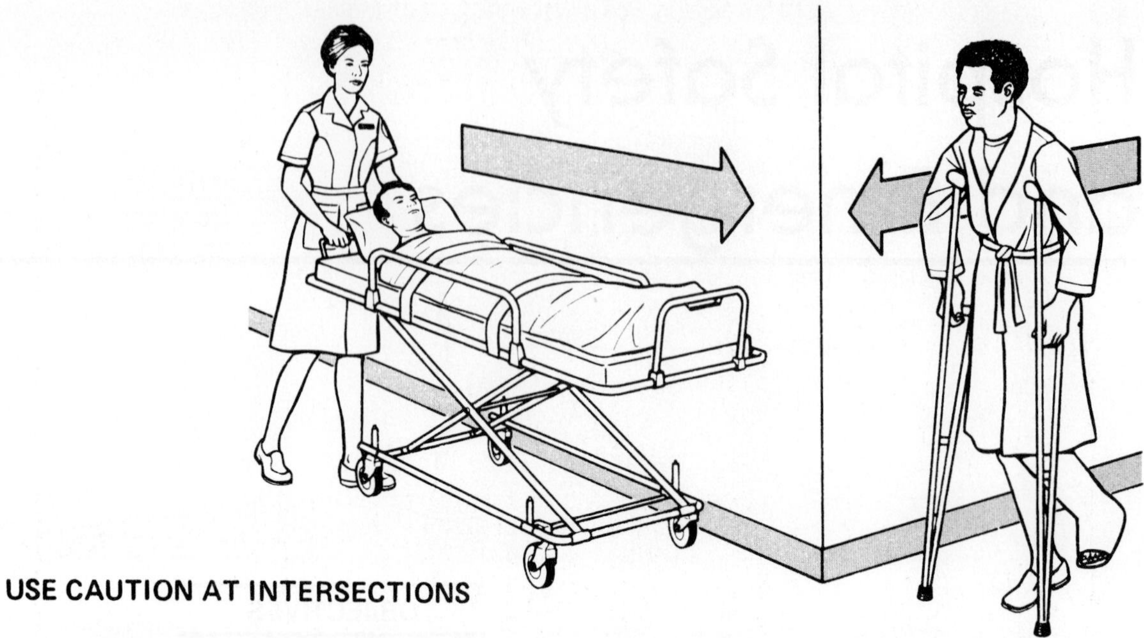
USE CAUTION AT INTERSECTIONS

Figure 9–1

KEY IDEA: OTHER SAFETY MEASURES

- Keep stairs and halls clear of equipment and obstructions. An apparatus that has been used for patient care should be returned to its proper place as soon as possible. Housecleaning equipment must not be left where people might trip over it.
- Wipe up spilled liquids or have wet floors mopped dry as necessary. (Fig. 9–4.)

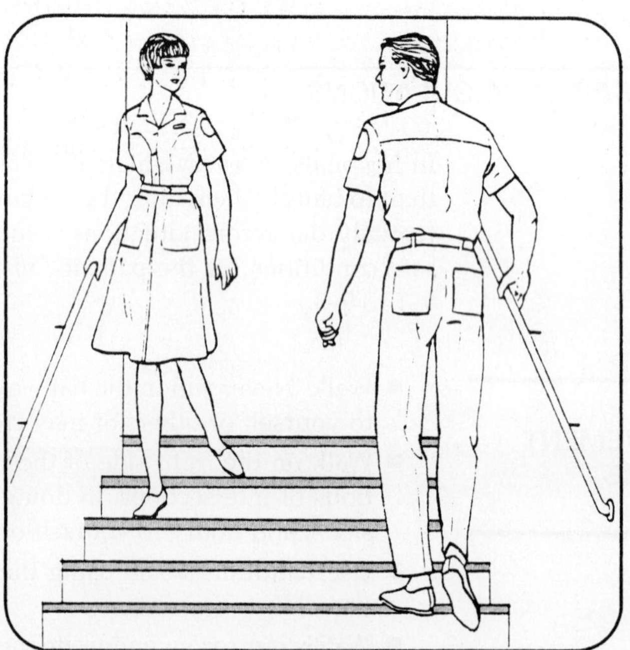
BE SAFETY CONSCIOUS AT ALL TIMES

Figure 9–2

WATCH OUT FOR SWINGING DOORS

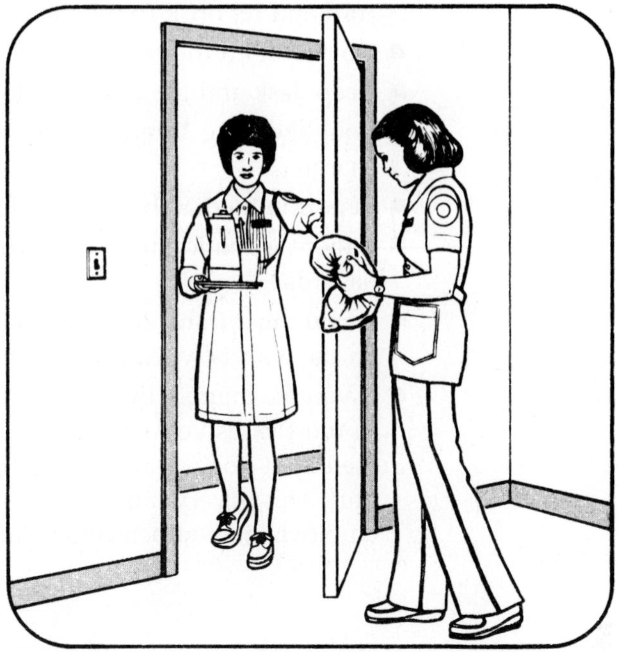

Figure 9–3

- Do not leave rubber bands, paper clips, or other objects lying on the floor.
- Have burned-out light bulbs replaced immediately.
- Never try to repair or adjust any electrical equipment yourself. Call the maintenance department. Stand away from light fixtures while they are being repaired or while bulbs are being changed.
- If an electric extension cord must be used, never suspend or drape the cord so that it hangs over steam pipes or sharp metal hooks. Lay it where it will not be pinched off by a closed door. Make sure it does not become a tripping hazard.
- Sweep up broken glass immediately; do not pick it up with your fingers. Wrap glass particles in heavy paper and label for disposal. Glass which shatters into fine pieces can be blotted up with damp toweling. (Fig. 9–4.)

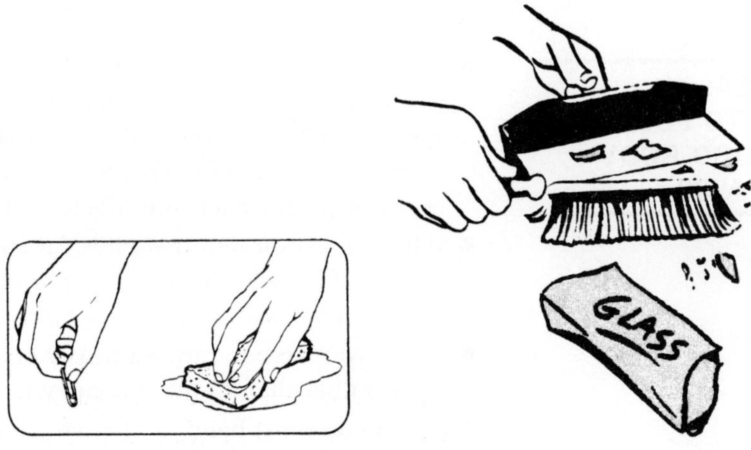

Figure 9–4

- Do not use electrical cords that are frayed or damaged. Disconnect the cord and report it to the maintenance department immediately.
- Do not sit on the edge of, or too far back in, your chair.
- Keep desk and file drawers closed when not in use.
- Roughhousing is not tolerated. Report any observed to the nurse in charge.
- Report immediately any unsafe conditions you may notice.
- If there are children on your nursing unit, be especially alert to potential hazards.
- If you must transport a patient by wheelchair, be sure to set the brakes on the wheels when moving the patient into or out of the wheelchair.
- If you are injured, even slightly, report the injury to the nurse in charge. In most cases you will be asked to visit the emergency room, be examined by a doctor, and complete a form called an employee accident report. This is very important to the hospital's safety program and for the employment compensation claims.

BODY MECHANICS

Body mechanics refers to ways of standing and moving one's body in order to make the best use of strength and avoid injury and fatigue. It is important to understand the rules of good body mechanics and to learn to apply them in your work. You will be less tired at the end of the day and will avoid injury to your body.

Before you lift, *think.* Plan every step before you lift physically:

1. Size up the load. Does it weigh more than would be safe for you to lift?
2. Check the pathways. Look for obstacles and choose a clear, safe route.
3. Solve repetitive problems. Think through your job tasks and find a smarter way. Try to lift less and save your back.
4. Find a better way. Get help from someone else or arrange for mechanical help.

KEY IDEA: RULES TO FOLLOW FOR GOOD BODY MECHANICS

- Use good posture. Keep your body aligned properly. Stand with your feet about six to eight inches apart to increase your base of support. Keep your head erect, put your shoulders back, and tuck in your abdomen and buttocks. This will tilt the pelvis forward, help straighten the curve of the back, and decrease muscle strain.
- When an action requires physical effort, try to use as many muscles or groups of muscles as possible. For example, use both hands rather than one hand to pick up a heavy object.
- When you have to move a heavy object, it is better to push it, pull it, or roll it rather than to lift and carry it.
- When you must bend, widen your base of support by putting your feet six to eight inches apart and one foot slightly forward. Bend at the

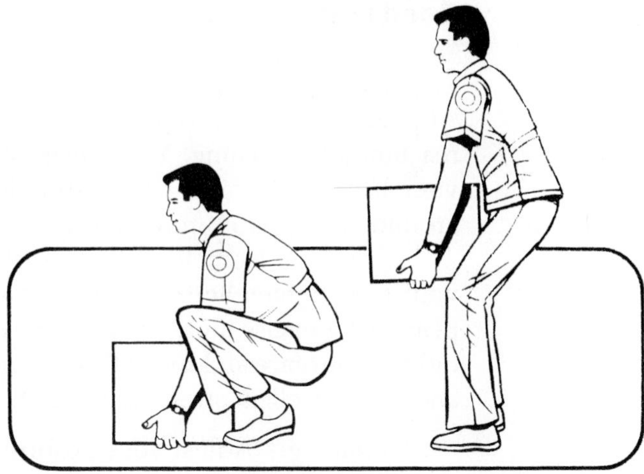

Figure 9–5

knees, keep your back straight, and balance your weight evenly on both feet. When you use this technique you will provide yourself with the stability to keep your balance. This technique makes use of the stronger thigh and leg muscles rather than weaker back muscles that are used if you bend at the waist.

- When you lift an object:
  - Squat close to the load
  - Keep your back straight
  - Grip the object firmly
  - Hold the load close to your body
  - Lift smoothly by pushing up with your strong leg muscles
  - If you think you may not be able to lift the load, get help.
  - When in doubt—don't! (Fig. 9–5.)
- When you want to change the direction of movement:
  - Pivot (turn) with your feet
  - Turn with short steps
  - Turn your whole body without twisting your back or neck. (Fig. 9–6.)

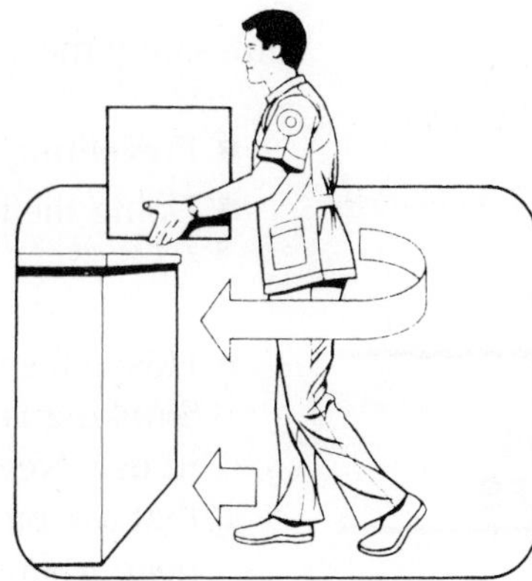

Figure 9–6

Good Posture Tips

Sitting: Try to avoid prolonged positions that put stress on your back. At your desk adjust your chair height so that you feel comfortable and aren't reaching or slouching. Your knees should be level with your hips. Support your back so you can sit up straight and every so often get up and walk around. Sitting is 1½ times harder on the back than walking or standing.

Use some isometric exercises that can be done at your desk. Begin at your toes, tighten your muscles for a couple of seconds, and then relax. Repeat this exercise until you've worked your way up to your head. Even tighten your face and relax. Done several times a day, this is hardly noticeable and is an excellent stress reducer.

Standing: Adjust your posture by placing your head and back against a wall. Move your pelvis forward and bend your knees a little so that your back touches the wall. Tighten your abdominal muscles. This is the posture you should assume when standing.

FIRE SAFETY AND PREVENTION

The common causes of fire are smoking and matches, heating and cooking equipment, electrical equipment and appliances, rubbish, trash, and flammable liquids. Each member of the hospital staff has a responsibility to see that proper care is taken in the use of equipment or materials which could cause fires. (Fig. 9–7.)

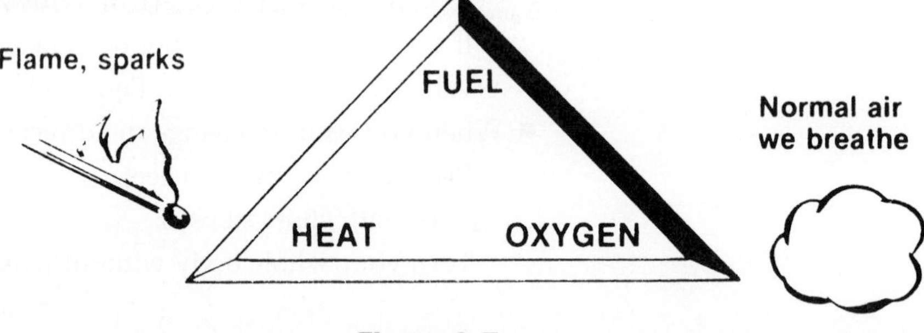

Figure 9–7

Fire safety means two things:

- Preventing fires
- Doing the right things if a fire breaks out.

KEY IDEA: GENERAL FIRE SAFETY RULES

- Hospital smoking regulations should be strictly observed and enforced. Smoking is permitted only in designated places; never when oxygen is in use. Never empty ashtrays into plastic bags or containers of rubbish that can burn. *Smoking is the number one cause of fires in health care institutions.* Many hospitals have a strict nonsmoking policy. (Fig. 9–8.)

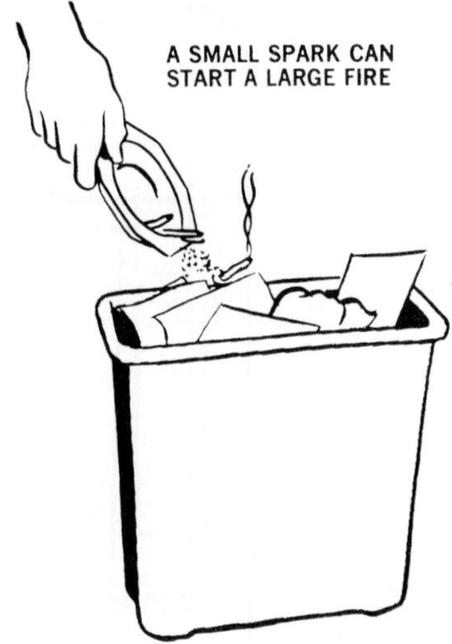

Figure 9–8

- Report any electrical equipment that does not seem to be functioning properly to the maintenance department. A small spark, dimming or flickering lights, the smell of smoke, or the sense of extreme heat are all warning signals that should not go unheeded. (Fig. 9–9.)
- Be sure flammable liquids are stored in the proper place with all caps or lids on tight. Keep all combustibles away from a potential source of heat.
- See that rubbish and trash are removed frequently. A small spark landing on an accumulation of paper, rags, or other combustible trash can start a fire immediately.
- Be familiar with your institution's fire plan. (Fig. 9–10.)

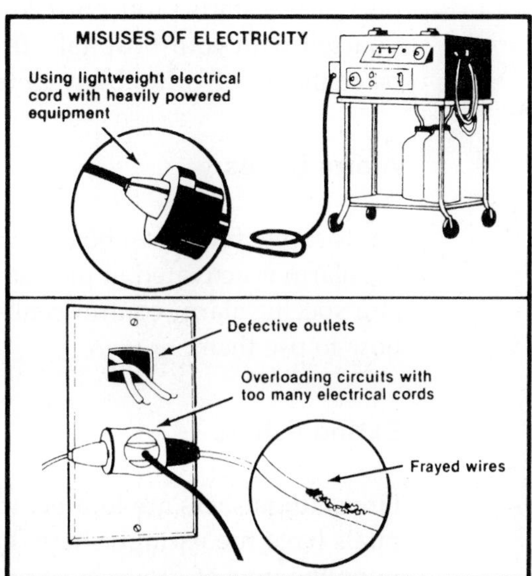

Figure 9–9

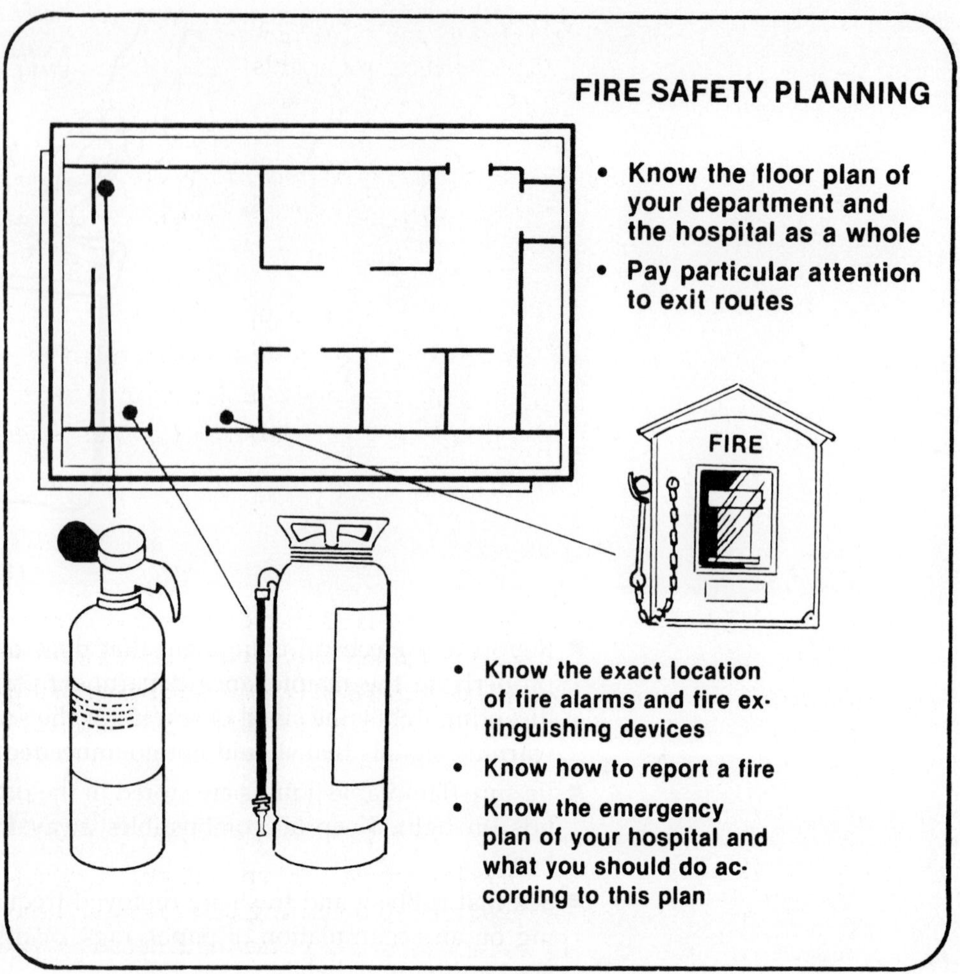

FIRE SAFETY PLANNING
• Know the floor plan of your department and the hospital as a whole
• Pay particular attention to exit routes
FIRE
• Know the exact location of fire alarms and fire extinguishing devices
• Know how to report a fire
• Know the emergency plan of your hospital and what you should do according to this plan

Figure 9–10

KEY IDEA: IN CASE OF FIRE

Fire strikes with a suddenness that demands immediate action. Part of your orientation program as a new employee will include information on what to do if a fire starts. You must know *what* to do and *how* to do it. Familiarize yourself with your hospital's fire policy so that in the event of a fire you will be confident of your ability to meet the crisis.

Alarm Boxes

At least one fire alarm box is located on the wall in your nursing unit. When the alarm is activated, it may sound automatically throughout the hospital or at a specific alarm control center. Know the location of your fire alarms and how to use them.

Extinguishers

Fire extinguishers are located at intervals throughout the hospital. Most hospitals have fire extinguishers that are rated A, B, and C, or ABC, depending upon the type of fire to be extinguished.

Type A—Wood, paper, and cloth fires
Type B—Burning liquids
Type C—Electrical fires

Type ABC extinguishers may be used on all types of fires.

The acronym PASS is used to help personnel remember the steps to take in using a fire extinguisher.

P Pull the pin on the upper handle.
A Aim low. The nozzle should be pointed at the base of the fire.
S Squeeze the handle of the extinguisher to release the fire retardant.
S Sweep the nozzle from side to side while aiming at the base of the fire.

Fire Doors

These are specially constructed doors to separate one unit from another and one floor from another, in order to contain a fire and prevent its spread. Fire doors are designed to close automatically and although they are used in normal passageways, they should never be wedged open.

Exit Routes

Somewhere on your unit, there will be a hospital map indicating the correct exit routes from your nursing unit in case it becomes necessary to evacuate the building or area. Learn these directions *thoroughly.*

KEY IDEA: YOUR PRIORITIES IN CASE OF A FIRE

Another acronym, RACE, can be used to help staff remember what steps to take in a fire.

R Remove the patient from the area of the fire.
A Activate the alarm and Alert other staff about the fire.
C Confine or contain the fire by closing doors in the area of the fire.
E Extinguish the fire if you can accomplish it safely.

Also:

- Follow the instructions of the nurse in charge. These may include checking the fire doors to be sure they are closed and closing the doors to patients' rooms.
- Return to the desk and remain alert for the signal to evacuate the patients from the unit.
- Keep the telephone lines open.
- Follow the fire emergency procedure for your hospital.
- Do not panic—lives could depend on your actions in an emergency.

MEDICAL EMERGENCIES

If a patient undergoes a sudden crisis such as hemorrhage, shock, prolonged convulsions, or severe trauma you may be asked to reach the doctor immediately. Follow the instructions of the nurse in charge. Keep the intercom open between your desk and the patient's room and prepare for emergency orders.

KEY IDEA: CARDIAC ARREST

Hospitals are equipped to handle cardiac arrest emergencies. When a patient's heart stops beating, it is called a cardiac arrest. When a patient stops breathing, it is called a respiratory arrest.

When a cardiac or respiratory arrest occurs in your nursing unit, you will be told to notify the switchboard to page the cardiac arrest team. Many hospitals have a special number you will dial (a hot line to the switchboard especially designated for cardiac arrests only); you will say "Code Blue," then the room and the number—i.e., "Code Blue, Room 100."

When this message is broadcast, a team of specially trained doctors, nurses, respiratory therapists, and other predesignated personnel will hasten to your unit. Within a short time the necessary equipment will be assembled and the cardiac arrest team will start to work to save the patient's life.

An emergency cart containing emergency supplies such as drugs, portable oxygen, resuscitation bags, and boards for external cardiac massage will be brought to the bedside. A machine called a defibrillator, designed to produce an electrical shock to restart the patient's heart, will be on the emergency cart and is frequently used in these emergencies. (Fig. 9–11.)

The health unit coordinator must remain at the desk, keep the intercom to the patient's room open for direction, be prepared for rapid emergency orders, and possibly direct visitors from the room in which the emergency is occurring. If the patient survives the cardiac arrest and is successfully resuscitated, the health unit coordinator should anticipate that the patient may be transferred to the coronary care unit.

KEY IDEA: CARDIOPULMONARY RESUSCITATION (CPR)

The American Red Cross and the American Heart Association offer classes on CPR—a method of saving lives. Most health care institutions require their employees to take these classes which are often available at the hospital. This is valuable training which may some day enable you, on or off the job, to save a life.

KEY IDEA: INTERNATIONAL HOSPITAL CODE SYSTEM

The International Hospital Code System is used to alert the staff to four major emergency situations. This system is used all over the world to report these emergencies. The four codes are:

1. **Code Red** means that there is a fire in the hospital.
2. **Code Blue** means that someone has stopped breathing (respiratory arrest), the heart has stopped beating (cardiac arrest), or both have happened.

"CODE" REPORT AND CPR FLOW SHEET

Date ______________

Est. Time of arrest ______________

Arrest observed: Yes No

CPR Started within one minute ________

CPR Stopped ______________

Cardiac Arrest: Yes No

Pulmonary Arrest: Yes No

Resuscitation Successful Yes No

Disposition of Pt. ______________
Place Time

Physician in charge ______________

Medication Nurse/Title ______________

Recording Nurse/Title ______________

Respiratory Therapist ______________

Intubation Yes No Et tube No. ________ Time ________ Intubation By: ______________

Time	Pulse	BP	Rhythm	ABG Sent	Defibrillation watts secs	NA HCO3 - 1meq /cc IV Push - 50 cc	Epinephrine 1:10,000 IV Push Amp 10cc	Epi 1:1000 or 1:10,000 ET/c/SL ____cc	Lidocaine 100 mg 10cc IV Push	Calcium Chloride 10% / 10cc	Atropine 1 mg/ 10cc IV Push			IV SOLUTIONS: Lidocaine ___6m ___cc	IV SOLUTIONS: Dopamine ___mg ___cc	IV SOLUTIONS: Isuprel ___mg ___cc			NURSE'S NOTES (Ph, PO_2, PCO_2, Color, Mental Status Temp, Pupils, procedures, ETC)

CARDIO – PULMONARY RESUSCITATION FLOW SHEET

Page ________ of ________

Figure 9–11

3. **Code Yellow** means there is an uncontrolled individual or a threatening situation.
4. **Code Green** means that a specially designated team of people in the hospital should report to the *triage area.* Each hospital has picked a particular area to use when a disaster occurs. Patients are sorted out for treatment according to the severity of their injury in the triage area.

The health unit coordinator must know the meaning of the International Codes and how to report the codes according to individual hospital policy.

INCIDENTS

An incident is any event which is not consistent with the routine operation of the hospital or the routine care of the patients. It may be an accident to a patient or to a visitor, a theft, or another unusual event involving patients, visitors, or members of the hospital staff. Some examples of incidents are:

- A patient or visitor is injured inside the hospital or an outlying hospital property such as sidewalks, parking lots, or entrances.
- There is a theft involving a patient, visitor, or hospital employee.
- A patient loses or misplaces property such as a hearing aid or false teeth.
- A nurse makes a medication error.

Whenever an incident occurs, a written report must be made. This is very important to the safety program of the hospital and so that the hospital can be prepared for possible lawsuits.

Incident or quality occurrence reports must be complete and accurate. They will be prepared under the direction of the nurse in charge. Nursing administration and the patient's physician are notified; a copy of the report is sent to the hospital's attorney. (Fig. 9–12.)

LEARNING ACTIVITIES

Complete the following:

1. List ten general rules of hospital safety.
   (a) ____________________
   (b) ____________________
   (c) ____________________
   (d) ____________________
   (e) ____________________
   (f) ____________________
   (g) ____________________
   (h) ____________________

I. **OCCURRENCE:**			(IF NO PLATE)	STATUS
DATE	TIME	LOCATION	NAME	☐ INPT ☐ OUT PT ☐ VISITOR ☐ OTHER

AGE	SEX ☐ M ☐ F	Diagnosis or Procedure	Witness Yes ☐ No ☐ Name ______ Dept. ______

Condition Prior to Occurrence	Meds Last 12 hrs (falls only)
☐ Alert ☐ Disoriented ☐ Asleep ☐ Anesthetized	

II. MEDICATION (all that apply)

- ☐ Wrong Medication
- ☐ Wrong Amount ☐ Wrong Date/Time
- ☐ Wrong Pt
- ☐ Wrong Route
- ☐ Transcription Error
- ☐ Allergic Reaction
- ☐ Omission
- ☐ Incorrect Narcotic Count
- ☐ Other ______

Name of Med

Consent:

- ☐ None written
- ☐ Mismatch
- ☐ Refused to sign
- ☐ Incomplete
- ☐ Other ______

AMA

- ☐ AMA signed
- ☐ Not signed
- ☐ AWOL
- ☐ Other

INTRAVENOUS (Note all that apply)

- ☐ Wrong Solution ☐ Wrong Medication
- ☐ Wrong Rate
- ☐ Wrong Time
- ☐ Infiltration
- ☐ Transcription Error
- ☐ PCA Error
- ☐ Blood Transfusion
- ☐ Hyperalimentation
- ☐ Other ______

Equipment

- ☐ Not available
- ☐ Disconnected
- ☐ Procedure not followed
- ☐ Nonsterile
- ☐ Malfunction
- ☐ Other ______
- ☐ Descript. of Item ______

Pressure Sore (complete both sides)

- ☐ On admission
- ☐ Hospital acquired
- ☐ Picture taken
- ☐ Stage I
- ☐ Stage II
- ☐ Stage III
- ☐ Stage IV

FALL (Complete both sides)

- ☐ Ambulating
- ☐ In BR
- ☐ Out of Bed
- ☐ To FRM B/R
- ☐ Other
- ☐ PT has fallen prev
- ☐ Restrained
- ☐ Side Rails up
- ☐ Side Rails down

Surgical — Please Comment

- ☐ Delay
- ☐ Consent Mismatch
- ☐ Unplanned Return
- ☐ Incorrect Count
- ☐ Unplanned repair / removal
- ☐ Arrest
- ☐ Death
- ☐ Anesthesia Related
- ☐ Other ______

Other

- ☐ Security ☐ Self abuse
- ☐ Engineering ☐ Lost/damage article
- ☐ Combative Pt. ☐ Hazardous Exposure
- ☐ Suicide Attempt ☐ Burn
- ☐ Fire ☐ Lab
- ☐ Respiratory ☐ X Ray
- ☐ Pharmacy ☐ Food Services
- ☐ Code blue, expired ☐ Housekeeping
- ☐ Code blue, survived ☐ Other (Comment)
- ☐ Complaint

III Severity of Outcome

☐ No Injury ☐ Inconsequential ☐ Consequential

IV Comments & Action

Name of MD notified	Date	Time	Seen by MD?
			Yes ☐ No ☐

X-ray / Lab / Tests Ordered?	Equipment
Yes ☐ No ☐ State ______	Sent for Repair ☐ Removed from service ☐

V Follow up (Director to complete)

- ☐ Communicated with ______
- ☐ Employee counseled
- ☐ Inservice
- ☐ Policy change / new
- ☐ Trend
- ☐ Other ______

Reported by — Date — Dept	Persons Involved Dept	Department Director Sign — Date

Ball Point Pen Only

QUALITY OCCURRENCE REPORT

- **Not Part of Medical Record •**
- **DO NOT Photocopy**
- **Complete all Sections and forward to QRS Immediately**

Figure 9–12

(i) ______

(j) ______

2. List three rules for lifting.
   (a) ______
   (b) ______
   (c) ______
3. List three rules for changing direction.
   (a) ______
   (b) ______
   (c) ______
4. List the five most common causes of fire.
   (a) ______
   (b) ______
   (c) ______
   (d) ______
   (e) ______
5. List five general fire safety rules.
   (a) ______
   (b) ______
   (c) ______
   (d) ______
   (e) ______
6. Define RACE.
   (a) ______
   (b) ______
   (c) ______
   (d) ______
7. If you discover a fire, you must attend to the safety of the ______.
8. List four responsibilities of the health unit coordinator in a medical emergency.
   (a) ______
   (b) ______
   (c) ______
   (d) ______

Match the International Code in column A with the description in column B.

Column A	*Column B*
(a) Code Red	____ There is a cardiac or respiratory arrest
(b) Code Blue	____ Triage
(c) Code Yellow	____ There is a fire in the hospital
(d) Code Green	____ There is an uncontrolled individual or threatening situation

CHAPTER 10

Introduction to Management at the Nurses' Station

OBJECTIVES

When you have completed this chapter, you will be able to:

- List three areas of health unit coordinator management.
- Discuss your responsibilities for medical and nursing supplies and equipment.
- Discuss your responsibilities for management of the nurses' station.
- List and explain the purpose of four clerical supplies or types of equipment used frequently at the nurses' station.
- List and define reference materials found at the nurses' station.
- Discuss the unit records and reports.
- State some of the ways you can better manage your time and health unit coordinator activities.

Now that you have learned about the hospital environment and your general duties, you are ready to become familiar with the management techniques which will help you organize and expedite your work.

In some areas of the country there is more than one position level for health unit coordinators, e.g., the beginning level or Unit Coordinator I, the next level or Unit Coordinator II, and Unit Managers. Unit Coordinator II's assume more responsibility and may act as assistant unit managers. However, the health unit coordinator, unless he or she has been promoted, does not supervise and manage other staff members. The health unit coordinator does manage other facets of the job through management of his or her own time and activities, the management of nursing and medical supplies and equipment, and the management of certain activities at the nurses' station.

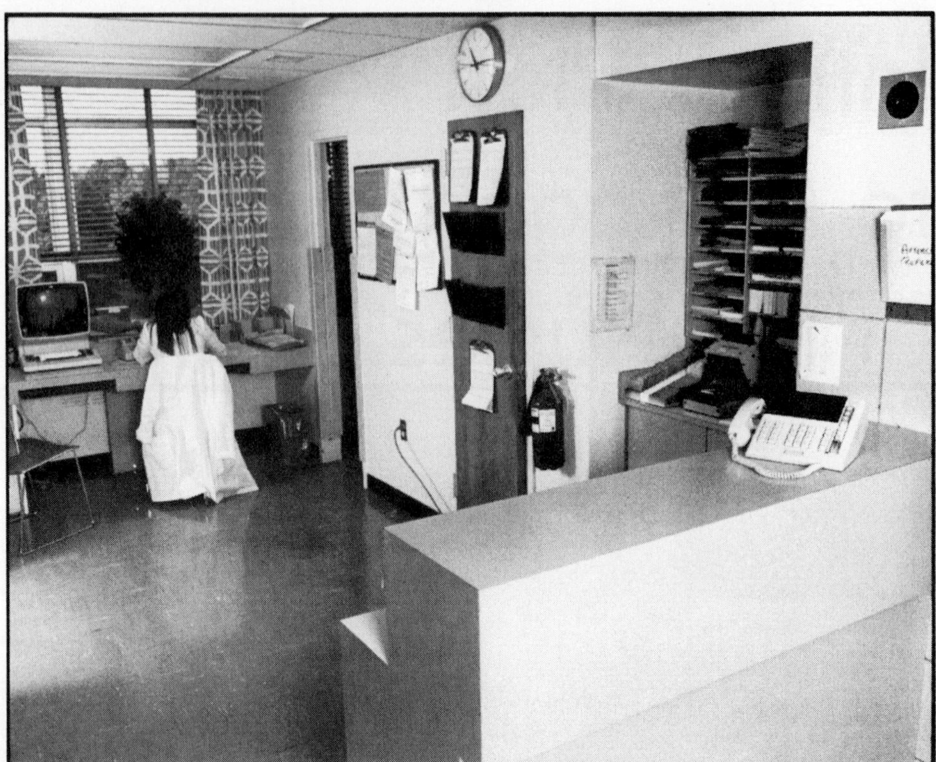

Figure 10–1

THE NURSES' STATION

Although most of your work is done at the nurses' station, it is not your private office. Doctors, nurses, aides, persons from other departments, and often student nurses come in and out freely to use the charts, computer, Kardex, and other forms and medical supplies. It will be largely your responsibility to keep the station neat and orderly and you should know what medical equipment and supplies you can expect to find there. (Fig. 10–1.)

KEY IDEA: OTHER WORK AREAS ON A NURSING UNIT

- **Treatment/examination room.** Patient physical examinations and treatments such as Pap smears, sigmoidoscopies and colonoscopies, certain biopsies, etc., are performed here.
- **Medication room.** Usually adjacent to the nurses' station—contains locked drugs such as narcotics, certain medications, refrigerator, and usually stock of intravenous solutions and supplies.
- **Utility rooms.**

  "Clean"—Contains nursing supplies from Central Supply.

  "Contaminated or Dirty"—Contaminated equipment and supplies are taken here for cleaning or for return to Central Supply.
- **Kitchen.** Patient snacks and sometimes meals are prepared here. Contains refrigerator, cupboards, sink, and usually a microwave oven.
- **Storage rooms.** Wheelchairs, guerneys, walkers, and other patient assistance equipment are stored here.

- **Dictation room.** Contains dictation equipment for physician and other professionals' use. Dictation is then transcribed by the medical transcriber in Health Information Services (Medical Records).
- **Waiting Room.** For visitors.
- **Nurse's lounge or office.** Area for conferences, change of shift report, and relaxation.

KEY IDEA: NURSING AND MEDICAL EQUIPMENT

Equipment used for physical examination of the patient is kept in the nurses' station. This may include:

- Stethoscopes
- Blood pressure machines (sphygmomanometer)
- Flashlights
- Percussion hammer
- Ophthalmoscope (for examining eyes)
- Otoscope (for examining ears)

If it is your responsibility to manage this equipment, always check it at the beginning of the shift. Replace any light bulbs that are not working and keep extra bulbs on hand. When the doctors and nurses have finished with the equipment be sure it is put in its proper place. (Fig. 10–2.)

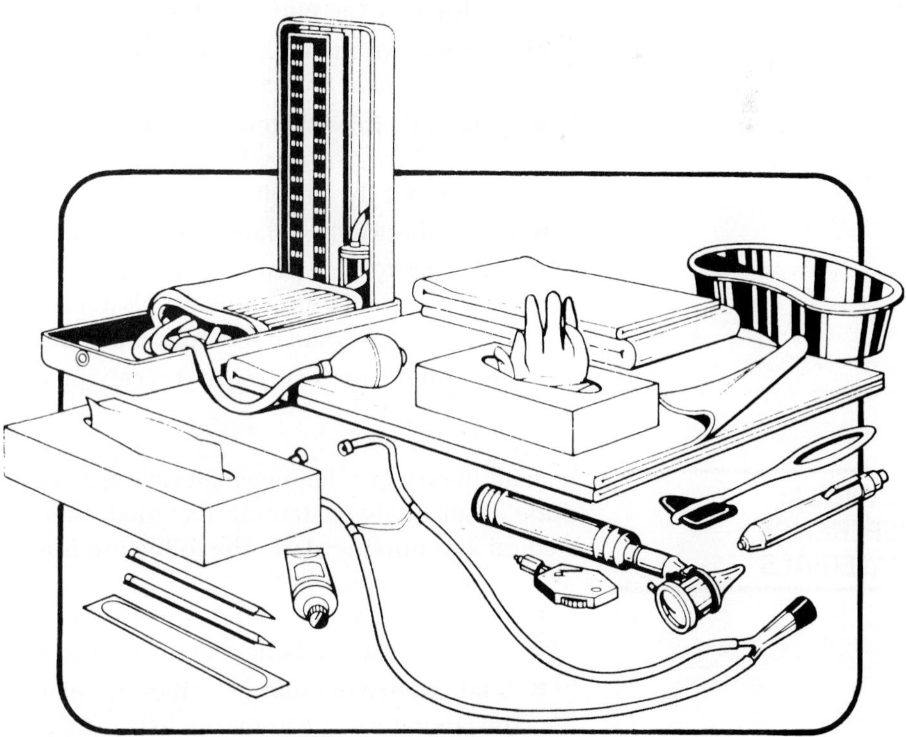

Figure 10–2

KEY IDEA: NURSING UNIT SUPPLIES

In order to properly manage supplies for the nursing unit, you must know what you have on hand and what you need. It will be necessary to regularly inventory the supplies for which you are responsible and keep a "want list" so that other nursing personnel can let you know when they are getting short of supplies.

You should order only what you need and reorder regularly. Overstocking is called hoarding and is discouraged.

Keep a list of desirable quantities of each supply and order properly so that you keep that amount on hand. For example:

- Physician's Orders forms—3 packages of 100 each.
- Telephone record pads—10.
- Black pens—25.

Certain clerical equipment and supplies will be of particular interest to you since the health unit coordinator uses them so frequently:

- **Imprinter (or addressograph machine)**—a small machine which, when used with the patient's imprinter card (addressograph plate), prints the patient's name, unit number, room number, doctor's name, and other pertinent information on all the chart forms and requisitions that pertain to the patient's care.
- **Imprinter or addressograph card holder**—a holder placed by the imprinter machine for each patient's card on the nursing unit. These cards, which originate in the admitting department, are usually filed by room number and must be returned to their proper space in the card holder. Improperly placed cards can result in a form or requisition being stamped for the wrong patient with resultant serious consequences.
- **Baskets**—for incoming and outgoing requisitions and test results. These should be neat and clearly labeled.
- **Pneumatic tube system**—the directions for use of this system should be *clearly visible* to all who use it. Incorrect use can disrupt the system throughout the hospital.
- **Files**—these will contain a supply of blank chart forms, blank requisitions, and other forms used frequently in your hospital. "Old Charts" (charts from a patient's previous admissions and sent from Medical Records) may also be kept in a file during the patient's current hospitalization.
- **Computer**—for sending and receiving a variety of information.

KEY IDEA: REFERENCE MATERIALS

A small library of reference materials are kept on the nursing unit. These include all manuals containing recorded material that might be of use to the medical and nursing staff. The following is a typical list:

- A **diet manual** lists and describes every type of diet the hospital kitchen provides (e.g., diabetic diet, ulcer diet, etc.).
- A **laboratory manual** describes in detail the various tests performed by the laboratory. It commonly lists the department regulations—when the laboratory is open, what constitutes an emergency laboratory test, etc. It may also include a list of "normal" values for each test.

- A **health unit coordinator manual** gives step-by-step descriptions of health unit coordinator procedures.
- A **nursing procedure manual** gives step-by-step descriptions of nursing procedures.
- A **hospital policy manual** gives administrative policies concerning such things as visiting hours, wage and salary scales, and smoking regulations.
- A **Physician's Desk Reference (PDR)** contains descriptions of medications in common usage.
- A **hospital formulary** lists and describes all medications stocked and used in the hospital.
- **General medical and nursing reference texts** often constitute a small reference library.
- An x-ray **procedure manual** gives pertinent data about the patient preparation required for each x-ray ordered.

Vital Signs Books or Sheets. As the nurse takes the vital signs, he/she records them in a special book to be graphed later by the health unit coordinator (see Chapter 13). You may fill in the skeleton form of this sheet by entering the patients' names, rooms, and bed numbers so that the nurse need only record the vital signs. (Fig. 10–3.)

Schedules. Working hours, vacations, tours, and days off for unit personnel are posted on the bulletin board. Most hospitals call this a "time sheet."

It is your responsibility, as a health unit coordinator, to know where the patients' charts are at all times. To some degree it is also your responsibility to know where the patients are. You must be able to locate nursing personnel on your unit, and you are frequently asked to find a doctor who is on the unit.

One method for keeping track of patients and their charts is a **patient activity log.** At the beginning of each shift, you would list each patient's room number and name; next to this note any pertinent data relating to their activity. (Fig. 10–4.) When a patient or chart has returned, draw a line through the notation.

Staff activity log. When you are asked to locate unit personnel, you will first refer to the assignment sheet to find the general location of their patient assignment. This sheet also frequently includes staff break and lunch times. If a staff member leaves the unit for a special purpose, jot it down. Keeping

Name	Room No.	8 a.m. TPR&BP	12 Noon TPR&BP	4 p.m. TPR&BP	8 p.m. TPR&BP
Jones, Wm.	449	97^6-78-20 120/80			
Clark, Geo.	450	99^2-80-20 110/70			

Figure 10–3

Patient Activity Log		
Room		Date
100	Brown, John	8A to surg c̄ chart
101A	Jones, Claire	
101B	Berol, Turquoise	10:15 to PT
102	Sevens, Dana	11:05 Chart c̄ Dr. in dictation room
103	Park, Perry	
104	Austin, Ryan	8:30 to X-ray; Rtd 10:05
105	Brayer, Nell	11:45 to OT
106	Siler, Linda	
107A		
107B	Dollar, Chris	7:35 to surg c̄ chart

Figure 10–4

notes on the location of staff members can be a great help on a busy day when your memory may fail you. (Fig. 10–5.)

KEY IDEA: MANAGEMENT OF YOUR TIME AND ACTIVITIES

Here are some rules of efficiency to help the health unit coordinator manage time and tasks more efficiently.

- Always put things back when you are through with them.
- Try never to run out of supplies.
- Complete one task before you move on to another. This may not always be possible but it is a good rule and something for which to strive.
- Learn to set priorities. Your ability to decide what to do first is important to your success as a health unit coordinator.

Stat (do immediately) orders and emergencies take precedence over other priorities. Assisting a doctor or nurse should come before your routine

STAFF ACTIVITY LOG

7:25 Mr Dean floated to 4W for day
12:15pm Miss Brown to staff meeting - due back 1:30
12:30pm Mrs Grey to help in O.B. for 1 hr.
1:15pm Dr. White to ER, back in about ½ hr.

Figure 10–5

health unit coordinator tasks. Patient and visitor requests should take priority over other health unit coordinator activities. Answering the telephone usually takes priority over other tasks.

Make good use of your time. If there is a period of the day when you are not busy, use this time to do some of your routine tasks. For example, you will learn that the chart of each new patient contains at least eight (and probably many more) different forms which must be arranged in a specific order. When you are not busy, you can arrange sets of these forms in the proper order. You will find this to be a great help to you on busy days when many admissions are expected.

- Make notes to yourself and lists of calls to make and things to do. When you have completed the task, draw a line through it on the list.
- Make out a daily work schedule.
- Look for ways to make your work more efficient. Avoid duplication of effort. Try to combine running errands with a coffee break or a lunch period. Don't waste energy by going to get a new supply of chart forms for your file, only to discover an hour later that you also needed a supply of dietary requisitions. Do not, however, confuse efficiency with short cuts. Meticulous attention to detail is part of your job.

KEY IDEA: TRAINING OTHERS

From time to time you will be asked to help train newly employed or student health unit coordinators. As you manage this part of your job responsibility, you truly can use your human relations and communications skills discussed in the first chapters of this book. In your role as teacher you become many things—role model, evaluator, and, if you try, a friend. When this time comes, think back to one of the main functions of a hospital—to provide education for health care workers. Look at this experience as a challenge. Show others that you know your job well enough to impart that knowledge to others. If you don't know what is expected of you, seek guidance from the Education Department, your head nurse, and the student health unit coordinator's instructor. Use empathy and remember when you, too, were a student.

LEARNING ACTIVITIES

Complete the following:

1. List three areas of health unit coordinator management.
   (a) ____________________
   (b) ____________________
   (c) ____________________
2. Define the following:
   (a) Sphygmomanometer ____________________
   (b) Ophthalmoscope ____________________
   (c) Otoscope ____________________
   (d) Imprinter or addressograph machine ____________________

3. State the purpose of each of the following reference materials:
   (a) Laboratory manual ______________________
   (b) Nursing procedure manual ______________________
   (c) Hospital policy manual ______________________
   (d) Physicians' Desk Reference ______________________
   (e) Hospital formulary ______________________
4. State the purpose of the following:
   (a) Change of shift report ______________________
   (b) Census record ______________________
   (c) Daily or summary report ______________________
   (d) Vital signs book or sheet ______________________
   (e) "Time sheet" ______________________
   (f) Patient activity log ______________________
5. List six rules of efficiency.
   (a) ______________________
   (b) ______________________
   (c) ______________________
   (d) ______________________
   (e) ______________________
   (f) ______________________

CHAPTER 11

The Patient's Chart

OBJECTIVES

When you complete this chapter, you will be able to:

- Explain the reasons for the patient's chart.
- Define terms used in this chapter that relate to the chart.
- List and explain the rules of charting.
- Describe the health unit coordinator's responsibilities in maintaining the chart and list the routine chart checks.
- List and discuss the standard chart forms.
- Assemble a patient's chart.
- List and describe the common supplemental chart forms.

The hospital keeps a vast collection of records for both medical and legal reasons. Probably the most important among these are those that make up the individual "patient's chart."

The Joint Commission on Accreditation of Health Care Organizations (JCAHO) has established a number of reasons why all patients should have charts.

KEY IDEA: PURPOSES OF CHARTS

1. To serve as a basis for the planning of patient care
2. To provide a practical means of communication between physicians and other members of the health team
3. To furnish documentation of the course of a patient's illness and care
4. For legal purposes in a court of law
5. To provide data for use in research (Fig. 11–1.)

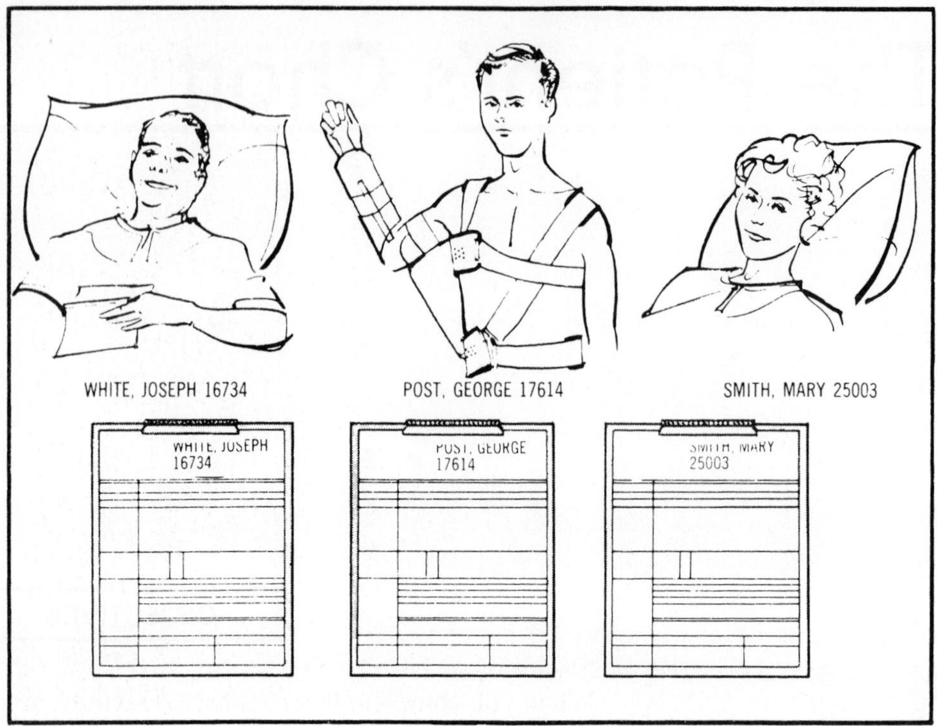

Figure 11–1

KEY IDEA: MAINTAINING PATIENT CHARTS

Each patient who enters the hospital has records kept on all phases of his medical progress. During the patient's hospital stay, all or most of these individual records are brought together, in proper order, and bound into loose-leaf metal or vinyl covers called "chart backs" or "chart holders." New sheets may be added as necessary. Or, if the patient's stay has been a long one, the chart may be "thinned" or "split" by removing certain chart forms and filing them on the unit. Your instructor will explain which forms you may take out of the chart and which you may not. One chart holder is available in every nursing unit for each hospital bed. When not in use by doctors or nurses, all chart holders are kept in special devices called "chart racks." The charts have special places in the rack, usually in the same order that the patients' rooms are located in the nursing unit. This arrangement makes them easy to find when needed. Each chart should be replaced in the rack after use.

After the patient is discharged, a health unit coordinator routes all record sheets relating to him to Health Information Services, where they are filed together, under a special "unit number" which was assigned to the patient on admission. All forms that were removed when the chart was "thinned" or "split" must be returned to the chart in proper sequence. If a patient is readmitted to the hospital at a later date, this "old" chart can be used as reference to patient's previous medical history. For each admission, a new chart is always started and kept in the unit, so that information can be continuously recorded. After the patient's discharge, this chart can be added to any previous records the hospital may have on the patient. (Fig. 11–2.)

STORAGE OF MEDICAL RECORDS

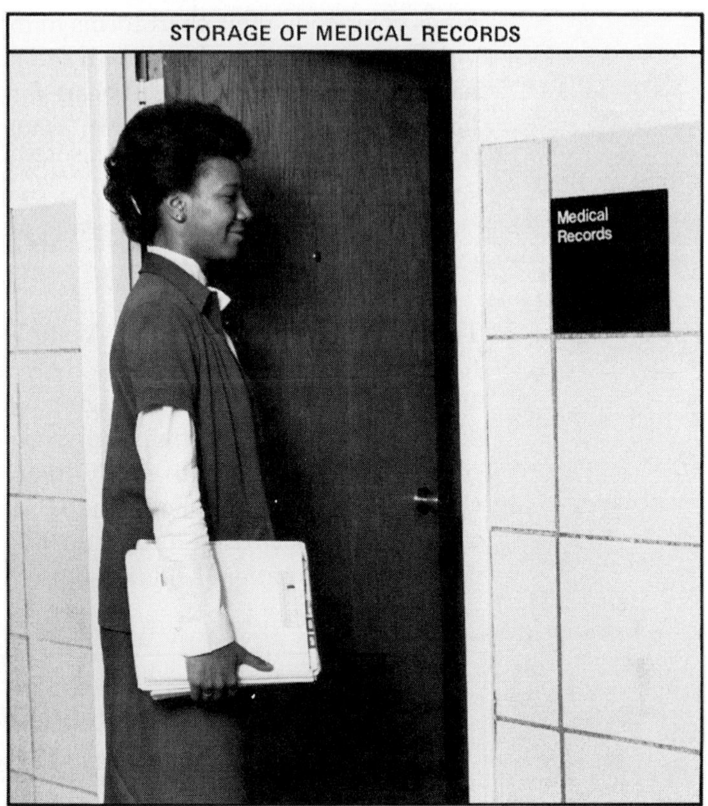

Figure 11-2

THE CHART FORM

The individual record forms that are assembled to make up the patient's chart have two things in common. The name of the hospital where it is used is printed on it and a space is provided on each for the patient's name. Most hospitals use some variation of the chart forms described in this lesson although the exact form varies from one hospital to another. Some hospitals print the forms according to their own needs and specifications.

The space which identifies the chart form with the patient is recorded by means of a mechanical device (an imprinter), which has been discussed in Chapter 6. One chart form varies in format from another according to the information to be recorded on it. Your instructor will help you to identify the forms among those listed below that are used in your hospital.

KEY IDEA: EXECUTION OF CHART FORMS

Health unit coordinators do not write on most chart forms. It is your responsibility to stamp these forms with the patient's imprinter card and place them in the proper sequence in the patient's chart. There are, however, several standard chart forms on which you may write or actually file diagnostic reports.

KEY IDEA: STANDARD CHART FORMS

There are at least nine chart forms that usually become part of every patient's chart upon admission. These are referred to as "standard forms." It is important that you learn to identify and describe each of these forms. Other chart forms, called "supplemental forms," are used only when required. Many hospitals color-code their chart forms to make them easy to identify and have dividers in the charts printed with the names of the forms. Your hospital may have different names for the chart forms other than those used here. Some hospitals or special units within a hospital may include other forms which they consider "standard" for their hospital or special unit. Following are descriptions of the nine standard chart forms. (Figs. 11–3 and 11–4.)

Conditions of Admission

The **conditions of admission** is completed by the Admitting Department. Information on this form includes the patient's name, date and time of admission, age, date of birth, sex, religion, address, telephone number, occupation, social security number, financially responsible party, type of insurance, next of kin, name of person to notify in an emergency, and admitting diagnosis. Other information may be included as well. The patient is assigned a hospital number, which is recorded on the form, and typically the form is sent along with the patient's addressograph plate to the nursing unit. The condi-

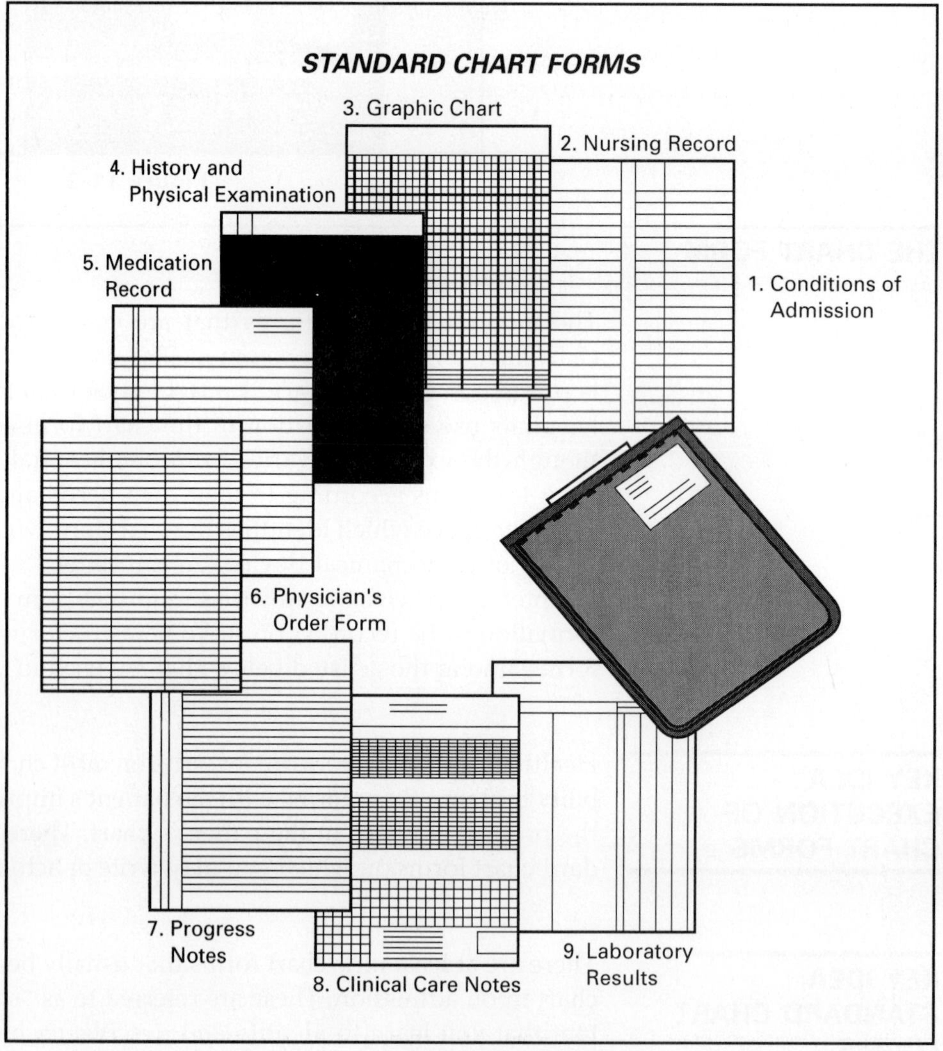

Figure 11–3

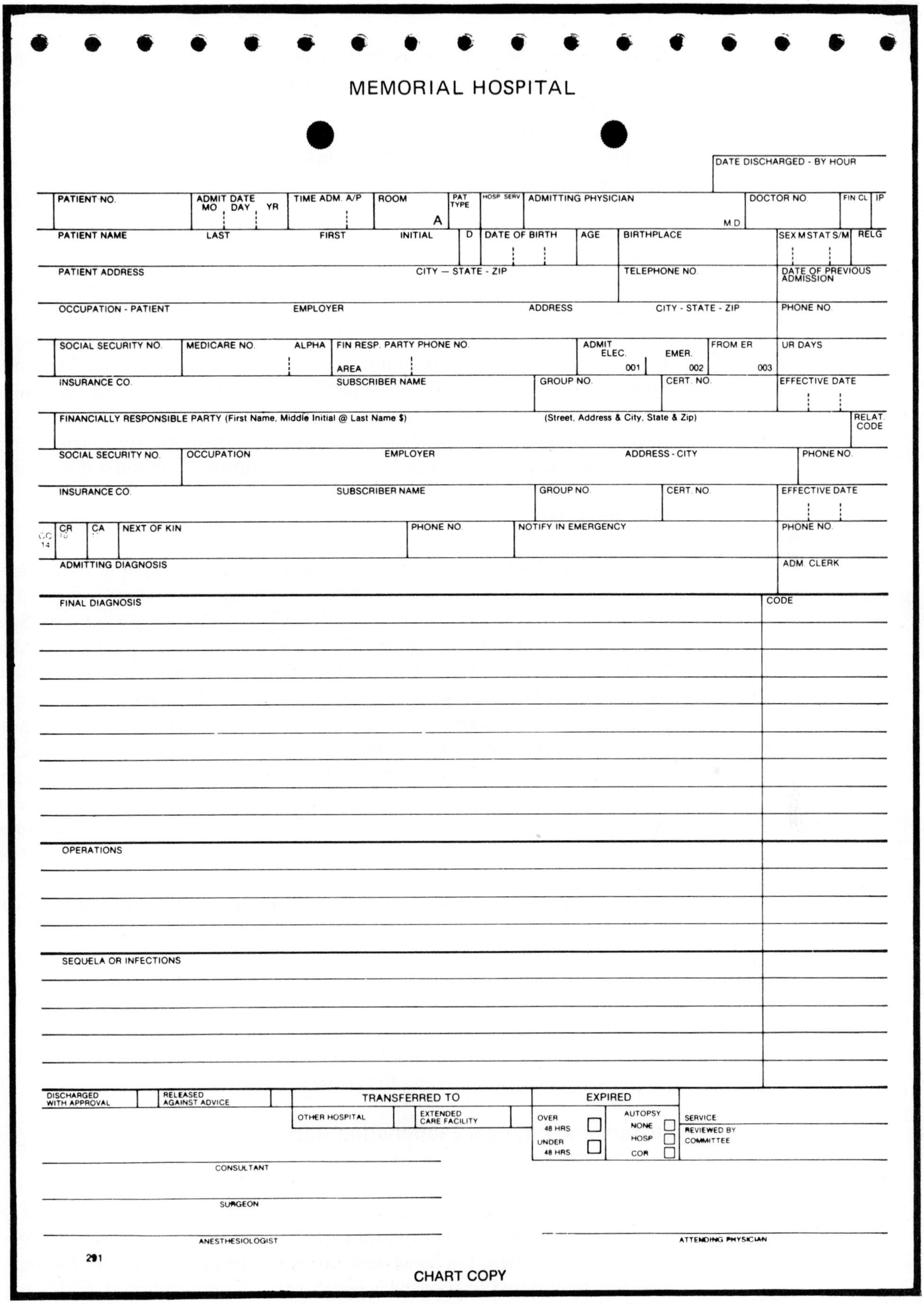

MEMORIAL HOSPITAL

DATE DISCHARGED - BY HOUR

PATIENT NO. | ADMIT DATE MO DAY YR | TIME ADM. A/P | ROOM A | PAT TYPE | HOSP SERV | ADMITTING PHYSICIAN M.D. | DOCTOR NO. | FIN CL | IP

PATIENT NAME LAST FIRST INITIAL | D | DATE OF BIRTH | AGE | BIRTHPLACE | SEX M STAT S/M | RELG

PATIENT ADDRESS CITY — STATE - ZIP | TELEPHONE NO. | DATE OF PREVIOUS ADMISSION

OCCUPATION - PATIENT EMPLOYER ADDRESS CITY - STATE - ZIP | PHONE NO.

SOCIAL SECURITY NO. | MEDICARE NO. | ALPHA | FIN RESP. PARTY PHONE NO. AREA | ADMIT ELEC. 001 EMER. 002 | FROM ER 003 | UR DAYS

INSURANCE CO. SUBSCRIBER NAME | GROUP NO. | CERT. NO. | EFFECTIVE DATE

FINANCIALLY RESPONSIBLE PARTY (First Name, Middle Initial @ Last Name $) (Street, Address & City, State & Zip) | RELAT. CODE

SOCIAL SECURITY NO. | OCCUPATION EMPLOYER ADDRESS - CITY | PHONE NO.

INSURANCE CO. SUBSCRIBER NAME | GROUP NO. | CERT. NO. | EFFECTIVE DATE

CC 14 | CR | CA | NEXT OF KIN | PHONE NO. | NOTIFY IN EMERGENCY | PHONE NO.

ADMITTING DIAGNOSIS | ADM. CLERK

FINAL DIAGNOSIS | CODE

OPERATIONS

SEQUELA OR INFECTIONS

DISCHARGED WITH APPROVAL | RELEASED AGAINST ADVICE | TRANSFERRED TO: OTHER HOSPITAL | EXTENDED CARE FACILITY | EXPIRED: OVER 48 HRS ☐ UNDER 48 HRS ☐ | AUTOPSY: NONE ☐ HOSP ☐ COR ☐ | SERVICE | REVIEWED BY COMMITTEE

CONSULTANT

SURGEON

ANESTHESIOLOGIST

ATTENDING PHYSICIAN

291

CHART COPY

Figure 11–4 Conditions of Admission form.

tions of admission is placed as the first page of the chart. When the patient is discharged, transferred, or expires (dies), the bottom portion is completed by the physician. This information includes the final diagnosis, any operations, and complications including infections. The completion of this information usually occurs after the chart has been sent to Health Information Services/Medical Records. (Fig. 11–4.)

Nursing Record

Special forms are provided for nurses to record their observations of the patient's condition and the care they give. The nurses' notes are their written communication with the physician. Hospitals have strict regulations regarding the frequency and the manner in which these notes are made. A comprehensive admission nursing assessment begins the nursing record, and there is usually a separate form for this purpose. The nursing diagnosis, ongoing assessment, intervention, daily care, and discharge planning are all components of the **nursing record.** Figure 11–5 shows examples of the nursing record.

Graphic Chart

The **graphic chart** is so called because it is primarily a graph; the patient's temperature, pulse, respiration (TPR), and frequently blood pressure are recorded on the graphic chart as soon as possible after they are taken. Space is usually provided for recording this data for a period of one week. Many hospitals use the graphic chart to record other information about the patient's daily condition and progress as well. Information such as the patient's appetite, total fluid intake and output, weight, height, and daily bowel movements may also be recorded on this sheet.

Temperature, pulse, and respiration rates of patients are taken at specified times during the day in most hospitals, and on certain patients more frequently as ordered. You may be responsible for entering this information on the graphic chart. Red ink may be used to record the temperature (although the trend is to use all black ink) and blue or black ink to record the pulse and respiration rates. To graph you will make a dot representing the value of each cardinal symptom (the cardinal symptoms are the temperature, pulse, and respiration) and the blood pressure, if required, in the column of the graph which indicates the day and hour it was taken. This dot is connected to the previous dot by a straight line similar to the one shown in Fig. 11–6. It is very important to be accurate when performing this task. The cardinal symptoms in some diseases have a characteristic pattern of rising and falling, and the graph is a visual aid in seeing the pattern at a glance.

History and Physical Examination Record

Every patient admitted to a hospital has a medical history taken and undergoes some sort of physical examination. Observations by the doctor are recorded in full on the **history and physical examination record.** The report may be handwritten, but most commonly the physician dictates the report, which is then typed (transcribed) by a medical transcriptionist. If this is the case, the report must be filed in the chart in the proper place when it arrives from the Medical Transcription Department, which is often a part of Health

NURSING RECORD

ADMISSION ASSESSMENT

PART I. ADMISSION BASELINE – (RN, LVN, NA)

DATE	TIME	DIAGNOSIS	ROOM	ID BAN VERIF

TRANSPORT MODE: ☐ W/C ☐ STR. ☐ AMB — ADMIT FROM: ☐ ER ☐ HOME ☐ SNF ☐ MD OFFICE ☐ OTHER HOSP. — VITAL SIGNS: TEMP. ____ PULSE ____ HT. ____ WT: STATED ____

EQUIPMENT WITH PT.: ☐ NONE ☐ DENTURES/PARTIALS ☐ U ☐ L ☐ CANE ☐ WALKER ☐ CONTACT LENSES ☐ GLASSES ☐ HEARING AID ☐ W/C ☐ OTHER:

ADVANCE DIRECTIVE: ☐ YES ☐ NO IF NO, INFORMATION GIVEN ☐

COPY TO CHART: ☐ YES ☐ NO

PART II. FUNCTIONAL HEALTH PATTERNS ASSESSMENT

INFORMATION DOCUMENTED BY: ☐ PATIENT ☐ SIGNIFICANT OTHER ☐ RN ☐ LVN

HEALTH PERCEPTION/HEALTH MANAGEMENT

☐ 1. REASON FOR HOSPITALIZATION (stated by patient/informant): ____

☐ 2. PERTINENT MEDICAL/SURGICAL HISTORY: ____

☐ 3. HOW DOES PATIENT DESCRIBE GENERAL HEALTH? ____

☐ 4. WHAT KIND OF THINGS DOES PATIENT DO TO KEEP HEALTHY? ____

☐ 5. USE OF TOBACCO: ☐ NO ☐ YES HOW MUCH? ____ HOW LONG?
ALCOHOL: ☐ NO ☐ YES HOW MUCH? ____ HOW LONG?
REC. DRUGS: ☐ NO ☐ YES DESCRIBE: ____

CURRENT MEDS	DOSE	FREQ.	LAST DOSE	CURRENT MEDS	DOS
				NON RX (LAX./ANALG.)	

☐ 6. HAS PATIENT BEEN ABLE TO FOLLOW PRESCRIBED MEDS/TREATMENTS: ☐ YES ☐ N

☐ 7. DISPOSITION OF MEDICATIONS: ☐ DID NOT BRING ☐ SENT HOME WITH FAMILY ☐

ALLERGIES

☐ NO KNOWN ALLERGIES ☐ YES ☐ ALLERGY BAND ON

	ALLERGY	TYPE OF
MEDS		
FOODS		
OTHER		

ACTIVITY/EXERCISE

☐ 1. MOBILITY STATUS: ☐ AMBULATORY ☐ AMBULATORY WITH ASSIST ☐ TRANSFER WI

☐ 2. ASSISTIVE DEVICES: ☐ NONE ☐ CRUTCHES ☐ CANE ☐ WALKER ☐ W/C ☐ C

☐ 3. LIMITATIONS: ☐ NONE ☐ WEAKNESS ☐ FATIGUE ☐ RECENT (6 MO. <) FALL?

☐ 4. ACTIVITIES OF DAILY LIVING: ☐ INDEPENDENT IN ALL ADL
FEEDING ___ TOILETING ___ GROOMING ___ DRESSING ___ BATHING ___ (A

☐ 5. EXERCISE REGULARLY? ☐ NO ☐ YES, DESCRIBE ____

SLEEP/REST

☐ 1. SLEEP: ☐ NO PROBLEM ☐ DIFFICULTY FALLING ASLEEP ☐ DIFFICULTY STAYING A
☐ DOES NOT FEEL RESTED AFTER SLEEP ☐ OTHER: ____

☐ 2. WHAT HELPS PATIENT SLEEP? ____

☐ 3. SLEEP ROUTINE: BEDTIME ____ NO. HOURS ____ ☐ NAPS ____ NO. PILLOWS ____

185 (10/93)

DAILY CARE RECORD - RN, LVN, CNA Shaded Areas

		02	04	06	08	10	12	14	16	18	20	22	24
VITAL SIGNS	Temperature: (R)ectal (A)xillary (T)ympanic												
	Pulse (A)pical												
	Respirations												
	Blood Pressure												
	Orthostatic Blood Pressure												
	Measurement: Type: ____												
SAFETY	Side Rails ↑, Bed ↓, Wheels Locked												
	Call Bell In Reach												
	Bands On: ID/ALLERGY (Circle)												
	Protective Device - Type: ____												
	Neuro-Vascular assessment q 2 h												
	Food-Fluid needs assessed q 2 h												
	Elimination needs assessed q 2 h												
	Released, ROM, reapplied q 2 h												
	Device removed												
	Device reapplied												
	Isolation - Category: ____												
	Protocol Maintained												
RESPIRATORY	Cough/Deep Breathing												
	Suction Frequency												
	Pulse Oximetry (% sat)												
	Incentive Spirometry												
	Oxygen ____ LPM per ____ Device												
HYGIENE	Bath: Type ____												
	AM, PM, HS Care												
	Linen Change												
	Perineal/Catheter Care												
	Denture/Oral Hygiene												
ACTIVITY/EXERCISE	Ambulate												
	Chair												
	Bedrest												
	BSC/BRP												
	Dangle												
	Position Change												
	ROM — Passive (P) Active (A)												
TREATMENTS	Dressing Change(s)												
	1. Site ____ 2. Site ____												
	Drainage *												
	Bowel Hygiene *												
	Antiembolic Treatment: Seq TEDS ____ Stockings ____												
IV MGT.	Type: 1. 2. 3.												
	Location: 1. 2. 3.												
	IV Site Checked — Clear, Without Complications												
	IV Patent & Infusing Well												
	Drsg Dry & Intact												
	IV(S) Discontinued—Without Difficulty-Catheter Intact												
	✔-Assessed/Completed *-See Nsg Note Blank-Does Not Apply	02	04	06	08	10	12	14	16	18	20	22	24

____, RN

DATE ___/___/___ ASSESSMENT / PROGRESS NOTES (RN)

PRIORITY #	NURSING DIAGNOSIS	PRIORITY #	NURSING DIAGNOSIS
	☐ Impaired Gas Exchange		☐ Potential for Infection
	☐ Ineffective Coping - Anxiety		☐ Potential for Physical Injury
	☐ Alteration in Comfort		☐ Impaired Communication
	☐ Alteration in Nutrition		☐ Knowledge Deficit
	☐ Impaired Skin Integrity		☐ Altered Mental Status
	☐ Activity Intolerance / Immobility		☐ Alteration in Elimination
	☐ Other:		☐ Other:

Time: Care Plan: ☐ Reviewed ☐ Revised Reviewed w/ ☐ Pt. ☐ SO RN Signature

Time: Care Plan: ☐ Reviewed ☐ Revised Reviewed w/ ☐ Pt. ☐ SO RN Signature

Time: Care Plan: ☐ Reviewed ☐ Revised Reviewed w/ ☐ Pt. ☐ SO RN Signature

TIME	FOCUS	D = DATA A = ACTION R = RESPONSE

MEDICAL / SURGICAL DAILY NURSING RECORD

ADDRESSOGRAPH

189 3/96

Figure 11–5

GRAPHIC CHART

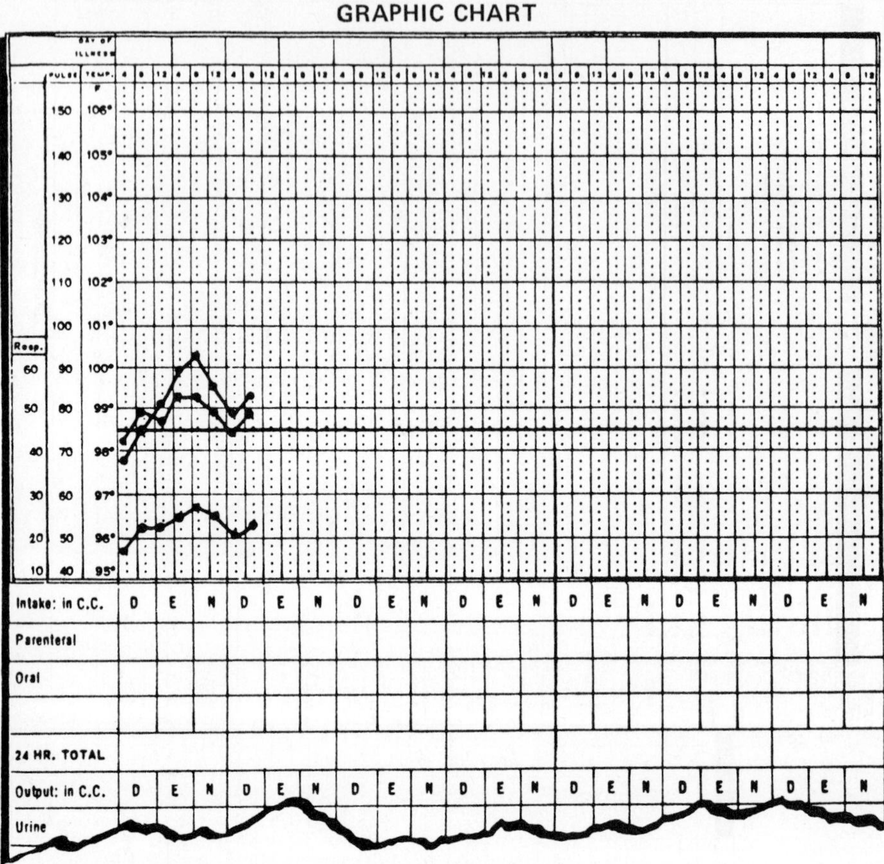

Figure 11–6

Information Services. Many hospitals use more than one type of history and physical record. Occasionally, a very long form may be used for research or educational purposes. An abbreviated form may be used for patients admitted for 48 hours or less or for certain outpatient procedures. (Fig. 11–7.)

Medication Record

The **medication record** is a chart form used for recording all medications given to the patient. Each time the nurse gives a medication, the nurse records that the prescribed medication was given at the appropriate time. A separate form may be used for intravenous (IV) medications.

If your hospital uses a record similar to the one described, you will have certain clerical duties to perform. When the **medication record** in progress has been filled, a new form must be stamped with the patient's name and unit number and placed in the chart. You may also be asked to transfer information, including the names of drugs currently being administered to the patient to the new chart form. Your instructor will explain the precise methods used in your hospital. (Fig. 11–8.)

Physician's Order Form

This chart form has primary importance and will be placed at the front of the chart in many hospitals. The doctor uses this standard chart form to write all orders for the patient. The form is dated and signed each time the physician

Chief Complaint; Present Illness
Past History; Family History
Systemic Review
Physical Examination

ALL POSITIVE AND IMPORTANT NEGATIVE FINDINGS

MEMORIAL HOSPITAL

PHYSICAL EXAMINATION & HISTORY

Patient Name: ______________________________

Chief Complaint:

History of Present Illness:

Past History:

- Illness & Injuries
- Operations
- Medications
- Habits
- Bleeding
- Allergies

Family History:

Review of Systems:

Physical Examination:

- General Appearance
- Head-Eye, Ear Nose and Throat
- Heart and Lungs
- Abdomen
- Genitourinary
- Extremities
- Neurologic
- Other

Pertinent Lab/Diagnostic Results:

Physician Signature ______________________________ Date__________

MEMORIAL HOSPITAL

SHORT HISTORY AND PHYSICAL
(To be used for patients in hospital less than 48 hours)

Figure 11–7

☐ ALLERGIC TO:
☐ NO KNOWN ALLERGIES

DIAGNOSIS

CONSENT DATES: LITHIUM ANTICHOLINERGICS ANTIPSYCHOTICS ANTIDEPRESSANTS

ROOM NO.

START / RE ORDER	RN	DRUG DOSE FREQ.	DATE DC	SCHEDULE RATE	DATE					
		PO IM IVPB IVP SQ. R			A.M.					
					SITE					
					P.M.					
					SITE					
		PO IM IVPB IVP SQ. R			A.M.					
					SITE					
					P.M.					
					SITE					
		PO IM IVPB IVP SQ. R			A.M.					
					SITE					
					P.M.					
					SITE					
		PO IM IVPB IVP SQ. R			A.M.					
					SITE					
					P.M.					
					SITE					
		PO IM IVPB IVP SQ. R			A.M.					
					SITE					
					P.M.					
					SITE					
		PO IM IVPB IVP SQ. R			A.M.					
					SITE					
					P.M.					
					SITE					
		PO IM IVPB IVP SQ. R			A.M.					
					SITE					
					P.M.					
					SITE					
		PO IM IVPB IVP SQ. R			A.M.					
					SITE					
					P.M.					
					SITE					
		PO IM IVPB IVP SQ. R			A.M.					
					SITE					
					P.M.					
					SITE					
		PO IM IVPB IVP SQ. R			A.M.					
					SITE					
					P.M.					
					SITE					
					7A					
					7P					

SLASH THROUGH TIME WHEN MEDICATION GIVEN.

CIRCLE MED NOT GIVEN & NOTE REASON:

NPO-FOR SURG/X-RAY REF-REFUSED
N/V-NAUSEA HELD-NOTE REASON

REFER TO MEDICATION SCHEDULE GUIDE TO DETERMINE APPROPRIATE ADMINISTRATION TIMES.

RECOPIED RN:

KEY
INJECTION SITE: (R or L)
D-Deltoid G-Gluteal
A-Abdominal T-Thigh
IC-Iliac Crest

Page ____ of ____

MEDICATION RECORD

☐ **ROUTINE** ☐ **PRN/NOW**

Figure 11–8

writes an order. All changes and cancellations of orders are written here as well. If a nurse takes a telephone or verbal order from the physician, it is recorded here. The doctor will sign those orders on the next visit. There is often a space on the **physician's order form** asking if another brand of drug identical in form and content may be dispensed by the pharmacy. If the doctor concurs, the space is checked.

Once written, doctor's orders are then "transcribed" to other hospital records. These orders guide the care that is given to the patient. The physician's order form serves as a "blueprint" of the care the patient is to receive.

Some of the clerical duties you will soon learn will require you to "take off" or transcribe the doctor's orders. You will then requisition the various tests, medications, procedures, treatments, services, supplies and equipment either by computer or by filling out order forms. (Fig. 11–9.)

Progress Notes

Progress notes contain the recorded observations, impressions, and recommendations of all physicians who examine and treat the patient during the patient's hospitalization. Entries are not always made after each visit by the physician, however, if the patient's condition is unchanged since the previous visit. Most hospitals require that a doctor's note appear on every patient's chart at designated intervals. Learn the regulations as to admission notes, postoperative notes, other progress notes, and discharge notes in effect in your hospital. (Fig. 11–10.)

Clinical Care Notes

The **clinical care notes** chart form is usually used by health care professionals other than doctors or nurses. It may be used by respiratory therapy, physical therapy, occupational therapy, nutrition services, etc. to describe the care and progress given to the patient by personnel from these departments. A supplemental form designed for a specific department may be used instead if available. (Fig. 11–11, pg. 210.)

KEY IDEA: SUPPLEMENTAL CHART FORMS

Supplemental chart forms may or may not be included in the individual patient's chart. Their use will depend on the tests, treatments, and procedures required to treat the patient's specific condition. The details of using supplemental chart forms vary among different hospitals. Learn to use the forms in your hospital. (Fig. 11–12, pg. 211.)

Laboratory Report or Clinical Pathology Record

All hospitals require certain laboratory tests to be performed on every patient admitted. The most common method of reporting the results is for the laboratory to send a computerized printout to the nursing unit. The results are then filed in the patient's chart.

Some hospitals have a system in which test results come back from the laboratory on special slips that are then attached to a type of **laboratory**

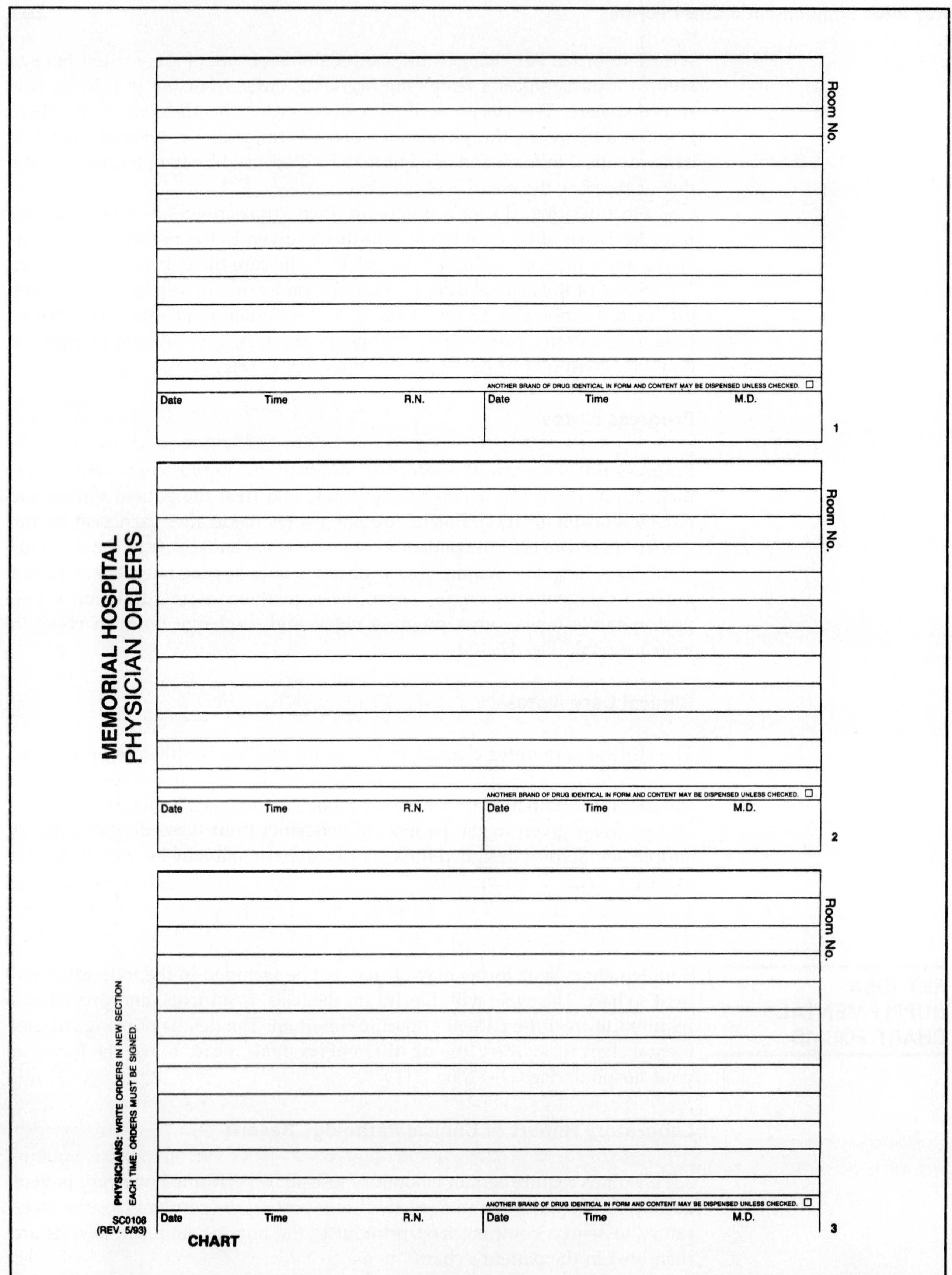
MEMORIAL HOSPITAL
PHYSICIAN ORDERS
Room No.
ANOTHER BRAND OF DRUG IDENTICAL IN FORM AND CONTENT MAY BE DISPENSED UNLESS CHECKED.
Date
Time
R.N.
Date
Time
M.D.
1
Room No.
ANOTHER BRAND OF DRUG IDENTICAL IN FORM AND CONTENT MAY BE DISPENSED UNLESS CHECKED.
Date
Time
R.N.
Date
Time
M.D.
2
Room No.
PHYSICIANS: WRITE ORDERS IN NEW SECTION EACH TIME. ORDERS MUST BE SIGNED.
ANOTHER BRAND OF DRUG IDENTICAL IN FORM AND CONTENT MAY BE DISPENSED UNLESS CHECKED.
SC0108 (REV. 5/93)
Date
Time
R.N.
Date
Time
M.D.
3
CHART

Figure 11–9

NOTE PROGRESS OF CASE, COMPLICATIONS, CONSULTATIONS, CHANGE IN DIAGNOSIS, CONDITION ON DISCHARGE, INSTRUCTIONS TO PATIENT.

DATE/TIME	

MEMORIAL HOSPITAL
PROGRESS NOTES

Figure 11–10

report form. (Fig. 11–13.) Hospitals have an established method for alerting the physician about abnormal test results. This is usually done by the laboratory. You will learn to follow the routine of your hospital before you are asked to post test results into the chart.

Surgical Records

A patient admitted to the hospital for surgery will have many specialized records in his chart before he is discharged. Prior to surgery, an **operation consent** must be signed by the patient, giving the surgeon and his assistants permission to perform the operation and a **consent for anesthesia** explaining the risks of anesthesia and giving consent for the procedure. Other preoperative forms such as a **preoperative check list** and **preanesthesia patient questionnaire** may be included at this time. At least two more records are added in the operating room—one to record the anesthesia given and the general progress of both the operation and the patient during surgery and

NOTE PROGRESS OF CASE, COMPLICATIONS, CONSULTATIONS, CHANGE IN DIAGNOSIS, CONDITION ON DISCHARGE, INSTRUCTIONS TO PATIENT.

DATE	

MEMORIAL HOSPITAL
Clinical Care Notes

Figure 11–11

another record which describes the operative procedures performed. When tissue is removed for laboratory examination, a third record, **surgical pathology,** is added to the chart. In the recovery room, a record is kept of the patient's condition while he is awakening from the anesthetic. This is often called the **post anesthesia care unit (PACU) record.** A **transfusion record** may be necessary for a patient who has received blood before or during the operation.

Special Therapy Records

Sometimes a patient receives special treatments from personnel in other hospital departments. When this occurs, special records are kept of these treatments. Examples of these records are:

- **Respiratory therapy records**—used when a patient has a condition requiring some type of inhalation therapy or pulmonary therapy. (Fig. 11–14, pgs. 213-14.)

SUPPLEMENTAL CHART FORMS

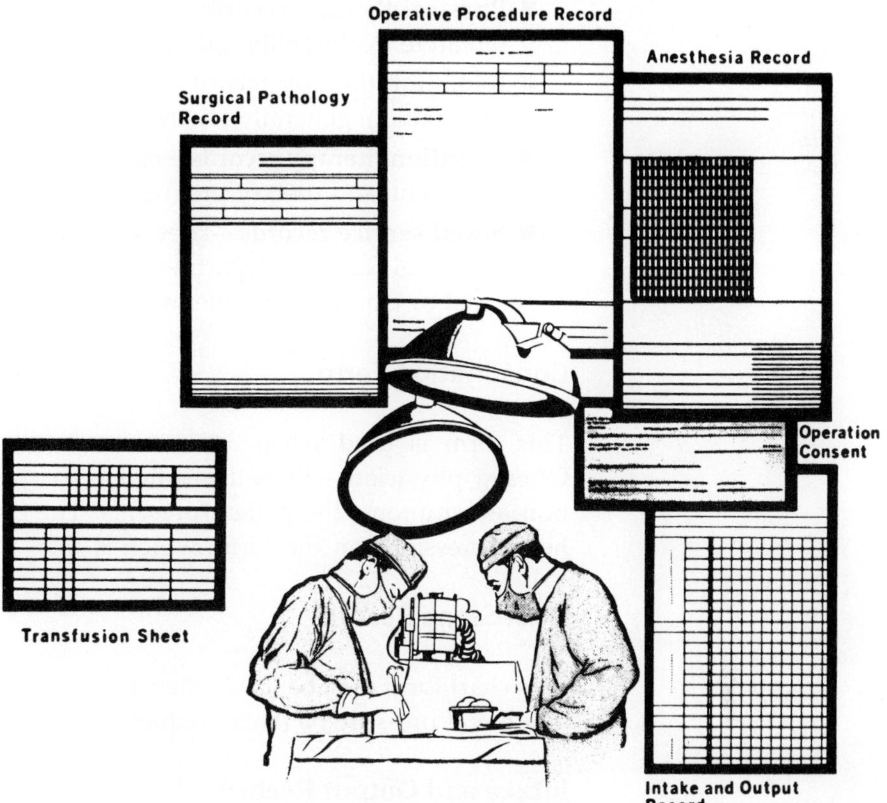

Figure 11–12

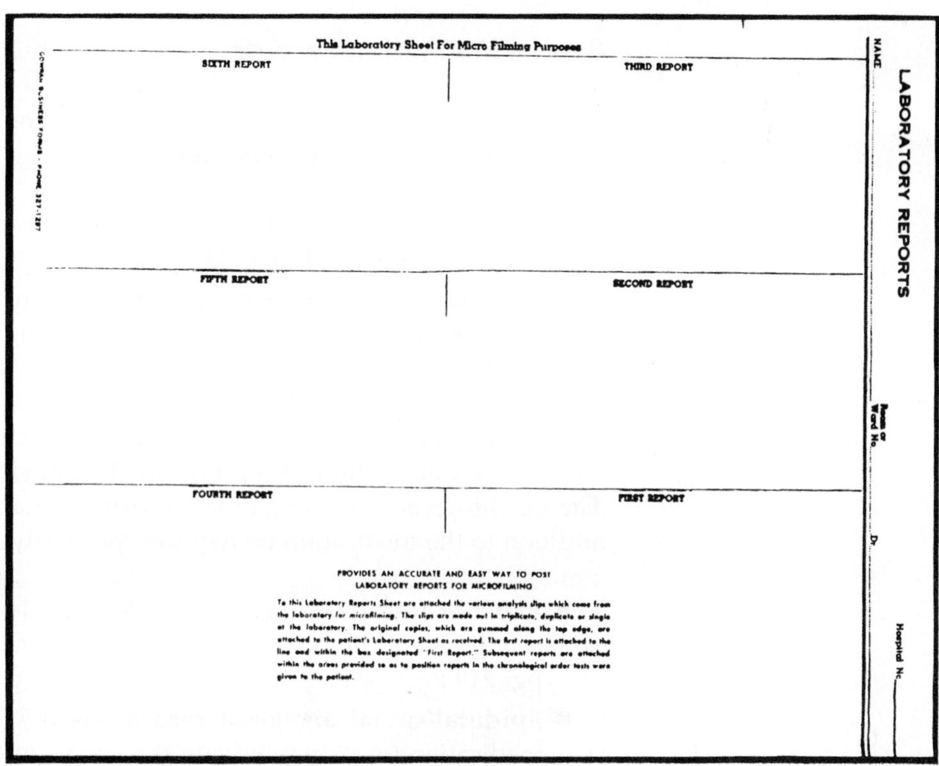

This Laboratory Sheet For Micro Filming Purposes

LABORATORY REPORTS

NAME

SIXTH REPORT	THIRD REPORT
FIFTH REPORT	SECOND REPORT
FOURTH REPORT	FIRST REPORT

Room or Ward No.

Dr.

Hospital No.

PROVIDES AN ACCURATE AND EASY WAY TO POST LABORATORY REPORTS FOR MICROFILMING

To this Laboratory Reports Sheet are attached the various analysis slips which come from the laboratory for microfilming. The slips are made out in triplicate, duplicate or single at the laboratory. The original copies, which are gummed along the top edge, are attached to the patient's Laboratory Sheet as received. The first report is attached to the line and within the box designated "First Report." Subsequent reports are attached within the areas provided so as to position reports in the chronological order tests were given to the patient.

Figure 11–13

- **Physical therapy records**—used when the patient is undergoing rehabilitative treatment because of injury or disease. (Fig. 11–15, pg. 215.)
- **Radiation therapy records**—used for patients who are receiving doses of radiation, generally for the purpose of killing cancerous cells.
- **Nutrition therapy records**—used to record a patient's nutritional status, treatment, and dietary progress.
- **Social service records**—kept on a patient being seen by personnel from the Social Services Department, who work to help patients adjust to personal or emotional problems brought on by illness.

Consultation Form

This form is used when a physician wants advice from another doctor. Often a physician will be consulted who specializes in the type of condition or symptoms the patient presents. The consulting doctor records his or her impressions on the form, which is then included in the patient's chart.

Vital Signs Record

This chart form may be used when a patient's condition requires that his TPR and blood pressure be taken frequently. (Fig. 11–16, pg. 216.)

Intake and Output Record

This form is used to measure all fluids taken into the body and all fluids leaving the body. (Fig. 11–17, pg. 217.)

Special Medication Records

Special records are kept when a patient is being given a particular type of medication. Some examples include:

- **Diabetic record**—used when a patient is receiving insulin and is being carefully monitored. (Fig. 11–18, pg. 218.)
- **Anticoagulant record**—used when a patient is receiving medications to keep the blood from clotting and is being carefully monitored. (Fig. 11–19, pg. 218.)

The anticoagulant record is used when a patient is taking medication such as Heparin or Coumadin to keep his blood from clotting as readily as normal. The insulin record contains much information about the diabetic patient in addition to the medication he requires, primarily insulin.

- **Patient-controlled analgesia (PCA) record**—used when a patient is receiving self-administered pain medication intravenously. (Fig. 11–20, pg. 219.)
- **Epidural/spinal analgesia record**—used when a patient is receiving medication for pain relief into the spaces of the spinal cord. (Fig. 11–21, pg. 220.)

RESPIRATORY THERAPY DEPARTMENT

Care Plan Date:________________ Ed Log Date:________________ Eval Due Date:________________

Date	HHN IS CPT/PD AERO	MODE MP MASK Blowby TRACH	Objective Complete ❑	MEDICATION ___ cc	Pulse 1. ___	Duration	Position HF ___ SF ___ LF ___	PEF 1.	❑ Cough ❑ Suction	SPUTUM Vol. ___	Adverse Reaction ❑ NO ❑ YES
Time			72° Eval ❑	___ cc ___ cc	2. ___ Resp. Rate	Volumes	___	PEF 2.	❑ Productive ❑ Non-Prod.	Vis. ___ Color ___	
Missed TX___	Initial s/u ❑	Circuit Δ ❑	Care Plan ❑ Ed Log ❑	___ ___ cc Nacl	1. ___ 2. ___	CPT: RUL RML RLL LUL LLL		Breath Sounds: ā ___ p̄ ___			

COMMENTS:

SIGNATURE:

Date	HHN IS CPT/PD AERO	MODE MP MASK Blowby TRACH	Objective Complete ❑	MEDICATION ___ cc	Pulse 1. ___	Duration	Position HF ___ SF ___ LF ___	PEF 1.	❑ Cough ❑ Suction	SPUTUM Vol. ___	Adverse Reaction ❑ NO ❑ YES
Time			72° Eval ❑	___ cc ___ cc	2. ___ Resp. Rate	Volumes	___	PEF 2.	❑ Productive ❑ Non-Prod.	Vis. ___ Color ___	
Missed TX___	Initial s/u ❑	Circuit Δ ❑	Care Plan ❑ Ed Log ❑	___ ___ cc Nacl	1. ___ 2. ___	CPT: RUL RML RLL LUL LLL		Breath Sounds: ā ___ p̄ ___			

COMMENTS:

SIGNATURE:

Date	HHN IS CPT/PD AERO	MODE MP MASK Blowby TRACH	Objective Complete ❑	MEDICATION ___ cc	Pulse 1. ___	Duration	Position HF ___ SF ___ LF ___	PEF 1.	❑ Cough ❑ Suction	SPUTUM Vol. ___	Adverse Reaction ❑ NO ❑ YES
Time			72° Eval ❑	___ cc ___ cc	2. ___ Resp. Rate	Volumes	___	PEF 2.	❑ Productive ❑ Non-Prod.	Vis. ___ Color ___	
Missed TX___	Initial s/u ❑	Circuit Δ ❑	Care Plan ❑ Ed Log ❑	___ ___ cc Nacl	1. ___ 2. ___	CPT: RUL RML RLL LUL LLL		Breath Sounds: ā ___ p̄ ___			

COMMENTS:

SIGNATURE:

Date	HHN IS CPT/PD AERO	MODE MP MASK Blowby TRACH	Objective Complete ❑	MEDICATION ___ cc	Pulse 1. ___	Duration	Position HF ___ SF ___ LF ___	PEF 1.	❑ Cough ❑ Suction	SPUTUM Vol. ___	Adverse Reaction ❑ NO ❑ YES
Time			72° Eval ❑	___ cc ___ cc	2. ___ Resp. Rate	Volumes	___	PEF 2.	❑ Productive ❑ Non-Prod.	Vis. ___ Color ___	
Missed TX___	Initial s/u ❑	Circuit Δ ❑	Care Plan ❑ Ed Log ❑	___ ___ cc Nacl	1. ___ 2. ___	CPT: RUL RML RLL LUL LLL		Breath Sounds: ā ___ p̄ ___			

COMMENTS:

SIGNATURE:

Date	HHN IS CPT/PD AERO	MODE MP MASK Blowby TRACH	Objective Complete ❑	MEDICATION ___ cc	Pulse 1. ___	Duration	Position HF ___ SF ___ LF ___	PEF 1.	❑ Cough ❑ Suction	SPUTUM Vol. ___	Adverse Reaction ❑ NO ❑ YES
Time			72° Eval ❑	___ cc ___ cc	2. ___ Resp. Rate	Volumes	___	PEF 2.	❑ Productive ❑ Non-Prod.	Vis. ___ Color ___	
Missed TX___	Initial s/u ❑	Circuit Δ ❑	Care Plan ❑ Ed Log ❑	___ ___ cc Nacl	1. ___ 2. ___	CPT: RUL RML RLL LUL LLL		Breath Sounds: ā ___ p̄ ___			

COMMENTS:

SIGNATURE:

MEMORIAL HOSPITAL
RESPIRATORY THERAPY TREATMENT RECORD

Figure 11–14a

Respiratory Therapy Continuous Flow Sheet

Date	Time	Physician's Orders

Date	Time	Cool/Htd Aerosol	Mask	NC	F102	Pulse Oximeter Sa 0_2	COMMENTS

MEMORIAL HOSPITAL

Figure 11–14b

DIAGNOSIS	
M.D. ORDERS	
REFERRING M.D.	CHIEF COMPLAINT
HISTORY	
TEST RESULTS/MED	COGNITION
PREVIOUS FUNCTION LEVEL	
SOCIAL HISTORY	

PRESENT FUNCTIONAL LEVEL

_____ BED MOBILITY
_____ SIT TO STAND
_____ BED TO CHAIR/COMMODE
_____DISTANCE
_____ SUPINE TO SIT
_____ STATIC STANDING BALANCE
_____ AMBULATION LEVEL SURFACE
_____ ASSISTIVE DEVICE
_____ STATIC SITTING BALANCE
_____ DYNAMIC STANDING BALANCE
_____ STAIRS
OTHER _________
_____ DYNAMIC SITTING BALANCE

KEY:

N	= NORMAL	*	= LIMITED BY PAIN
G	= GOOD	MIN	= MINIMAL ASSIST
F	= FAIR	MOD	= MODERATE ASSIST
P	= POOR	MAX	= MAXIMAL ASSIST
I	= INDEPENDENT	U	= UNABLE
S	= SUPERVISED	NT	= NOT TESTED
C	= CONTACT GUARD		

STRENGTH
(0 - 5)

ROM: WITHIN NORMAL LIMITS	LIMITATIONS	ABNORMAL MOTOR FINDINGS (INCLUDING TONE, COORDINATION, ETC.)
LUE		
RUE		
LLE		
RLE		
TRUNK		
OTHER		

MEMORIAL HOSPITAL
PHYSICAL THERAPY
INITIAL EVALUATION PAGE 1 of 2

Figure 11–15

MEMORIAL HOSPITAL V.S. CHECKLIST						
DATE	TIME	ARM B.P.	PULSE	RESP.	TEMPERATURE	LEVEL OF CONSCIOUSNESS

Figure 11–16

There are many supplemental chart forms. The preceding examples will help you recognize some of the more common types used in your hospital.

CHARTING RESPONSIBILITIES

KEY IDEA: CONFIDENTIALITY AND THE PATIENT'S CHART

In your work with patients' charts, you will have access to information of a very personal nature. Always remember that this information, as well as all data related to the patient's medical condition, *must* be kept confidential. You are not permitted to reveal this information to the patient or to his visitors, nor should you discuss it with your fellow workers or friends. You may only discuss the patient's chart with hospital personnel who are directly involved with the care of that patient. Charts are the legal property of the hospital. It is the health unit coordinator's responsibility to protect all charts and the information they contain from loss, damage, alteration, or use by unauthorized persons.

Information in the chart cannot be released to another physician without written consent of the admitting doctor. Charts can be inspected at any time by court order and can be removed from a hospital only if requested by court order.

Members of the nursing and medical staff will have occasion to inspect or record in the charts. As a health unit coordinator, in fairly constant attendance at the desk, you will be expected to keep track of the charts which are used by others. Always remember to do the following:

FLUID / ELECT. / NUTRITION

Date: ______

IV SOLUTION / RATE — PUMP
A. ______ ❑
B. ______ ❑
C. ______ ❑
D. ______ ❑
I.V. Site ______ ❑

TUBE FEEDING SOLUTION — PUMP — TUBE FDG. BAG CHANGE — TIME
______ ❑ ❑ ______
______ ❑ ❑ ______

N/G TUBE TYPE: ______ DATE LAST B.M.: ______
PLACEMENT VERIFIED: ______ SUCTION: N Y LIS LCS

TIME	PO	KEY (Credit / Absorbed) TUBE FEEDING	INTAKE IV Solutions – Absorbed					TOTAL INTAKE	OUTPUT URINE	NG	IRRIG	B.M.	O.B.	TOTAL OUTPUT
0700														
0800														
0900														
1000														
1100														
1200														
1300														
1400														
8-HR TOTAL														
1500														
1600														
1700														
1800														
1900														
2000														
2100														
2200														
8-HR TOTAL														
2300														
2400														
0100														
0200														
0300														
0400														
0500														
0600														
8-HR TOTAL														
24-HR TOTAL														

7A SIGNATURE ______
3P SIGNATURE ______
11P SIGNATURE ______

FLUID RESTRICTION? Y N
24° Amount:

DAILY MEASUREMENT

ADMISSION WEIGHT	DIET TYPE Breakfast % | Lunch % | Dinner % | Snacks
TODAY'S WEIGHT ST. CH. BED	

MEMORIAL HOSPITAL
INTAKE-OUTPUT

Figure 11–17

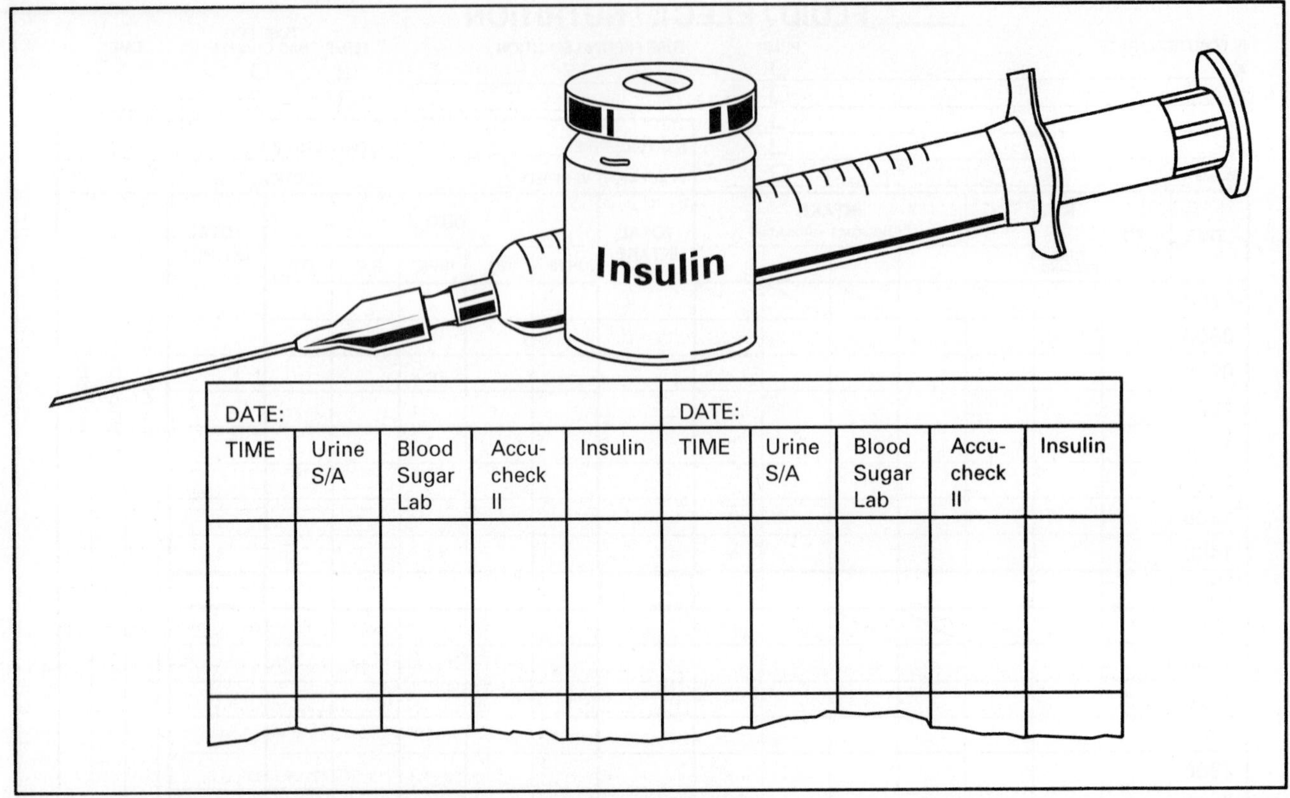

DATE:					DATE:				
TIME	Urine S/A	Blood Sugar Lab	Accu-check II	Insulin	TIME	Urine S/A	Blood Sugar Lab	Accu-check II	Insulin

Figure 11–18

ANTICOAGULANT RECORD

DATE	PROTHROMBIN X	COUMADIN	HEPARIN	PTT

Figure 11–19

- Replace all charts in the rack after use.
- Take care to replace the chart in its designated position in the chart rack.
- Keep a written record of all charts removed from the general nurses' station area by medical personnel.
- Before reporting off-duty each day, check to see that all charts are at the nurses' station, in the rack, or in use.

KEY IDEA: ROUTINE CHART CHECKS

Now that you are familiar with the chart forms used in your hospital you are ready to learn what facts to look for in all patients' charts at specified intervals throughout the day.

PCA

Date:____________________

Drug:____ Concentration: ____________________

Time	# DOSES Given	# DOSES Attempted	Clinician Activated Bolus (mg)	Total GIVEN (mg)	Assessment: LOC	Assessment: Respiratory Rate / Quality	Assessment: Level of Pain	Assessment: Side Effects
7-8								
8-9								
9-10								
10-11								
11-12								
12-13								
13-14								
14-15								
Total								
15-16								
16-17								
17-18								
18-19								
19-20								
20-21								
21-22								
22-23								
Total								
23-24								
24-01								
01-02								
02-03								
03-04								
04-05								
05-06								
06-07								
Total								
24 Hr Total								

TIME	AMT. IN SYRINGE	SIGNATURES IN	OUT
7A			
3P			
11P			
SYRINGE/CHANGE:			

DOSAGE/CHANGES TIME:

Drug:

Incremental Dose (mg)

Basal Rate (   )

One Hour Limit

ASSESSMENT

Before and after the first dose, then
Every hour X 4 hours, then
Every 2 hours X 4, then
Every 4 hours until PCA discontinued
or as ordered
PRN as indicated
- Level of consciousness
- Respiratory rate & quality
- Level of pain
- Side effects
- IV Site check every shift

LEVEL OF CONSCIOUSNESS CODE

1. awake
2. drowsy, dozing intermittently
3. only awakens when aroused
4. difficult to awaken / lethargic
5. non-responsive

RESPIRATORY QUALITY CODE

S - Shallow   A - Absent
O - Obstructive   NL - Normal

LEVEL OF PAIN

1-10
Scale

SIDE EFFECTS CODE

1. Nausea
2. Vomiting
3. Pruritius
4. Respiratory depression
5. Urinary Retention
6. Other

MEMORIAL HOSPITAL
PCA FLOW SHEET

Figure 11–20

EPIDURAL/SPINAL
Analgesia

Date: ____________________

Drug: ____________________ Concentration: ____________________

Time	Continuous RATE (ml/hr)	Clinician Activated Bolus (ml)	Total GIVEN (ml)	Assessment: LOC	Assessment: Respiratory Rate / Quality	Assessment: Level of Pain	Assessment: Side Effects
7-8							
8-9							
9-10							
10-11							
11-12							
12-13							
13-14							
14-15							
Total							
15-16							
16-17							
17-18							
18-19							
19-20							
20-21							
21-22							
22-23							
Total							
23-24							
24-01							
01-02							
02-03							
03-04							
04-05							
05-06							
06-07							
Total							
24 Hr Total							

TIME	AMT. IN BAG ML	SIGNATURES IN	SIGNATURES OUT
7A			
3P			
11P			
BAG CHANGE:			

DOSAGE/CHANGES

Continuous Dose (ml/hr)

Titrate from to ml/hr

Bolus Dose (ml)

Accelerated Infusion Dose

ASSESSMENT

Level of consciousness qh
Respiratory rate & quality qh
Level of pain as indicated
Side effects as indicated
Site check every shift

LEVEL OF CONSCIOUSNESS CODE

1. awake
2. drowsy, dozing intermittently
3. only awakens when aroused
4. difficult to awaken / lethargic
5. non-responsive

RESPIRATORY QUALITY CODE

S - Shallow A - Absent
O - Obstructive NL - Normal

LEVEL OF PAIN

1-10 Scale

SIDE EFFECTS CODE

1. Nausea
2. Vomiting
3. Pruritius
4. Urinary Retention
5. Other__________

ADDITIONAL COMMENTS: __________

MEMORIAL HOSPITAL
EPIDURAL FLOW SHEET

Figure 11–21

- All forms included in the chart must be checked to be sure that the patient's name and unit number are entered correctly.
- Each chart must be checked for the proper sequence of pages.
- Each chart must be reviewed for forms that are completed; new forms must be stamped properly and added to the chart as necessary.
- All charts belonging to new admissions must be checked routinely for inclusion of laboratory reports and completed medical history and physical examinations. If any reports have been omitted, appropriate personnel should be requested to supply the missing information.
- All preoperative charts must be checked on the morning of surgery to make certain all prescribed laboratory tests have been completed and the results posted in the chart. They are also checked for inclusion of blank surgical records.
- Charts must be reviewed periodically to see that "progress notes" have been recorded at required intervals. If any of these have been omitted, physicians responsible must be notified.
- Doctor's "order sheets" from all charts must be reviewed frequently for orders that need transcription and for orders calling for requisitions.

KEY IDEA: RULES OF CHARTING

Four basic rules should guide all the charting you do, not only on patients' charts, but on other hospital forms as well.

1. **Recording information on charts must be done accurately.** Data recorded incorrectly can lead physicians to wrong conclusions about their patients. Treatments ordered on the basis of incorrect conclusions can significantly retard or otherwise affect the patients' medical progress. You must not be responsible for errors of this sort. **BE ACCURATE.**
2. **Your handwriting must be neat and legible.** If a doctor or nurse is unable to read what has been recorded, both your time and theirs has been wasted: **WRITE LEGIBLY.**
3. **The patient's chart is considered a legal document.** It can be admitted as evidence in a court of law in the case of a suit against the hospital or

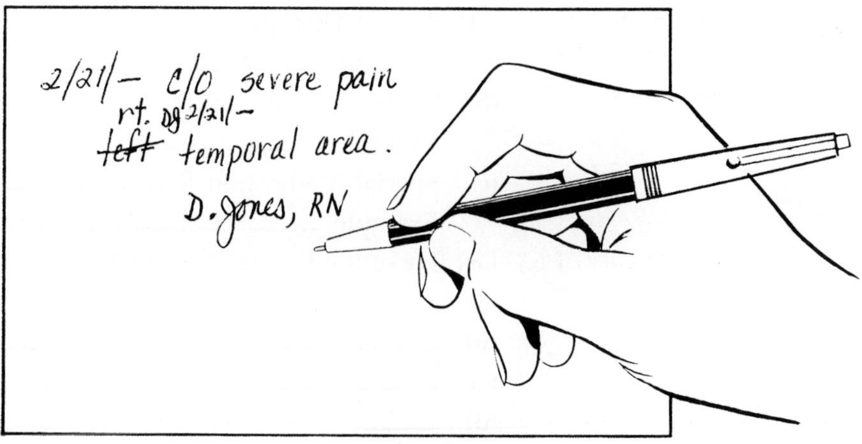

Figure 11–22

physician. Any chart with erasures will not be admitted as legal evidence: **DO NOT ERASE.** Despite all precautions, recording errors will occasionally be made. One accepted way to make corrections is to draw a single line through the error, write in the correction, initial and date. Some hospitals will want the word error written as well. (Fig. 11–22.)

4. To further strengthen the status of chart records in court as legal documents, hospital regulations require that all recording be done in ink. **WRITE ALL ENTRIES IN INK.**

LEARNING ACTIVITIES

Complete the following:

1. Define:
   (a) Chart holder or chart back ____________________.
   (b) Chart rack ____________________.
   (c) Chart ____________________.
   (d) Unit number ____________________.
   (e) "Old" chart ____________________.
   (f) Splitting or thinning ____________________.
2. List the purposes of the chart.
   (a) ____________________.
   (b) ____________________.
   (c) ____________________.
3. In keeping track of the charts always remember to do the following:
   (a) ____________________.
   (b) ____________________.
   (c) ____________________.
   (d) ____________________.
4. Before use, each chart form must be ____________________.
5. Define and give an example of each of the following categories of supplemental chart forms.
   (a) Special Therapy Records ____________________.
   Example ____________________.
   (b) Surgical Records ____________________.
   Example ____________________.
   (c) Special Medication Records ____________________.
   Example ____________________.
6. List five of the Routine Chart Checks.
   (a) ____________________.
   (b) ____________________.
   (c) ____________________.
   (d) ____________________.
   (e) ____________________.

Match the standard chart forms in the left column with the definitions in the right.

Column A	*Column B*
(a) Doctor's order sheet	____ X-ray reports
(b) Progress notes	____ Nurses' communication with doctor
(c) Nurses' notes	____ Face sheet
(d) Graphic chart	____ Laboratory test results
(e) Summary sheet	____ Inhalation therapy reports
(f) Clinical pathology report	____ Regular medications
(g) Medication record	____ "Blueprint" of care
(h) Surgical records	____ Operative consent
(i) Special therapy records	____ TPR
(j) Diagnostic examination	____ Recorded observations of physician

CHAPTER 12

The Health Unit Coordinator and Computers

OBJECTIVES

When you complete this chapter, you will be able to:

- List and describe types of computers.
- List the basic components of all computer systems.
- Identify the single technology that has contributed to the growth of computerization.
- Identify input devices.
- Identify output devices.
- Name the working unit of the computer system.
- Describe what computers do.
- Name the functions of computers in hospital patient care areas.
- Identify the most important computer key.
- Describe possible ethical concerns of using computers in hospitals.
- Recognize computer terminology.
- List rules of computer confidentiality.

INTRODUCTION

Computers have been used in some hospital departments for many years. For example, Central Supply has used them to keep track of inventories and the Accounting Department to itemize statements sent to patients or prepare paychecks for employees. It was only a matter of time before the computer appeared in the patient care areas, and today computers are widely used there. There is no doubt that health unit coordinators entering the job market today will encounter a computer in their job environment.

The health unit coordinator is a primary operator of the computer system in the patient care area. Computers are designed to help you do your job more efficiently, consistently, and easily. Computers soon lose their mystique as you learn what they can do, what they can't do, and how you can operate them.

KEY IDEA: GLOSSARY OF COMPUTER TERMS

- **Cathode ray tube (CRT)**—viewing screen
- **Central processing unit**—working unit of the computer, "the brain"
- **Command**—user's instruction to tell the computer to process information
- **Cursor**—flashing indicator that denotes where information input will begin
- **Debug**—remove problems in a computer program that keep it from working
- **Enter key**—key that gives the computer the command to process information
- **Ergonomics**—the science of fitting a job to workers' physical and psychological needs in terms of their bodily position and ability to see in relation to the equipment they are using. This is done to make the work safer and more comfortable for the worker.
- **Hard copy**—printed page of computer information
- **Input**—to enter information into computer
- **Keyboard**—computer typewriter
- **Light pen**—input device that looks like a pencil but is capable of sensing information typed on screen
- **Machine language**—the computer's language, comprised of binary digits. Does not require translation to work.
- **Mainframe**—the largest of all computers. Capable of performing multiple tasks at rapid speeds.
- **Menu**—list of computer functions available
- **Microcomputer**—the smallest of computers. Also called a personal computer.
- **Minicomputer**—a medium-size computer that is capable of stand-alone functions or auxiliary to a mainframe
- **Monitor**—viewing screen or CRT
- **Mouse**—a device used for data input that serves as a pointer and moves the cursor around the screen so that different items may be selected
- **On-line**—used to identify that computer is being used
- **Output**—what comes out of the computer as processed information
- **Password**—secret code that allows access to a computer system
- **Program**—instructions given to computer that cause it to perform functions
- **Terminal**—computer station that is capable of sending and receiving information to the mainframe via telephone lines

KEY IDEA: COMPUTERS IN GENERAL

Since the 1950s, computer technology has seen growth at an unbelievable rate. The early computers were comprised of vacuum tubes and required large, environmentally controlled rooms. Even then they often overheated and became inoperable for many hours. Repairing them was time consuming. Large systems were very expensive, and only the largest organizations were able to afford them. Today's computers are comprised of large-scale-integration (LSI) devices or microprocessor chips that are often as small as ⅛ inch square. Each LSI allows thousands of microscopic electronic circuits to be crowded together to do what tons of equipment did in the early years. This technology has allowed computers to become smaller, more powerful, and less expensive.

Today, computers come in three basic sizes: small, medium, and large. The small computers, known as **microcomputers** or personal computers, have become very popular with individuals who have learned they can be helpful to them in organizing their work at home or in a small business. Schools have introduced the microcomputer into the curriculum from elementary grades through high school. Such computers are self-contained and can do all of the things a larger computer can do but on a limited scale. They are easy to use, just like typing on a typewriter. Programs have been written for the microcomputer that can be used by anyone, even without knowledge of programming or how the computer works. Microcomputers can even connect with larger computer systems over telephone lines with a device called a modem. (Fig. 12–1.)

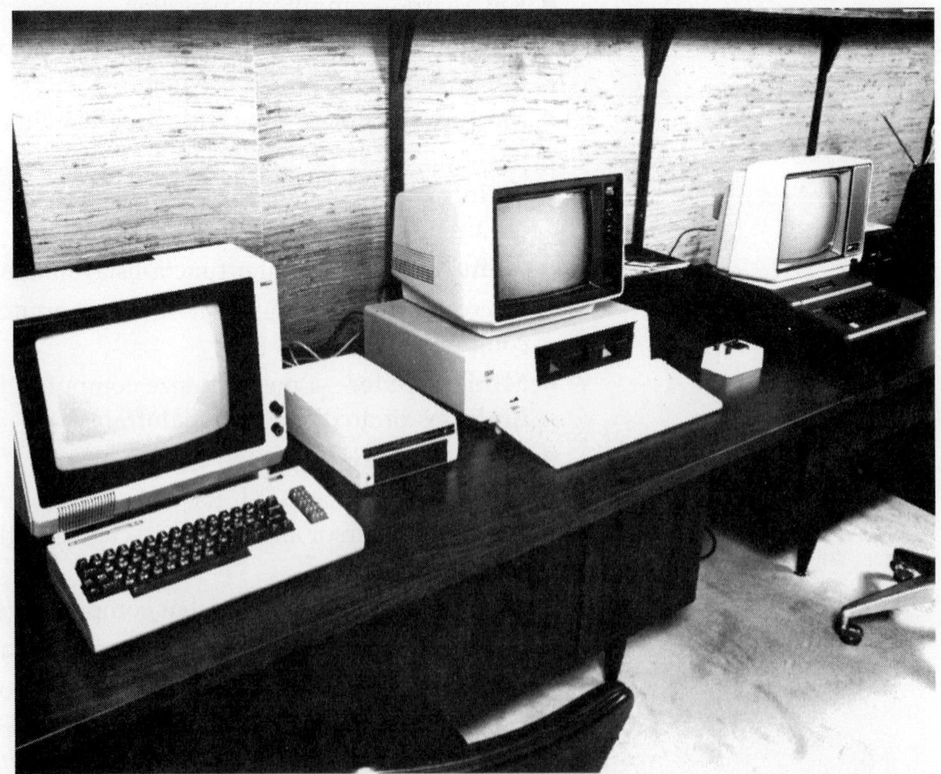

Figure 12–1

The medium-sized computer is called the **minicomputer.** The minicomputer is a desktop or stand-alone computer that is capable of processing data like a large computer but does not need a special environmentally controlled room or heavy electrical wiring. They were first used for a specific or predefined function such as a front-end machine in data-entry editing but today have become complete data-base systems or main systems. Minicomputers operate on high-level languages within their system and are not dependent on the larger system.

The largest of all the computer systems is called a **mainframe system.** It is capable of processing large amounts of information at unbelievable speeds. Mainframe computer systems can access information from auxiliary storage devices as well as send information to other computers or terminals located in remote sites. Most large organizations have their own mainframe computer; some smaller businesses "purchase" computer time from the large organizations.

In the hospital, you will most likely be working on a minicomputer system that may or may not be connected to a mainframe system or on a remote terminal connected to a minicomputer or a mainframe system. Regardless of the system, operating it is basically the same.

BASIC COMPUTER SYSTEM

Whether you operate a small microcomputer or interact with a large mainframe computer, you are working on a computer system with three basic components. All computers must have a means to "input" information, a means to "process" information, and a means to "output" information.

KEY IDEA: INPUT

There are several ways to put information into the computer. The most common one used by the health unit coordinator is the **keyboard.** The keyboard looks like a typewriter with the exception of a few extra keys. One key plays a very important function—the **ENTER** key. When you are finished putting your information into the computer, you must signal the computer "I'm done, now it's your turn." You do this with the ENTER key. Some computer companies color this key red because of its importance. It is not absolutely necessary to have typing skills to operate the computer keyboard; however, being familiar with the keyboard will help you develop computer keyboard skill. (Fig. 12–2.)

A second common input device is the **light pen.** The light pen looks like a pencil, but it is designed to sense the writing on the computer screen. The operator selects a choice, moves the light pen across the choice and then across the ENTER statement. The information is entered into the computer's processing unit.

A **mouse** is an input device used for pointing that moves the cursor around the screen so that a selection can be made from items listed on the screen. The **cursor** (flashing light or lighted mark of some sort) is a symbol that indicates where the user is on the screen. It takes some practice to become competent at using a mouse. The clicking of mouse buttons and

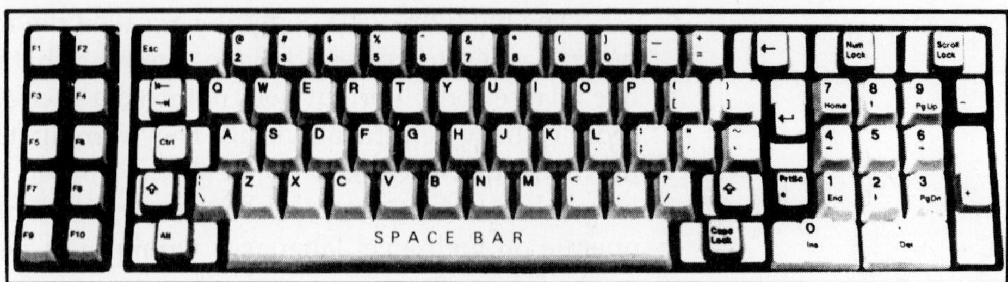

Figure 12–2

movements of the mouse elicit various commands and require some eye-hand coordination.

Other input devices of computer systems include keypunch cards, floppy diskettes, or magnetic disks or tapes. These become storage devices of the hospital computer system and are "behind the scene" of the health unit coordinator using the computer. Stored information must be retrieved from the computer and input with current information. This is usually not done at the keyboard of a hospital system.

KEY IDEA: PROCESS

A computer processes information that is input to it and returns that processed information to the person putting it in or to someone else in another department. This **Central Processing Unit (CPU)** is the working unit of the computer and often consists of many electronic components and microchips. The computer performs its processing function in computer or machine language based on arithmetic logic. It is given instructions to do a specific task in a program. The person using the computer does not have to understand the computer's language nor the program in detail but must understand the commands the computer needs to initiate its functions. The processing unit can only process information it receives; if it receives wrong information, it processes wrong information. So it is very important for the health unit coordinator to input only correct information. So far computers have not been designed to "think" as we do, they just process information in a logical, rapid, and consistently accurate manner.

KEY IDEA: OUTPUT

What goes in must come out. Such is also true for computers. Just as there are several ways to put information into the computer, there are several ways to get it out. The most common ways are **visually on the monitor** or **video screen** and **printed copy via a printer.** The health unit coordinator will work with these two methods equally. A monitor or video screen is also called a **cathode ray tube or CRT.** It looks much like a television. As you input information, the information can be seen on the screen of the monitor. When it is processed, it returns to you and can be seen on the screen. Information that is stored can also be called to the screen. If you need a printed copy of the results of the processing, a printer is used to type information on paper. Information printed on paper is called **hard copy** and can be subsequently filed with the patient's record. Information can also be output to keypunch cards, floppy diskettes, or magnetic disks or tapes. In these cases, you would need to request to see this information on your screen or printer. (Fig. 12–3.)

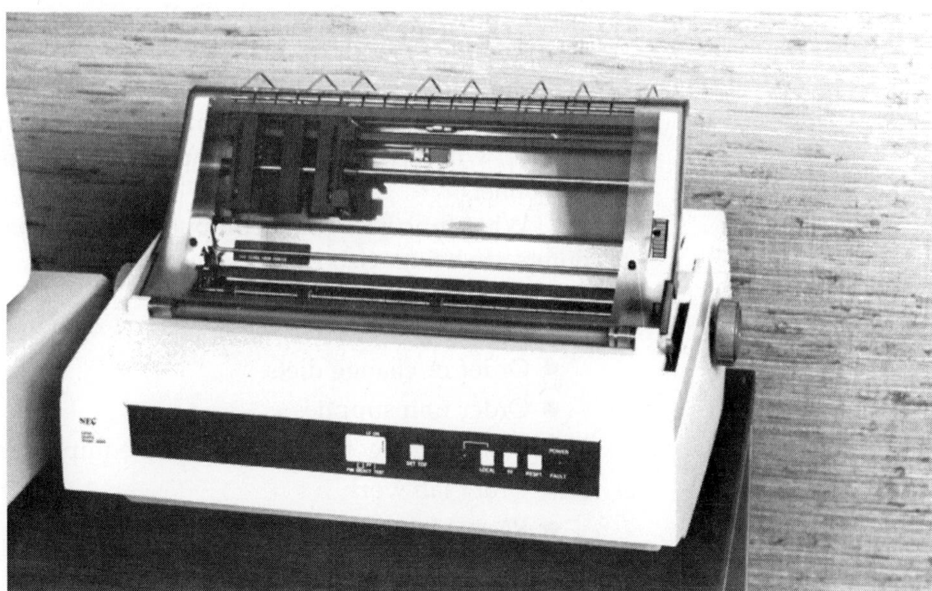

Figure 12–3 Printer.

There is no mystery in the computer. Information to be used must first be input, it is then processed via electronic components in arithmetic logic, and it is returned as output. The health unit coordinator will be involved in inputting information and receiving the output for the patient's record.

WHAT COMPUTERS DO IN HOSPITALS

By now you are aware that hospitals process information (i.e., records, charges, charts, supplies, and files). Today virtually all accounting and purchasing functions are done with computers. Some hospitals even have computer diagnostic services where individuals can have their complete physical examination analyzed by a computer and be told the results at the end of the examination. Depending upon the hospital and its needs, the hospital may either own its own computer system or purchase computer services. It may design its own program to meet its needs or purchase a computer system from a supplier of programs. Computers are widely used in patient care areas as well as in accounting and purchasing. The health unit coordinator has become a processor of information via the computer. Using a computer helps health unit coordinators with their job responsibilities, cuts down the required writing and potential errors, and increases the speed with which orders can be carried out.

KEY IDEA: COMMON SYSTEMS IN PATIENT CARE AREAS

It is not possible to describe each computer system that may be found in the hospital, since many companies have designed systems. Some of the systems today are IBM, EDS, SMS, TDS, and Med-Pro. Computer systems can be designed solely for one hospital, or they can be designed with general applications to a variety of hospitals. Much research goes into selecting a computer system. Putting a hospital "on-line" can often take months or years. Problems often develop that have to be worked out. This process is called **debugging.**

Those individuals who work with the system often develop new skills in identifying computer problem areas and can be very helpful to the computer department. The department in the hospital responsible for computers is often called **Information Systems.** It is staffed with specialists in computer science, who often plan and implement the computer training of hospital personnel.

What functions can a computer perform in the patient care area? Computers are being used to:

- Order medications
- Order or change diets
- Order unit supplies
- Process charges for nursing care equipment
- Order lab work
- Record lab results for patient records
- Schedule x-rays, special tests, or surgery
- Process discharges

Computers can obtain a census listing names of patients, room numbers, bed assignments, and conditions. They can transfer patients to another unit and even send appropriate departments a message of the change (e.g., pharmacy, the business office, and dietary). They can print out a complete record of all the patient's orders since admission. Computer systems can even print routine preparation or procedure orders that can be used to instruct patients or notify a department with a sound when a stat request has been ordered or a stat report is available. If this list sounds like what you do, you are correct. Remember, we said computers process information. (Fig. 12–4.)

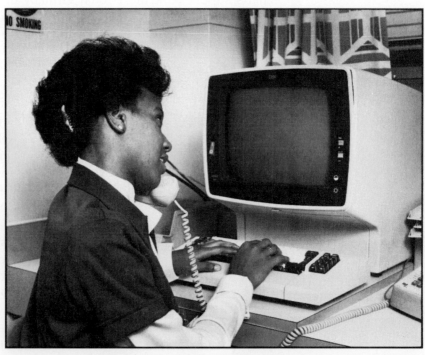

Figure 12–4

KEY IDEA: THE HEALTH UNIT COORDINATOR AND THE COMPUTER

In many of the tasks you will be performing, you will be using the computer. There are some general skills you can learn now that will be useful regardless of the computer system you must use. If you have a computer in your school, you should practice these skills.

1. Signing on
2. Cursor movement
3. Entering data
4. Verifying orders
5. Inquiring about orders
6. Correcting mistakes
7. Deleting orders
8. Notifying other departments
9. Contingency planning

Signing On

Although a computer is easy to operate, access is limited to special persons. When you have been cleared, you will be given a security ID and/or a password. It will identify you as an eligible user of the computer. This should never be given to anyone.

Most systems require a sequence of operations to sign on. You will learn the required sequence for your hospital's sytem. When requested, enter your security ID and/or password. When you have completed your sign-on (if it is correct), you will see a "menu" displayed, showing all of the possible requests you can make of the computer. Both a main menu and submenus are available.

Cursor Movement

Somewhere on the screen you will see a flashing indicator called a **cursor,** which identifies the starting point of your request. The cursor can be moved right and left or up and down. When an order is sent to the computer, the cursor will automatically reset itself to the point where you will begin to enter an order. You should practice moving the cursor around the screen.

Entering Data

The most important key on the computer keyboard is the enter key. Once you have selected the function you wish the computer to perform, you must press the ENTER key. This signals the computer processor to process your order. If you use a light pen, you must pass the pen over the ENTER command. THE COMPUTER AWAITS YOUR COMMAND; YOU ARE IN CONTROL! If you make a spelling or a selection error, it can be easily corrected with cursor movement prior to entering your order. You should always check what you have typed to be sure it is correct. Once you press ENTER, the computer tries to process your order. If it does not recognize the request, it will tell you so; if it recognizes the request it will process it, even if it is wrong. For example, you request a barium enema procedure for a patient. In typing your order you spell "barium" as "bareum." The computer will not recognize the spelling and will tell you so. If you request a barium enema when a barium swallow is really wanted, the computer will schedule the barium enema. REMEMBER, IT IS POSSIBLE TO CORRECT ERRORS EVEN AFTER THEY ARE ENTERED.

Inquiring about Orders

Requesting "order inquiry" will allow you to see all orders or orders placed on a certain day (like today). You can trace orders to see where they were lost. You can even learn the identification of the person who entered the order as well as if another department placed an order. This function also allows you to perform a similar inquiry order to allow you to locate patients by their name should a visitor be looking for someone in the hospital.

Correcting Mistakes

All computer systems have ways to correct mistakes. There is one procedure to use prior to entering the order, such as cursor movement and backspace, and another after the order has been entered such as deleting orders. You will want to become familiar with both of these ways. Some computers use order verification, a second ENTER step, to allow a review of the order to be sure it is correct.

Verifying Orders

After an order has been placed, the request will appear on the screen. If the information is correct, you should press the ENTER key. If it is not correct, correct it at this time. When you have entered all orders, you can request an inquiry of the orders as another check.

Deleting Orders

If, after you have entered an order, you find it is not correct, you can request that the computer delete the order. This command is also used when an order is canceled, such as when a new medication is ordered and the old one is no longer needed.

Notifying Other Departments

Many times an order request affects another department such as dietary, laboratory, radiology, accounting, or admitting. Hospital computers are designed to forward messages to departments that need this information. For example, when an x-ray is ordered that requires the patient to be NPO, the dietary request to hold the next meal is made at the same time. The charge for the procedure is then sent to accounting. This is what makes the computer so special. All this can be done through the computer without additional paperwork or phone calls.

Contingency Planning

Whenever humans depend on machines, contingency plans need to be made in case the machine is out of order. When a computer is not functioning, it is **down.** Down time can be scheduled to allow a new program to be entered into the computer's memory or to make changes. Down time can also be unexpected—power failure or component failure. Hospitals have learned the importance of an alternate plan in case failure occurs. Despite modern technology, you still need to know manual methods of entering orders. You will probably still prefer the computer once you have mastered the technique.

The computer will perform many functions for you to make you more efficient in your job. Only a few general ones have been discussed. With time, you will learn all of the things the computer can do and you will learn how to do them. Practice is important in learning how to use the computer to its fullest capability.

KEY IDEA: ETHICS AND CONFIDENTIALITY

By now you should be able to see how important ethics and confidentiality are when using a computer. Your identification code or password in the hands of the wrong person could be disastrous to patients. If you were tempted to alter patient information, serious consequences would result. Although there are many safeguards built into the computer system, they can be bypassed by an unethical person knowledgeable of computers. More than anything, ethics and confidentiality are essential when computers are used. Maintaining privacy is always a concern.

RULES OF CONFIDENTIALITY

1. The type and amount of information gathered and recorded about a patient, caregiver, employee, etc., will be limited to that information required for legitimate purposes.
2. All individuals engaged in the collection, handling, or dissemination of information shall be specifically informed of their responsibility to protect confidential data and of the penalties for violation of this trust. Proven violation of confidentiality of private information may be cause for disciplinary action or termination of employment. Breach of confidentiality is considered to be a very serious employment offense.
3. Access to material which contains confidential information will be limited to situations in which legitimate need and purpose can be demonstrated.
4. Access to areas where confidential information may be discussed, e.g., patient treatment areas, will be limited to only those individuals whose presence is required for a legitimate purpose.
5. Confidential information will be protected from access by unauthorized individuals in both manual and automated systems.
6. Computerized information and access codes are authorized by directors based upon the "need to know" concept.
7. All caregivers who receive a computer access code are required to read and sign a Confidentiality Statement at the completion of the system training period.

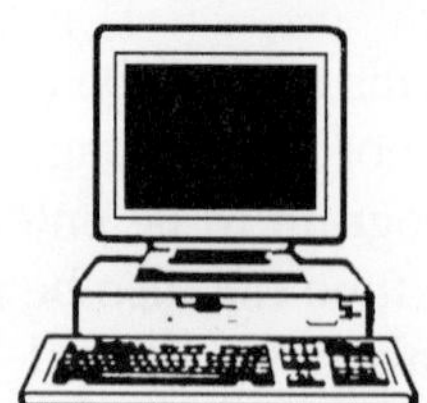

MEMORIAL HOSPITAL
Computer User's Access Codes (Log-ins) Confidentiality Statement

Obtaining access to the Hospital's computerized information system requires a clear understanding of your responsibilities regarding access and adequate training on the system. The following statements will provide an understanding of the significance of the User Access Code you receive following your training. Please, read them **carefully.**

1. **My User Access Code (password) is confidential. It identifies me in a *unique* manner. I am responsible for all data entered into Merlin under my code.**
2. **I will not disclose my User Access Code to anyone, nor will I attempt to learn another person's access code.**
3. **I will not use another person's access code to enter, update, or retrieve data on Merlin.**
4. **If I have reason to believe the confidentiality of my code has been compromised, I will notify Information Systems Services immediately so that my code can be deleted and a new code issued to me.**
5. **I understand that all patient data viewed, printed, or entered is confidential patient data and part of the medical-legal record. I will not access data on patients for whom I have no responsibilities and for whom I have no "need to know."**
6. **I understand that any misuse of my confidential User Access Code is a violation of Hospital policy, and will subject me to disciplinary action up to and including termination of employment.**

Your signature below acknowledges agreement with and understanding of these statements.

Signature ______________________ Name Printed ______________________

Department ______________________ Date ______________________

Trainer's Initials/ I.S. Issuer ______________________ Date ______________________

DISTRIBUTION: ORIGINAL - HUMAN RESOURCES, Employee File PHOTOCOPY - DEPT. DIRECTOR

- -

Employee# ______________ **Access Code** ______________________
(if known) (PRINT password CLEARLY)

Please Note: If you have not received a certificate of class completion and/or access is not available within 4 days, please notify your director.

8. Special confidentiality/security procedures for sensitive records, e.g., payroll records, will be documented in the individual department policy and procedure manual.

SUMMARY

Not all hospitals have installed computers in their patient care areas where the health unit coordinator will be working, but most have done so or are moving in this direction. You may be one of the pioneers in your hospital as computer technology helps you do your job more efficiently and consistently. Computers are machines and only that. They were designed by humans and help humans. Humans are in control of the computer.

Sample Computer Use for Laboratory Order

Screen	*Input*
Step #1 - PASSWORD	
return	
ENTER FUNCTION	**ORDER ENTRY (F2) (will select from menu of many functions, each with own letter).**
return	
PATIENT NUMBER(#), e.g., #123456	**FROM ADDRESSOGRAPH PLATE**
return	**Will echo name**
DEPARTMENT PRESS "HELP" TO CHOOSE FROM CRC-CV-CAR-CT-CS-EPI- LAB-MIC-NEU-NUC- NCS-OT-PT-RAD-RT-SS- US-ST-PF-MRI. Enter one group of initials	
Example: LAB	
COLL BY LAB?	**If yes, press return**
DATE TO COLL	**If today, press return**
TIME TO COLL (RETURN)	**If tomorrow, press T + 1 IT WILL SHOW THE APPROPRIATE DATE**
PRIORITY (HELP)	**ROUTINE—STAT, ASAP, PREOP, AM DRAW (If press R, will show routine)**
TEST	• **In this system at this point HUC must go to book of codes to select valid item number and will enter that number. *For example:* #1020 = CBC**
ORDER DR. NAME	**If same as chart, push Return Will echo name**
COMMENTS	**Type in anything special**
ENTER	**Press return**
ORDER ENTRY #	• **Screen shows number which is to be copied on Physician's Order Sheet next to order and on Kardex.**
PUSH EXIT TO GET OUT	

This is an example of computer use in one hospital to order laboratory work.

Sample Computer Abbreviations

Abbreviations	*Departments*
CRC	Cardiac Rehabilitation
CV	Cardiovascular
CAR	Cardiology
CT	Cat Scan
CS	Central Supply
EPI	Epidemiology
LAB	Laboratory
MIC	Microbiology
NEU	Neurology
NUC	Nuclear Medicine
NCS	Nutrition Care Services
OT	Occupational Therapy
PT	Physical Therapy
RAD	Radiology
RT	Respiratory Therapy
SS	Social Services
US	Ultrasound
ST	Speech Therapy
PF	Pulmonary Function
MRI	Magnetic Resonance Imaging

Sample Computer Functions

Codes	*Function*
F1	NAME INQUIRY SELECT
F2	ORDER ENTRY
F3	CANCEL REQUEST
F4	ORDER INQUIRY
F5	PATIENT FILE REVISION
F6	INPATIENT DISCHARGE
F7	TRANSFER/SWAP SELECT
F8	POST BED STATUS
F9	MAINTENANCE SELECT
F10	SEND/RECEIVE MESSAGE SELECT
F11	FACE SHEET INQUIRY
<NBM>	NEWBORN MINI-ADMIT
<ORS>	ORDER SET ENTRY
S1	NAME INQUIRY - HELD OUTPATIENT
S2	VERIFY HELD OUTPATIENT
S7	CORRECT DISCHARGE
S8	CENSUS SELECT
S9	PRINT CENSUS UTILITIES (Diets, Nursing Worksheets, etc.)
S10	VACANT BED LIST
S11	PRINTER UTILITIES
S12	REQUEST CHART PULL
<PC3>	PRINT CENSUS UTILITIES

LEARNING ACTIVITIES

Complete the following:

1. List and describe three types of computers.
   (a) ______________________________
   (b) ______________________________
   (c) ______________________________

2. List the three basic components of all computer systems.
   (a) ____________
   (b) ____________
   (c) ____________
3. List two input devices.
   (a) ____________
   (b) ____________
4. List two output devices.
   (a) ____________
   (b) ____________
5. Describe what computers do. ____________
6. Name eight functions computers perform in hospital patient care areas.
   (a) ____________
   (b) ____________
   (c) ____________
   (d) ____________
   (e) ____________
   (f) ____________
   (g) ____________
   (h) ____________
7. Name the most important function key on the computer keyboard. ____________
8. What is the significance of the cursor? ____________
9. List four rules of computer confidentiality.
   (a) ____________
   (b) ____________
   (c) ____________
   (d) ____________

Match the word in column A with the definition in column B.

Column A	*Column B*
(a) Cursor	____ An input device
(b) Debug	____ Secret code
(c) Light pen	____ Listing of available functions
(d) CRT	____ Flashing indicator
(e) Program	____ Viewing screen
(f) Command	____ Instructions
(g) Menu	____ Request
(h) Password	____ Problem solving

CHAPTER 13

Introduction to Order Transcription

OBJECTIVES

When you complete this chapter, you will be able to:

- State two reasons for doctors' orders and the three methods by which they may be obtained.
- List and discuss the "tools of transcription."
- List and explain the seven steps of order transcription.
- State the purpose of symbols in order transcription.
- List and define the six general classifications of doctors' orders.
- List and discuss the four categories of doctors' orders.

GENERAL INFORMATION

All medical and many nursing services performed in a hospital for the patient require written orders from the patient's doctor. There are two main reasons for this:

1. Only the doctor knows what medical treatment will best meet the needs of the patient.
2. Legal safeguards are necessary to protect the patient from incorrect medical treatment.

Often the doctor will give the nurse orders over the telephone. The nurse will write these on the physician's order sheet, write T.O. (telephone order) Dr. ____________________, and sign his/her name. The physician must sign these orders when he/she comes to the hospital. Occasionally, you will see doctors' orders written by the nurse and followed with V.O. (verbal order) Dr. ____________________ and the nurse's signature. This means the doctor has told the nurse to do something (often in an emergency) and will sign the order later.

Sometimes doctors will have their routine orders printed to reduce the need for handwriting, make individual corrections as necessary, and sign these when they visit. But most frequently, doctors will write their own orders in handwriting and sign them at that time.

For both medical and legal reasons, then, medical care orders for the patient originate and are given with the doctor's direction and consent.

Once an order has been written by the doctor, the responsibility for seeing that the order is carried out rests with the nurse. As a health unit coordinator, you will share this responsibility with the nurse by performing the clerical task called "transcription of orders." For purposes of carrying out a doctor's orders, equipment or services often must be ordered from other departments. The orders themselves must be transferred to other records which will be available to all nursing staff members who will care for the patient. In transcribing doctor's orders, you are simply ordering by computer or rewriting them on requisitions, patient chart forms, and special records.

The most important hospital records are those concerning the doctor's orders for the treatment of patients. Errors in these records, and resulting errors in treatment, may have immediate as well as long-term effects on the condition of a patient. Consider, for example, what may happen to a patient who is given the wrong dosage of a potent medicine because the written order was copied incorrectly on a medicine sheet. Consider a newly admitted patient with bleeding ulcers who, by clerical error, has a regular diet ordered for him and begins to hemorrhage violently after eating the meal. As you learn the principles and methods of transcribing orders, **always remember that any error can have disastrous effects.** If you do not understand an order or are unable to read the doctor's writing, the nurse is present to answer your questions.

- Always **ASK** when in doubt.
- Always be **ALERT** when transcribing doctor's orders.
- Always be **ACCURATE.**

TOOLS OF TRANSCRIPTION

KEY IDEA: DOCTOR'S ORDER SHEET

The tools of transcription are the doctor's order sheet and the Kardex. Review the discussion of the doctor's order sheet in Chapter 11. Then study the figure below until you have a general understanding of what the term "doctor's order" means. Note that the doctor does not indicate how or where you should transcribe the order, nor identify the type of order for you. When you finish learning transcription of orders, you will know these facts solely by what is actually written. (Fig. 13–1.)

KEY IDEA: KARDEX (PATIENT CARE RECORD CARD)

You already know that the Kardex is used for consolidating information about the patient and the treatment prescribed. Nursing personnel use this form to learn their specific duties regarding a patient without having to refer constantly to the chart or order sheet. You have probably used it too, to an-

DATE	ORDER	SIGNATURE
6-1-xx	*Hot soaks to elbow q4h*	
	Aspirin 600 mg. p.o. q4h for Temp > 103°F.	
	Out of bed ad. lib.	
	Allow shower in A.M.	
	Electrolytes in A.M.	
	IVP	
	Transfer to semiprivate in P.M.	
	Remove restraints. Replace if necessary.	

Figure 13–1

swer some of the many questions about patients directed to you during the day. As a health unit coordinator, you will be engaged in much of the actual recording of information on the Kardex. You will need to understand fully the information it contains and how this information is recorded.

Kardex systems vary widely from one hospital to another. The example used in this chapter consolidates nearly all the information that is ordinarily included. Your hospital will use a Kardex best suited to its needs and will have other methods of consolidating any information not included on its card.

The Kardex holder is usually a vinyl or metal-backed rectangle with a series of graduated inserts. (Fig. 13–2.)

The Kardex, one for each patient, is placed in the inserts with the identifying information (patient's name, room number, etc.) visible at the bottom of the card. Each card can be flipped upward to expose the additional information on a particular patient. The cards are filed by room number.

- Permanent recording on the Kardex, such as the patient's name and doctor's name, is usually done in ink.
- Different colors of ink may be used to record certain data, such as a patient's allergies, so that such information will be easy to see.

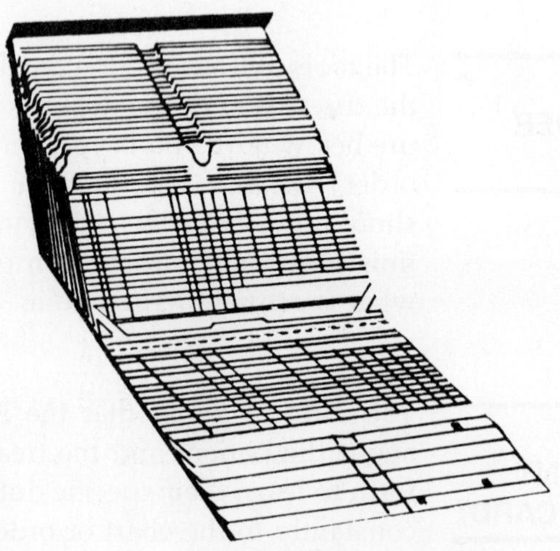

Figure 13–2

- Some of the recording is done in pencil, so it can be erased and replaced with new orders when the original orders are cancelled.
- Sometimes small "throw-away" cards are used with the more permanent Kardex for recording orders to be carried out only once. These cards are kept primarily to provide information to the nursing staff through one 24-hour period and are discarded on a daily basis or when full.
- If a Kardex becomes mutilated after long use or many erasures, the orders currently in effect may be recopied on a new card and the old card destroyed or marked "copied" and kept behind the new card.
- The Kardex is removed when the patient is discharged, and a blank card, to be used for the next patient to occupy the bed, is then inserted.
- The Kardex is often used to construct staff patient care assignments, to give change-of-shift reports, and to check on specific orders for a patient.

Sample Construction of Kardex

On Side 1, as indicated in Fig. 13–3, a place is provided to list all diagnostic tests and special procedures on the patient. These may include laboratory tests, x-rays, cardiograms, internal visualizations, isotopic examinations, etc. Surgical procedures might be recorded in red ink for emphasis. With this

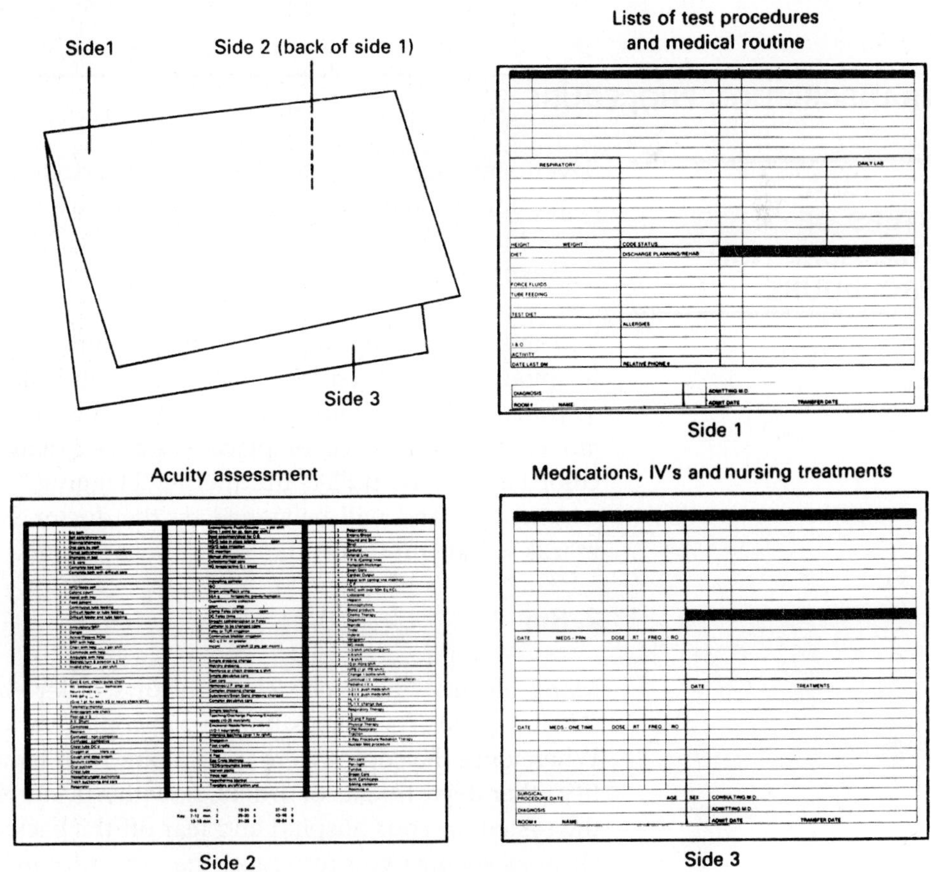

Figure 13–3

record, the doctor is able to tell at a glance what tests have been ordered and performed; the nursing staff is able to order necessary preparations of patients for medical and surgical procedures and to see that all ordered procedures have been performed. Side 2 is an acuity assessment used to plan staffing. Side 3 shows medications, IVs, and treatments, as carried out by nursing personnel. At the very bottom of this page, visible on each card when the file is closed, is the summary information for identification of the patient.

The Computer-Generated Kardex

Many hospitals are using computers in the patient care areas and many no longer use the Kardex just described. Instead, the computer prints out a Kardex for each patient on demand. This means that instead of handwriting all of the orders into the various spaces on the Kardex each time an order is transcribed, all the work is done for you at the time the orders are entered into the computer. The printout is the most up-to-date information available on the patient and is used by nursing in the same way that the older Kardex was used. The individual Kardexes may be kept in a notebook or on a clipboard at the nurse's station, but the Kardex holder will no longer be used. Figure 13–4 shows a three-page computer-generated Kardex for a patient on the medical floor. All of the information that would have been on the handwritten Kardex is available; it simply looks different.

Step 4 in the transcription procedure described below will be deleted if a computer-generated Kardex is used.

TRANSCRIPTION PROCEDURE

KEY IDEA: STEPS OF TRANSCRIPTION PROCEDURE

Seven steps are necessary for the transcription of each order. Learn these steps, and use them as a checklist when performing this task.

1. Recognize

You must first recognize and note that an order needs transcription. Every hospital has a method by which doctors indicate to the nursing and clerical staff that new orders have been written. The patient's chart, or the order sheet alone, may be marked or placed in a designated container. A red or other color tag may be pulled up; this is "Flagging." A new order will show the current date and will be signed by the doctor. No other writing, initials, or marks will be present.

2. Rip

Many hospitals have chosen a doctor's order sheet that has several copies (NCR copies). The disposition of the copies varies widely with the hospital. Where once the copies were used along with handwritten requisitions to notify other departments of orders, now this is largely done by computer. Know the system in your hospital and tear off the back copies of the doctor's order sheet as soon as you recognize that an order exists. Always be sure that all

```
                              KARDEX            Pg. 1 of 3

41001  EXAMPLE, IMA        1234567890 66 F  ADM-042197 053097 16:49 4MS
DX ADM BRONCHITIS             ADM  000022  GOODDOCTOR, GEO. AL1 pcn
DX CUR pneumonia              ATT  000022  GOODDOCTOR, GEO. AL2 asa
   DX1 ARDS                   CON1 000023  ALSOGOOD, ALVIN  AL3 codeine
   DX2                        CON2 000024                   AL4
   DX3                        CON3 000026                   AL5
   DX4                        CON4 000027                   AL6
  SUR1 lobectomy 1995         CON5 000000                    HT 64
  SUR2                        CON6 000000                    WT 150
  SUR3                        CON7 000000
  SUR4                        INVS LNE
 HIST1                        DIAB
 HIST2                                                    IV
 HIST3                        IS TY                       OXYGEN
 HIST4                        COMM                             MRN-00219218


----- SKIN ASSESSMENT -----------------!----- ALLERGY/HT/WT -----------------
___ Assess skin q shift.              ! ___ Allergies/Ht/Wt entered in Merlin
                                      !     (If ht/wt/allergies do not show in
___ Begin Pressure Ulcer Protocol.    !     upper right hand corner of this
                                      !     Kardex, then they still need to be
                                      !     entered.)
----- LABORATORY ----------------------!----- NUTRITION SERVICES -------------
   483 053097 ROUTINE URINE, CREATI-   !   186 042197 CAFFEINE,BLAND,RESIDUE
       NINE RANDOM COLLECT BY NURSE    !       OR FIBER CONT BLAND LOW RESIDUE
   717 053097 ROUTINE TYPE & SCREEN    !   296 042197 ORAL NUTRITION /
       COLLECT BY LAB                  !       SUPPLEMENTS - SUSTACAL PLUS
   718 053097 ROUTINE TYPE AND         !       FLUID RESTRICTION
       CROSSMATCH PACKED RBCS          !   385 042197 STANDARD TUBE FEEDING
   719 053097 STAT CSF PANEL (INCL.    !       FORMULA T.F.PRO CONTINUOUS 40CC
       CELL CT., GLUC, T.P.)           !       HR
   720 053097 STAT CSF IMMUNOSUPPRES-  !   387 042197 STANDARD PROTOCOL: REG.
       SED PANEL                       !       DIETITIAN TUBE FEEDING CONSULT
   737 053097 STAT INDIA INK PREP (CSF)!  1057 051497 STANDARD TUBE FEEDING
   738 053097 STAT CRYPTOCOCCUS        !       FORMULA T.F.PRO CONTINUOUS 40CC
       ANTIGEN (CSF)                   !       HR
   739 053097 STAT CULTURE/GM. STAIN   !  1058 051497 STANDARD PROTOCOL: REG.
       (CSF)                           !       DIETITIAN TUBE FEEDING CONSULT
   740 053097 STAT CULTURE, FUNGUS     !       TESTING SORT SORTING TEST
       (CSF)                           !   313 052897 STANDARD TUBE FEEDING
   741 053097 ROUTINE CULTURE, BLOOD - !       FORMULA T.F.PRO CONTINUOUS 60CC,
       IMMUNOSUP (HIV) COLLECT BY NURSE!       HR
   742 053097 ROUTINE CULTURE,         !   315 052897 STANDARD PROTOCOL: REG.
       RESPIRATORY (BRONCH-IMMUNOS)    !       DIETITIAN TUBE FEEDING CONSULT
       COLLECT BY NURSE                !   484 053097 PROTEIN CONTROLLED DIET-
   743 053097 COLLECTION OF AUTOLOGOUS !       RENAL,HEPATIC 35 GM PRO 2.5 GM
       BLOOD                           !       K+ FLUID RESTRICTION 700 CC
```

Figure 13–4 Example of computer-generated Kardex.

KARDEX Pg. 2 of 3

41001 EXAMPLE, IMA 1234567890 66 F ADM-042197 053097 16:49 4MS

----- CARDIOPULMONARY -----

192 042197 ROUTINE OXYGEN ORDER 4L

204 042197 ROUTINE COLOR FLOW

205 042197 STAT COMPLETE ECHO

206 042197 STAT HOLTER MONITOR

485 053097 VENTILATOR ORDER 100% 14 SIMV

486 053097 VENTILATOR CHANGES ORDER 90%

487 053097 Q6H IPPB TERBUTALINE

488 053097 ROUTINE CAROTID DUPLEX ULTRASOUND CARDIZEM

713 053097 ROUTINE ELECTROCARDIO-GRAM DIGOXIN

714 053097 ROUTINE TREADMILL BETA BLOCKERS

----- DISCHARGE/SOCIAL SERVICES -----

----- RADIOLOGY/NUC MED -----

482 053097 STAT ENTIRE SPINE LTD PAIN

----- PHYSICAL THERAPY -----

201 042197 PHYSICAL THERAPY EVALUATION REQUEST

225 042197 GAIT TRAINING

226 042197 PHYSICAL THERAPY EVALUATION REQUEST

227 042197 THERAPEUTIC EXERCISE

228 042197 TRANSFER TRAINING

715 053097 GAIT TRAINING S/P TOTAL HIP

----- REHAB SERVICES -----

----- BEHAVIORAL MEDICINE -----

----- NURSING ORDERS -----

231 042197 14H ACCUCHECKS BY NURSING

275 042197 Q6HR ACCUCHECKS BY NURSING

276 042197 BATH NURSING ORDER PARTIAL BATH

277 042197 DIET NURSING ORDER CALORIE COUNT

278 042197 DRESSINGS NURSING ORDER SUBCLAVIAN/SWAN DRESSING CHANGE

279 042197 GASTRO NURSING ORDER COLOSTOMY CARE

289 042197 Q6H ACCUCHECKS BY NURSING

292 042197 Q8GR STANDARD PROTOCOL: CHECK GASTRIC RESI 500CC OR MORE, HOLD TUBE FEEDING X 1 HOUR AND RECHECK RESIDUAL. NOTIFY M.D. IF TUBE FEEDING HELD MORE THAN 2 CONSECUTIVE HOURS.

293 042197 STANDARD PROTOCOL: RECORD WEIGHT Q 3 DAYS FIRST WEEK, THEN Q WEEK

386 042197 HYDRATION/TUBE FEEDING ORDER: IRRIGATE TUBE WITH 50 CC OF H2O AT LEAST Q 8 HRS

388 042197 STANDARD PROTOCOL: TUBE CONFIRMATION: CHECK FEEDING TUBE PLACEMENT PRIOR TO BEGINNING TUBE FEEDING

389 042197 STANDARD PROTOCOL: TOLERANCE EVAL: ADVANCE TUBE FEEDING AS ORDERED IF RESIDUAL NO GREATER THAN 100 CC OR ABOVE SPECIFIED LEVEL, NO ABDOMINAL DISTENTION, NO GREATER THAN 5 LIQUID STOOLS PER 24 HOURS.

390 042197 STANDARD PROTOCOL: ELEV. HEAD OF BED > 30 DEGREES DURING FEEDING & 30 MIN. AFTER DELIVERY

391 042197 TUBE ORDER: INITIATE FEEDING THROUGH CURRENT NASOENTERIC TUBE

1063 052897 Q6HRS STANDARD PROTOCOL:

Figure 13–4 ***(Continued)***

KARDEX Pg. 3 of 3

41001 EXAMPLE, IMA 1234567890 66 F ADM-042197 053097 16:49 4MS

CHECK GASTRIC RESI 400CC OR MORE, HOLD TUBE FEEDING X 1 HOUR AND RECHECK RESIDUAL. NOTIFY M.D. IF TUBE FEEDING HELD MORE THAN 2 CONSECUTIVE HOURS.

1064 052897 STANDARD PROTOCOL: RECORD WEIGHT Q 3 DAYS FIRST WEEK, THEN Q WEEK

314 052897 HYDRATION/TUBE FEEDING ORDER: IRRIGATE TUBE WITH 50 CC OF H2O AT LEAST Q 8 HRS

316 052897 STANDARD PROTOCOL: TUBE CONFIRMATION: CHECK FEEDING TUBE PLACEMENT PRIOR TO BEGINNING TUBE FEEDING

317 052897 STANDARD PROTOCOL: TOLERANCE EVAL: ADVANCE TUBE FEEDING AS ORDERED IF RESIDUAL NO GREATER THAN 100 CC OR ABOVE SPECIFIED LEVEL, NO ABDOMINAL DISTENTION, NO GREATER THAN 5 LIQUID STOOLS PER 24 HOURS.

318 052897 STANDARD PROTOCOL: ELEV. HEAD OF BED > 30 DEGREES DURING FEEDING & 30 MIN. AFTER DELIVERY

319 052897 TUBE ORDER: INITIATE FEEDING THROUGH CURRENT NASOENTERIC TUBE

481 052897 ANY MISCELLANEOUS NURSING ORDER ANY FURTHER INFORMATION ANY REMARKS ANY MORE REMARKS

745 053097 Q6HR ACCUCHECKS BY NURSING

----- CENTRAL SUPPLY -----------------

270 042197 AIR MATTRESS DAILY

----- MEDICATIONS --------------------

232 042197 SQ Q4H SLIDING SCALE REGULAR INSULIN

280 042197 SQ Q4H REGULAR HUMAN INSULIN 3U

290 042197 75 ML/HR IV ORDER D5NS 10MEQKCL

291 042197 PO MED: DIGOXIN

744 053097 SQ Q6HR REGULAR HUMAN INSULIN 4UNITS ACCUCHECKS Q 6 HRS

746 053097 SQ Q4HRS SLIDING SCALE REGULAR INSULIN IF <150=0 U; IF 151-200 = 2 U; IF 201-250 = 4U; IF >251, CALL IF >251, CALL MD.

747 053097 75 ML/HR IV ORDER D5W 20MEQ KCL

----- MESSAGES RE THIS PATIENT -------

716 053097 TO ADMITTING - ADMITTING INFO FORM ADMITTING CLERK MAY COME & SEE PATIENT NOW FAMILY IS HERE TO INTERPRET

----- HOME HEALTH SERVICES -----------

Figure 13–4 (*Continued*)

doctor's orders are stamped with the correct addressograph plate before tearing off the copies.

3. Prioritize

Now you must read the doctor's orders and do those orders first that have the highest priority. When you see words like **stat, now, immediately,** this A.M., etc., you should call the nurse's attention to it at once, i.e., **without delay.** Sometimes the order will simply make a statement such as D.C. IV (discontinue intravenous) or electrolytes (a blood test). If you have several charts and all have orders, you must prioritize the orders on each chart.

4. Kardex

The order must then be transferred to the special records and forms from which the nursing staff will carry out the order or make sure that it has been done if that remains the process in your hospital. As stated earlier, this step will be omitted if your hospital uses the computer-generated Kardex. Most orders are copied directly from the doctor's order sheet to the patient care record card. This process is called Kardexing.

5. Requisition

All equipment and services necessary to carry out the order must then be requisitioned. You will select and complete the requisitions you need to order the various laboratory tests, x-rays, treatments, diet changes, etc., which the doctor may order for the patient. If you are ordering by computer, it is still termed requisitioning. You just don't have to fill out all those forms! (Fig. 13–5.)

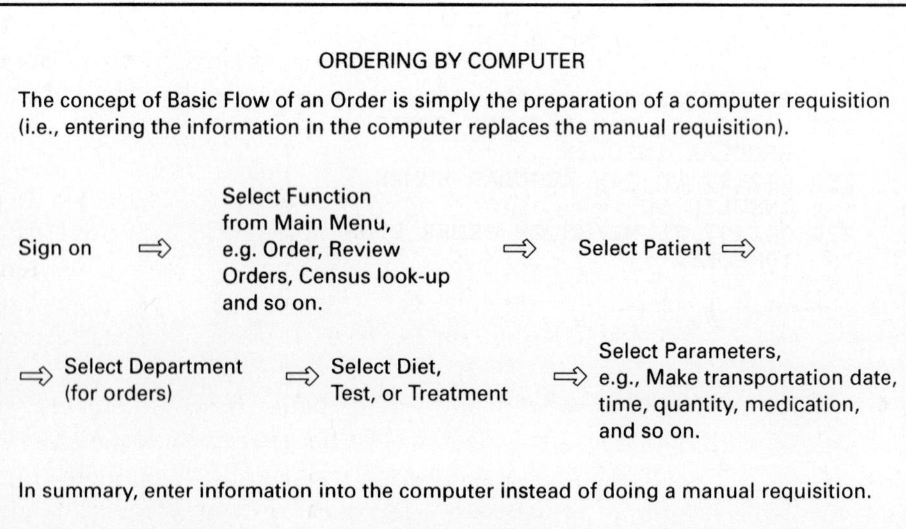

ORDERING BY COMPUTER
The concept of Basic Flow of an Order is simply the preparation of a computer requisition (i.e., entering the information in the computer replaces the manual requisition).
Sign on
Select Function from Main Menu, e.g. Order, Review Orders, Census look-up and so on.
Select Patient
Select Department (for orders)
Select Diet, Test, or Treatment
Select Parameters, e.g., Make transportation date, time, quantity, medication, and so on.
In summary, enter information into the computer instead of doing a manual requisition.

Figure 13–5

Steps of Order Transcription

1. Recognize
2. Rip
3. Prioritize
4. Kardex
5. Requisition or Computer Order
6. Symbols
7. Nurse Checks

Figure 13-6

6. Symbols

At this point, the order itself is in the process of being carried out. Before the transcription procedure is complete, however, you must indicate in writing on the doctor's order sheet what you have done to set the order in motion. Symbols—which you will learn more about in the next section—may be used for this purpose.

7. Nurse Checks

The final step in transcribing orders is designed to protect both you and the patient. Because your knowledge of medicine is often limited to the instructions you receive in this course, and because you are directly responsible to the registered nursing staff on your floor, **all orders you have transcribed must be checked by the nurse.** All requisitions, tickets, and special records, as well as the orders themselves will be checked for accuracy and completeness. The nurse will then sign the orders he/she has checked. This procedure saves the nurse's time and effort in transcribing the order and the accuracy of the transcription will be doubly assured by the efforts of two persons. In this way, too, the nurse is kept informed of the orders in effect for his/her patients.

REMEMBER: Be sure the nurse sees any **stat** orders without delay. Do not wait until he or she checks your transcription. (Fig. 13–6.)

KEY IDEA: TRANSCRIPTION SYMBOLS

Letters and symbols can be used to indicate to the nurse the work you have completed. The example below shows one set of symbols and letters; those used in your hospital might be entirely different. The important lesson to be mastered is that you thoroughly learn and use those indicators applied in your hospital to show that the work has been accomplished. (Fig. 13–7.)

To simplify the nurse's checking task, you may be asked to write these symbols in red ink, because most orders are written in blue or black ink. It may sometimes be necessary to include other information besides the symbols alone, as in connection with appointments. After the nurse checks your order transcription, she or he will sign, state the time, and date the orders.

Figure 13–8 shows how the doctor's orders would look after they had been transcribed, using the proper symbols.

O or S to indicate that	**A slip or requisition for equipment or services has been filled out.**
K to indicate that	**An order has been transcribed to the Kardex.**
T to indicate that	**A ticket has been filled out.**
AP to indicate that	**An appointment has been made. The date of the appointment should accompany this symbol on the doctor's order sheet.**
P or Called to indicate that	**The appropriate department or persons have been notified of an order by telephone.**
✓ to indicate that	**All activities necessary to complete transcription, and not indicated by any of the symbols included above, have been carried out.**

Figure 13–7

DATE	ORDER	
6-1-xx	K Hot soaks to elbow q4h	
	K Aspirin 600 mg. p.o. q4h for Temp 103°F.	
	K Out of bed ad. lib.	
	K Allow shower in A.M.	
	K Electrolytes in A.M.°	
	K IVP Ap 6-3	
	K Transfer to semiprivate in P.M. Called	
	K Remove restraints. Replace if necessary.	

Date Time R.N.	Date Time M.D.	Date Time H.U.C.
6-1-XX-2100 L. Bowman	6-1-XX-2100 J. Stevens	6-1-XX-2100 D. Jones

Figure 13–8

KEY IDEA: SIGNATURES

When the doctor writes an order, he/she signs it in the space provided. As previously stated, if the nurse takes a telephone or verbal order, he/she signs it and the doctor signs it later.

After the registered nurse has carefully checked your transcription, he/she will sign off the orders as shown above.

It is recommended that the health unit coordinator also sign off as the person who transcribed the order. Use the first letter of your first name, your last name, your title, and HUC for health unit coordinator or CHUC if you are a certified health unit coordinator. Example:

Date	Time	
6-1-xx	2100	D. Jones, CHUC

Be very careful when writing anything on the physician's order sheet, that you do not write over the doctor's orders. It is very important, from a legal standpoint, that the orders are completely visible.

GENERAL CLASSIFICATION OF ORDERS

Doctor's orders can be classified according to the subject of the order. You will probably encounter the general types of orders discussed below.

Medication Orders

All medication orders on a patient are written in a similar form and are a major class of orders in themselves. The orders will be discussed in Chapter 14, Understanding Medication Orders.

Treatment/Monitoring Orders

Treatment orders include a wide variety of procedures to be performed for a patient with his cooperation. Such diverse activities as oxygen administration and ice pack applications are all treatments. Monitoring orders include orders for vital signs, circulation check, etc. Nursing treatment and monitoring orders will be discussed in Chapter 15. Radiation, Respiratory, and Physical Therapy orders are covered in Chapter 16.

Diagnostic Procedure Orders

All laboratory tests, x-rays, isotopic procedures, electrocardiograms, etc., fall into this category. The orders are discussed in Chapter 16.

Diet Orders

These include orders that refer to any nourishment to be given to the patient by any method. Special fluid restrictions, tube feeding, as well as meal orders, are all part of this category of orders. Diet orders are covered in Chapter 16.

Intravenous Orders

These include the various types of intravenous fluids given to the patient. These are discussed in Chapter 15.

Activity Orders

These refer to orders governing the level or type of activity the patient is to be allowed. A sub-category of activity orders are POSITION ORDERS. These are also found in Chapter 15.

Miscellaneous Orders

This group is a catchall term for all orders not included above. Miscellaneous orders are alike in that they generally indicate quite precisely a special task to be performed or limitation to be accepted and understood. As examples: The doctor may request, by order, that a patient's family be informed of impending surgery or that x-rays be sent with the patient to the operating room. The doctor may place a patient on the critical list, in isolation, or sign an order for his discharge. The doctor may order special permissions, such as "may go on pass," restrictions such as orders for side rails on the patient's bed, or protection orders such as restraints. These are discussed in Chapter 15.

KEY IDEA: FOUR MAIN CATEGORIES OF DOCTOR'S ORDERS

There are four main categories of doctor's orders:

1. **Standing routine orders.** Once these orders are written, they will remain unchanged until done so by the physician. Standing routine orders are done on a regular basis. Examples of standing routine orders are:
   - V.S. q.i.d. (vital signs four times a day)
   - P.T. ROM b.i.d. (physical therapy with range of motion twice a day)
   - O.O.B. in W.C. 30 min. t.i.d. (out of bed in wheel chair 30 minutes three times a day)
   - BS q AM (blood sugar every morning)
2. **Standing PRN orders.** These orders stand as written until changed but the order is carried out on an as-needed basis. For example, SSE q.o.d. prn (soap suds enema every other day as needed); may wash hair prn.
3. **One time or limited orders.** For example:
   - Remove NG (nasogastric) tube this morning
   - ECG today (electrocardiogram today)
   - Hct X 3 days (hematocrit to be drawn for 3 days only)
4. **STAT orders.** These orders are to be carried out immediately. For example, D.C. IV Stat (discontinue the intravenous immediately), tracheal suction now; FC/SD stat (Foley catheter (retention catheter), to straight drainage immediately).

In order for you to intelligently transcribe doctor's orders you must learn many medical abbreviations. A glossary of abbreviations is included in Chapter 4, Medical Terminology, for easy reference.

LEARNING ACTIVITIES

Complete the following:

1. The primary reasons for doctor's orders are

   (a) ______________________________

   (b) ______________________________

2. The three methods of obtaining doctor's orders are
   (a) ________________
   (b) ________________
   (c) ________________
3. No matter what the method of obtaining orders, they must always be ________________ by the doctor.
4. The tools of order transcription are
   (a) ________________
   (b) ________________
5. List the seven steps of order transcription.
   (a) ________________
   (b) ________________
   (c) ________________
   (d) ________________
   (e) ________________
   (f) ________________
   (g) ________________
6. List the seven general classifications of doctor's orders.
   (a) ________________
   (b) ________________
   (c) ________________
   (d) ________________
   (e) ________________
   (f) ________________
   (g) ________________
7. Doctor's orders fall into four main categories, which are
   (a) ________________
   (b) ________________
   (c) ________________
   (d) ________________

CHAPTER 14

Understanding Medication Orders

OBJECTIVES

When you complete this chapter, you will be able to:

- Define the terms antimicrobial, pharmacodynamic, and chemotherapeutic drugs.
- Recognize common drug names and state their purpose.
- Discuss your responsibilities in relation to anticoagulants and antidiabetic drugs and the laboratory tests to monitor these drugs.
- Discuss intravenous medication orders.
- Demonstrate knowledge of the abbreviations used in this chapter.
- Demonstrate the ability to transcribe medication orders.

Before you learn to transcribe orders for medication, you must learn more about the medications themselves and how they are ordered. Understanding a new set of medical terms will be necessary. In this chapter you will learn about the general types of medication used in hospitals. Then you will study specific drug names and preparations, drug dosages, and routes and times of administration.

You will also learn about the types of medication orders and how to transcribe these orders.

Remember that errors in medication transcription may have disastrous effects for the patient. Pay close attention to the material presented in this chapter.

Remember too that there is much to learn about medications and that new or different medications will frequently come to your attention. Be inquisitive and listen and learn about medications whenever you can.

KEY IDEA: CLASSIFICATIONS OF MEDICATIONS

Medication is one of the most effective methods of treating many diseases. Drugs may be categorized in different ways.

1. They may destroy or render harmless microorganisms in the body which cause disease. Drugs acting in this manner are called **antimicrobial drugs.**
2. They may either stimulate or depress normal body functions in such a way that the nature or course of a disease is altered. These drugs are called **pharmacodynamic drugs.**
3. They may treat neoplastic disease and have a selective effect on the invading cells or organisms. These are called **chemotherapeutic drugs.**

Drugs are ordinarily grouped according to the disease or symptom they treat or the body function they affect. You will often hear drugs referred to by category and should be familiar with the most common groups of medications. However, some drugs, because they affect different body parts and functions, can be used to treat a number of different diseases. Table 14–2 describes the major drug categories. This is not a complete list of categories, nor does it include all the possible uses for each drug.

Antimicrobial Drugs

Many types of microorganisms, by definition too small to be seen without a microscope, can cause disease. In addition to viruses and bacteria, there are others such as fungi, protozoa, rickettsiae, and spirochetes. Many of them can be destroyed by drugs. (Fig. 14–1, pg. 256.) The most common groups of antimicrobial drugs are listed in Table 14–1.

Pharmacodynamic Drugs

Diseases may be caused by the malfunction of an organ or body part. Such malfunctions can usually be traced to either an excess or a decrease in the normal activity of the organ concerned. For this reason, pharmacodynamic

TABLE 14–1

Antimicrobial Drugs That Affect Disease-Causing Organisms

Category	*Description*
Antiseptics	**Chemicals that kill or inhibit the growth of microorganisms and are used on living tissue.**
Disinfectants	**Chemicals that kill or inhibit the growth of microorganisms and are applied to inanimate objects.**
Antibiotics	**Drugs produced by microorganisms that prevent the growth of, or destroy, other microorganisms.**
Antifungals	**Drugs that inhibit or stop the growth of fungus.**
Antivirals	**Drugs that inhibit or stop the growth of viruses.**
Sulfonamides	**Chemical substances that weaken susceptible bacteria; commonly called "sulfa drugs."**
Tuberculostatics	**Drugs that inhibit the growth of the bacteria which cause tuberculosis.**

TABLE 14–2

Pharmacodynamic Drugs and the Body Systems Which They Affect

Category	*Description*
	Nervous System
Stimulants	Drugs that produce increased functional activity. They are often used to counteract mental depression.
Analgesics	This type of medication is given primarily fir relief of pain without loss of consciousness.
Narcotic Analgesics	Habit-forming analgesics which, when withdrawn from the addicted patient, produce certain uncontrollable physical symptoms.
Nonnarcotic Analgesics	This group differs from narcotics in not being habitforming. In addition to relieving pain, some of the drugs in this group also reduce fever (antipyretics).
Nonsteroidal antiinflammatory (NSAIDs)	Inhibit prostaglandins synthesis and reduce inflammation and fever.
Hypnotics and sedatives	Compounds that exert a general depressant effect on the central nervous system and are defined based on the dose and degree of effect.
Barbiturates	A group of compounds structurally related to barbituric acid. They include amobarbital, aprobarbital, butabarbital, mephobarbital, pentobarbital, phenobarbital, and secobarbital. The body may develop a strong dependence upon barbiturates.
Nonbarbiturate hypnotics	These drugs are used as sleeping medications when the doctor chooses not to order barbiturates.
Tranquilizers or antianxiety	Reduce anxiety or tension; however, this group of drugs differs from the hypnotics in that they are not usually given to produce sleep.
Antidepressants	Drugs that elevate the mood and relieve depression.
Anesthetics	Drugs that produce loss of sensation and an inability to perceive pain.
General	General anesthetics produce loss of sensation and muscle relaxation accompanied by loss of consciousness. They are administered by inhalation of a gas or by intravenous injection.
Local	Local anesthetics produce loss of sensation in a limited area of the body by "deadening" the nerves in that area and are usually administered by injection. *Topical* anesthetics are applied to the skin, usually to mucous membranes.
Anticonvulsants	Drugs that suppress convulsions or seizures.
	Endocrine System
Insulin	Hormones that aid in the metabolism of sugars; used primarily in the treatment of diabetes.
Oral hypoglycemics	Chemicals taken by mouth to lower blood sugar in certain types of diabetes, such as non-insulin-dependent diabetes (NIDDM) Type II, and as an adjunct to insulin therapy.
Corticosteroids	Hormones produced by the adrenal glands; often used to treat inflammatory conditions.
Other hormones	Examples are estrogen and thyroid replacement used when the individual gland is not producing enough of its hormone.

TABLE 14–2 (*Continued*)

Category	*Description*
	Respiratory System
Antitussives	Given for the purpose of relieving coughs.
Expectorants	These drugs increase or modify mucus secretions in the bronchi and aid the expulsion of sputum.
Bronchodilators	Drugs which widen the bronchial tubes.
Antihistamines	These drugs help relieve allergic symptoms by counteracting the effect of histamine in the body. Also relieve allergic symptoms of the skin such as hives and other reactions of the body due to allergy.
	Gastrointestinal System
Antacids	Drugs which lower the acidity of the gastric secretions. Commonly used to treat the symptoms of "indigestion."
Antiemetics	Drugs that stop vomiting and relieve nausea.
Antiflatulents	Drugs that decrease amount of gas in gastrointestinal tract.
Emetics	Drugs to produce vomiting.
Cathartics	These drugs aid in causing bowel movements.
Antidiarrheals	Drugs used in the treatment of diarrhea.
Antispasmodics	Drugs used to relieve spasm of the digestive tract.
	Circulatory System
Antiarrhythmics	Drugs such as calcium channel blockers and beta blockers help correct abnormal heart rhythms.
Cardiotonics	These are drugs that affect the heart, usually improving the quality of the heart's action.
Diuretics	These drugs increase the flow of urine. They are used primarily to reduce the blood pressure by reducing fluid retention.
Antihyperlipidemic	Drugs that lower cholesterol levels in the blood.
Vasoconstrictors	These drugs cause the blood vessels to constrict or narrow. They are often used in emergencies to counteract shock by raising the blood pressure.
Vasodilators	These drugs cause the blood vessels to dilate or widen. They may be used to treat hypertension and other diseases of circulatory impairment, where the blood vessels have narrowed.
Anticoagulants	These drugs inhibit the clotting of blood. In disease, they are used most frequently on patients with abnormal clotting within blood vessels.
Hematinics	Iron supplements.
	Musculoskeletal System
Antiarthritics	To treat symptoms of arthritis and other related diseases.
Antigout medications	To treat gout.
Muscle relaxants	To reduce painful spasms of the muscles.

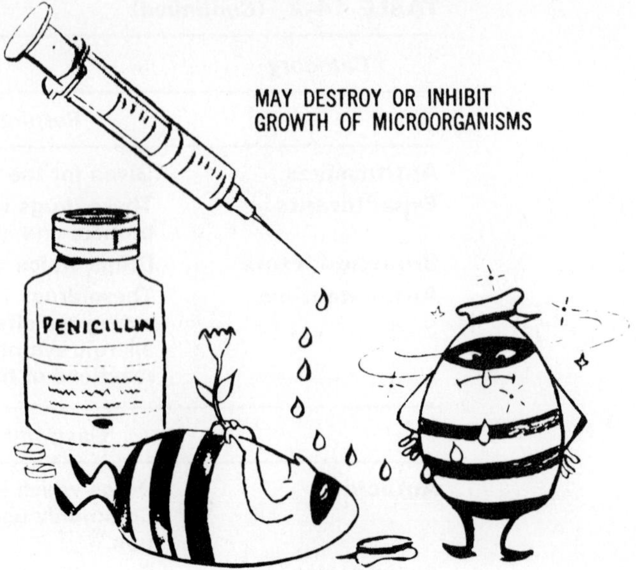
MAY DESTROY OR INHIBIT
GROWTH OF MICROORGANISMS
PENICILLIN

Figure 14–1

drugs serve either to depress specific body functions or to stimulate them. Table 14–2 lists drugs commonly used for various conditions of the different body systems, and Table 14–3 lists chemotherapeutic drugs.

KEY IDEA: COMMONLY ORDERED DRUGS

There are many drugs which doctors commonly order. Add any medications used frequently in your health care institution to the appropriate categories. Examples of these drugs are listed by category below; generic names (which are not capitalized) follow in parentheses. If a drug is a combination of drugs, only one name (brand or generic) will be given. Keep in mind that this is not a complete list of all the drugs a doctor may order and that you will want to become most familiar with the drugs approved to be used in your hospital. (*Note:* Asterisk indicates those categories of drugs that are usually "Automatic Stop" and must be reordered by the doctor within a hospital-specified time period to be continued.)

Analgesics

NONNARCOTIC

Aspirin (acetylsalicylic acid)
Bufferin
Darvon (propoxyphene)

TABLE 14–3
Chemotherapeutic Drugs

Category	*Description*
Antineoplastics	**These drugs are used to kill cancerous body cells.**
Antiparasitics	**These drugs are used to treat diseases caused by such animal parasites as helminths (worms), amoeba, and protozoa.**

Fiorinal
Advil, Naprosyn, Motrin (ibuprofen)
Norgesic
Ovuvail (ketoprofen)
Percogesic
Talwin (pentazocine)
Tylenol (acetaminophen)

NARCOTIC*

Codeine
Codeine in combination with other drugs such as:

- Tylenol c̄ codeine (*Note:* Numbers are assigned to analgesics containing codeine to designate the amount of codeine found in the medication.)
    - #1 = ⅛ grain of codeine (7.5 mg)
    - #2 = ¼ grain of codeine (15 mg)
    - #3 = ½ grain of codeine (30 mg)
    - #4 = 1 grain of codeine (60 mg)
- Aspirin or Empirin c̄ codeine—*Example:* Emp. #3 po q4h prn headache *means* Empirin with ½ grain of codeine.

Demerol (meperidine)
Dilaudid (hydromorphone)
Duragesic (fentanyl)
Empracet c̄ codeine
MSIR, MS Contin, Roxanol, MS, (morphine)
Pantopon
Percocet
Percodan
Vicodin

Anesthetics—Local

Dermoplast (benzocaine)
Marcaine (bupivacaine)
Xylocaine (lidocaine)—with or without epinephrine

Anorexiants

Dexatrim
Obe-Nix (phentermine)
Pre-lu (phendimetrazine)
Redux, Tenuate (dexfenfluramine diethylpropion)

Antacids

Aluminum hydroxide gel
Alphojel

Gelusil
Maalox
Mylanta
Riopan (magaldrate)

Antianxiety (Tranquilizer)

Atarax, Vistaril (hydroxyzine)
Ativan (lorazepam)
Buspar (buspirone)
Compazine (prochlorperizine)
Equanil (mebrobamate)
Librium (chlordiazepoxide)
Mellaril (thioridazine)
Sinequan (doxepin)
Stelazine (trifluroperazine)
Thorazine (chlorpromazine)
Xanax (alprazolam)

Antiarthritics

Ascriptin (aspirin)
Butazolidin (phenylbutazone)
Feldene (piroxicam)
Motrin (ibuprofen)
Naprosyn (naproxen)
Tolectin (tolmetin)

Antibiotics*

Achromycin, Panmycin, Tetrex (tetracycline)
Amikin (amikacin)
Amoxil (amoxicillin)
Bicillin (penicillin G benzathine)
Cipro (ciprofloxacin)
Floxin (ofloxacin)
Garamycin (gentamicin)
Ilosone (erythromycin)
Kantrex (kanamycin)
Keflex (cephalexin)
Keflin (cephalothin)
Kefzol, Ancef (cephazolin)
Mefoxin (cefoxitin)
Monurol (fostomycin tromethamine)
Mycifradin (neomycin)

Nebcin (tobramycin)
Principen, Omnipen, Polycillin (ampicillin)
Prostaphlin (oxacillin)
Rocephin (ceftriaxone)
Staphcillin (methicillin)
Streptomycin
Terramycin (oxytetracycline)
Vantin (cefpodoxime proxetil)
Vibramycin (doxycycline)
Wycillin (procaine penicillin G)
Zinacef (cefuroxime)
Zovirax (acyclovivir)

Anticoagulants*

Coumadin (warfarin sodium)
Dicumarol
Heparin

Anticonvulsants

Cerebyx (fosphenytoin)
Dilantin (phenytoin)
Mysoline (primidone)
Phenobarbital

Antidepressants

Aventyl (nortriptyline)
Elavil (amitriptyline)
Nardil (phenelzine)
Norpramin (desipramine)
Paxil (paroxetine)
Prozac (fluoxetine)
Sinequan (doxepin)
Tofranil (imipramine)
Triavil (perphenazine and amitriptyline)
Zoloft (sertraline)

Antidiabetics

ORAL HYPOGLYCEMICS

Diabinese (chlorpropamide)
Dymelor (acetohexamide)
Glucotrol (glipizide)

Micronase (glyburide)
Orinase (tobutamide)
Precose (acarbose)

INJECTABLE HYPOGLYCEMICS

Humulin R
Iletin: regular, lente, semilente, NPH
Insulin: regular, lente, semilente, NPH
Isophen insulin (NPH)
Novolin R
Protamine zinc and iletin (PZI)
Ultralente

Antidiarrheals

Donnagel
Imodium (loperamide)
Kaopectate
Lomotil (diphenoxylate and atropine)
Paregoric (opium)

Antiemetics/Antinauseants

Antivert (meclizine)
Compazine (prochlorperazine)
Dramamine (dimenhydrinate)
Emete-Con (benzquinamide)
Phenergan (promethazine)
Thorazine (chlorpromazine)
Tigan (trimethobenzamide)
Torecan (thiethylperazine)
Vistaril (hydroxyzine)

Antiflatulents

Ilopan (dexpanthenol)
Mylicon, Flatulex (simethicone)

Antigout

Anturane (sulfinpyrazone)
Benemid (probenecid)
Colabid
Col-Probenecid
Colchicine
Indocin (indomethacin)
Zyloprim (allopurinol)

Antihistamines

Actifed
Allegra (fexofenadine)
Benadryl (diphenhydramine)
Chlor-Trimeton (chlorpheniramine)
Claritin (loratadine)
Dimetane Extentabs (brompheniramine)
Ornade
Triaminic

Antihyperlipidemics

Lipitor (atorvastatin)
Mevacor (lovastin)
Pravachol (pravastatin)
Questran (cholestyramine)
Zocor (simvastatin)

Antineoplastics

Adrucil (fluorouracil)
Cytoxan (cyclophosphamide)
Methotrexate
Nitrogen mustards
Platinol AQ (cisplatin)

Antisecretory Agents

Prevacid (lanisoprazole)
Prilosec (omeprazole)
Tagamet (cimetidine)
Zantac (ranitidine)

Antispasmodics

Bentyl (dicyclomine)
Clindex (clidinium)
Daricon (oxyphencyclimine)
Donnatal
Probanthine (propantheline)

Antitussives

Benylin DM (dextromethorphad)
Codeine
Hycodan (hydrocodone bitartrate)

Sudafed, Dorcol (pseudoephedrine)
Terpin hydrate
Tessalon (benzonatate)

Antivirals

Cytovene (ganciclovir)
Epivir (lamivudine)
Famvir (famciclovir)
Flumadine (rimantadine)
Foscavir (foscarnet)
Hivid (zalcitabine)
Invirase (saquinavir)
Retrovir (zidovudine)
Symadine (amantadine)
Valtrex (valacyclovir)
Videx (didanosine)
Virazole (ribavirin)
Zerit (stavudine)
Zovirax (acyclovir)

Bronchodilators

Adrenalin (epinephrine)
Atrovent (ipratropium)
Brethaire (terbutaline)
Bronkosol (isoetharine)
Choledyl (oxytriphylline)
Ephedrine
Isuprel (isoproterenol)
Metaprel, Alupent (metaproterenol)
Phyllocontin (aminophylline)
Proventil (albuterol)
Theolair (theophylline)

Cardiotonics

Incor (amrinone)
Lanoxin (digoxin)
Primacor (milrinone)

Cardiovasculars

ANTIANGINALS

Cardene (nicardipine)
Cardizem (diltiazem)

Isordil (isosorbide dinitrate)
Nitrobid, Nitrostat (nitroglycerin)
Procardia (nifedipine)
Vascor (bepridil)

ANTIARRHYTHMICS

Calan (verapamil)
Inderal (propranolol)
Pronestyl (procainamide)
Quinidine
Xylocaine (lidocaine)

ANTIHYPERTENSIVES

Aldomet (methyldopa)
Apresoline (hydralazine)
Calan, Isoptin (verapamil)
Capoten (captopril)
Cardura (doxazosin)
Catapres (clonidine)
Diovan (valsartan)
Ismelin (quanethidine)
Lexxel (enalapril)
Lopressor (metoprolol)
Minipress (prazosin)
Norvasc (amlodipine)
Plendil (felodipine)
Tenormin (atenolol)
Zestril (lisinopril)

VASODILATORS

Apresoline (hydralazine)
Loniten (minoxidil)
Priscoline (tolazoline)
Vasodilin (isoxsuprine)
Vasotec (enalapril)

Cathartics, Laxatives, and Stool Softeners

Cascara
Colace, D-S-S (docusate)
Dulcolax (bisacodyl)
Metamucil (psyllium)
Milk of Magnesia (magnesium hydroxide)
Mineral oil

Peri-Colace
Senokot (senna)

Diuretics

Aldactazide
Aldactone (spironolactone)
Bumex (bumetanide)
Diamox (acetazolamide)
Diuril (chlorothiazide)
Dyazide
Edecrin (ethacrynicacid)
Esidrix (hydrochlorothiazide)
HydroDIURIL
Hygroton (chlorthalidone)
Lasix (furosemide)
Midamor (amiloride)

Emetics

Ipecac syrup

Hematinics

Imferon
Ircon-FA (ferrous fumarate)
Feosol (ferrous sulfate)

Hormones

Delestrogen (estradiol)
DES (diethylstilbestrol)
Norplant (levonorgestrel)
Prednisone
Premarin (conjugated estrogens)
Provera (medroxyprogesterone)
Solu-Cortef (hydrocortisone)
Solu-Medrol (methyprednisolone)
Synthroid (levothyroxine)
Tace (chlorotrianisene)
Thyroid

Muscle Relaxants

Flexeril (cyclobenzaprine)
Paraflex, Flexaphen (chlorzoxazone)

Robaxin (methocarbamol)
Soma (carisoprodol)
Valium (diazepam)

Nasal Decongestants

Afrin (oxymetazoline)
Neo-Synephrine (phenylephrine)
Otrivin (xylometazoline)

Potassium Replacements

K-Dur, K-lyte (potassium chloride)
Kaon (potassium gluconate)
Slow-K (potassium)

Vitamins

Centrum
Optilets
Solu-B $\bar{c}$ C
Theragran

Sedatives/Hypnotics

Chloral hydrate
Dalmane (flurazepam)
Halcion (triazolam)
Luminal (phenobarbital)
Nembutal (pentobarbital)
Placidyl (ethchlovynol)
Restoril (temazepam)
Seconal (secobarbital)

KEY IDEA: DRUG MONITORING

Anticoagulants

Anticoagulant drugs require careful monitoring. They are given to reduce the potential for the formation of blood clots. If a patient receives too little of the medication, dangerous blood clots may form. If the patient receives too much, hemorrhage may occur. Therefore, patients on anticoagulants will frequently have daily blood tests to monitor the effects of the drug. Two common laboratory tests are **prothrombin time** and **partial thromboplastin time (PTT)** or **activated partial thromboplastin time (APPT).**

The doctor will decide to increase, continue, decrease, or discontinue the anticoagulant based on the results of the laboratory tests.

The health unit coordinator must understand the significance and extreme importance of these orders. Often an **anticoagulant record** will be added to the chart to help monitor the results of each blood test and the amount of the anticoagulant given. This is a *supplemental chart form* (see page 218). Results of the PTT may be telephoned to the doctor before the next dose of anticoagulant is ordered.

Insulin

Insulin is given to reduce the amount of sugar in the blood. Careful monitoring of both the urine and blood of the diabetic is necessary to ensure that the patient is receiving the correct amount of insulin. The **Diabetic Record** (a supplemental chart form) is often added to the patient's chart to help monitor the results of blood and urine tests and record insulin dosages (see page 218).

The doctor will select the type of insulin based on how quickly or slowly it acts and how long that action lasts. Some patients will receive more than one type of insulin. Here are two types:

- Regular insulin is quick-acting and of short duration.
- NPH insulin is slower to act but of longer duration.

Other types of antidiabetics or hypoglycemics are ordered for their intermediate action. Each diabetic condition is individual and requires a careful decision by the doctor.

Sliding Scale Insulin Orders

Sliding scale is a term indicating the amount of insulin to be given according to the results of a test to measure the amount of sugar in the urine or in the blood. These tests are done on the nursing unit by the nursing staff and not by the laboratory. No requisition or computer-generated order to the laboratory is necessary.

Urine Test: Using a chemically treated test strip, the nurse will test the patient's urine. A common order would require this test done a.c. & h.s.

Blood Test: Most commonly, however, the nurse performs a simple bedside blood test, using a device to prick the patient's finger and then analyze the results on a glucometer such as an Accucheck or Glucometer. Insulin is given to the patient based on the results of the blood test, using an **insulin sliding scale order** such as the one shown below.

If Accucheck	< 150	=	0 U regular insulin
	151–200	=	2 U regular insulin
	201–250	=	4 U regular insulin

If > 260, notify physician.

Other medications which are monitored by blood testing include

- Lithium
- Digitalis
- Barbiturates

KEY IDEA: MEDICATION ORDER FORM

The nurse must have precise directions from the physician for each medication he/she is to administer to a patient. For this reason, every medication order is written according to a specific form which includes all necessary directions. There are four primary categories in this form and often one additional category.

1. **Name of drug**—what is the name of the drug to be given?
2. **Dosage of drug**—how much of the drug should be given at one time?
3. **Route of administration**—by what means is the drug to be introduced into the patient's body?
4. **Frequency of administration**—how often is this drug to be given?
5. **Qualifying phrase**—the doctor may want to qualify the order. For example, he may specify that the medication be given "with milk," or "for pain in feet."

A typical form a medication order takes is shown below.

Aspirin 1	600 mg 2	p.o. 3	q4h p.r.n 4	for headache 5

KEY IDEA: NAMES OF DRUGS

You will soon become familiar with the names of drugs frequently ordered by the doctors in your hospital. At first many names will sound alike to you, and you will need to pay close attention to spelling variations. Each drug usually has at least three names and *may* have many more. (See Table 14–4 for example.)

- **Chemical Name:** This is a precise description of the chemical constitution of a drug. It is rarely, if ever, used in writing a doctor's order.
- **Generic name:** This is usually proposed by the company that has developed the drug. Generic names are established by the U.S. Adopted Name Council. Once the generic name is agreed upon, it is never changed. It cannot be used as a name for a new drug, and it can be used

TABLE 14–4

Examples of Drug Names for Single Preparation

	Drug	*Manufacturer*
Chemical name	4-dimethyl-amino-1, 4, 4a, 5, 5a, 6, 11, 12a-octahydro-3, 6, 10, 12, 12a-pentahydroxy-6-methyl-1, 11-dioxo-2-naphthacene-carboxamide.	
Generic name	tetracycline	
Brand name	Achromycin®	Lederle
	Panmycin®	Upjohn
	Sumycin®	E.R. Squibb & Sons

in all countries. The generic name is often derived from the chemical name but it is much simpler. It is never capitalized. Many hospitals require their pharmacies to label all medications with their generic names.

- **Trade or brand name:** This is the special name given to a drug by each company manufacturing it.

In addition to the name of the drug itself, the way in which it is pharmaceutically prepared is often indicated. Examples are: Zinc Oxide *Ointment; Enteric-Coated* Aspirin; Darvon® *Capsules;* and *Spirits* of Ammonia.

Pharmaceutical preparations are usually indicated by abbreviations. Table 14–5 lists the English names and their usual abbreviations. These abbreviations are important for at least two reasons:

1. You are much less likely to make errors, particularly when deciphering difficult handwriting, if you *know* the meanings of the abbreviations.
2. Many of the abbreviations are used, not only with medication orders, but as parts of other orders and frequently in conversation.

KEY IDEA: DOSAGES OF DRUGS

Drug dosages are measured either by weight or by volume. There are two systems of weights and measures used in hospitals today:

1. **Apothecaries' system:** Because the United States originated as a colony of England, their system was widely used here until modern times. Weight equivalents in this system are erratic; for example, 8 drams = an ounce, and 12 ounces = a pound by weight.
2. **Metric system:** This system, like our money system, is based on multiples of 10 and is a simpler system in which to compute dosages.

Unless your hospital has strict rules about the use of one system or the other, you will have to be familiar with both. You will not be required to convert dosages from one system to another. However, you must be able to rec-

TABLE 14–5

Names and Abbreviations of Pharmaceutical Preparations

Name	*Abbreviation*	*Name*	*Abbreviation*
Ampules	Amp.	Oil	Ol.
Capsules	Caps.	Ointment	Ung.
Compound	Comp.	Pills	Pil.
Elixir	Elix.	Powder	Pulv.
Emulsion	Emul.	Solution	Sol.
Enteric-coated	E.C.	Spansules	Spans.
Extract	Ext.	Spirits	Spt.
Fluidextract	Fldext.	Suppository	Supp.
Liniment	Lin.	Syrup	Syr.
Liquid	Liq.	Tablets	Tab.
Lotion	Lot.	Tincture	Tr., Tinct.
Mixture	Mixt.	Troches, lozenges	Troch.

TABLE 14–6

Measures in the Apothecaries' and Metric Systems

	Apothecaries' System		*Metric System*	
	Terms	*Abbreviations*	*Terms*	*Abbreviations*
Measures of weight	Grain	gr.	Microgram	mcg.
	Dram	ʒ	Milligram	mg.
	Ounce	oz. or ℥	Gram	Gm.
	Pound	lb.	Kilogram	kg.
Measures of volume	Minim	min. or ♏	Milliliter (Cubic centimeter)	ml. (c.c.)
	Fluidram*	fl. ʒ		
	Fluidounce*	fl. oz. or fl℥		
	Pint	pt.	Liter	L.
	Quart	qt.		
	Gallon	gal.		

*In practice, the "fluid" in these two terms is not commonly used.

ognize the abbreviations and copy them accurately from the doctor's order sheet (see Table 14–6).

Other variations in recording drug dosages exist between the two systems, as shown in Table 14–7.

Other abbreviations for measures of drug dosages you will occasionally encounter are shown below.

Term	*Abbreviation*
Drop	gtt.
Teaspoon	tsp. or t.
Tablespoon	tbsp. or T.
Unit	U.
Milliequivalent	mEq.

TABLE 14–7

Variations in Drug Dosages

Apothecaries' System	*Example*	*Metric System*	*Example*
1. Quantities less than one are written as common fractions; one half is designated by the symbol $\overline{\text{ss}}$.	gr. 1/4 gr. $\overline{\text{ss}}$	1. Quantities less than one are written as decimal fractions, with a zero placed in front of the decimal point, if no number precedes it.	0.25 mg. 0.6 mg.
2. Lowercase Roman numerals are used to indicate whole numbers.	ʒ iii ♏ v gr. ii $\overline{\text{ss}}$	2. Arabic numerals are used to indicate whole numbers.	3 mg. 5 c.c.
3. Labels designating measurements are placed before the numerals.	As above	3. Labels designating measurements follow the numerals.	As above

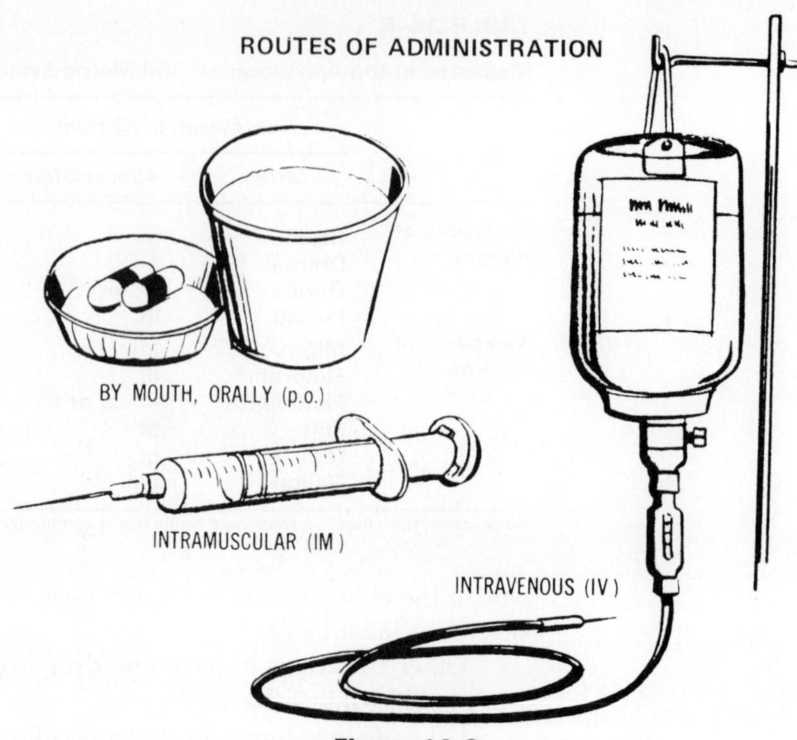

Figure 14–2

KEY IDEA: ROUTE OF ADMINISTRATION

The same drug can often be prepared in different ways and administered to patients by different routes. (Fig. 14–2.) For example, codeine comes in tablet form and can be given to a patient by mouth, but if the doctor wants his patient to have much faster pain relief he/she may order codeine solution to be given by injection. Most routes of administration are abbreviated in the written order, as indicated below.

Route	*Abbreviation*
by mouth—orally	**p.o.**
subcutaneous	**s.c., subcut.**
hypodermic	**H.**
intramuscular	**IM**
intravenous	**IV**
intravenous push	**IVP**
in right eye	**OD**
in left eye	**OS**
in both eyes	**OU**
in right ear	**AD**
in left ear	**AS**
in both ears	**AU**
sublingual—under the tongue	**subling.**

KEY IDEA: INTRAVENOUS MEDICATION ORDERS

Types of intravenous orders are discussed in detail in Chapter 15, Nursing Procedure Orders. In that chapter it is explained that doctors often order medications to be placed directly into the IV bottle or bag. The most common orders are for potassium chloride (KCl) or for vitamins, although other medications are also ordered.

1000 cc 5% DW c̄ 20 mEq. KCl
1000 cc 5% DW c̄ 1 amp. solu B c̄ C.

These types of orders mean that the medication, dissolved in the IV fluid, will drip into the patient's vein at the rate of flow of the existing IV.

Intravenous Push (IVP)

When the doctor orders medication by IVP, it is given directly into the vein by syringe and needle or into the IV tubing via a special part of the tubing designed for this purpose.

Lanoxin 0.5 mg. IVP
Demerol (meperidine) 25 mg IVP

Some IVP medications may be injected into a minibag and allowed to drip into the patient's vein rather than by actual injection into the tubing (discussed further in Chapter 15).

IV Heparin Lock

There are times when the doctor wishes a patient to receive IV medication on a regular basis. However, the doctor does not want the patient to suffer the inconvenience of being attached to IV tubing or the patient has no need for an IV, so a Heparin lock is ordered. A needle with a small length of tubing is inserted into the vein. The end of the tubing has a resealable stopper. The ordered IV medication is instilled into this stopper and the needle is kept open (unclogged by clotted blood) by flushing a small amount of heparin solution (an anticoagulant which prevents the blood from clotting) into the tubing each time after the medication is injected into the stopper.

PCA Device

Heparin lock flush solution, USP, may be ordered for this purpose. It allows a patient to administer his/her own pain medication (see p. 308, Chapter 15).

KEY IDEA: TIMES OF ADMINISTRATION

The nurse must be given special directions concerning *when* a medication is to be given. Some drugs, such as sleeping medications, should be given only at night before bedtime. Others, given to affect digestion, are best administered before meals. Some must be given three or four times a day to produce the desired level of medication in the blood. Abbreviations are often used to denote how often a drug is to be given. Most hospitals have a precise schedule of hours equivalent to each of these expressions. For example, q.i.d. may mean that a medication should be given at 10 A.M., 2 P.M., 6 P.M., and 10 P.M. In other hospitals, q.i.d. may indicate that the medication be given at 9 A.M., 1 P.M., 5 P.M., and 9 P.M. (see Table 14–8).

European or Military Time

Many hospitals prefer to use this designation of time to eliminate the need for A.M. or P.M. The clock in Fig. 14–3 illustrates military time.

Each nursing station will have a schedule of medication times posted. An example of medication times using military time is shown in Table 14–9. Your hospital will provide a schedule of medication times, which will be posted at your desk at the nurses' station. Table 14–10 shows examples of working shifts in military and standard time. Table 14–11 shows examples of medication times.

KEY IDEA: QUALIFYING PHRASES

Most phrases in doctor's orders which qualify the administration of a drug will be written out in longhand. They need only be copied as written when you are transcribing the order. Sometimes, however, you will encounter the abbreviations shown below and you should know what they mean.

Phrase	*Abbreviations*
of each	$\overline{aa}$
with	$\bar{c}$
without	$\bar{s}$
freely, as desired	ad lib.
do not repeat	non rep.

TABLE 14–8

Typical Times of Administration and Their Common Abbreviations

Times	*Abbreviations*
every other day	q.o.d.
every day	q.d.
twice a day	b.i.d.
three times a day	t.i.d.
four times a day	q.i.d.
every hour	q.h.
every ____ hours	q.____h.
at hour of sleep (once only)	h.s.
at hour of sleep (when necessary)	h.s. p.r.n.
before meals	a.c.
after meals	p.c.
at once, without delay	Stat.
when necessary or required	p.r.n.
may be repeated once if necessary	s.o.s.

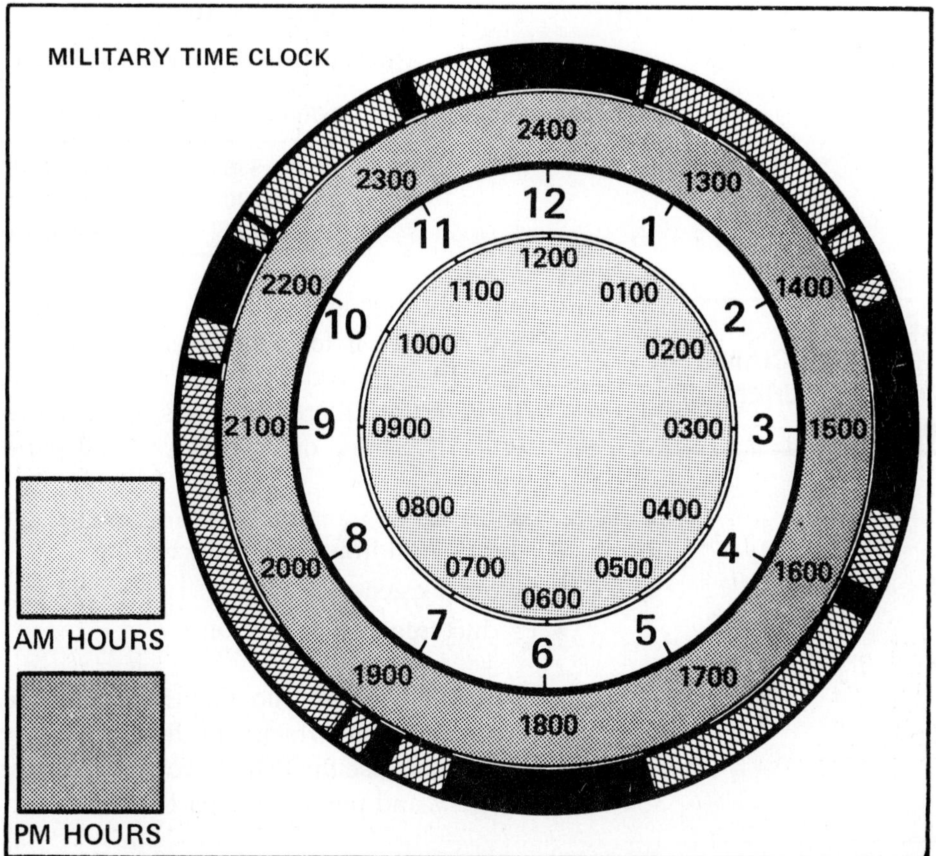

Figure 14–3

TABLE 14–9

Hours of Day

Military Time	*Standard Time*	*Military Time*	*Standard Time*
0030	12:30 A.M.	1230	12:30 P.M.
0100	1:00 A.M.	1300	1:00 P.M.
0130	1:30 A.M.	1330	1:30 P.M.
0200	2:00 A.M.	1400	2:00 P.M.
0300	3:00 A.M.	1500	3:00 P.M.
0400	4:00 A.M.	1600	4:00 P.M.
0500	5:00 A.M.	1700	5:00 P.M.
0600	6:00 A.M.	1800	6:00 P.M.
0700	7:00 A.M.	1900	7:00 P.M.
0800	8:00 A.M.	2000	8:00 P.M.
0900	9:00 A.M.	2100	9:00 P.M.
1000	10:00 A.M.	2200	10:00 P.M.
1100	11:00 A.M.	2300	11:00 P.M.
1200	12:00 P.M. (NOON)	2400	12:00 A.M. (MIDNIGHT)

TABLE 14–10

Shifts in Military and Standard Time

Military Time	*Standard Time*
0700–1530	7:00 A.M.–3:30 P.M.
1500–2330	3:00 P.M.–11:30 P.M.
2300–0730	11:00 P.M.–7:30 A.M.

KEY IDEA: THE PHYSICIAN'S DESK REFERENCE (PDR)

The PDR, published by Medical Economics each year, is a very helpful reference. You can use it for clarifying drug dosages, drug usage, and correct spelling of drugs for order transcription.

The PDR has different sections listed under the Table of Contents, and each section is printed on different colored paper. The sections you will use most often are:

- Alphabetical index by product name
- Section by generic name
- Product information section

A page number is listed following the drug name. On this page you will find product identification which will describe and explain the drug. It is recommended that you use the PDR as you study drugs for knowledge of spelling, drug category, and purposes of each.

KEY IDEA: THE HOSPITAL DRUG FORMULARY

This resource lists all the drugs that are approved for use in your hospital. There is an ongoing review of the formulary by a committee such as a Pharmacy and Therapeutics Committee. Drugs are added to or deleted from the formulary based on efficacy; existence of other (more or less effective) drugs; cost; demand or usage; bioavailability; and drug availability. If a doctor orders a drug that is not in the formulary, the pharmacist will contact the physician to see if a formulary item could be substituted without compromising

TABLE 14–11

Examples of Medication Times

Order	*Military Time*	*Order*	*Military Time*
DAILY	0900	c̄ MEALS	0800–1200–1700
BID	0900–1700	a.c.	0800–1200–1700
TID	0900–1300–1700	p.c.	0900–1300–1800
QID	0900–1300–1700–2100		
Q2H	0100–0300–0500–0700–0900–1100 1300–1500–1700–1900–2100–2300	COUMADIN	1800
Q3H	2400–0300–0600–0900 1200–1500–1800–2100	HEPARIN	
		•BID	0900–2100
Q4H	0100–0500–0900–1300–1700–2100	•Q6H	0300–0900–1500–2100
Q6H	0600–1200–1800–2400	•Q8H	0100–0900–1700
Q8H	0600–1400–2200		
Q12H	0900–2100		

patient care. The Pharmacy Department is responsible for keeping the formulary up to date and relaying formulary changes to physicians and nurses. Unless the physician indicates otherwise on the Physician's Order Form, the pharmacist will substitute a generic drug as long as the generic product meets the standards required. There will be a copy of the hospital formulary at each nursing station.

KEY IDEA: TYPES OF MEDICATION ORDERS

There are three main types of medication orders, identified by the time and frequency of administration. Your responsibilities in transcribing each of these will vary, so you must be able to tell them apart. The three main types are:

- Standing—Routine and PRN
- Single Dose
- Stat

Standing Orders

This most common type of medication order designates that medication should be given to the patient on a regular schedule for a predetermined number of days or until further notice by the physician. In other words, the order stands as written until it is changed or canceled.

A special category of standing order is the "p.r.n." order. As you have learned, p.r.n. is an abbreviation of Latin words meaning "whenever necessary." The p.r.n. order is transcribed like routine standing orders but differs in that there is no specific time schedule designated for administration. A sample of standing orders is shown below:

Aspirin gr. $\bar{x}$ p.o. q.i.d.
Procaine Penicillin 600,000 U. IM q8h
Codeine 30 mg. p.o. q4h p.r.n. for headache

Single-Dose Orders

Occasionally, the doctor wants his patient to have just one dose of a medication for a specific purpose. Preoperative medications would be examples of this type of order. Often, before being sent to the operating room, the patient is given an injection containing a narcotic, a barbiturate, or perhaps another medication. Since this is to be given once only, it qualifies as a single-dose order.

The time of administration is the factor that generally identifies an order as a single-dose order. No time of administration may be indicated at all; or a specific time of day or date may be written; or an abbreviation such as "h.s." or tonight (which indicates the drug is to be given once only) will identify single-dose orders.

Other medications, commonly ordered as a short series of injections of various dosages—for example, anticoagulants—may also be classified as single-dose orders according to the methods used to transcribe them in your hospital. Examples of single-dose orders are shown below:

> ***Resperine 50 mg. IM at 2 p.m.***
> ***Heparin 40,000 U. IM a.c. noon***
> ***Nembutal 100 mg. p.o. h.s***

Stat. Orders

"Stat." is an abbreviation for the Latin word "statim," meaning "immediately." In serious or emergency situations, a medication may be ordered "stat." This requires that the nurse administer the medication as soon as possible. Typical stat. orders are shown below:

> ***Morphine sulphate gr. 1/6 SC stat.***
> ***Nitroglycerine 0.9 mg. p.o. stat.***
> ***Compazine 50 mg. IM stat.***

KEY IDEA: BASIC TRANSCRIPTION PROCEDURE

Transcribing a standing order entails a number of specific tasks. The seven-step procedure described in Chapter 13 may help to simplify your duties.

First, Recognize the Order

Remember: Standing orders can be identified by the time-of-administration schedules accompanying them. Any medication of a specific dosage ordered for an unstated period of time or for longer than 24 hours will generally qualify as a standing order. Refer again to the example of standing orders on p. 275.

Second, "RIP"

Tear off the NCR copy and route to Pharmacy if this is your hospital's method for obtaining patient drugs. Another NCR copy may go to the nurse to notify him or her of the medication order. Hospitals have different ways of letting the Pharmacy Department know about medication orders. In hospitals with integrated computer systems, the entering of the orders into the computer will be the form of notification. Some hospitals FAX the new orders to the pharmacy. Learn your hospital's rules regarding this procedure.

Third, Prioritize

Always select those orders of highest priority to transcribe first.

Fourth, Transfer the Order to Special Records (Kardex)

There may be as many as three special records on which a medication order should be noted—Kardex, medication records, and medication ticket.

Kardex. The order must be transcribed, exactly as written, to the appropriate section of the Kardex. It must be written legibly and accurately. The order is often recorded in pencil so it can be erased when canceled. Often, you are required to specify the time schedule of administration in terms of hours.

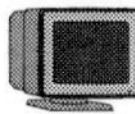

When computer-generated Kardexes are used, orders are entered into the computer and a printout is obtained. No handwriting is necessary. If the noncomputerized method is used, the order must be transcribed exactly as written, to the appropriate section of the Kardex.

Medication Record. All hospitals have some kind of medication record, which is one of the standard chart forms. When orders for a newly admitted patient are received, it is usually the nurse who transcribes the orders onto the Medication Administration Record (MAR). In a computerized system, pharmacy usually prints out an MAR for every hospitalized patient, and these are distributed at a designated time to each nursing unit (usually at night). The night nurse then compares the computerized sheet with the initial sheet that was completed upon admission, updates the computerized sheet, places a copy in the chart, and returns a copy to pharmacy. This serves as a double check of all medication orders. The copy given back to pharmacy is also used for charging purposes. (Fig. 14–5.)

As new orders come in, the health unit coordinator inputs them into the computer and they are printed out onto the Kardex. The nurse (or the health unit coordinator if specially trained) writes the new orders on the medication administration record, pharmacy receives the new information via the computer or FAX, and the cycle repeats.

If it is your responsibility to record medications on the medication record, you must be particularly careful to demonstrate your skill of accuracy. Be sure when writing a dosage that includes a decimal to always write a zero before the decimal point to exclude any possibilities of a fraction being interpreted as a whole number (see Fig. 14–4—digitoxin **0.2 mg**).

DATE	MEDICATION	5/30 MON.	5/31 TUES.	6/1 WED.	6/2 THUR.	6/3 FRI.	6/4 SAT.	6/5 SUN.
5-27-XX	Digitoxin 0.2 mg. p.o. qd.	A.J.T. 10 a.m.	A.J.T. 10 a.m.	10 a.m.				
6-1-XX	Aspirin gr. $\bar{x}$ p.o. q.i.d.			10-2 6-10				
6-1-XX	Procaine Penicillin 600,000 U IM q8h			4P. 12Mn.	8 a.m. 4 p.m. 12 Mn			

Figure 14–4

M.A.R. VERIFIED

BY:

MEDICATION ADMINISTRATION RECORD

M.A.R.

Name: EXAMPLE, IMA   Allergies ==> PENICILLINS   MEMORIAL HOSPITAL
Room: 000   Patient ID: 12345
Sex: F Age: 62 Hgt: 149cm Wgt: 49.09kg MR#:
Diagnosis: DEPRESSION

CONSENT DATES: LITHIUM ANTIPSYCHO ANTICHOLINERGICS ANTIDEPRESSA

Physician: JOHN GOODDOCTOR   MD Phone: 000-0000
Comments: OWN CALCIUM

ADMINISTRATION PERIOD: 05/30/9 @ 2301 thru 05/31/5 @ 2300			s1	s2	s3
Medication	Start	Stop	2301 thru 0700	0701 thru 1500	1501 thru 23
CALCIUM CARBONATE TAB 500MG TUMS PO 1 TAB x 500MG/EA BID LOT #: EXP DATE: **CHEWABLE TABLET**	2000 05/22 JML			0900	1700
ESTROGENS, CONJUGATE TAB 1.25MG PREMARIN PO 1 TAB x 1.25MG/EA DAILY	1800 05/21 RS			0900	
NEFAZODONE TAB 200MG SERZONE PO 2 TAB x 100MG/EA BID	1800 05/21 RS			0900	1700
PATIENT'S OWN MED 1 PT OWN MED PO UD OTC CALCIUM SUPPLEMENT	2000 05/21 RS				
RISPERIDONE TAB 1MG RISPERDAL PO 1 TAB x 1MG/EA HS	1800 05/21 RS				2100
TRIMETHOPRIM/SULFAME 800-160 TAB 1 SEPTRA DS PO 1 TAB BID Total Doses: 20 X 10 DAYS	2000 05/22 JML	1701 06/01		0900	1700

RESPONSE	MEDS NOT GIVEN	INJECTION SITES	SIGNATURE	INITIALS	SIGNATURE	INITIA
A. Relief in 30 Minutes B. Relief in 60 Minutes C. No Relief	B. BP Changes N. Med Not Avail. P. Patient Asleep Q. Off of Unit R. Refused S. NPO/Studies T. NPO/Surgery	INDICATE INJECTION SITE – R OR L 1. Deltoid 2. Abdominal 3. Iliac Crest 4. Thigh = 1-10 Scale Pre & Post Analgesic Pain Assessment 1 = Least Pain 10 = Most Pain				
			Printed: 13:02 on 05/30/9		Page 1 of	

SCHEDULED

Figure 14–5

Medicine Ticket. In many hospitals with the unit dose system, the medicine ticket is no longer used. However, medicine tickets are sometimes used in long-term care or psychiatric facilities. The purpose is to guarantee the nurse's accuracy. The nurse refers to this ticket as the medication is prepared, keeps each ticket with the appropriate medication, and makes a final check just before it is administered to the patient. Medicine tickets vary in form but will ordinarily include the type of information shown. (Fig. 14–6.)

Standardized rules almost always apply to the filling out of medicine tickets:

- *All* information included in the order must be transferred to the ticket *accurately, legibly, and exactly as written.* Abbreviate where the doctor has done so; write out any words or phrases the doctor has written out. This rule should apply whenever orders are transcribed.
- If any information in the order, such as qualifying phrases, cannot be included on the front of the ticket for reasons of space, show *clearly in large, bold letters* that the ticket must be turned over for further inspection.
- Medicine tickets may be color-coded or size-coded to distinguish among different types of medications (e.g., hypnotics, narcotics) or different types of orders (e.g., standing, single dose). Your instructor will explain any variations of this type used in your hospital.

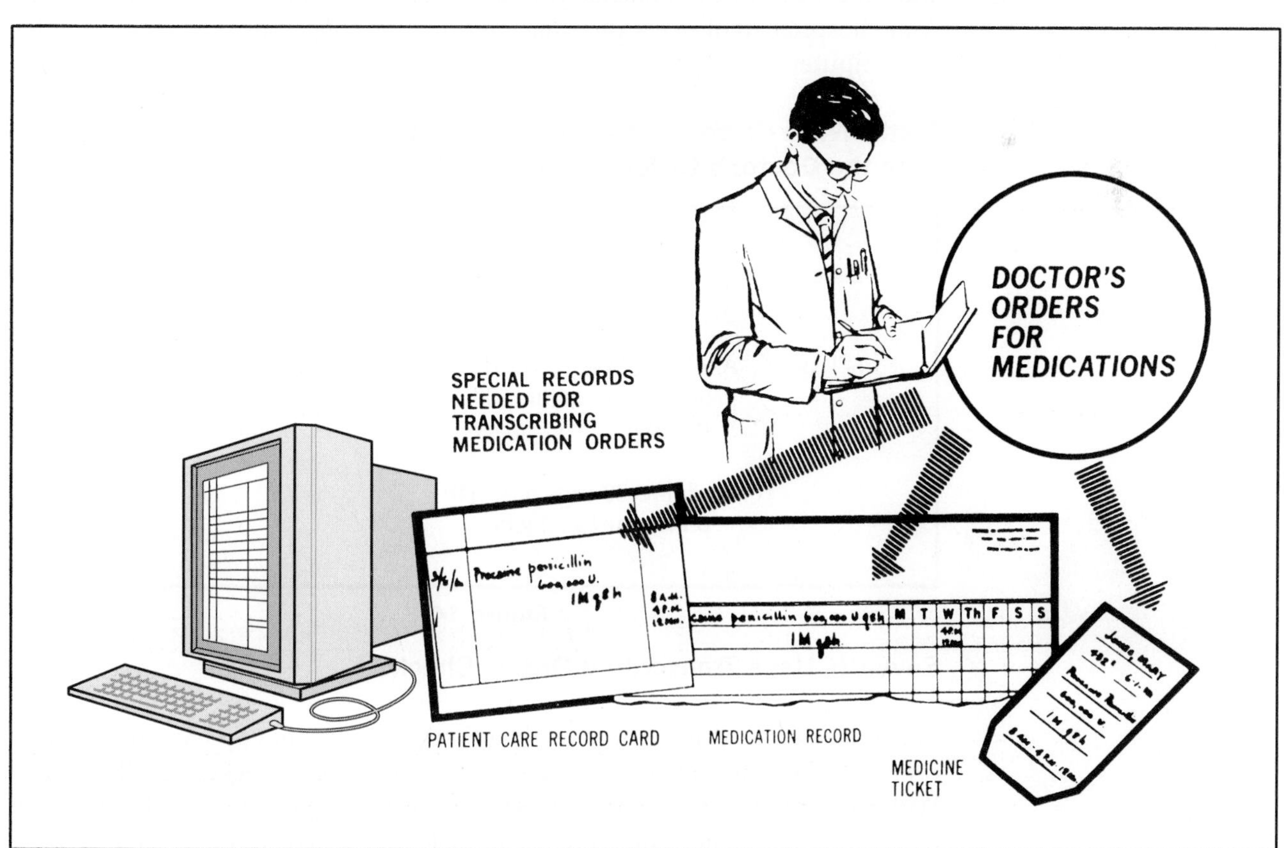

Figure 14–6

Memorial Hospital
PHARMACY — DRUGS Requisition and Charge

Date ______	Are drugs to be taken home? ☐Yes ☐No
Room No. ______	Signature (R.N.) ______
Name ______	Prescribed by ______
Hosp. No. ______	Rx No. ______
Doctor ______	

Order filled and charged by

QUANTITY	ITEM	STRENGTH OR DOSAGE	DIRECTIONS FOR USE	ORAL OR HYPO	CHARGE
				TOTAL CHARGE	

Figure 14–7

Fifth, Requisition Equipment and Services

To carry out a medication order, the nurse must have the medication on hand. Step two, tearing off the appropriate NCR copy from the doctor's order sheet and sending it to the pharmacy, is the common method of obtaining drugs. Some hospitals will use a pharmacy requisition. (Fig. 14–7.) Many will order by computer.

Sixth, Write Correct Transcription *Symbols* on the Doctor's Order Sheet (Fig. 14–8.)

Date	*Order*	*Signature*
6-1-xx	K Aspirin gr. $\overline{x}$ p.o. q.i.d.	
	K Procaine Penicillin 600,000 U. IM q8h	
	K Codeine 30 mg. p.o. q4h p.r.n. for headache	AJ Stahl

Figure 14–8

Seventh, Have Transcribed Orders Checked

This final step is as important as the others. The orders you have transcribed cannot be put into effect until your work has been checked by the nurse. With the help of the nurses with whom you work, you will be able to work out a method of accomplishing this task that is convenient for everyone concerned.

KEY IDEA: STANDING ORDER VARIATIONS

Once a medication has served its purpose and is no longer indicated for the patient in his treatment, the doctor may cancel the order. Also, certain drugs being given to a patient may cancel automatically after a designated number of hours or days and must be renewed by the doctor if the patient should continue to receive them.

Sometimes the physician may wish to increase or decrease the dosage of a particular medicine or to change its route of administration or preparation. If so, a new order will have to be written to that effect. You will learn how to transcribe medication orders for cancellations, renewals, and changes.

Cancellations

> ***Discontinue order for Procaine Penicillin 600,000 U IM q8h $\overline{p}$ 4 p.m. dose***
> ***Cancel Aspirin gr. $\overline{x}$ p.o. q.i.d.***
> ***Discontinue Streptomycin 0.5 gm. IM b.i.d. after today***

When the doctor writes an order for a specific medication to be canceled, several things must be done (Pharmacy will be notified by NCR copy or computer, and the nurse by NCR copy of orders or by health unit coordinator (Fig. 14–9):

- First, the canceled order must be erased from the Kardex (or lined through).
- Next, the medication must be canceled on the medication record.
- If medicine tickets are used, they must be destroyed.

If the patient has been charged for more of the drugs than he actually used before the cancellation order, the remainder must be sent to the phar-

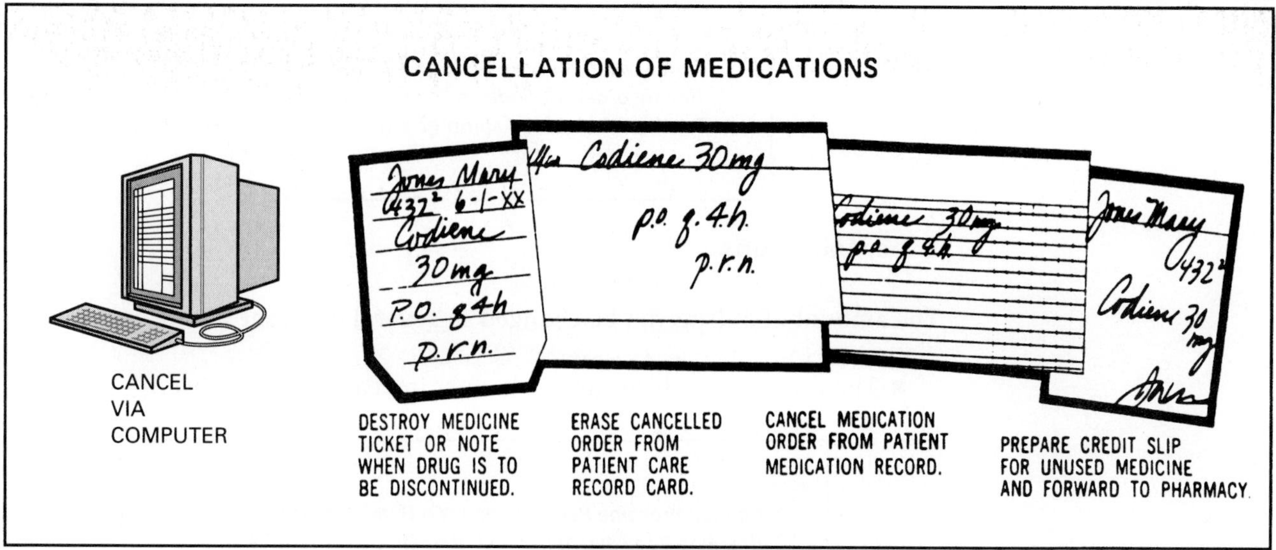
CANCELLATION OF MEDICATIONS
CANCEL VIA COMPUTER
DESTROY MEDICINE TICKET OR NOTE WHEN DRUG IS TO BE DISCONTINUED.
ERASE CANCELLED ORDER FROM PATIENT CARE RECORD CARD.
CANCEL MEDICATION ORDER FROM PATIENT MEDICATION RECORD.
PREPARE CREDIT SLIP FOR UNUSED MEDICINE AND FORWARD TO PHARMACY.

Figure 14–9

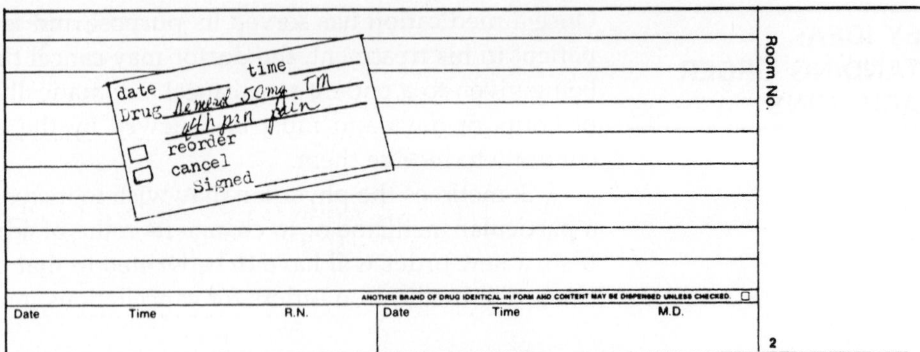

Figure 14–10

macy, where it can be credited to the patient's account. In many hospitals this is taken care of by the pharmacy.

Automatic Stops

In most hospitals, certain medications cancel automatically after being in use for a specified, generally limited number of hours (48 to 72). The continued administration of hypnotics, narcotics, antibiotics, and anticoagulants might result in addiction, habituation, or serious side effects. Orders for such medications usually specify a limited number of times for administration. Many hospitals have established routines by which a patient's doctor is notified that an order for a particular medication has run out. If the doctor wishes the order to be continued, he/she must write an order for renewal. Many hospitals use a stamp on the doctor's order sheet to indicate that an automatic-stop drug must be cancelled or reordered. (Fig. 14–10.)

Renewals

If the doctor wishes an order to continue unchanged, the order may be written as follows:

Renew Streptomycin 0.5 Gm. IM b.i.d. order.
Renew order for Codeine 30 mg. p.o. q4h p.r.n.
Continue order for Aspirin gr $\bar{x}$ p.o. q.i.d.

Other Variations

The amount of a drug can be changed in several different ways:

- The dosage of a drug can be directly increased or decreased.

Change Procaine Penicillin 600,000 U. IM q8h order to read
Procaine Penicillin 300,000 U. IM q8h.

- Or, the same dosage can be given to the patient more or fewer times during the day. Over a period of time, this method may have the same effect as an increase or decrease in dosage.

Change Procaine Penicillin 600,000 U. IM q8h. to Procaine Penicillin 600,000 U. IM q.d.

The route of administration may also be changed.

- If the patient has difficulty swallowing large pills, the doctor may change the order to a liquid preparation. If the patient is nauseated and vomits medication given by mouth, the doctor may order that it be given by injection.

Dilantin 100 mg. p.o. t.i.d. If pt. refuses give IM as ordered previously.

The type of medication may be changed.

Change sleeping medication from Seconal 100 mg p.o. h.s. to Nembutal 100 mg. p.o. h.s. p.r.n.

The preparation of medication may also be changed.

Change Aspirin gr $\bar{x}$ p.o. q.i.d. to E.C. Aspirin tabs gr $\bar{x}$ p.o. q.i.d.

In these kinds of situations, the doctor is always responsible for writing the order for a change in medication on the doctor's order sheet.

KEY IDEA: TRANSCRIBING SINGLE-DOSE AND STAT. ORDERS

Procedures for handling these orders vary widely among hospitals, so specific guidelines will necessarily come to you from your instructor.

KEY IDEA: CONTROLLED DRUGS

The manufacture, distribution, and utilization of medications is the subject of a large body of federal and state laws. The general regulation of drugs by the federal government started with the Food and Drug Act of 1906. Certain drugs have a high potential for abuse. The Controlled Substances Act of 1971 contains the laws regarding these drugs. Controlled substances are classified into five categories called **schedules.** Schedule I drugs are experimental. Schedule II drugs have the highest potential for abuse and schedule V the least. Prescriptions of these drugs are regulated, and the containers are labeled with a "C" followed by the Roman numeral (II–V) indicating the schedule of the drug. As dispensers of controlled substances for medicinal purposes, hospital pharmacies are required by law to be registered with the Drug Enforcement Administration, and careful records must be kept on certain drugs.

Controlled substances are kept locked on the nursing unit, and the nurse or nurses who give medications carry the key to this locked cupboard or drawer of a medicine cart.

When a controlled substance from the locked cupboard is given to a patient, the nurse must record the patient's name and dosage on the sheet for that drug. The nurse's signature must also be on the sheet. When the sheet is completed, it is returned to the pharmacy. The nurse responsible for medications must count each of the controlled drugs at the end of each shift with the nurse coming on duty, who will receive the key and assume the responsibility for the drugs during the next shift. Each drug must be accounted for. Any inaccuracy is serious and must be resolved. No controlled drug may go unaccounted.

The pharmacy is responsible for the replacement of controlled drugs, which are delivered in person by pharmacy personnel. The nurse receiving the new supply of drugs must sign the sheet accompanying the drug at the time of delivery. Clearly, very strict controls of these drugs, mainly narcotics and barbiturates and other hypnotics, are maintained.

When transcribing orders for medications, the health unit coordinator must be aware that drugs in the category of controlled substances are already on the nursing unit in the locked cupboard or drawer. Learn the names of the controlled substances kept on the nursing unit of your hospital.

LEARNING ACTIVITIES

Complete the following classifications of medications:

1. Drugs that destroy or render harmless microorganisms are called ______________________________ drugs.
2. Drugs which alter disease by stimulating or depressing normal body functions are called ______________________________ drugs.
3. Drugs which treat neoplastic disease are called ______________________________ drugs.

Match the category of antimicrobial drugs in column A with the description in column B.

	Column A		*Column B*
(a)	Sulfonamides	____	Produced by microorganisms that prevent the growth of or destroy other microorganisms.
(b)	Antiseptics	____	Chemicals used on inanimate objects that kill or inhibit the growth of microorganisms.
(c)	Antibiotics	____	Drugs that inhibit the growth of the bacteria which cause tuberculosis.
(d)	Disinfectants	____	Commonly called "sulfa drugs."
(e)	Tuberculostatics	____	Chemicals used on living tissue that kill or inhibit the growth of microorganisms.

Match the category of pharmacodynamic drugs in column A with the description in column B.

	Column A		*Column B*
(a)	Anesthetic	____	Produces vomiting
(b)	Stimulant	____	Lowers blood sugar
(c)	Hypoglycemic	____	Increases urine output
(d)	Emetic	____	Treats cancer
(e)	Antitussive	____	Inhibits blood clotting
(f)	Antacid	____	Relieves cough
(g)	Anticonvulsant	____	Relieves allergic symptoms
(h)	Antihistamine	____	Improves quality of heart action
(i)	Cardiotonic	____	Produces loss of sensation
(j)	Antineoplastic	____	Produces increased functional activity
(k)	Diuretic	____	Lowers acidity of gastric secretions
(l)	Anticoagulant	____	Suppresses seizures

Complete the following:

4. List three common anticoagulants.
   (a) ____________________
   (b) ____________________
   (c) ____________________
5. Explain why anticoagulant drugs require careful monitoring.
   ____
   ____
   ____
6. Name two common laboratory tests for monitoring anticoagulants.
   (a) ____________________
   (b) ____________________
7. What does the term "sliding scale" mean?
   ____
   ____

8. List the four main categories of the medication order form.
   (a) ______
   (b) ______
   (c) ______
   (d) ______
9. What is the additional category?
   ______
10. Drugs have at least three names, which are:
    (a) ______
    (b) ______
    (c) ______
11. The generic name is never ______.
12. What does it mean when a medication is ordered IVP?
    ______
    ______
13. What is an IV Heparin lock? ______
    ______
    ______
14. The three main types of medication orders, identified by the time and frequency of administration, are:
    (a) ______
    (b) ______
    (c) ______
15. A special category of the standing order is the ______ order.
16. Give two examples of types of single-dose orders.
    (a) ______
    (b) ______
17. The factor that generally identifies an order as a single-dose order is the ______ of administration.
18. Give two reasons why a medication may be canceled.
    (a) ______
    (b) ______
19. State two ways the dosage of a drug can be changed.
    (a) ______
    (b) ______
20. List two reasons why the route of administration of the medication may be changed.
    (a) ______
    (b) ______
21. The Controlled Substances Act of 1971 contains laws regarding those drugs that have a ______ for abuse.
22. Where are controlled substances kept on the nursing unit?
    ______

23. Which schedule of controlled substances has the highest potential for abuse—II or V? ____________________

24. Define the following medical abbreviations:

(a) a.c. ____________________

(b) OS ____________________

(c) b.i.d. ____________________

(d) mEq. ____________________

(e) $\bar{s}$ ____________________

(f) Gm. ____________________

(g) gr. ____________________

(h) gtt. ____________________

(i) H. ____________________

(j) h.s. ____________________

(k) cc. ____________________

(l) U ____________________

(m) t.i.d. ____________________

(n) stat. ____________________

(o) s.o.s. ____________________

(p) $\bar{c}$ ____________________

(q) q.i.d. ____________________

(r) q.h. ____________________

(s) q.d. ____________________

(t) OD ____________________

(u) p.r.n. ____________________

(v) p.c. ____________________

(w) I.M. ____________________

(x) I.V. ____________________

(y) P.D.R. ____________________

(z) A.U. ____________________

CHAPTER 15

Nursing Procedure Orders

OBJECTIVES

When you complete this chapter, you will be able to:

- Describe nursing treatment orders for suction, bowel care, heat and cold applications, and urinary catheterization.
- Discuss monitoring orders for vital signs, circulation, neurological checks, and blood and urine tests done by nursing.
- Describe the various types of intravenous orders.
- Give examples of activity, positioning, comfort, and safety orders.
- Give examples of miscellaneous orders.
- Demonstrate the ability to transcribe treatment orders.
- Show knowledge of the abbreviations used in this chapter.

A treatment can be loosely defined as any medical or nursing procedure intended to keep a record of, improve, or in any way treat a patient's condition. It would be impossible to describe every type of treatment a doctor might order for his patient. It is even difficult to categorize them effectively. You should be familiar with treatments most frequently ordered. The following descriptions are given for that purpose. As you study this chapter, note the list of abbreviations and definitions for the various orders included in this chapter. Add to the list any other terms in general use in your hospital.

This chapter will include information regarding the following types of orders:

- Suction
- Bowel care
- Heat and cold applications
- Urinary catheterizations
- Vital signs
- Circulation checks
- Craniotomy or neurological checks
- Intake and output
- Capillary blood glucose testing
- Urine tests by nursing for glucose and acetone
- Intravenous therapy
- Activity
- Positioning
- Comfort and safety
- Miscellaneous orders
- Transcription procedure

TREATMENT ORDERS

KEY IDEA: SUCTION ORDERS

Fluids or air are removed from the patient's body through tubes or catheters. The methods used are either **gravity** or **suction.** When fluids are removed by **gravity,** the collecting container is placed near the patient at a level that is lower than his body. The fluids drip into the container. Suction is most commonly ordered to remove fluids from the throat, stomach, intestines, chest, or wounds. Suction apparatus includes various tubes and machines. The doctor will write orders for the establishment, maintenance, and removal of the suction equipment. There may also be orders for irrigation of the various tubes in order to keep them **patent** (draining).

Throat suction is ordered when a patient's throat is blocked by mucus secretions. A catheter and a continuous type of throat suction machine are used.

Deep tracheal suction is a sterile procedure requiring sterile catheters and the use of sterile gloves. The instillation of sterile saline to loosen secretions precedes this procedure. If a patient has a **tracheostomy** (an artificial opening into the windpipe), suctioning is often ordered. This is also a sterile procedure.

Gastric suction is ordered to remove gastric fluids and air from the patient's stomach. This is a low, intermittent type of suction machine quite different from that used for throat suction. It may be portable (Gomco) or built into the wall at the patient's bedside. (Fig. 15–1.)

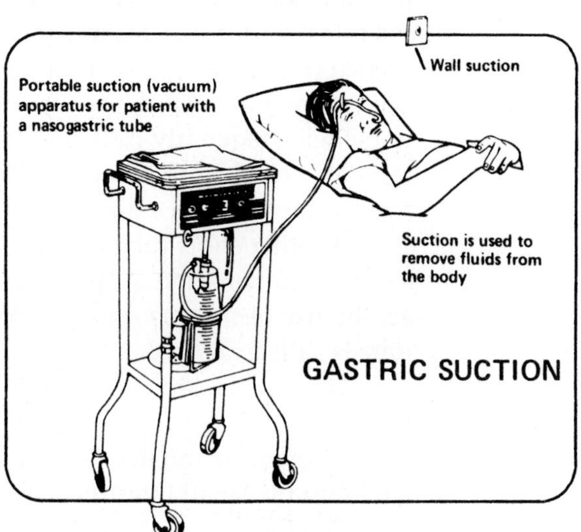
Wall suction
Portable suction (vacuum) apparatus for patient with a nasogastric tube
Suction is used to remove fluids from the body
GASTRIC SUCTION

Figure 15–1

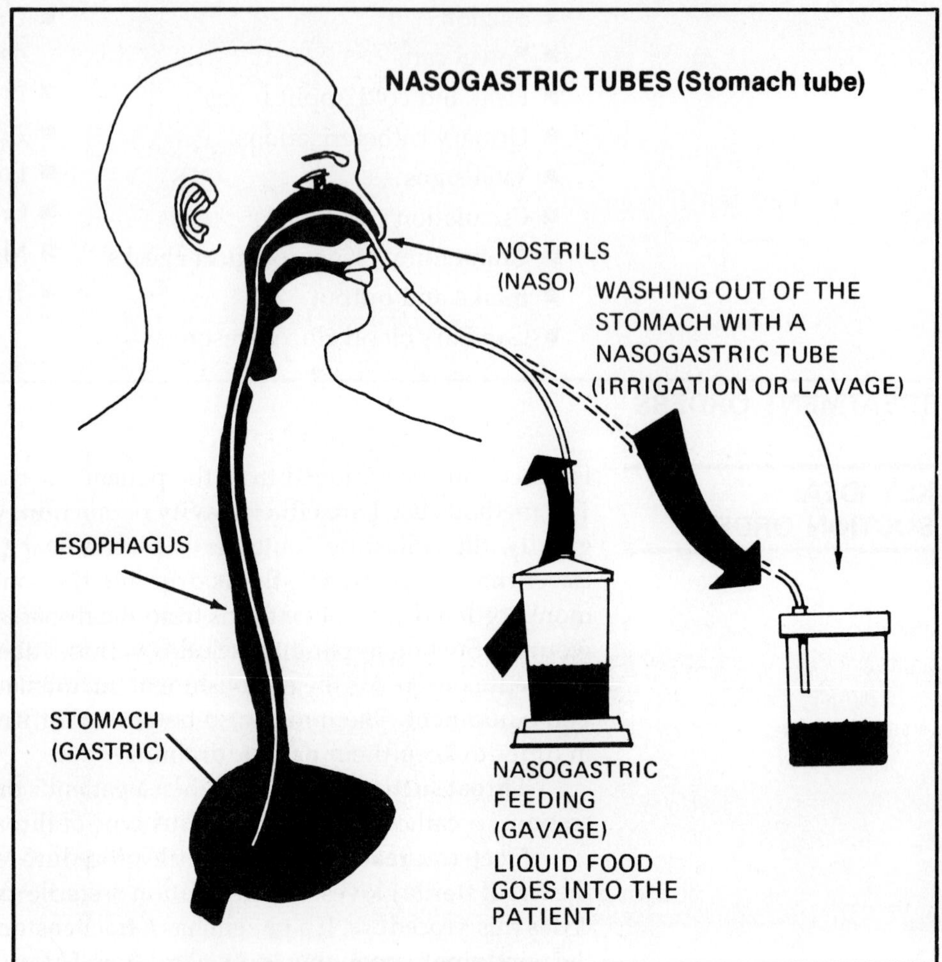

Figure 15–2

To accomplish gastric suction a *nasogastric tube* (also called *Levin tube* or just *NG tube*) is inserted through the patient's nose and into the stomach by the nurse or doctor. This is a single-lumen tube that comes in several sizes: 16 French (Fr) is used most commonly for adults, 6 Fr to 12 Fr for children. This tube is then attached to a tube leading to the gastric suction machine. The nurse will frequently milk and/or irrigate the N/G tube with normal saline (NS) to keep the tube draining. An irrigation tray, usually disposable, will be needed for this procedure. (Fig. 15–2.)

Another short tube is a *gastric sump tube* (e.g. *Salem* or *Ventrol*), which is a double-lumen tube. A special procedure that washes out the patient's stomach by use of the nasogastric tube is called *lavage* (feeding through the N/G tube is called *gavage*).

Long tubes are used to decompress the bowel and are usually 6 to 10 feet long. The *Miller-Abbott tube* is a double-lumen tube with a balloon that, once inserted, is inflated with air, or partially filled with mercury, to help it pass into the small intestine.

The *Cantor tube* is a single-lumen tube with a small rubber bag at the distal (far) end that is filled with mercury before insertion.

Gastric suction may also be accomplished via a gastrostomy tube. This tube leads directly from the stomach and has been sutured in place by a doctor. It is connected to the gastric suction machine.

Thoracic drainage is accomplished when chest tubes are inserted by the physician into the chest cavity to remove air or fluid. This is usually done in surgery, often as an emergency procedure. These tubes are then attached to a water-sealed bottle system or disposable plastic unit (e.g., Pleur-evac), and either gravity drainage or suction such as an Emerson pump is used to drain air and fluids from the pleural cavity.

> ***Chest tube to Emerson pump c̄ 20 cm (centimeters) pressure.***

Hemovac suction. A Hemovac is a small, disposable suction apparatus attached to a drain (tube) during surgery that leads from a patient's wound. It is used frequently with mastectomies. The throat, gastric, and chest suction machines must be plugged into an electrical outlet for operation. The Hemovac is *not electrical* and is manually compressed at intervals and allowed to expand to create suction.

The health unit coordinator should know that the tubes or catheters utilized in throat, gastric, and chest suction are disposable. The machines are not disposable. The kind of catheter and suction machine is different with each type of suction, and the machine will be returned to central supply for cleaning and reissue. It is the licensed nurse (RN or LVN/LPN) who carries out the various types of suction orders. In many hospitals deep tracheal suction is done by the inhalation or respiratory therapists.

KEY IDEA: WOUND REINFUSION

In wound reinfusion or autoreinfusion, a drain from a wound (usually an orthopedic wound), instead of being attached to a Hemovac, is put into a sterile collector where blood and other wound drainage is collected (usually about 100 to 200 cc). This then drops into a sterile blood bag and reinfuses as an IV. The Stryker Autovac and CBC II are examples of these devices.

KEY IDEA: BOWEL CARE ORDERS

The doctor will frequently write orders dealing with the patient's intestinal elimination. Orders for enemas are often written prior to surgery, certain x-ray procedures, delivery, or during the patient's hospitalization to relieve flatus (intestinal gas) or constipation. Common types of enemas are:

- **TWE**—tap water enema
- **SSE**—soap suds enema
- **NSE**—normal saline enema
- **OR enema**—An oil retention enema inserts oil into rectum to soften stool
- **Fleet or Travad enema**—disposable enema (Fig. 15–3.)

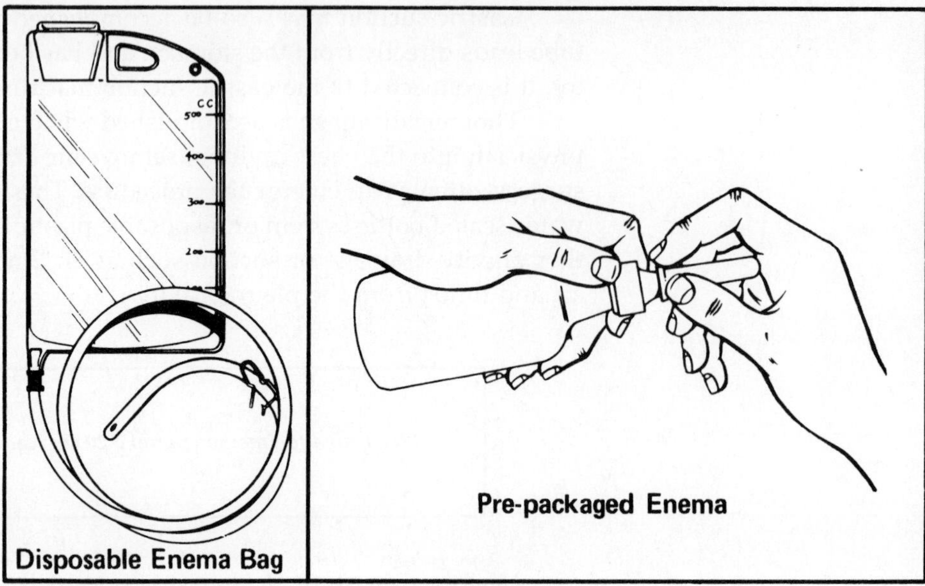

Figure 15–3

Other Intestinal Elimination Orders

Harris Flush. An irrigation of the rectum in which water is run in and out of the rectum for about 10 minutes is called a Harris Flush. The purpose of the Harris Flush is to relieve the patient of uncomfortable intestinal gas.

A **rectal tube** (flatus bag) is a tube attached to a bag and inserted into the rectum for the purpose of removing intestinal gas.

Colostomy Irrigation. A **colostomy** is an artificial opening into the patient's large intestine to allow for bowel movements. An order for a colostomy irrigation is an order for an enema. The difference between an enema and an irrigation is that the irrigating tube is inserted into the **stoma,** or surgically created opening, to change the path of the patient's feces from the rectum. This is done when the colon is diseased or injured. (Fig. 15–4.)

SIGMOID COLOSTOMY

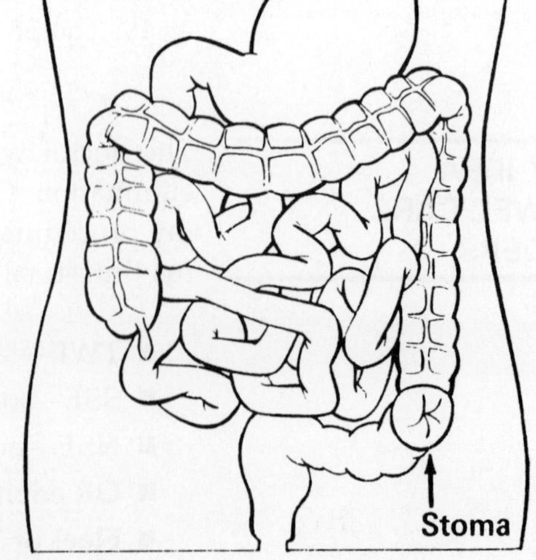

Figure 15–4

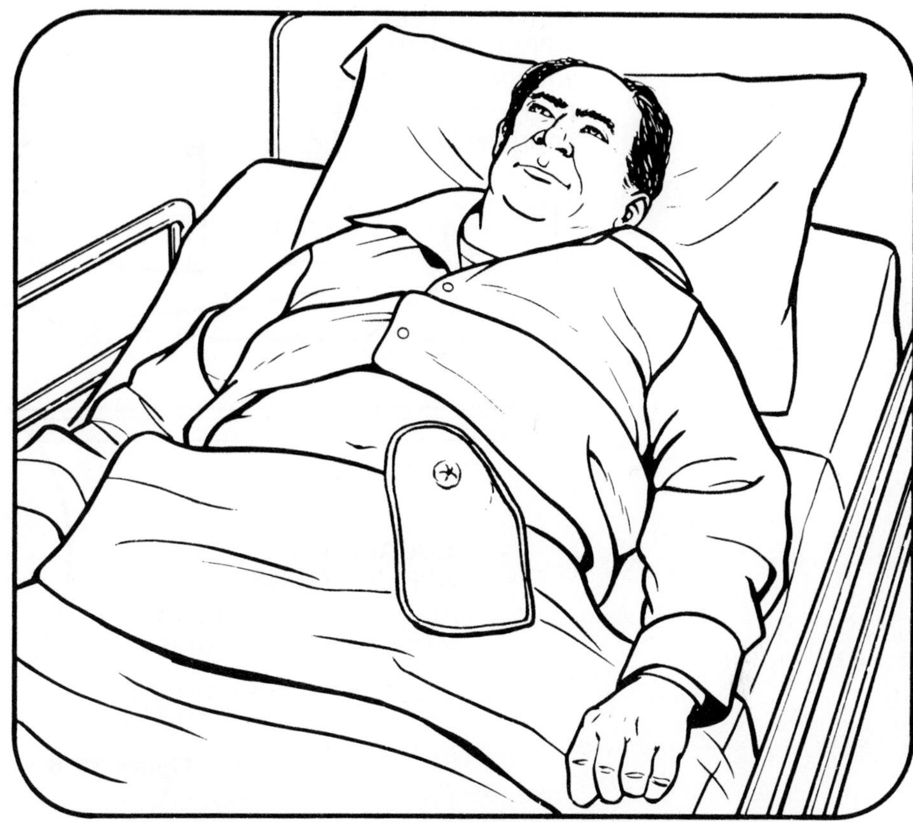

OSTOMY APPLIANCE IN PLACE OVER THE STOMA

Figure 15–5

A person with a stoma often must wear an ostomy appliance to collect fecal matter released through the stoma. (Fig. 15–5.)

KEY IDEA: HEAT AND COLD APPLICATION ORDERS

Heat may be applied to an area of the body to speed up the healing process or to ease the pain caused by inflammation and congestion. A **generalized application** is applied to the patient's entire body. A **localized application** is applied to a specific part or area of a patient's body. (Fig. 15–6.)

Cold applications are applied to prevent or reduce swelling and pain or to control bleeding. Cold may also be applied to a patient's entire body. This is usually done to lower a patient's body temperature when he has a fever. Orders for special equipment and procedures used to help lower the body temperature include those for:

- An oxygen tent with a temperature regulator
- Hypothermia blanket and refrigeration machine
- Alcohol sponge baths

KEY IDEA: MOIST AND DRY APPLICATIONS

All applications are either moist or dry. A **moist application** is one in which water touches the skin. A **dry application** is one in which no water touches the skin. (Fig. 15–7.) There are several types of moist and dry application:

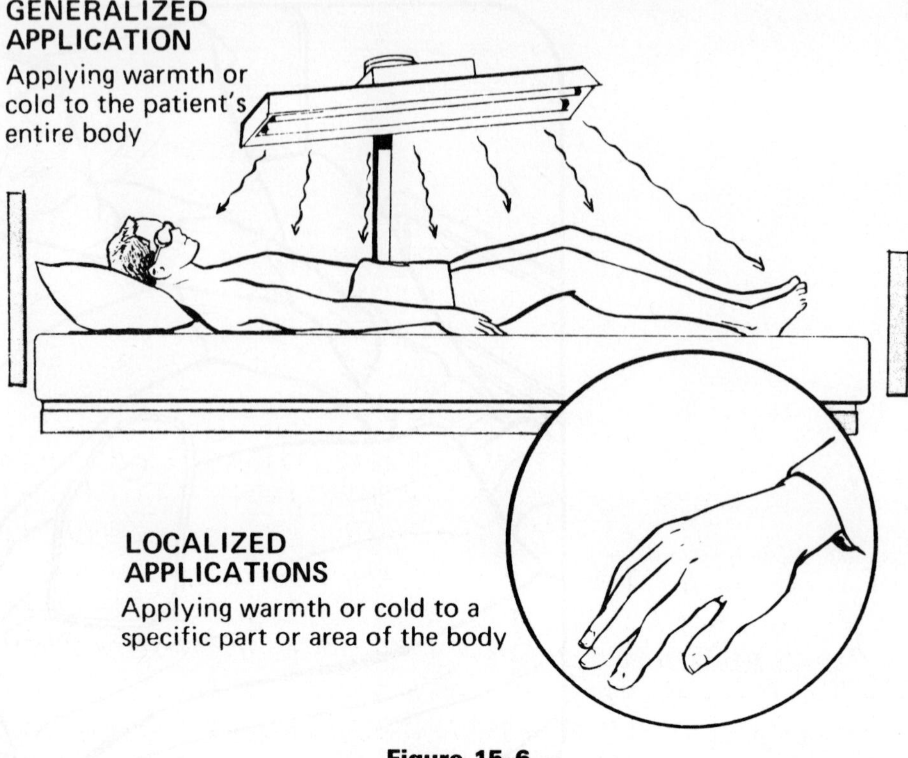

GENERALIZED APPLICATION
Applying warmth or cold to the patient's entire body
LOCALIZED APPLICATIONS
Applying warmth or cold to a specific part or area of the body

Figure 15–6

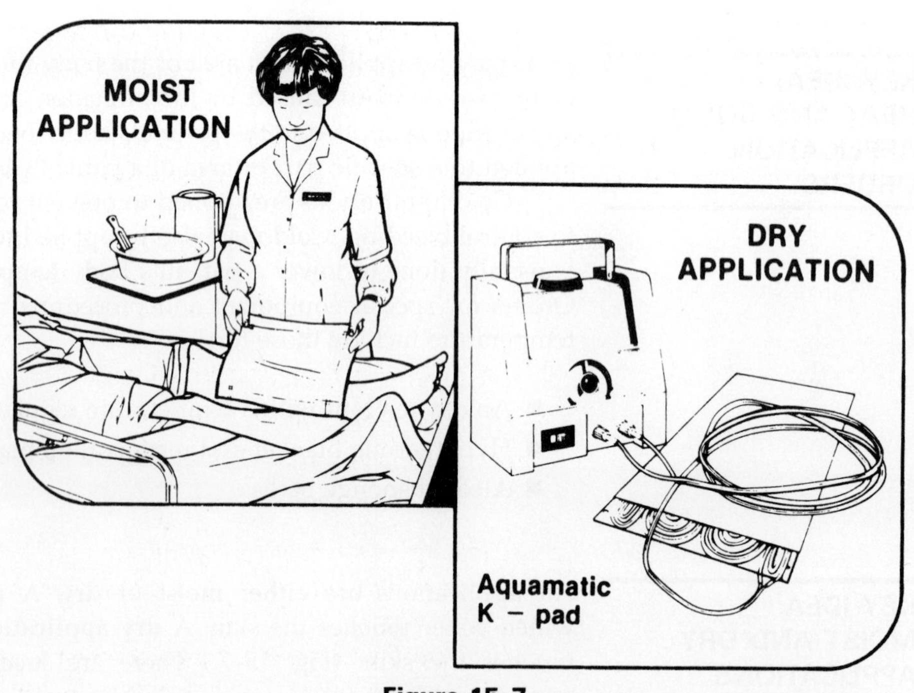

Figure 15–7

MOIST	DRY
■ Soak—warm or cold	■ Ice pack and ice collar
■ Compress—warm or cold	■ Heat lamp
■ Tub	■ Aquamatic K-pad
■ Alcohol sponge bath	■ Thermal blankets
■ Sitz bath	■ Electric heat cradle
■ Cool wet packs	■ Commercial unit cold pack
■ Commercial unit warm pack	

Two of these applications require further definition.

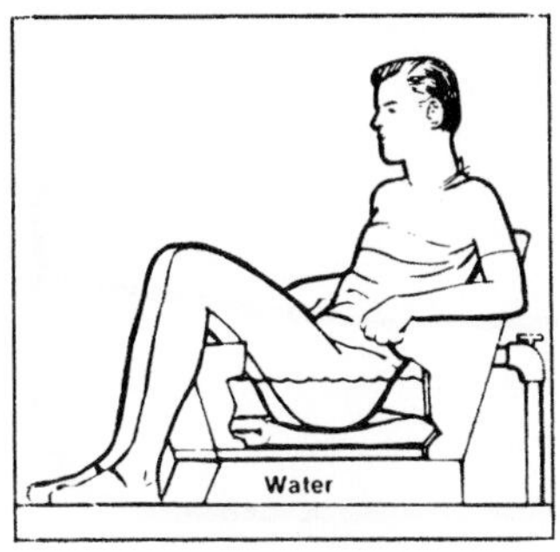

SITZ BATH

Figure 15–8

- A **sitz bath** is ordered when the doctor wishes warm water applied to the rectal and perineal area (genital area to anus). Special tubs and disposable units are used for this procedure. (Fig. 15–8.)
- **K-pads** (thermal units) are used for application of continuous dry heat to various parts of the body and especially to the limbs. In the K-pad the water which is electrically heated circulates throughout the pad. The pad comes in several sizes and for safety, the temperature is preset in Central Supply.

Thermal Blankets or Hypothermia Machines

These are reusable pieces of equipment which circulate fluid through tubes in a patient-sized pad. They may be used for **hypothermia** (reduction of body temperature) or **hyperthermia**—elevation of body temperature. Patients receiving either of these treatments will be monitored very closely by the nursing staff.

KEY IDEA: URINARY CATHETERIZATION ORDERS

Urinary catheterization is ordered to remove urine from the body. A **urinary** catheter is a tube made of latex or silicone and inserted through the patient's urethra into the bladder. This is a sterile procedure and is done by the doctor or nurse. Intermittent self-catheterization is taught to some patients when feasible. Urinary catheters vary in size and are designated by number. The higher the number, the larger the catheter. For adults, the catheter size will usually be #14, #16, or #18 Fr. (French). The two types of catheterization—nonretention and retention—are discussed below. (Fig. 15–9.)

The purposes of catheterization are:

- To remove urine when the patient is unable to **void** (urinate)
- To obtain a **sterile urine specimen** to be sent to the laboratory
- To measure the amount of urine left in the bladder after a patient voids **(residual)**

These types of catheterization are called **nonretention.** The catheter is inserted and then removed. A nonretention catheter is sometimes called a straight catheter.

A **retention catheter** is ordered when a patient is unable to control his urine **(incontinence)** or when a patient is unable to void over a period of

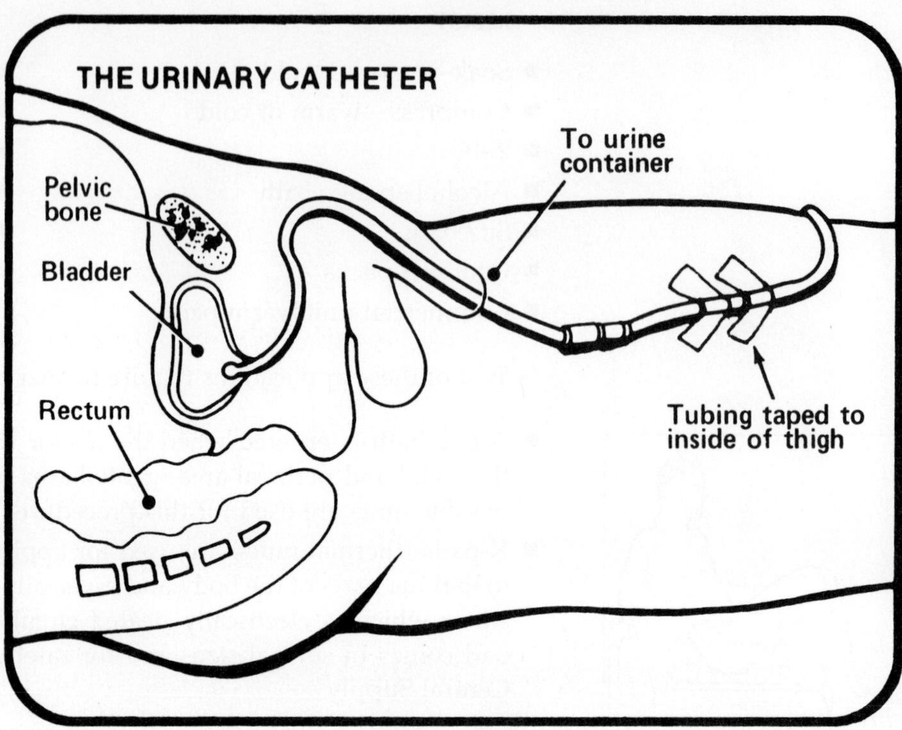

Figure 15–9

PLASTIC URINE CONTAINER HUNG ON BED FRAME

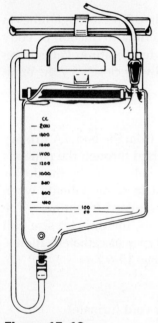

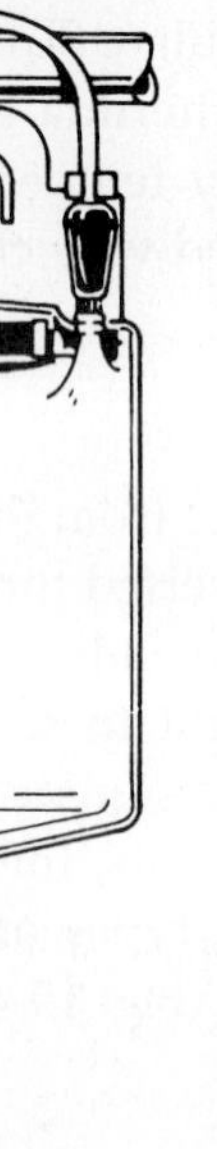

Figure 15–10

time. Retention catheters are also called **indwelling** or **Foley catheters** which remain in the bladder and are connected to a tube which drains into a urine-collecting bag attached to the bed frame. (Fig. 15–10.) A urine meter, as part of the drainage system, makes hourly measurement of urine output possible. A smaller, leg bag may be worn by the ambulatory patient.

The health unit coordinator must know that the two types of catheterization require different types of catheters plus a catheterization tray. These items are disposable and are ordered from Central Supply.

As with other types of tubes or catheters left in the patient's body, there may be orders for irrigation. This requires another special disposable tray ordered from Central Supply. This procedure is always performed by the doctor or nurse.

Sometimes the doctor will order continuous or intermittent irrigation of an indwelling catheter. A Hoffman or Nesbit-Young irrigation set-up may be ordered from Central Supply for this purpose. A three-way catheter and antimicrobial solution are used.

Normal saline solution (NSS) is most commonly ordered for catheter irrigation, although other solutions, such as acetic acid, may be ordered.

Vital Signs

KEY IDEA: MONITORING ORDERS

When the body is not functioning normally, changes happen in the measurable rates of the vital signs. **Temperature, pulse, respiration, and blood pressure** make up the vital signs. (Fig. 15–11.) Common abbreviations for these signs are:

- Temperature = T
- Pulse = P
- Respiration = R
- Blood Pressure = BP
- Vital Signs = TPR and BP

> **Average Normal Adult Rates**
> ***Temperature:*** **98.6°F or 37°C**
> ***Pulse:*** **72–80 beats per minute**
> ***Respiration:*** **16–20 per minute**

The Temperature

Body temperature is a measurement of the amount of heat in the body. The body creates heat in the process of changing food into energy. The body can also lose heat—through perspiration, respiration (breathing), and excretion. The balance between the heat produced and the heat lost is the body temperature. The normal adult body temperature is 98.6° Fahrenheit or 37° Centigrade. There is a normal range in which a person's body temperature may vary and still be considered normal. (Table 15–1).

Types of Thermometers. The body temperature is measured by an instrument called a thermometer. There are several types of thermometers (Figs. 15–12 and 15–13):

- **Glass thermometers**—oral, rectal, and security for infant temperatures
- **Battery-operated electronic thermometers**
- **Chemically treated paper or plastic thermometers**

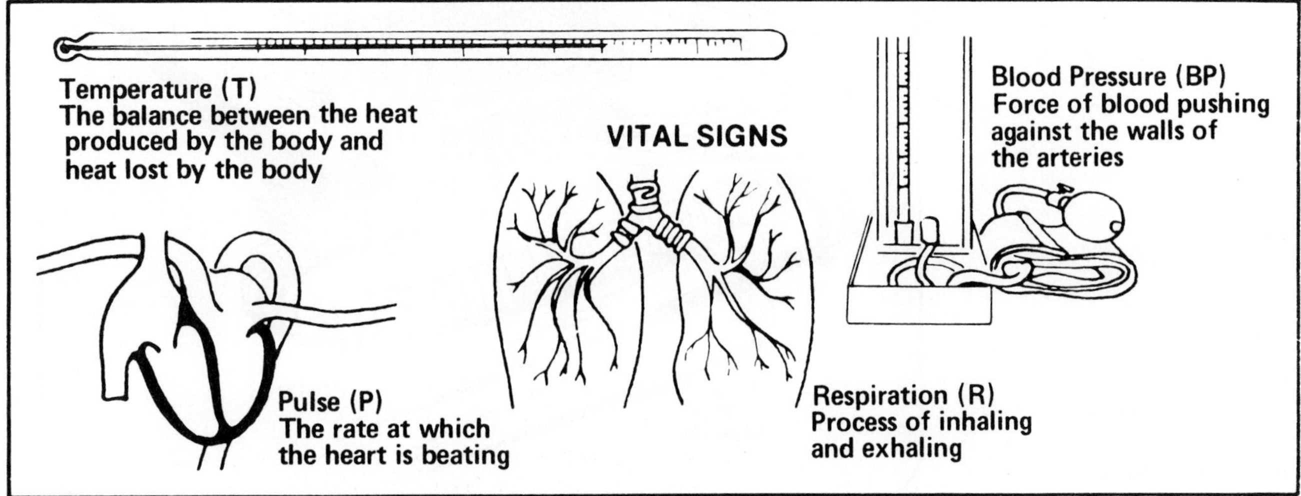

Figure 15–11

TABLE 15–1

Normal Ranges of Body Temperature

	Centigrade	*Fahrenheit*
Oral	36.4 to 37.2°C	97.6 to 99°F
Rectal	37.0 to 37.8°C	98.6 to 100°F
Axillary	35.9 to 36.7°C	96.6 to 98°F

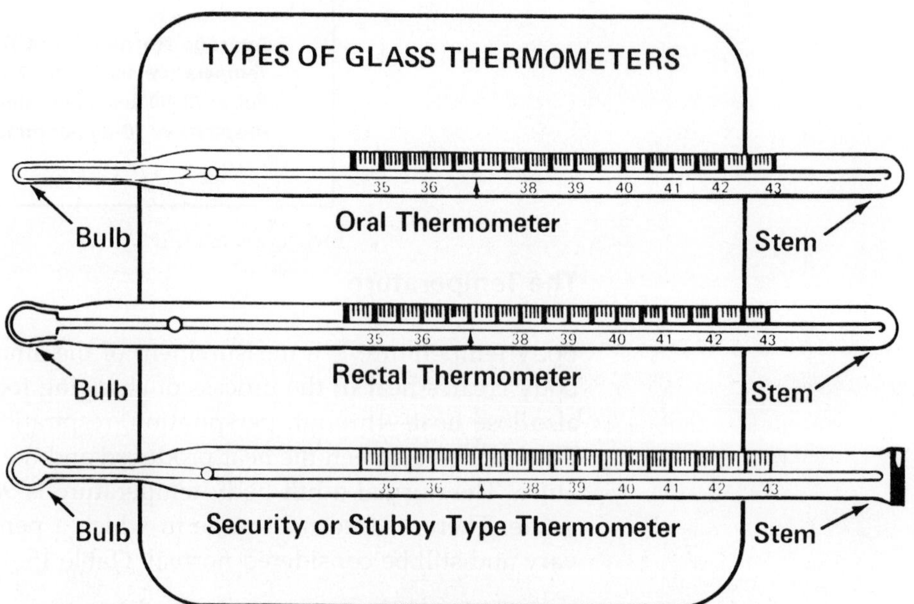

Figure 15–12

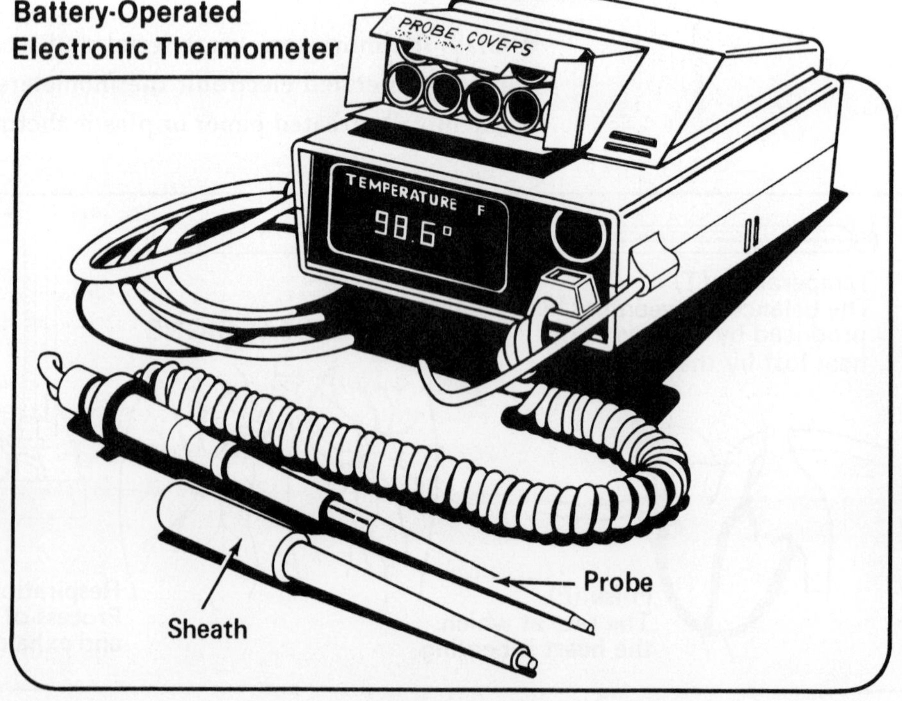

Figure 15–13

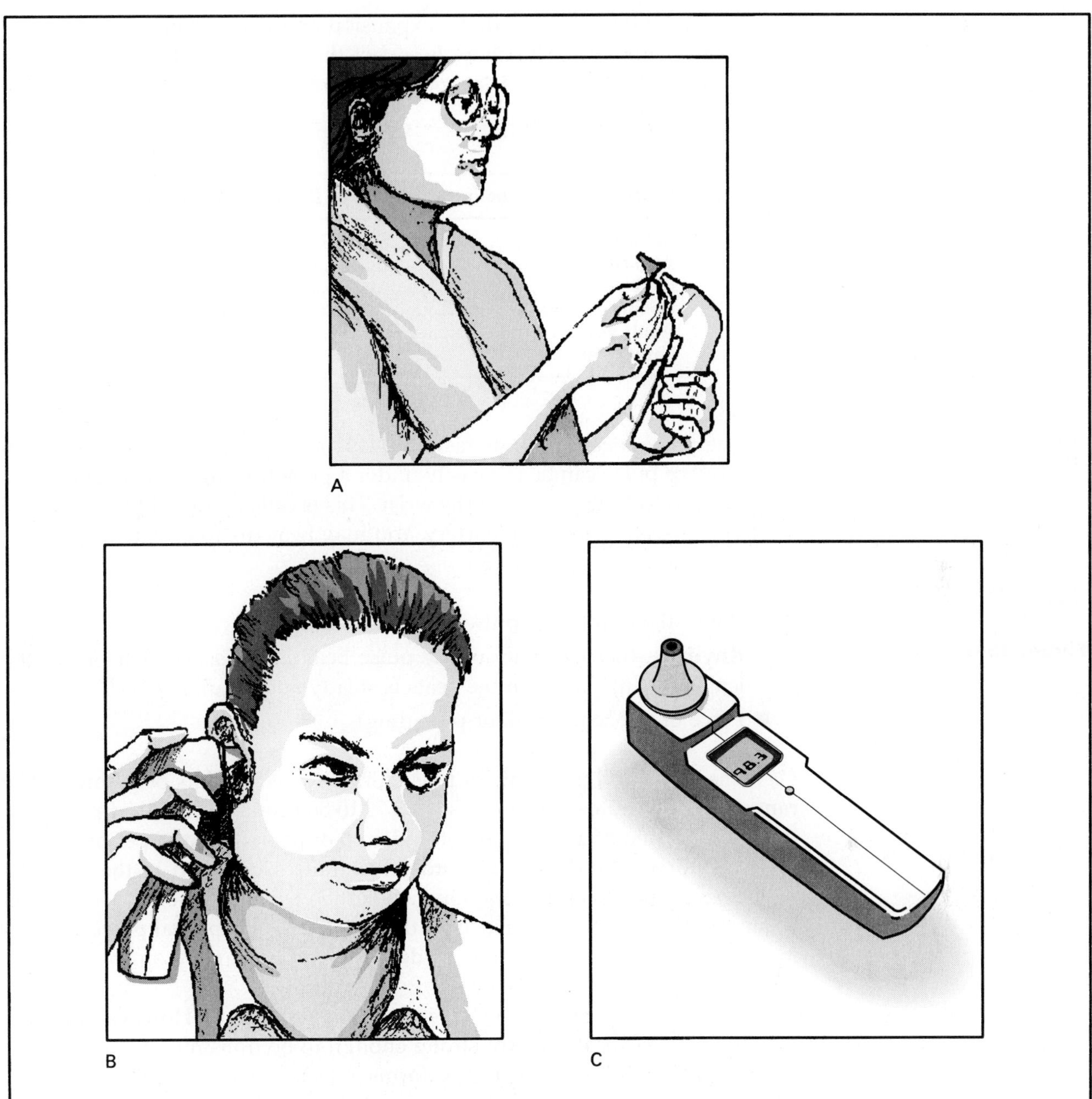

Figure 15–14 The tympanic membrane thermometer.

- **Tympanic membrane thermometer**—also known as an aural thermometer, this device is fast becoming one of the most widely used. A disposable sheath is placed over the end of the thermometer, which is then inserted into the ear. In a matter of seconds an electronic reading is obtained. (Fig. 15–14.)

The Pulse

Each time the heart beats, it pumps a certain amount of blood into the arteries. This causes the arteries to expand (get bigger). Between heartbeats, the arteries contract and return to their normal size. The heart pumps the blood in a steady rhythm. The rhythmic expansion and contraction of the arteries, which can be measured to show how fast the heart is beating, is called the pulse. Measuring the pulse is a simple method of observing how the circulatory system is functioning.

Normal Pulse Rates (per minute) for Different Age Groups	
Before birth	140–150
At birth	130–140
First year	115–130
Childhood years	80–115
Adult years	72–80
Later years	60–70

MEASURING THE RADIAL PULSE

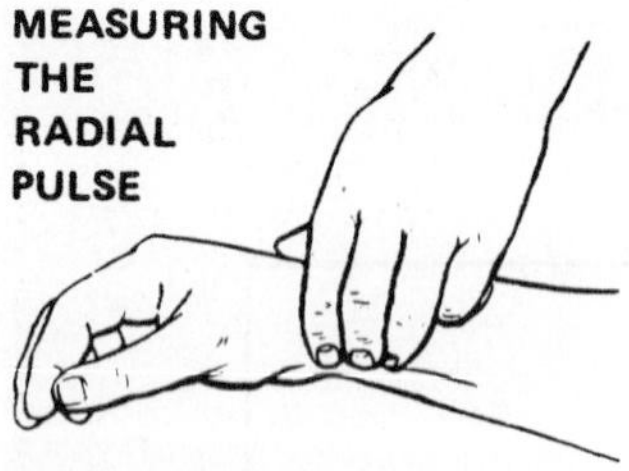

Figure 15–15

The pulse measures how fast the heart is beating. At certain places on the body, the pulse can be felt easily under a person's fingers. One of the easiest places to feel the pulse is at the wrist. This is called a **radial pulse** because the nurse is feeling the radial artery. You may hear the following terms used to describe a pulse. (Fig. 15–15.)

- **Rate**—the number of pulse beats per minute
- **Rhythm**—the regularity of the pulse beats, that is, whether or not the length of time between the beats is steady and regular
- **Force** of the beat (weak or pounding)

The normal average rate of pulse for adults is 72 beats per minute. The range of normal rates for adults is from 72 to 80 beats per minute. Special notice will be taken of a pulse rate of under 60 or over 100 beats per minute.

Sometimes the doctor will order that pulses be taken in the patient's lower extremities. This is often done when there is concern for the circulation to this area. Common orders include those for taking **popliteal pulses,** pulses in arteries behind the knee, and **pedal pulses** (from artery on top of foot). (Fig. 15–16.)

The pulse rate should be the same as the heart rate. However, in some patients the heartbeats are not strong enough to be transmitted along the arteries. This may be because of some forms of heart disease. For these patients, an **apical pulse** would be taken. An apical pulse is a measurement of the heartbeats at the apex of the heart. The apex of the heart is located just under the left breast.

Sometimes the patient has a **pulse deficit.** This means that there is a difference between the apical heartbeat and the radial pulse rate. To determine this, the apical pulse (heart rate) is counted with a stethoscope over the apex of the heart. At the same time, the pulse rate is counted at the radial pulse. The two figures are compared. The difference between the apical heartbeat and the radial pulse beat is the pulse deficit. (Fig. 15–17.)

Pulse oximeter. The pulse oximeter is a device that electronically measures the oxygen concentration of the arterial blood. It is attached most commonly to the tip of a finger and sometimes to the earlobe or the bridge of the nose.

MEASURING THE PULSE

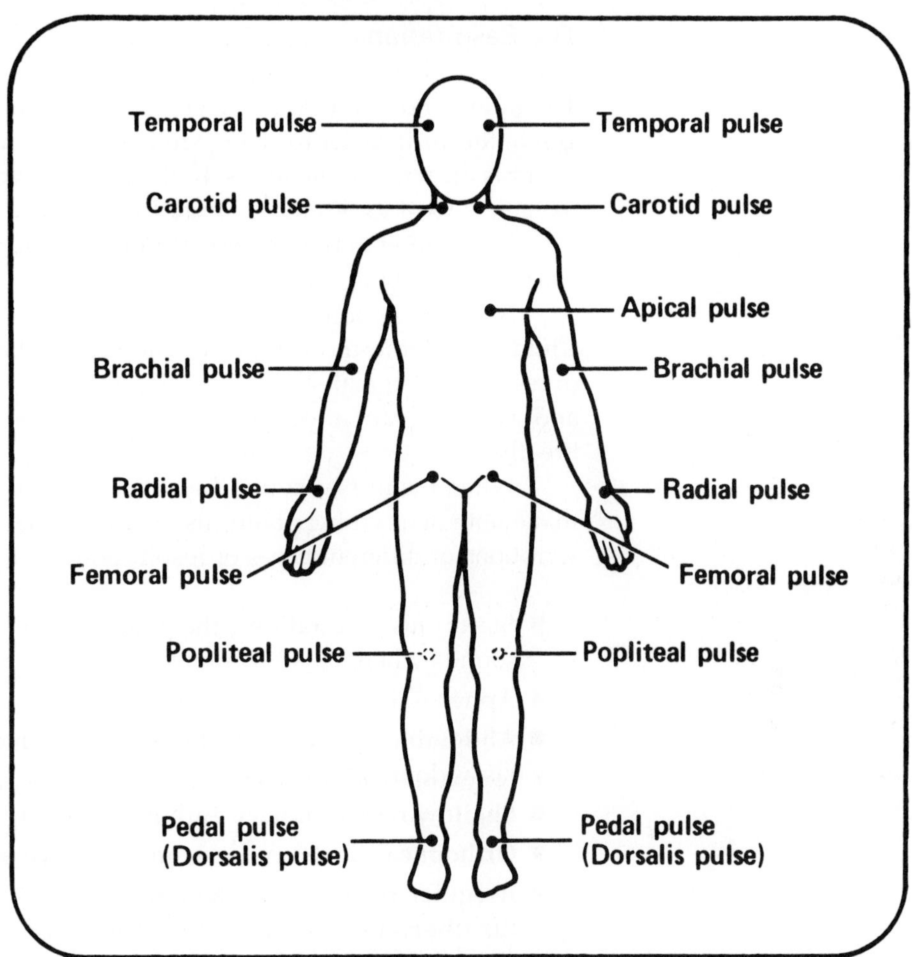

Figure 15-16

MEASURING APICAL PULSE DEFICIT

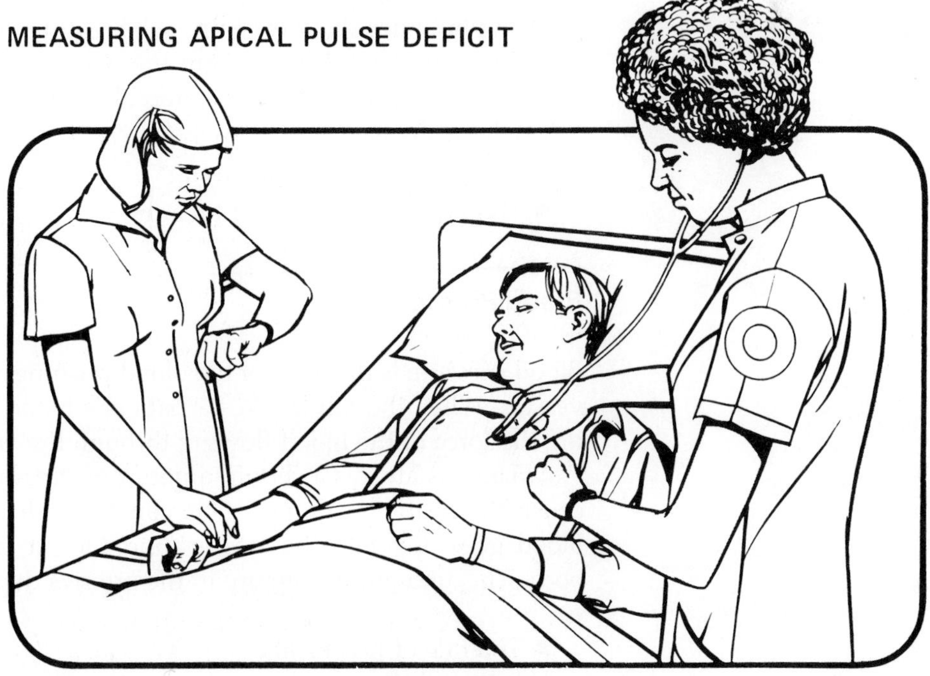

Figure 15-17

The Respiration

The human body must have a steady supply of air. The body needs the oxygen in the air in order to change food into heat and energy. When you breathe in, air is drawn into the lungs. In the lungs, oxygen is taken out of the air. The oxygen is used to produce energy for the body.

Respiration is the process of inhaling and exhaling. One respiration includes breathing in once and breathing out once.

Normally, adults breathe at a rate of from 16 to 20 times per minute. Children breathe more rapidly. The elderly breathe more slowly. Exercise, digestion, emotional stress, disease conditions, some drugs, stimulants, heat, and cold all can affect the number of times per minute that a person breathes.

When the nurses count the patient's respirations, they will observe and make note of anything about his breathing that appears to be **abnormal.** Descriptions of different types of respirations include:

- **Stertorous respiration**—the patient makes abnormal noises like snoring sounds when he is breathing
- **Apnea**—absence of respirations
- **Abdominal respiration**—breathing in which the patient is using mostly his abdominal muscles
- **Shallow respiration**—breathing with only the upper part of the lungs
- **Orthopnea**—inability to breathe well when lying flat
- **Irregular respiration**—the depth of breathing changes and the rate of the rise and fall of the chest is not steady
- **Cheyne-Stokes respiration**—one kind of irregular breathing. At first the breathing is slow and shallow; then the respiration becomes faster and deeper until it reaches a kind of peak. The respiration then slows down and becomes shallow again. The breathing may then stop completely for about 10 seconds and begin the pattern again. This type of respiration may be caused by certain cerebral (brain), cardiac (heart), or pulmonary (chest) diseases.
- **Dyspnea**—difficult breathing
- **Hyperpnea**—very rapid breathing

Blood Pressure

Blood pressure is the force of the blood pushing against the walls of the blood vessels. When the nurse takes a patient's blood pressure, he/she is measuring the force of the blood flowing through the arteries.

There is always a certain amount of pressure in the arteries. This is because the heart, by pumping, is constantly forcing blood to circulate. The blood goes first into the arteries and then it circulates through the whole body. The amount of pressure in the arteries depends on two things:

- The rate of heartbeat
- How easily the blood flows through the blood vessels

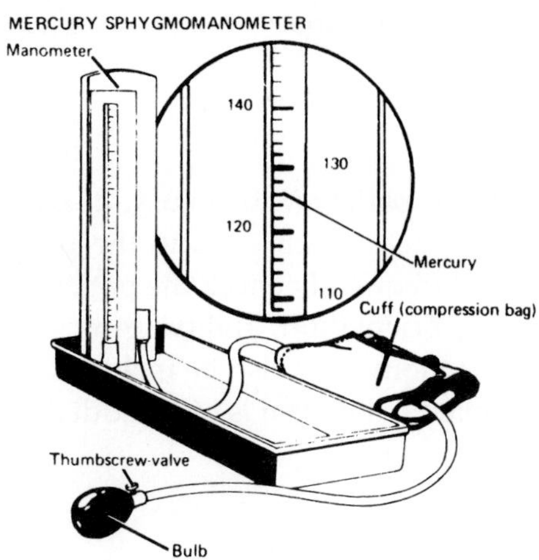

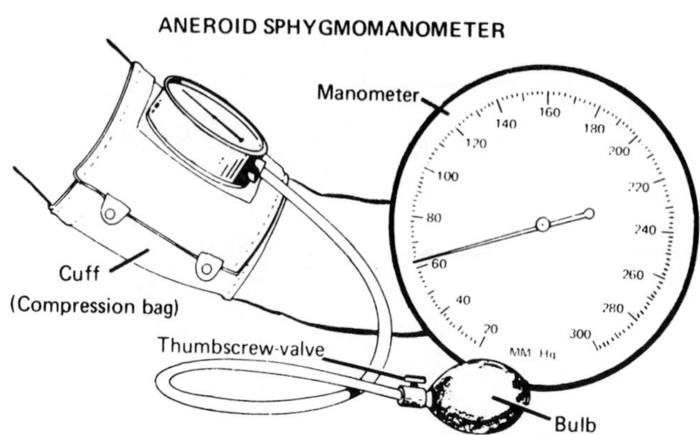

Figure 15–18

The heart contracts as it pumps the blood into the arteries. When the heart is contracting, the pressure is highest. This pressure is called the **systolic pressure.** As the heart relaxes between each contraction, the pressure goes down. When the heart is most relaxed, the pressure is lowest. This pressure is called the **diastolic pressure.** When the nurse takes a patient's blood pressure, he/she is measuring these two rates—the systolic pressure and the diastolic pressure.

In young, healthy adults, the blood pressure range for systolic pressure is between 100 and 140 millimeters (mm) mercury (Hg). Diastolic pressure is between 60 and 90 millimeters (mm) mercury (Hg). These figures are written as follows:

$$120/80 \text{ or } \frac{120}{80} \begin{array}{l} = \text{Systolic} \\ = \text{Diastolic} \end{array}$$

When a patient's blood pressure is higher than the normal range for his age and condition, it is referred to as high blood pressure or **hypertension.** When a patient's blood pressure is lower than the normal range for his age or condition, it is referred to as low blood pressure or **hypotension.**

Instruments for Measuring Blood Pressure. When the nurse takes a patient's blood pressure, he/she will be using an instrument called a **sphygmomanometer.** (Fig. 15–18.) Sphygmomanometer is a combination of three Greek words:

- **Sphygmo**—meaning pulse
- **Mano**—meaning pressure
- **Meter**—meaning measure

This instrument, however, is usually called simply the blood pressure cuff.

KEY IDEA: CIRCULATION CHECK

A circulation check is most commonly ordered for patients with a limb in a cast. The nurse will check (among other things) warmth, color, and sensation in the patient's fingers or toes. If the nurse feels the circulation check is abnormal, she/he will notify the doctor who may choose to adjust or remove the cast.

KEY IDEA: CRANIOTOMY CHECK (NEUROLOGICAL CHECK)

A craniotomy check is done to monitor the patient with injury, disease, or surgery of the head and/or brain. Because serious changes in the patient's condition may occur rapidly, the nurse will frequently check the patient's VS, level of consciousness, grip of each hand, orientation, ability to move, and pupil of the eye reaction to light. Other reactions may also be included in the craniotomy or neuro check. A special supplemental form is often added to the chart for this purpose.

KEY IDEA: INTAKE AND OUTPUT

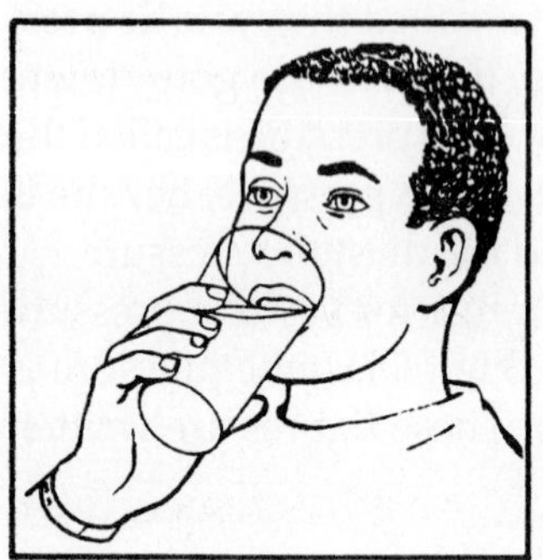

Figure 15–19

Water is essential to human life. Next to oxygen, water is the most important thing the body takes in (Fig. 15–19). A person can be starving, can lose half of his body protein and almost half of his body weight, and can still live. But losing only one-fifth of the body's fluid will result in death.

Through eating and drinking, the average healthy adult will take on about 3½ quarts of fluid every day. This is his **fluid intake.** The same adult also will eliminate about 3½ quarts of fluid every day. This is his **fluid output.** Fluid is discharged from the body of a healthy person in several ways:

- Most of the fluid passes through the kidneys and is discharged as urine.
- Some of the fluid is lost from the body through perspiration.
- Some fluid is evaporated from the lungs in breathing.
- The remaining fluid is absorbed and discharged through the intestinal system.

It is difficult to measure accurately the amount of fluid discharged through evaporation and breathing. Therefore, a person may seem to have a greater fluid intake than output. There is, however, a fluid balance in the normally functioning body. Fluid balance means that just about the same amount of fluid taken in by the body is also eliminated.

An imbalance of fluids in the body occurs when too much fluid is kept in the body or when too much fluid is lost. In some medical conditions, fluid may be held in the body tissues and make them swell. This is called **edema.** In other conditions, much fluid may be lost by vomiting, bleeding, severe diarrhea, or excessive sweating. (Fig. 15–20.)

When a patient's body loses more fluid than he is taking in or retains more than he is putting out, a doctor can treat the condition in various ways. A specific method is prescribed to meet the needs of the individual patient. The only way a doctor can know when a patient's fluids are imbalanced is by knowing the patient's measurable intake and output. Therefore, it is very important for members of the nursing staff to keep accurate records of fluid intake and output. The record of the patient's intake and output is kept for a full 24-hour period.

The amounts of intake and output are written on a special sheet called the **Intake and Output (I&O) sheet,** kept near the patient's bed. (Fig. 15–21.)

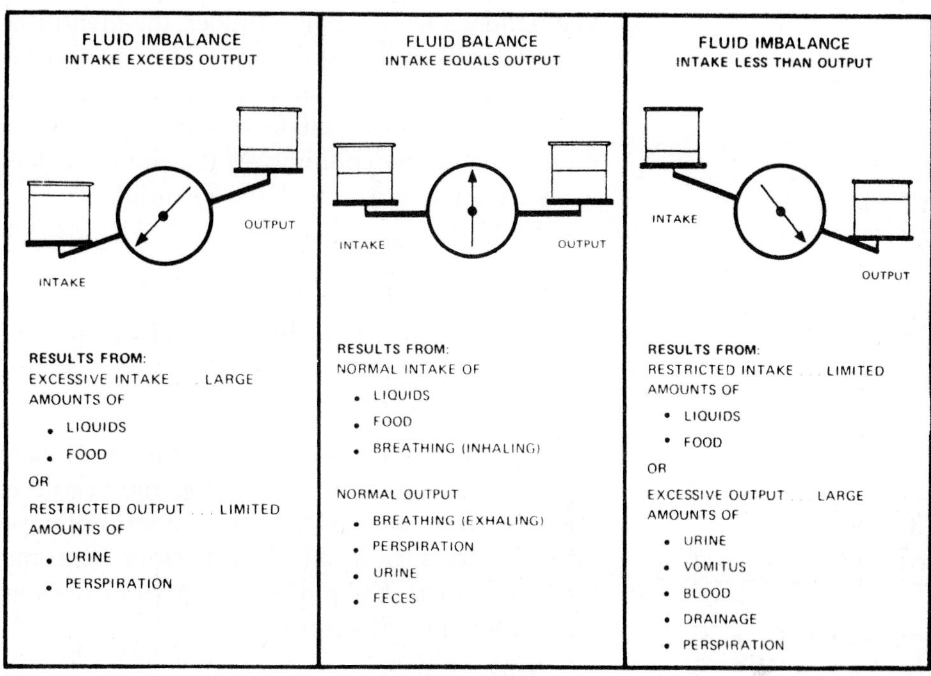

Figure 15–20

INTAKE AND OUTPUT SHEET

Hospital # ____________ Patient Name ____________

Date ____________ Room # ____________

INTAKE				OUTPUT			
				URINE		GASTRIC	
Time 7-3	BY MOUTH	TUBE	PARENTERAL	VOIDED	CATHETER	EMESIS	SUCTION
TOTAL							
Time 3-11							
TOTAL							
Time 11-7							
TOTAL							
24 HOUR TOTAL							
24 Hour Grand Total • Intake				24 Hour Grand Total • Output			

Figure 15–21

The patient's name, room number, the identification institution number, and the date are recorded at the top of the page. The intake and output sheet is divided into two parts—intake on the left side and output on the right.

After measuring intake or output, the nurse will record the amount and time in the proper columns. At the end of each eight-hour shift, the amounts in each column are totaled and recorded.

KEY IDEA: DIABETIC TESTING

When the diabetic is hospitalized, he or she is carefully monitored for the amount of glucose in the blood, and insulin is ordered based on the results of the tests. Two methods of testing done by nursing are capillary puncture and urine testing.

Capillary Puncture. This test requires that the nurse prick the patient's finger with a specially designed sterile needle or lancet. A drop of blood is then placed on a chemically treated strip of paper, and the paper is inserted into a device such as an AccuCheck or Glucometer that electronically reads the blood sugar. The nurse then gives or does not give insulin based on the written orders of the physician.

S & A TEST

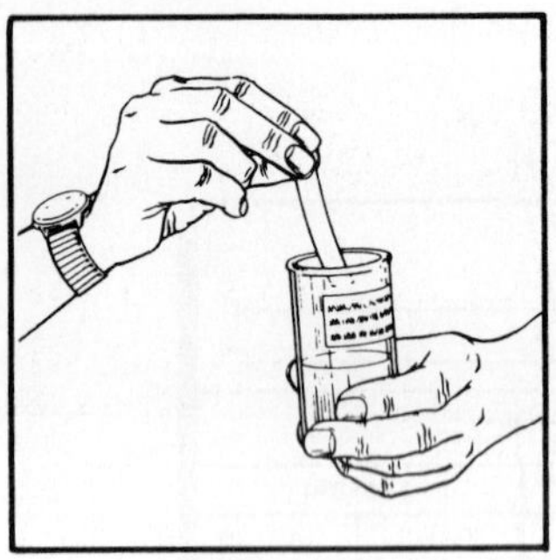

Figure 15–22

Urine Testing. This test for sugar and acetone (S&A) requires the nurse to place a chemically treated strip of paper into fresh urine and then compare the results to a color chart. (Fig. 15–22.) These tests, called fractionals, are usually done four times a day, a half-hour before each meal and at bedtime. The capillary puncture previously described is considered a more accurate test.

An older test for sugar in the urine is called the clinitest. This test, which is rarely ordered any more, involves dropping tablets into urine, adding water, and observing any color change.

Remember, the foregoing are not considered laboratory tests and are done on the nursing unit, not by laboratory personnel. Other, more sophisticated tests for diabetic monitoring are ordered through the laboratory.

Urine Fractionals for Glucose and Ketones
S&A q.i.d. ac and hs
C&A q.i.d. ac and hs

KEY IDEA: INTRAVENOUS ADMINISTRATION ORDERS

Orders for the administration of fluids by vein are extremely common and important forms of patient therapy. IVs are ordered when:

- The patient, because of illness or surgery, is unable to swallow or tolerate fluids by mouth.
- The patient is unconscious.
- The patient is dehydrated (lacking in fluid intake).
- Medications must be given into a vein.
- The doctor feels the patient's condition is such that he may require emergency medications by vein.

- The patient's condition is such (e.g., shock) that the doctor wishes to measure the pressure in the venous system. This is called the **CVP (central venous pressure)** and is a special procedure requiring special equipment and often done in the Intensive Care Unit.

To start central venous pressure monitoring, an IV catheter is inserted by the physician into a vein and then into the superior vena cava or right atrium. The catheter is connected to IV tubing that is attached to a manometer and three-way stopcock. The CVP readings, usually taken with the patient lying flat, measure the pressure in the venous system and the efficiency of the right ventricle of the heart. Too low a reading may mean hypovolemia (not enough blood volume); too high a reading hypervolemia (too much fluid) or right ventricular failure. The changes indicate the blood volume, the need for more or less fluid replacement, and the effect of certain cardiac drugs on the heart.

When measurements are not being taken, the IV runs at a KVO (keep vein open) rate.

Parenteral Nutrition

- When the patient requires **parenteral nutrition therapies.** Parenteral nutrition support encompasses two modalities: Peripheral parenteral nutrition (PPN) and total or central parenteral nutrition (TPN).

Peripheral parenteral nutrition (PPN) is administered intravenously to provide nutrients. PPN is used often in conjunction with oral feedings or in the absence of gastrointestinal function for a shorter period of time. This therapy is limited in the amount of dextrose and amino acid concentration in the solution that can be administered, because the infusate may damage the vessel.

Total parenteral nutrition (TPN), on the other hand, is usually administered through the central vein via a catheter. The dextrose and amino acid solution concentrates can be higher, because the larger vein can dilute the infusate rapidly. This allows for greater amounts of nutrients to be given and therefore meet the nutritional needs of the patient. Candidates for TPN are those patients who have a nonfunctioning gut and require support for longer periods of time. Lipids are an important nutrient to prevent fatty acid deficiencies and can be given intravenously in TPN as fat emulsions that are caloric dense; they are a very useful energy source when volume is restricted. The amounts and types of additives may change frequently and are prepared by the pharmacist, based on the physician's orders. The dietitian works in conjunction with the pharmacist and other team members to assure that the nutritional needs of the patient are met.

Patients on TPN or hyperalimentation therapy generally have a surgically placed indwelling central venous catheter. An infusion-control device delivers the TPN at a controlled prescribed rate. The solutions are kept refrigerated until used.

Patients receiving TPN are monitored carefully and have their temperatures and fractional urines measured every six hours, as glucose imbalances and sepsis (infection) are potential risks. (Fig. 15–23.)

TOTAL PARENTERAL NUTRITION "HYPERALIMENTATION"

1. ☑ PHYSICIAN TO PLACE CATHETER IN CENTRAL VEIN
1A. ☐ PERIPHERAL INFUSION (CHECK ONE)

2. CHEST X–RAY FOR POSITION OF CATHETER. (CENTRAL LINE)

3. KEEP I.V. OPEN WITH D5W UNTIL INSTRUCTED TO BEGIN TPN INFUSION.

4. NOTE: STANDARD TPN SOLUTION CONTAINS; 8.5% FREAMINE 500 ml, 50% DEXTROSE 500 ml, (CENTRAL LINE) 5 mEq SODIUM, 10 mEq PHOSPHATE 36 mEq ACETATE AND 875 NON–PROTEIN CALORIES PER LITER.

5. SPECIAL ORDERS AS FOLLOWS:

BASE SOLUTION:
DEXTROSE 50 % 500 ml
AMINO ACIDS 8.5% 500 ml

ADD:
NaCl 50 mEq
KCl 25 mEq
K PHOSPHATE 10 mEq
Ca GLUCONATE 4.6 mEq
$MgSO_4$ 8.1 mEq
MVI - 12 (1 amp. daily)
TRACE ELEMENTS (once daily)

STANDARD ADDITIVES
50 mEq NaCl
25 mEq KCl
4.6 mEq Ca Gluconate
10 mEq K acid phosphate
8.1 mEq $MgSO_4$

6. WEIGH PATIENT Daily

7. INTAKE AND OUTPUT q 8h

8. TEST SUGAR/ACETONE OF URINE Q6H. CALL M.D. IF 3+ – 4+

9. TEMPERATURE Q6H. CALL M.D. FOR NEW FEVER OVER 101°

10. SMA-14, EVERY MONDAY, WEDNESDAY AND FRIDAY.

11. CBC, Mg EVERY MONDAY.

12. START TPN WHEN INSTRUCTED AT INITIAL RATE OF 100 ml/hr WITH INFUSION PUMP TPN SOLUTION SHOULD BE GIVEN AT A CONSTANT RATE THROUGHOUT 24-HOUR PERIOD.

13. CONSIDER ADDING IV LIPIDS PERIODICALLY IF PATIENT IS TO BE ON HYPERALIMENTATION FOR MORE THAN 2 WEEKS.

10% 500 ml Q ______ INFUSE OVER ______ HOURS (550 KCAL/500ml)

(20% 500 ml) Q 2 d. INFUSE OVER 10 HOURS (1000KCAL/500ml)

FOR FURTHER INFORMATION – CALL PHARMACY

Nurses Signature	DATE	TIME	TRANSCRIBER	PHYSICIA

TOTAL PARENTERAL NUTRITION
"HYPERALIMENTATION"

Figure 15–23

Note: If special procedures such as CVP or TPN are ordered, the health unit coordinator must check with the nurse to determine which special equipment will be needed.

IV Infusions of Analgesic via Syringe Pump with PCA Device

PCA, or patient-controlled administration, of an analgesic allows the patient to administer his or her own pain medication within limits prescribed by the physician. The pump is obtained from central supply and the orders are written by the doctor and instituted and monitored by the nurse. (Fig. 15–24.)

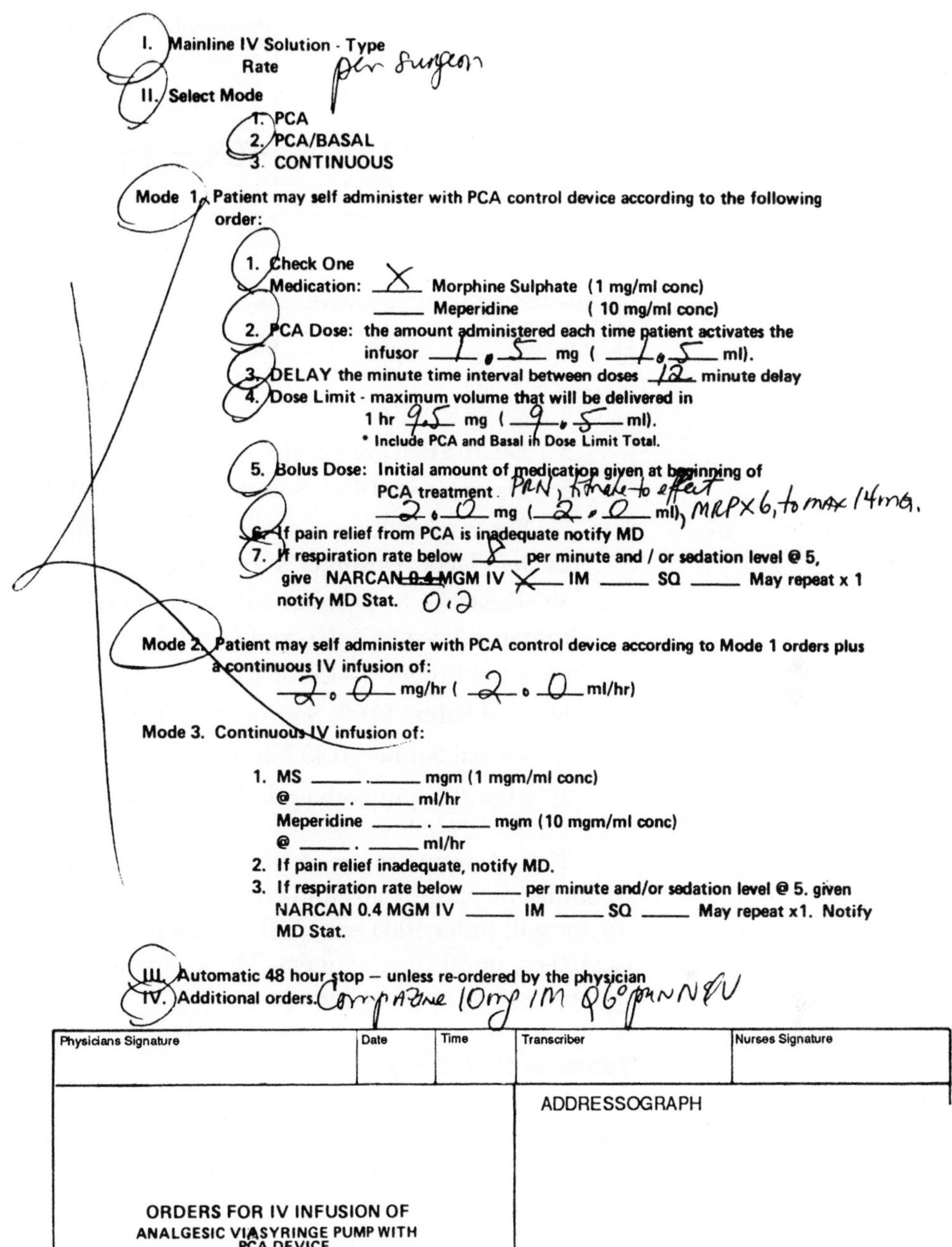
I. Mainline IV Solution - Type
Rate per surgeon

II. Select Mode
1. PCA
2. PCA/BASAL
3. CONTINUOUS

Mode 1. Patient may self administer with PCA control device according to the following order:

1. Check One
Medication: X Morphine Sulphate (1 mg/ml conc)
____ Meperidine (10 mg/ml conc)
2. PCA Dose: the amount administered each time patient activates the infusor 1.5 mg (1.5 ml).
3. DELAY the minute time interval between doses 12 minute delay
4. Dose Limit - maximum volume that will be delivered in 1 hr 9.5 mg (9.5 ml).
* Include PCA and Basal in Dose Limit Total.
5. Bolus Dose: Initial amount of medication given at beginning of PCA treatment. PRN, titrate to effect
2.0 mg (2.0 ml), MRPx6, to max 14mg.
6. If pain relief from PCA is inadequate notify MD
7. If respiration rate below 8 per minute and / or sedation level @ 5, give NARCAN ~~0.4~~ MGM IV X IM ____ SQ ____ May repeat x 1 notify MD Stat. 0.2

Mode 2. Patient may self administer with PCA control device according to Mode 1 orders plus a continuous IV infusion of:
2.0 mg/hr (2.0 ml/hr)

Mode 3. Continuous IV infusion of:

1. MS ____.____ mgm (1 mgm/ml conc)
@ ____.____ ml/hr
Meperidine ____.____ mgm (10 mgm/ml conc)
@ ____.____ ml/hr
2. If pain relief inadequate, notify MD.
3. If respiration rate below ____ per minute and/or sedation level @ 5. given NARCAN 0.4 MGM IV ____ IM ____ SQ ____ May repeat x1. Notify MD Stat.

III. Automatic 48 hour stop – unless re-ordered by the physician
IV. Additional orders. Compazine 10mg IM Q6° prn N&V

Physicians Signature	Date	Time	Transcriber	Nurses Signature

ORDERS FOR IV INFUSION OF ANALGESIC VIA SYRINGE PUMP WITH PCA DEVICE

ADDRESSOGRAPH

Figure 15–24

IVs are started by doctors or registered nurses. The supplies required for this procedure include the bag of prescribed IV fluid (from the pharmacy), the tubing which is connected to the bag (IV tubing), and the needle or catheter which is inserted into the patient's vein. (Fig. 15–25.)

Types of Intravenous Fluid

There are many types of intravenous fluids supplied by the pharmacy. The doctor will specify the type he/she wishes the nurse to administer. Some common orders include:

PHARMACY CHARGE SLIP

I.V. SETS

✓	DESCRIPTION	✓	DESCRIPTION	✓	DESCRIPTION	✓	DESCRIPTION
	ACCUSET		ANS SAFTISET		HEPARIN LOCK		
	ABBO CATH 22		BUTTERFLY		INTERCATH		SAFTI-TANDEM
	ABBO CATH 16		CATHETER PLUG		IV LOOP		SEC. ADD SET
	ABBO CATH 18		CHEX SET Y		PRIMARY ADD SET		SUBCLAVIAN
	ABBO CATH 20		EXTENSION SET		SAFTIFILTER		VOLUTROLE

DRUGS

DOSE	DESCRIPTION

I.V. SOLUTIONS

QTY	DO NOT USE	DESCRIPTION (TYPE & SIZE)	QTY	DESCRIPTION
				PLASMANATE 250cc
				PLASMANATE 500cc
				SALT POOR ALBUMIN 50cc
				SALT POOR ALBUMIN 100cc

DO NOT WRITE BELOW THIS LINE | DO NOT WRITE BELOW THIS LINE

	PRICE OVERRIDE	MISC.	CODE	PRICE OVERRIDE
☐ DRUGS TO DATE		☐	417	
☐ DRUGS CLOSING		☐	417	

DEPARTMENT COPY

Figure 15–25

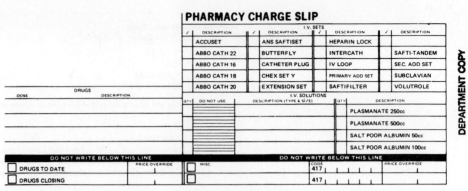

5% Dextrose in water—D5/W or D5W

5% Dextrose in 0.45% Sodium Chloride—D5/0.45NaCl or D5/½NS

5% Dextrose in Ringer's—(Ringer's has higher concentrations of Na and Cl than lactated Ringer's solution)

5% Dextrose in lactated Ringer's—D5/LR or D5LR (lactated Ringer's contains Na, K, Ca, Cl, and lactate)

Lactated Ringer's—LR or RL

Normal Saline (0.9% Sodium Chloride)—NS or NSS

½ Normal Saline—0.45 NS or ½ NS

10% Dextrose in Water—D 10/W or D10W

These various types of sterile fluids are supplied, as previously stated, in bottles or plastic bags and come in several quantities. Most commonly the doctor will order 1000 cc or 500 cc. Smaller quantities may be ordered in 250-cc, 100-cc, or 50-cc containers. These smaller amounts would most often be ordered for children or infants.

Types of IV Tubing

The tubing required for IV administration is usually ordered from the pharmacy. The tubing is a prepackaged, sterile, disposable item. One end is inserted into the container of the IV fluid and the other into the needle, which is inserted into the patient's vein.

The three most common types of IV tubing are:

- **Straight tube**—tube without special modification which leads from bag or bottle to needle. (Fig. 15–26.)
- **Tube with mini-bag or volume control chamber**—modified straight IV tubing with addition of small bag of its own. This is located several inches below point of insertion into IV fluid bag or bottle and can be filled and then shut off by a clamp from the main IV bag. The purpose of a mini-bag type of IV tubing is:
  1. To allow the nurse to carefully limit the amount of fluid a patient may receive at one time. Most mini-bags hold 100 cc. The nurse can fill the mini-bag from the 1000-cc bag with 100 cc, clamp the mini-

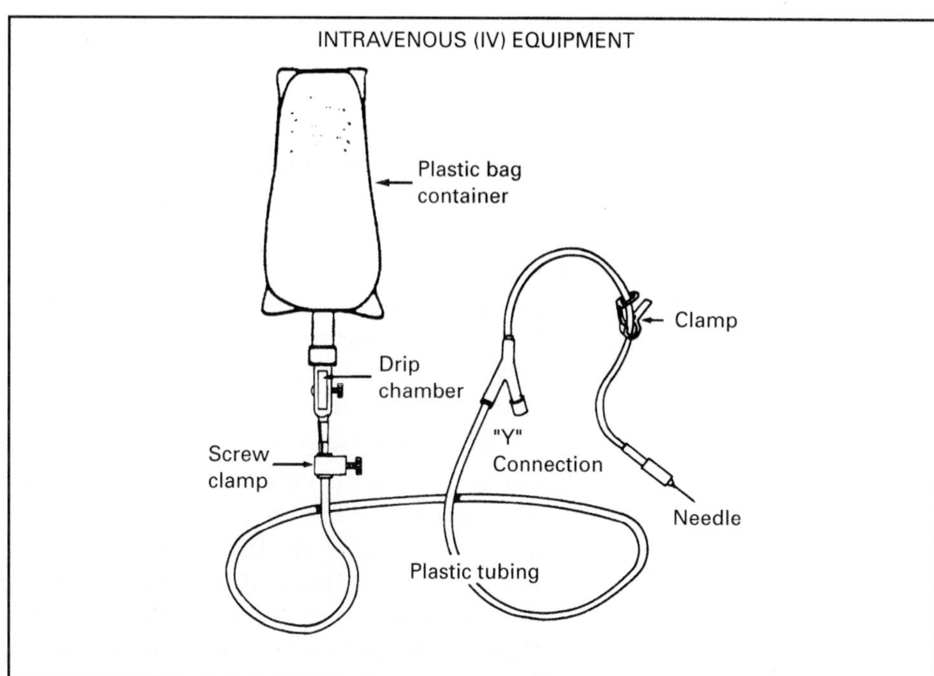

Figure 15–26

bag off above the mini-bag, and then be assured that the patient will receive only 100 cc of fluid at a time. This is especially important when administering fluids to small children or to adults with conditions which may be seriously jeopardized by receiving too much fluid at one time.

2. To provide a receptacle (container) for the administration of IV medications. Very often the doctor wishes the patient to receive medication into the vein. The mini-bag type of IV tubing is a safe and convenient method of administering many types of IV medication. The nurse allows some IV fluid to run into the mini-bag, clamps the bag off, and then injects the prescribed medication into the fluid in the mini-bag, which slowly drips into the patient's vein and circulation. When the mini-bag with the medication is nearly empty, the nurse will open the clamp and allow the IV fluid to flow again as prescribed by the physician.

- **Y tubing for blood administration**—a special type of IV tubing. One point of the Y tube will be inserted into a bag of IV fluid (usually normal saline solution [NSS] or a variation of a saline solution), and the other point of the Y will be inserted into the bag containing blood. Another important feature of blood tubing is that there is a special part which serves as a filter for the blood that will be transfused into the patient's vein.

The nurse or doctor will always start the blood transfusion by clamping off the part of the Y tube that leads to the bag of blood and opening the clamp that allows the other IV solution to run in first. When the IV is established, the clamp to the NSS will be closed and the clamp on the Y tubing to the blood will be opened to allow the blood transfusion to occur.

Types of Needles

IV therapy requires a container (most commonly sterile bag) of IV fluid, the proper tubing, and a means of piercing the skin and entering the vein. The latter requires the use of some type of needle. The most common types of needles include:

- **Intracaths**—sterile, prepackaged, disposable items from pharmacy or central supply. Intracaths have a needle attached to a very narrow tube. The nurse or doctor inserts the needle into the vein and then threads the intracath through the hole of the needle. The plastic tube remains in the vein; the needle does not. The IV tubing leading from the IV bottle is attached to the intracath.
- **Butterfly or scalp vein needle**—a short tiny needle with flaps resembling wings for taping to the skin which comes in various sizes. The higher the number, the thinner the needle. Common sizes are #18, 20, 21, and 22 G (or gauge). A #18 needle would be the thickest—#22 the thinnest. The length of the needle is usually ½ to 1 inches.

  NOTE: A cutdown is a small incision the doctor makes into the vein to insert a catheter. This is done when venipuncture becomes too difficult.
- **Indwelling central venous catheters**—these are more common than cutdowns and do away with the need for repeated venipunctures.

Rate of Flow

In order to ensure that the patient will receive the proper amount of IV fluid, the doctor will order the rate of flow of the solution.

The nurse controls this by adjusting the clamp on the IV tubing to regulate the flow of drops from the drip chamber. A tape is often placed vertically on the IV bottle with calibrations that tell the nurse where the fluid level should be each hour. The nurse checks the IVs frequently and adds bottles as necessary so that the patient will receive the fluids as ordered.

If the patient's condition is such that exact fluid intake must be constant, or if certain medications must be infused (put into the vein) at an exact rate, an infusion-control device such as an **IVAC** is obtained from central supply.

Remember, IVs are supplied most commonly in 1000-cc or 500-cc quantities. If the doctor wishes the patient to receive one liter, or 1000 cc of fluid in a specified number of hours, he or she will write 1000 cc or 1 L, the name of the solution, and the rate of flow (number of drops per minute or number of hours over which the IV is to be given).

- To convert drops to minutes:

  Order—1000 cc D51/2S @ 100 cc hr

  1 cc = 15 drops

  100 × 15 = 1500 drops/hr (60 min.)

  1500 ÷ 60 = 25 drops/min.
- To convert number of hours to cc per hour:

  Order—1000 cc 5% DW over next 8 hours

  1000 ÷ 8 = 125 cc/hr

Examples of doctor's orders:

1000 cc 5% DW over next 8 hrs.
1000 cc D5W @ 100 cc per hr.
1L 5% D/RL @ 50 gtts/min.
500 cc 0.45 NS over next 6 hrs.

The doctor may order several different IVs over a 24-hour period:

#1) 1000 D5W
#2) 1000 cc D5/NS
#3) 1000 cc D5/R

Here each liter would run eight hours, or three liters (1000 cc ea) per 24 hours. If the IV is only to keep the vein open, the order will read:

IV D5W TKO or KVO

The nurse will set the drip at a very slow rate to accomplish this.

Sometimes the doctor wishes more than one IV to run at the same time. The common term for this is **piggyback.** One IV will be started and a second will be hung and run through the tubing of the first. This is usually done when special medications are contained in the piggybacked IV.

IV Medications

Medications are discussed in Chapter 14. However, to understand IV orders, the health unit coordinator must know that when medications are to be added to the bottle of IV fluid, that order must be a part of the original IV order. The example that follows shows such an IV order:

1000 cc 5% DW c̄ 40 mEq KCl (Potassium Chloride)
1000 cc 5% D½S. Add 1 amp Solu. B c̄ C (Vitamins B&C)

When medications are to be run "piggyback" or are to be added to the IV bag itself, this will be done by the nurse or, more commonly, in the pharmacy (IV Admixture).

This is not considered the same as an IV medication order, which is discussed in Chapter 14.

IV Team

Because of the importance of IV therapy, many hospitals have special teams of nurses whose main responsibility is starting, maintaining, and discontinuing IVs throughout the hospital.

As you can see, orders for intravenous therapy are complex. You must understand IV orders and be careful to transcribe these orders exactly as written by the physician. As always, when you have any question about an order, you must ask a nurse.

KEY IDEA: ACTIVITY ORDERS

The nursing staff must always know how much or how little activity a doctor wants his patients to have. A seriously ill patient may be confined to bed. A convalescent patient may be allowed out of bed at will, without restrictions. Some of the common phrases and their abbreviations follow:

ORDER	MEANING
Out of bed (OOB)	No restriction
Ambulate ad. lib. (Amb)	No restriction
Complete bed rest (CBR)	The patient is to remain in bed at all times
May use bedside commode (BSC)	May use a portable commode or toilet at bedside
Stand to void	Male on bedrest may stand at bedside to urinate
Bathroom privileges (BRP)	May go to bathroom only
May shower or take a bath	A doctor's order is necessary for this activity
Progressive ambulation (prog. amb.)	Ambulation allowed in following progressive stages: ■ Dangle—sit on bed with feet dangling over side ■ Stand—may stand at bedside ■ Chair—move to chair with help ■ Walk c̄ help ■ Walk alone

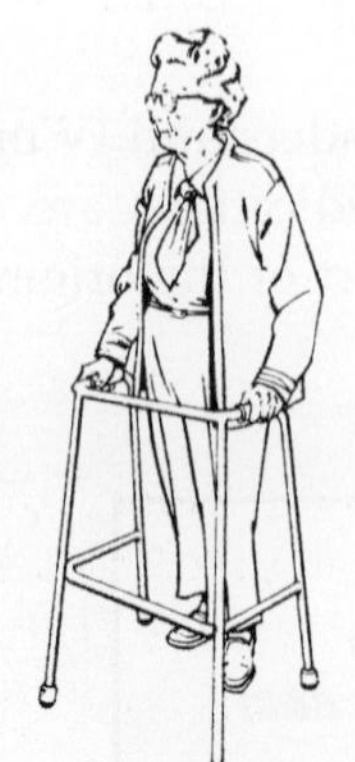

Figure 15–27

Orders allowing increased activity may also specify the length of time and/or number of times per day this activity will occur:

Up in hall c̄ help 5 min. b.i.d.
May sit in chair 15 min. t.i.d.

Certain devices to aid ambulation may also be ordered, such as wheelchairs, walkers, and crutches.

KEY IDEA: POSITIONING ORDERS

If the doctor, for medical reasons, requires that a patient's body or body part be placed in a special position, orders will be written to indicate this. The patient's head may be elevated to facilitate breathing or as a position of choice following a head injury or certain diagnostic procedures or kept flat because of other conditions or procedures. The patient may be turned to a specified side or a limb may require elevation. Certain positions may be utilized for examinations or for comfort. Patients may require certain types of special beds to facilitate turning. There are endless reasons for orders which require special patient positions. Some examples include:

- Elevate head of bed (↑ head of bed) and may include height (e.g., 20°—30° c̄ 2 pillows etc.)
- Fowler's position (patient is placed in a semi-sitting position and the patient's knees are slightly bent)
- Elevate rt. foot on 2 pillows (↑ rt. ft. on 2 pillows)
- Keep flat for 2 hrs.—the patient is not allowed to raise head for specified time
- Turn, cough, and deep breathe (TCDB)—the patient is to do this activity under the supervision of the nurse; the frequency will often be ordered also, such as TCDB q 2°. (Fig. 15–28.)

Stryker Frame

This special device is frequently used for patients with burns or injuries to the neck to facilitate turning and maintain body alignment when patients cannot be lifted or moved. It will be used in place of the usual hospital bed.

A circle bed may be ordered for the same purpose. (Figs. 15–29 and 15–30.)

Traction

Traction means the exertion of pull by means of weights and pulleys. Traction is used to promote and maintain alignment of broken (fractured) bones and for other orthopedic conditions. It may be applied to the skin externally or to the bone internally through surgery. It is maintained by the use of a special frame on the bed. Buck's traction is commonly used for a fractured leg. (Fig. 15–31.)

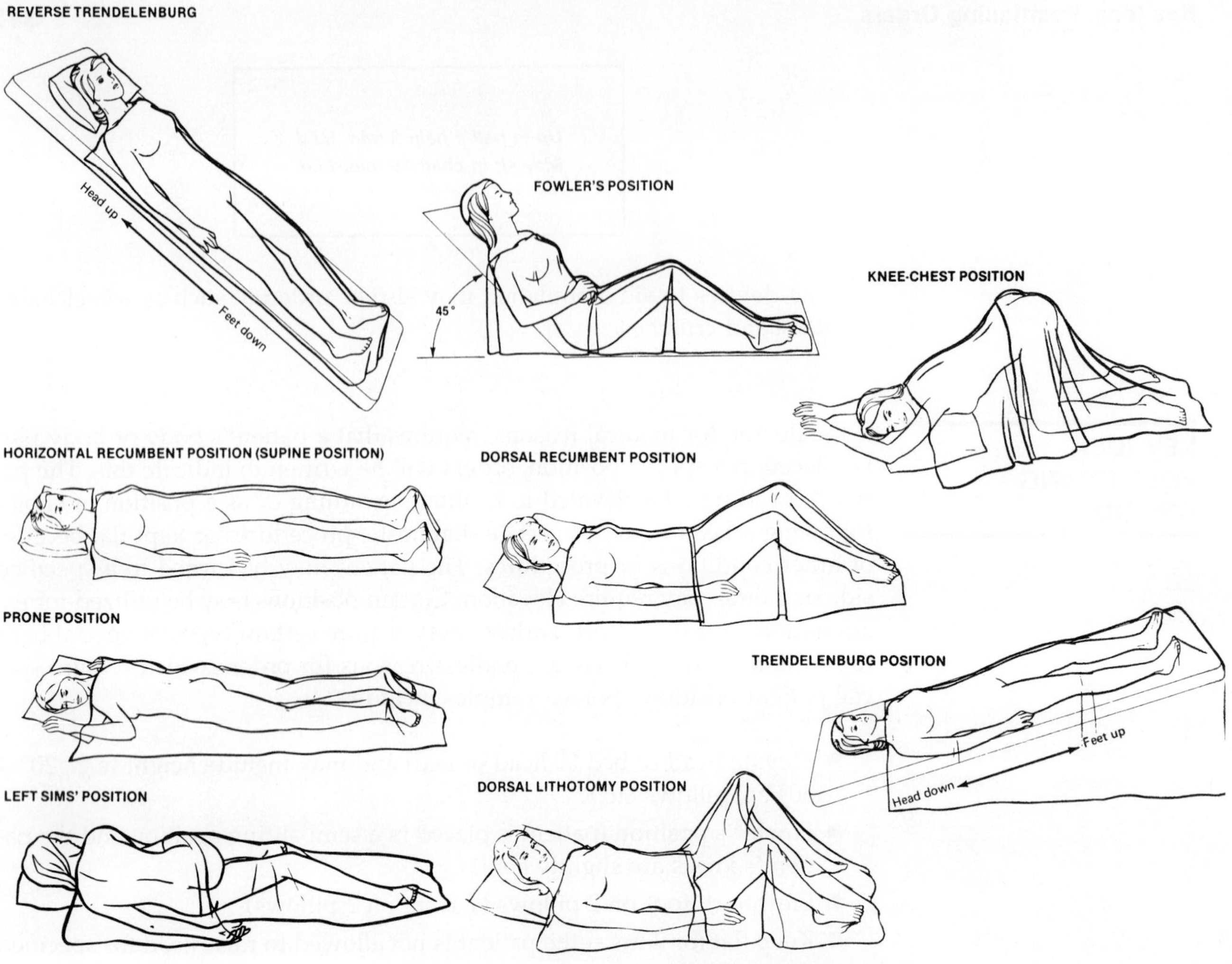

REVERSE TRENDELENBURG

Head up

Feet down

FOWLER'S POSITION

45°

KNEE-CHEST POSITION

HORIZONTAL RECUMBENT POSITION (SUPINE POSITION)

DORSAL RECUMBENT POSITION

PRONE POSITION

TRENDELENBURG POSITION

Feet up

Head down

DORSAL LITHOTOMY POSITION

LEFT SIMS' POSITION

Figure 15–28

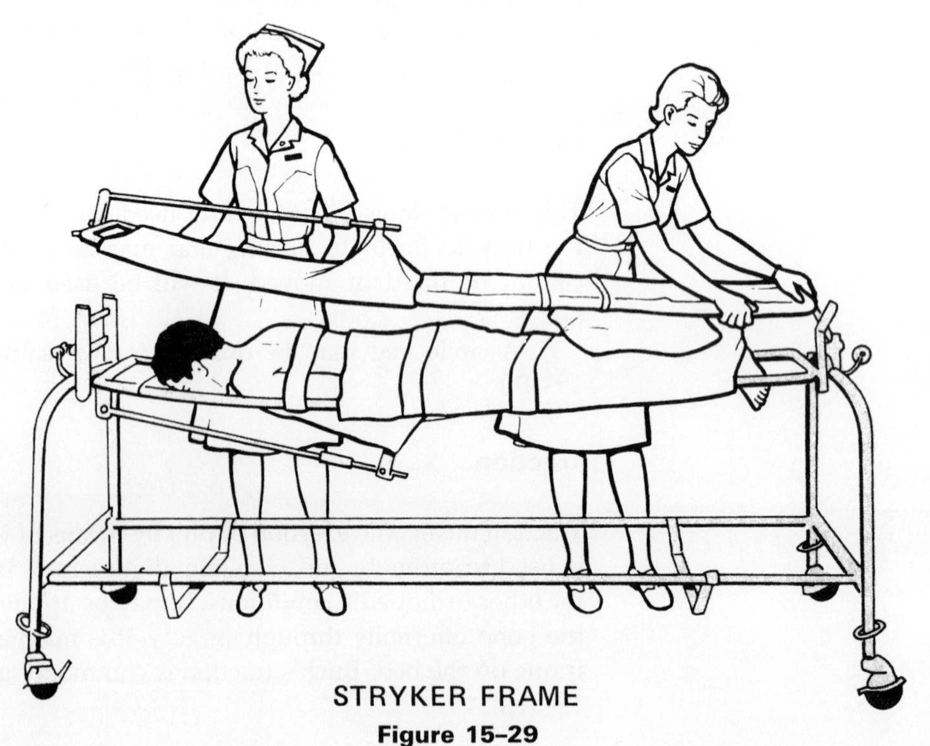

STRYKER FRAME

Figure 15–29

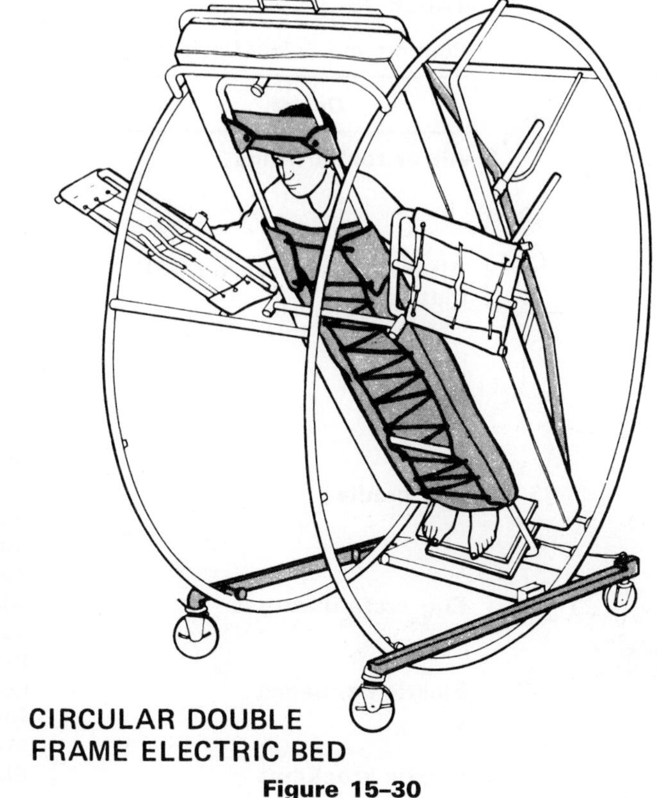

CIRCULAR DOUBLE FRAME ELECTRIC BED

Figure 15–30

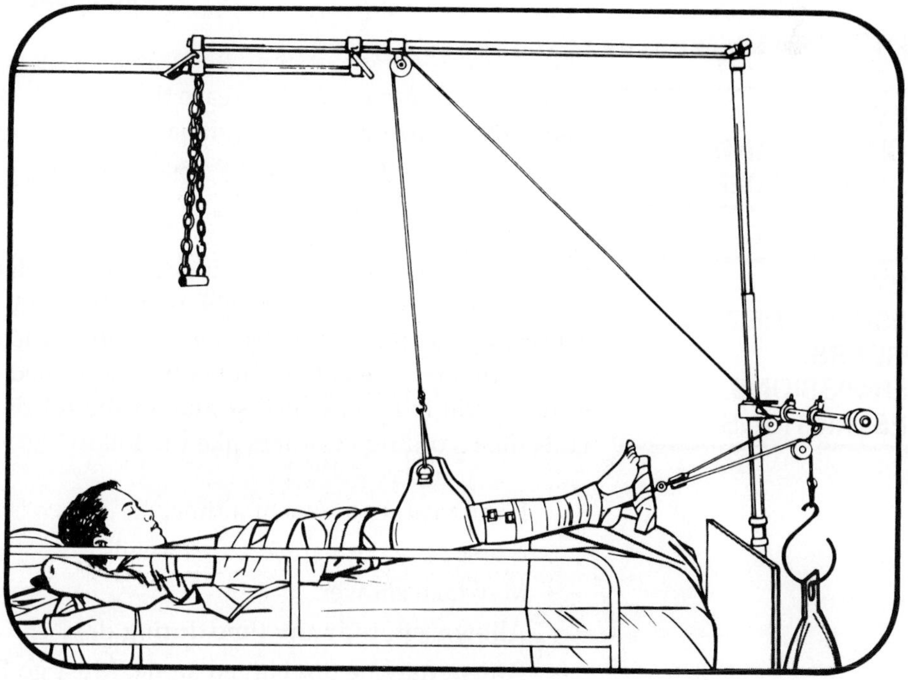

TRACTION

Figure 15–31

TABLE 15–2

Comfort and Safety Devices

Device	Description
Air or rubber rings	Devices that look like small inner tubes, used to relieve pressure over the lower back or buttocks, to prevent or treat decubiti (bedsores).
Alternating-pressure (A-P) mattress	A device like an air mattress placed beneath the bedridden or elderly patient to prevent pressure on the shoulders, back, heels, and elbows.
Bed board	A large board placed beneath the mattress to provide additional support for patients with back or bone involvement.
Bed cradle	A device placed over the patient's body in bed to raise the bedclothes away from him to prevent pressure on sore or chafed areas.
Egg crate mattress	All-foam mattress that looks like underside of egg carton. To help prevent pressure sores.
Elastic bandages	Long strips of elasticized cotton, used for the same purposes as elastic stockings.
Elastic stockings	Elasticized stockings that extend from toes to knees to improve circulation or to provide support after strain or sprain at the ankle joint; also called TED or antiembolism hose.
Foot board	A small board placed perpendicular to the bed springs at the foot of the bed; used to keep the feet in proper alignment.

KEY IDEA: COMFORT AND SAFETY ORDERS

Many devices are used to increase the patient's comfort or safety during hospitalization. Most of these require a doctor's order. Table 15–2 gives examples of some of the most commonly used devices.

KEY IDEA: MISCELLANEOUS ORDERS, PERMISSIONS, RESTRICTIONS

Sometimes the doctor believes it necessary to place specific restrictions on the patient or to reinforce hospital regulations by written order (Fig. 15–35). These permissions and restrictions are all written on the doctor's order sheet and, with a few exceptions, must be transcribed only to the Kardex. Your instructor will tell you which section of the Kardex used in your hospital best suits the recording of orders like the following:

Limit visitors to one at a time.

Nurse may cut patient's fingernails.

May take shower.

Allow visitors at any time during day.

Patient may be discharged alone. Must go home by taxi.

TABLE 15–2 (*Continued*)

Device	*Description*
Sheepskins or lamb's wool	**Wide strips of lamb's wool or soft synthetic materials used for the same purpose as air or rubber rings**
Restraints	**Devices, generally made of cotton, that restrain a patient's arms, legs, or body to prevent him from injuring himself.**
Roto-Rest Bed	**Used to eliminate pressure points and prevent bedsores. (Fig. 15–32)**
Pneumatic hose or boots	**Placed on patient's feet/legs to compress vessels by way of intermittent air pressure delivered by a device attached to boots.**
Portable patient lift	**A mechanical device used to move the patient from bed to chair and back again; it is used when the patient needs full assistance.**
Sandbags	**Reusable and made in various sizes to maintain a body part in a certain position.**
Stretcher	**This is a narrow table on wheels used to transport patients; also called a litter or gurney.**
Slings	**A disposable bandage used to support an arm (Fig. 15–33).**
Walker	**An aluminum frame used by the patient to help himself walk.**
Wheelchair	**A chair with wheels used to transport patients (Fig. 15–34).**

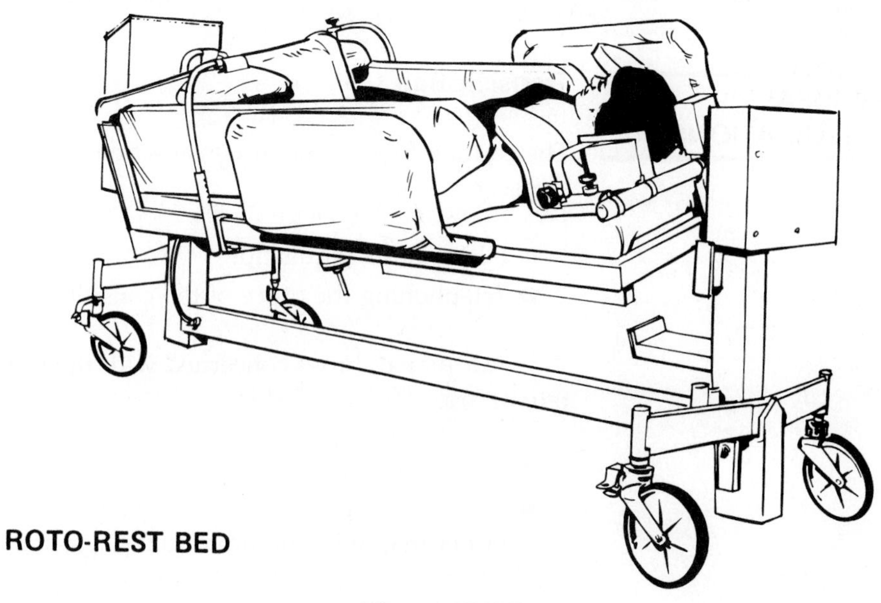

ROTO-REST BED

Figure 15–32

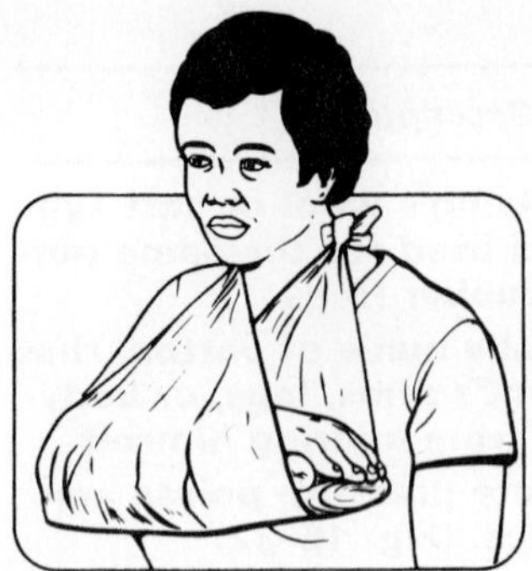

Figure 15–33

EQUIPMENT

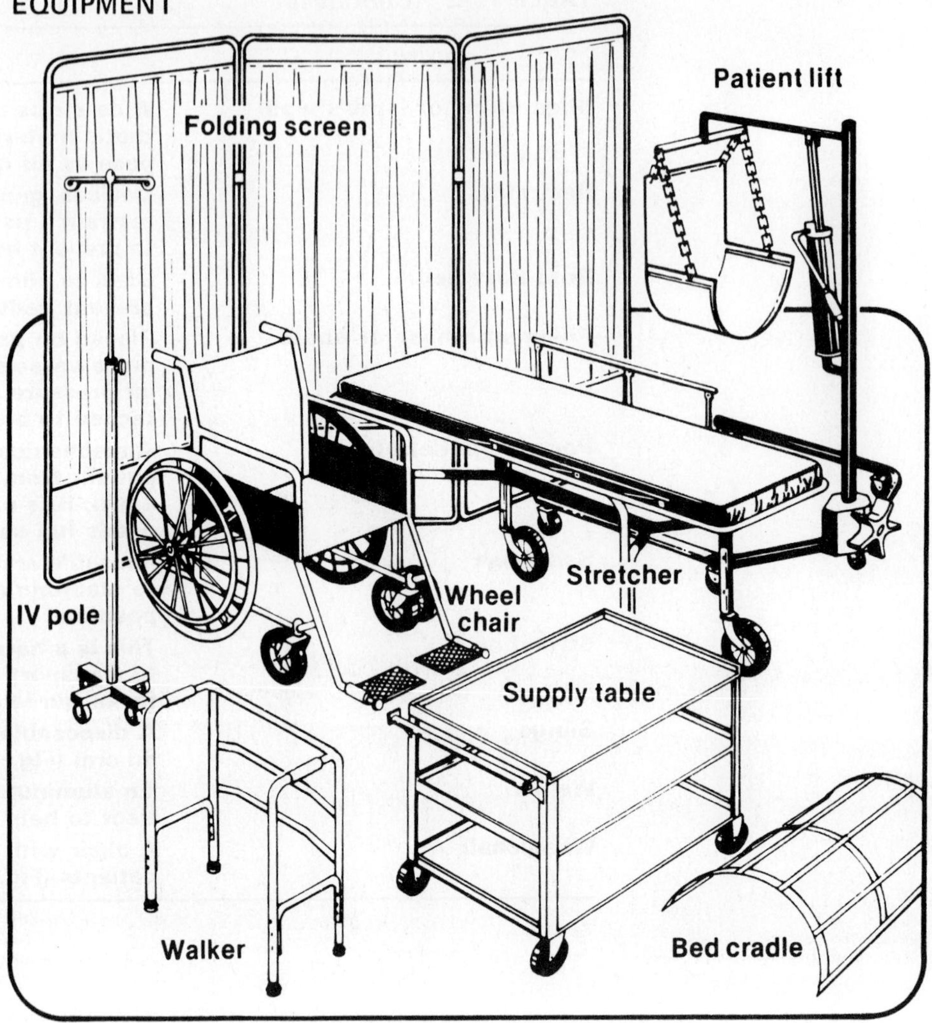

Figure 15–34

KEY IDEA: CONSULTATIONS

Transcription

The routine for arranging consultations normally requires these immediate steps:

- Filling out a requisition
- Telephoning the office of the consultant whose services are requested

Additional duties concerned with the transcription of orders for consultations are:

- Transcribing the order to the patient care record card
- Making an appointment if the consultation is to be with a department rather than with an individual physician

Typical orders for consultation are shown on the next page.

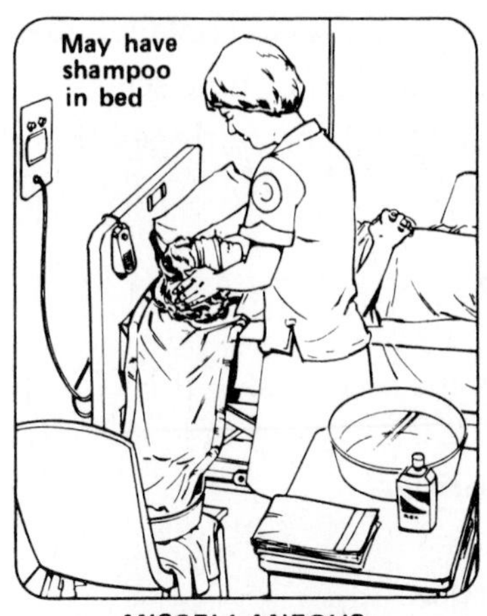

MISCELLANEOUS
PERMISSION ORDER

Figure 15-35

> *G-U consultation—Dr. Biers.*
> *Physical therapy consultation.*
> *Contact Social Service.*
> *Consultation c̄ Dr. Ainsley on heart murmur and EKG abnormalities.*

KEY IDEA: CRITICAL CONDITION LIST

A written order from the doctor is usually required to place a patient on the critical condition list or remove him from it. The orders are written simply and are generally transcribed only to the Kardex. The nursing office, information desk or switchboard, and the patient's family are notified of this change.

> *Place on Critical Condition List.*
> *Discontinue Critical Condition List.*

KEY IDEA: ISOLATION TECHNIQUE

The isolation of one patient from the others may also be referred to as "precautions." The type of precaution varies with the patient's disease and the reasons for the isolation. Isolation is discussed in detail in Chapter 6—Diseases & Diagnoses.

TRANSCRIPTION PROCEDURE

KEY IDEA: STANDING ORDERS

Step 1—Recognize

As you can see from all the preceding examples, the form of a treatment order is not as standardized as that of a medication order. Three factors will help you recognize a treatment order:

1. The order will always contain a mention of the treatment itself.
2. Usually, some sort of time schedule or limitation will be included.
3. Often, there will be fairly specific directions on how to carry out the order.

Step 2—RIP

RIP is always the second step if NCR copies are used.

Step 3—Prioritize

Step 4—Kardex

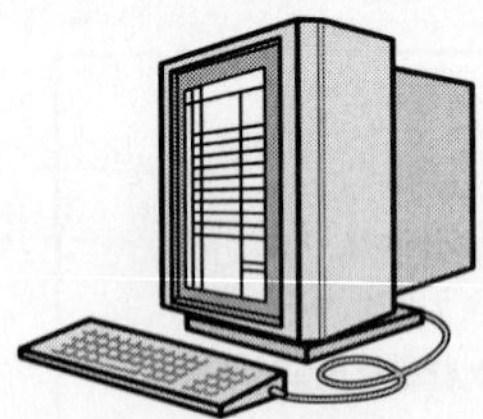

- **Kardex.** All standing orders for treatments must be transcribed exactly as written to the treatment section of the patient care record card.
- When done by computer, all orders will be printed on a computer-generated Kardex.
- **Treatment tickets.** Some hospitals provide treatment tickets similar to medicine tickets. They are not ordinarily used for all standing-order treatments but only for those to be repeated at specific intervals during the day. Compare the two orders shown in Fig. 15–36.

Hot soaks to right elbow continuously.
Irrigate Foley catheter c̄ 10 cc. saline q.i.d.

PATIENT'S NAME
Jones, Mary

ROOM
432^2

TIME
9-5-1-9

TREATMENT
Irrigate Foley
Catheter c̄
10cc. Saline
q.i.d.

Figure 15–36

The first order is a continuous one; the nurse caring for the patient is responsible for changing the soak whenever necessary. The second order is to be carried out only at specified intervals throughout the day. The time schedule on a treatment ticket would serve as a reminder to the nurse that this task must be performed.

Step 5—Requisition

Specialized equipment must be requisitioned for carrying out many treatments. You should already be familiar with much of the frequently used medical and hospital equipment. By now you should know where different types of equipment are stored or stocked in your hospital. If a treatment order requires equipment *not* stocked in the nursing unit, a requisition form may be necessary. A sample request-charge slip for equipment is shown in Fig. 15–37. More and more, items are requisitioned by computer.

- **Special records and forms.** Treatment orders may need to be transcribed to certain other chart records or special forms. For example, a diabetic being tested for urinary sugar throughout the day requires the addition of a diabetic summary sheet to his chart.

  Also, many nursing units compile daily lists of patients for whom blood pressures or temperatures have been ordered on a special basis. In such cases, a new order might require that the patient's name be transcribed to these records.

Step 6—Symbols

Utilize the symbols used in your hospital.

CENTRAL SUPPLY DEPARTMENT		IMPRINT SPACE
REQUEST-CHARGE SLIP		
Description of Service		
Requested by:	Chg. by:	$

Figure 15–37

Step 7—Nurse Checks

Treatment orders must be checked by the nurse after you have completed the transcription process. Use the same methods that were described or decided upon for checking medication orders.

KEY IDEA: STAT AND SINGLE-TIME ORDERS

A STAT treatment order is a fairly rare occurrence. When encountered, it must be carried out without delay as in the case of STAT medication orders.

A few treatments—e.g., enemas—are ordered on a single-time basis. These are transcribed differently from standing orders. Your instructor will describe the procedure to be used for transcribing single-time orders.

ORDER VARIATIONS

The orders described above are concerned solely with starting a treatment. As with medication orders, orders for treatments can also be canceled or altered according to the patient's needs and the doctor's wishes.

KEY IDEA: CANCELED TREATMENT ORDERS

Canceled treatment orders usually read in the straightforward way as shown below:

Discontinue nasal oxygen or 5/min p.r.n.
Discontinue hot soaks continuously® elbow.
Remove NG tube in A.M.
Discontinue q.i.d. temperature.

Qualified Canceled Treatment Orders

However, sometimes a canceled order will include additional instructions, requiring notification and transcription, described on the next page.

D.C. IV—Call Dr. Smith if unable to tolerate oral fluids.
Remove Foley catheter in A.M.; replace if pt. has not voided within 8 hrs.

KEY IDEA: CHANGED TREATMENT ORDERS

Sometimes the doctor will change the original treatment order. Changed treatment orders ordinarily can be considered and handled as new orders, since the original (or old) order has in effect been canceled. Orders below show changed treatment orders.

> ***Continue dressing change on leg q.d., but omit wash and powder.***
> ***Apply DSD (dry sterile dressing).***
> ***Clamp Foley 1 hr. on, 1 hr. off × 24 hrs. Then clamp continuously, emptying at q4h intervals × 24 hrs. Then remove.***

KEY IDEA: CANCELED TREATMENT ORDER TRANSCRIPTION

Most of your duties in connection with canceled treatment orders are simply the reverse of the steps taken when the order was started.

- Reusable equipment must be removed from the patient, cleaned, and returned to the proper department.
- The order must be erased from the Kardex, shown as canceled in the computer, and all indications of it removed from special records.
- If tickets have been made out, they must be discarded.

The changing of an order may require that certain equipment be returned or other equipment be ordered. The order should be changed in the computer, on the Kardex, on the ticket (if any), and on all other pertinent record forms.

LEARNING ACTIVITIES

Complete the following:

1. A treatment can be loosely defined as ____________________.
2. Define the following:
   (a) Gravity suction (or drainage) ____________________
   ____
   (b) Catheter ____________________
   (c) Patent ____________________
   (d) Throat suction ____________________
   (e) Gastric suction ____________________
   (f) Tracheostomy ____________________
   (g) Nasogastric tube ____________________
   (h) Lavage ____________________
   (i) Gastrostomy tube ____________________
   (j) Chest suction ____________________
   (k) Hemovac suction ____________________
3. Give the meaning of the following terms and abbreviations relating to bowel care orders.
   (a) TWE ____________________
   (b) SSE ____________________
   (c) NSE ____________________

(d) Harris Flush ______
(e) Colostomy ______
(f) Stoma ______

4. List two purposes for the application of heat to an area of the body.
   (a) ______
   (b) ______
5. List two purposes for the application of cold.
   (a) ______
   (b) ______
6. A generalized application is applied to the patient's ______.
7. A localized application is applied to ______.
8. Define the following:
   (a) Sitz bath ______
   (b) K-pad ______
   (c) Thermal blanket ______
   (d) Hypothermia ______
   (e) Hyperthermia ______
9. List three purposes of urinary catheterization.
   (a) ______
   (b) ______
   (c) ______
10. When a urinary catheter is inserted and removed, this is called a nonretention or ______ catheterization.
11. Urinary catheters vary in size and are designated by number. The ______ the number, the larger the catheter.
12. Urinary catheters sized #14, 16, and 18 Fr. are available on the unit. Which is the smallest (in diameter)? ______
13. Retention catheters are also called ______ or ______ catheters.
14. Give the common abbreviation for each of the following vital signs.
    (a) Temperature ______
    (b) Pulse ______
    (c) Respiration ______
    (d) Blood Pressure ______
15. The temperature measures ______ and the average normal adult temperature is ______.
16. The pulse measures ______ and the average normal adult rate is ______.
17. The respiration measures ______ and the average normal adult rate is ______.
18. The blood pressure measures ______ and in young healthy adults is between ______ and ______ millimeters of mercury systolic pressure and ______ to ______ mm Hg diastolic pressure.

19. The patient's BP is 134/82—the top reading is the systolic or diastolic pressure? ______
20. Define the following:
    (a) Radial pulse ______
    (b) Apical pulse ______
    (c) Hypertension ______
    (d) Hypotension ______
    (e) Sphygmomanometer ______
    (f) Dyspnea ______
    (g) Apnea ______
21. Define the following:
    (a) Circulation check ______
    (b) Craniotomy check ______
    (c) Intake and output ______
22. Two devices used by nursing to measure the glucose in the blood are:
    (a) ______
    (b) ______
23. The doctor will often write an order for the medication ______ based on the results of these tests.
24. Define the following abbreviations:
    (a) CVP ______
    (b) TPN ______
    (c) D5W ______
    (d) D5½NS ______
    (e) D5 0.45 NaCl ______
    (f) D5/R ______
    (g) D5 0.45 NS ______
    (h) D10W ______
    (i) TKO ______
25. Explain the following IV orders:
    (a) 1000 cc D5½S @ 100cc per hour ______
    (b) 1L D5W at 60 gtts/min. ______
    (c) 1000cc 5% DW c̄
        20 mEq KCI TKO ______
    (d) 1000cc D5W @ 40 gtts/min. Add 1 amp Solu B c̄ C
        ______
26. True or False. Circle T if the statement is true and F if it is false.
    T F (a) All IV tubing is the same.
    T F (b) Intracaths are sterile tubes inserted into the vein for IV fluid administration.
    T F (c) When an IV order includes the statement "with" or "add," and a medication and dosage, it means this medication is to be added to the IV bottle or bag.

T F (d) The term *piggyback* means a second IV is running in conjunction with the existing IV.

T F (e) A PCA device allows patient's to administer an analgesic to themselves by IV.

Match column A with column B.

Column A	*Column B*
(a) Slings	____ Foam mattress that looks like underside of egg carton.
(b) Bed board	____ Wide strips of soft synthetic material used for the same purpose as air or rubber rings.
(c) Egg crate mattress	____ Reusable and made in various sizes to maintain a body part in a certain position.
(d) Elastic bandages	____ Devices that look like small inner tubes, used to relieve pressure over the lower back or buttocks, to prevent or treat decubiti (bedsores).
(e) Sheepskins or lamb's wool	____ A device placed over the patient's body in bed to raise the bedclothes away from him to prevent pressure on sore or chafed areas.
(f) Sandbags	____ Elasticized stockings that extend from toes to knees to improve circulation or provide support after strain or sprain at the ankle joint. Also called TED hose.
(g) Air or rubber rings	____ A disposable bandage used to support an arm.
(h) Bed cradle	____ A large board placed beneath the mattress to provide additional support for patients with back or bone involvement.
(i) Elastic stockings	____ Long strips of elasticized cotton, used for the same purpose as elastic stockings.

CHAPTER 16

Diagnostic and Therapeutic Department Orders

OBJECTIVES

When you complete this chapter, you will be able to:

- Understand how to work with the following departments:
  - Laboratory
  - Radiology
  - Cardiology
  - Respiratory Therapy
  - Physical Therapy
  - Endoscopies
  - Electroencephalography
  - Dietary
- State the general purpose of each of the departments discussed.
- Recognize abbreviations and define the terms listed specific to each department.
- Discuss the health unit coordinator's responsibilities to each department.
- Demonstrate an ability to transcribe orders relating to each department.
- Describe a well-balanced diet and the four basic food groups.
- Define and describe the therapeutic diets.

In this chapter you will be introduced to some of the most important diagnostic and therapeutic departments in the hospital. You will learn the names of many tests and treatments ordered for patients by their doctors and will learn about your responsibilities as a health unit coordinator.

This is a complicated study and you will continue to add to your knowledge throughout your career. As technology advances, new diagnostic examinations are developed and some others discarded. New forms of therapy are constantly being devised to improve patient care. Be alert and inquisitive as you come across orders for tests and treatments which are new to you and make an effort to learn about them.

THE LABORATORY

KEY IDEA: PURPOSE OF LABORATORY TESTING

There are several important reasons the doctor orders laboratory tests.

1. **To help in making a diagnosis.** The doctor may suspect a certain diagnosis, but needs the results of the laboratory tests to be certain he/she is correct.
2. **To evaluate the success of certain medications or other treatments.** For example, a patient receiving an anticoagulant such as heparin would have a blood test called a PTT done daily to assess if the patient needs more, less, or the same amount of the drug.
3. **To establish a normal baseline for an individual patient.** Individuals will have somewhat different normal levels based on such factors as age, sex, race, and geographic location. It is important to know what is normal for each patient.
4. **To provide early detection of disease and therefore reduce the severity.** Diabetes and anemia are examples of diseases which can be detected by routine blood examination. Prompt and proper treatment are required to control these conditions and help prevent serious complications.
5. **To meet the requirements of the law.** Many states require premarital screening for syphilis. Most also require this test done on pregnant women. The scope of AIDS screening is yet to be determined. (Figs. 16–1 and 16–2.)

In most hospitals, the tests performed by the laboratory personnel are divided into several broad categories.

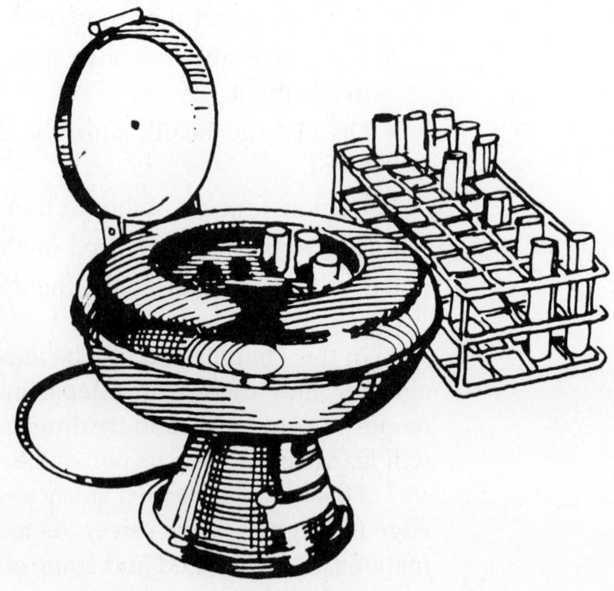

Figure 16–1

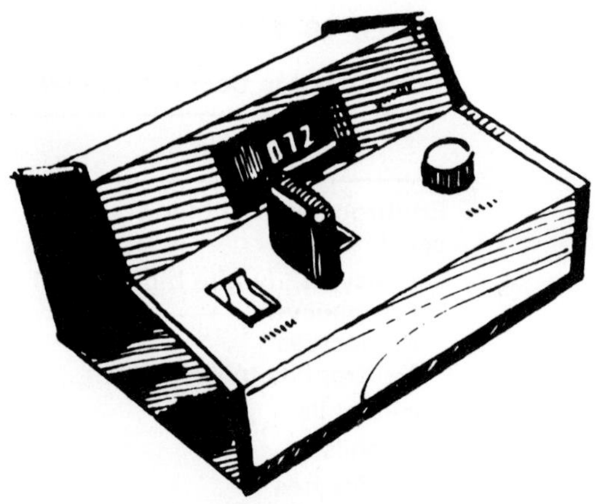

Figure 16–2

KEY IDEA: HEMATOLOGY

This division performs tests which analyze specimens of blood for its basic physical properties. For example, the number, size, shape, and microscopic appearance of red blood cells may be important to know when a patient has anemia. This department also performs tests related to clotting and bleeding disorders and coagulation studies to monitor patients on anticoagulant therapy.

Hematology Orders

Complete Blood Count (CBC). The CBC is done routinely on most admissions preoperatively and at any other time the doctor deems it necessary. Actually, the CBC is a combination of many tests. Any of these tests can be ordered separately. The specimen is analyzed in the hematology division of the hospital laboratory. It is important that you recognize certain terms related to the results of the complete blood count. These are listed in Table 16–1.

Hemoglobin (Hgb). The hemoglobin is the oxygen-carrying portion of the blood and is found within the red blood cells. The Hgb is frequently ordered to determine the need for blood following injury, surgery, or disease to diagnose anemia.

Hematocrit (Hct) or Packed Cell Volume (PCV). The Hct or PCV is a measurement of the volume percentage of red blood cells in the blood. In anemias and in polycythemia after hemorrhage the hematocrit reading is lowered, and in dehydration it is raised.

White Blood Cells (WBC). This test examines and counts the number of white blood cells (leukocytes) in the blood. WBCs increase in number in the presence of infection. There are a number of different kinds of white blood cells. The **differential** counts the number of each of the WBCs.

Some of the different WBCs are:

- Myelocytes
- Lymphocytes
- Monocytes
- Bands—also called stabs—are immature neutrophils
- Neutrophils

TABLE 16–1

Terms Used in Connection with Complete Blood Count Test

Examination	*Abbreviations*	*Normal Value*
Erythrocytes (red blood cells)	Eryths., RBCs	M 4.6–6.2 million/cu.mm. F 4.2–5.4 million/cu.mm.
Leukocytes* (white blood cells)	Leukos., WBCs	4,800–10,800/cu.mm.
Lymphocytes	Lymphs.	20%–40%
Monocytes	Monos.	2%–8%
Neutrophils (polys, segs.)	Neutros.	40%–60%
Eosinophils	Eos.	1%–3%
Basophils	Basos.	0%–1%
Reticulocytes	Retics.	0.5%–1.5%
Bands (stabs)		2%–6%
Platelets		150,000–350,000/cu.mm.
Erythrocyte Sedimentation Rate	ESR	M_1O mm.–8 mm. in 1 hr or F_2O mm.–15 mm. in 1 hr
Hemoglobin	Hb., Hgb.	M14 GM–18 Gm or F12 Gm–16 Gm
Hematocrit	Hct.	M 42%–52% F 37%–47%
Mean cell hemoglobin	MCH	M & F 20 ± 2 μμ g
Mean corpuscular hemoglobin concentration	MCHC	M & F 34% ± 2%
Mean cell volume	MCV	M & F 87 ± 5 μM^3

**Note:* Normal values vary somewhat with different laboratories. M = male; F = female.

- Eosinophils
- Basophils

Red Blood Cells (RBC). This is a measurement of the number of RBCs (erythrocytes) in the blood. The size and shape (morphology) of the RBC will also be studied.

Reticulocytes (Retics). This is a count of the reticulocytes (immature red blood cells) to determine bone marrow activity.

RBC Indices. Measure done to indicate the amount of Hgb and help diagnose anemia. Results may be stated as:

- MCH = **mean cell hemoglobin.** Hemoglobin content in average red blood cell. Is reported in micromicrograms (μμg).
- MCHC = **mean corpuscular hemoglobin concentration.** Average hemoglobin concentration per 100 ml of packed red cells. Reported as percentage.
- MCV = **mean cell volume.** Average volume or size of individual red cells. Reported in cubic microns (μm^3).

Sedimentation Rate (ESR or Sed Rate). Determines how fast red blood cells settle out of the liquid portion of the blood and is used to determine the progress of inflammatory diseases. Is usually markedly increased during pregnancy.

Platelets (Thrombocytes). Platelets are a type of cell in the blood necessary for blood coagulation (clotting). This test counts the number of platelets in the blood.

Prothrombin Time (Pro Time). Measures the clotting ability of the blood. This test may be ordered daily when a patient is receiving anticoagulant therapy—usually Coumadin®—so the doctor may be sure the correct dose is being administered. The normal value is 12–14 seconds.

Activated Partial Thromboplastin Time (APTT or PTT). This is another example of a coagulation study. This test is often used when a patient is receiving an anticoagulant such as heparin. The normal value is 35–45 seconds.

Clotting or Coagulation Time. This test measures how long it takes the blood to clot.

Bleeding Time. This is a test to denote how long it takes a capillary puncture (fingerstick) to stop bleeding.

Lupus Erythematosus (LE) Cell Test. A test to help diagnose LE, a serious chronic inflammatory disease involving multiple organ systems and producing widespread damage to connective tissues, blood vessels, etc.

An example of the hematology laboratory results sent from the lab to your nursing unit to be filed on the appropriate patient's chart is shown in Fig. 16–3.

Urinalysis

The urinalysis is often done by the hematology division of the laboratory, although it is not a blood test. A urinalysis is ordinarily done on every hospital admission and consists of a physical, chemical, and microscopic examination of the urine. A sample chart showing results is given in Table 16–2.

The **physical examination** will include a determination of the color, transparency (clarity), and specific gravity (weight of the urine compared with the weight of an equal volume of distilled water). There may even be a comment regarding the odor of the urine.

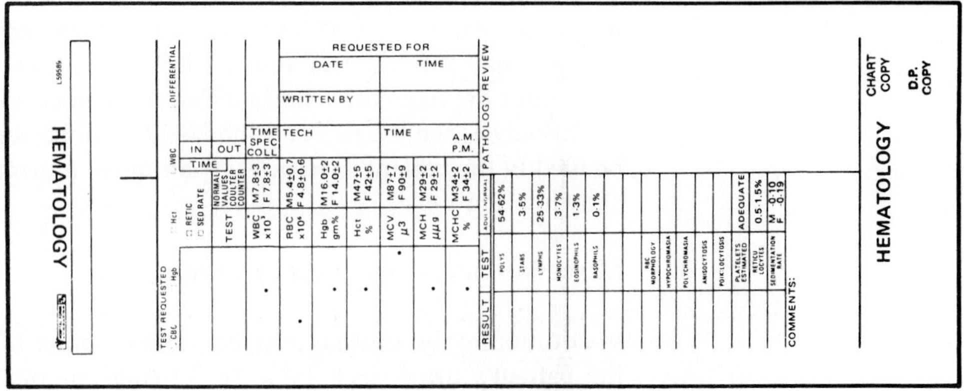

HEMATOLOGY

L59586

TEST REQUESTED: ☐ CBC ☐ Hgb ☐ Hct ☐ RETIC ☐ SED RATE ☐ WBC ☐ DIFFERENTIAL

TIME: IN | OUT

REQUESTED FOR: DATE | TIME

WRITTEN BY

TIME SPEC COLL | TECH | TIME A.M. P.M.

TEST	NORMAL VALUES COULTER COUNTER
WBC $\times 10^3$	M 7.8±3 F 7.8±3
RBC $\times 10^6$	M 5.4±0.7 F 4.8±0.6
Hgb gm%	M 16.0±2 F 14.0±2
Hct %	M 47±5 F 42±5
MCV μ^3	M 87±7 F 90±9
MCH $\mu\mu g$	M 29±2 F 29±2
MCHC %	M 34±2 F 34±2

PATHOLOGY REVIEW

RESULT	TEST	ADULT NORMAL
	POLYS	54-62%
	STABS	3-5%
	LYMPHS	25-33%
	MONOCYTES	3-7%
	EOSINOPHILS	1-3%
	BASOPHILS	0-1%
	RBC MORPHOLOGY	
	HYPOCHROMASIA	
	POLYCHROMASIA	
	ANISOCYTOSIS	
	POIKILOCYTOSIS	
	PLATELETS ESTIMATED	ADEQUATE
	RETICULOCYTES	0.5-1.5%
	SEDIMENTATION RATE	M 0-10 F 0-19

COMMENTS:

HEMATOLOGY

CHART COPY

D.P. COPY

Figure 16–3

TABLE 16–2

Sample Chart Showing Results of a Routine Urinalysis

Examination	Abbreviation	Normal Values
Color		Yellow/amber
Characteristics		Clear
Reaction	pH	4.6–8.0
Specific gravity	Sp. Gr./SG	1.025–1.035
Protein (albumin)	Prot./Alb.	0–trace
Glucose		None
Acetone		None
Blood		None
Microscopic:		
Red blood cell casts	RBC casts	None
White blood cell casts	WBC casts	None
Hyaline casts		Few, possibly
Crystals	X1s	None
Renal tubular casts		None

The **chemical examination** of the urine includes tests for pH, glucose, protein, ketone bodies, blood, bilirubin, urobilinogen, and perhaps nitrite.

The **microscopic examination** studies the urine sediment (solid materials contained in the urine). RBCs, WBCs, epithelial cells, casts, and crystals may be seen during the microscopic portion of the urinalysis. Other structures which may be reported include mucus threads, bacteria, yeast cells, parasites, and spermatozoa.

There are several types of urine specimens. These include:

- **Voided**—the patient urinates into a clean container
- **Clean catch or midstream**—nursing uses a special cleaning procedure and the patient starts his or her urine stream to wash away germs on the outside of the urinary tract. The urine is then collected "midstream."
- **Catheterized**—a sterile specimen obtained through urinary catheterization; is sent to the lab in a sterile container

The health unit coordinator should know that the requisition for any urinalysis is not sent to the laboratory until the specimen is obtained.

Urine specimens must be sent *directly* to the laboratory. If the urine is allowed to stand over 30 minutes, several changes can take place. These changes may alter the true results of the urinalysis.

After the requisition and labeled urine specimen are received in the lab, the urinalysis will be run and the results will be sent to your nursing unit to be filed in the patient's chart. An example of a urinalysis laboratory report is shown in Fig. 16–4.

Miscellaneous Specimen Examinations

In addition to the routine urinalysis, many other tests may be performed on the patient's urine. (See Table 16–3.) Analysis of the urine for a particular chemical or mineral element, such as chlorides or ammonia, may be made on a single specimen or on a 24-hour collection of the patient's urine. The doctor

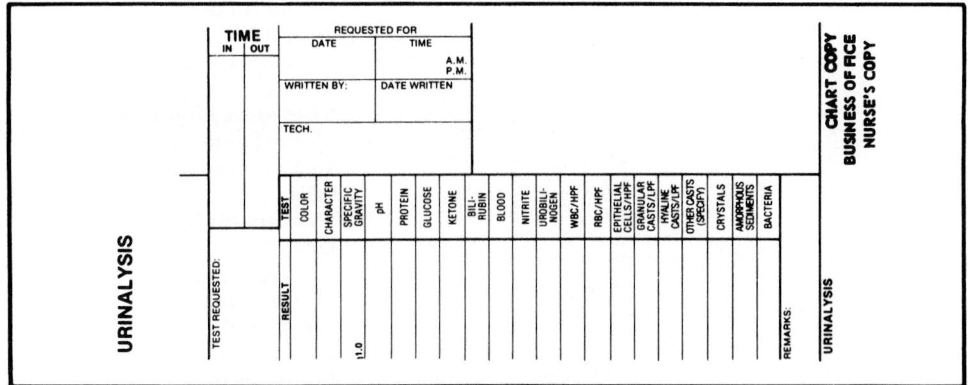

URINALYSIS
TIME
IN | OUT
REQUESTED FOR
DATE | TIME
A.M.
P.M.
WRITTEN BY: | DATE WRITTEN
TECH.
TEST REQUESTED:
TEST | COLOR | CHARACTER | SPECIFIC GRAVITY | pH | PROTEIN | GLUCOSE | KETONE | BILI-RUBIN | BLOOD | NITRITE | UROBILI-NOGEN | WBC/HPF | RBC/HPF | EPITHELIAL CELLS/HPF | GRANULAR CASTS/LPF | HYALINE CASTS/LPF | OTHER CASTS (SPECIFY) | CRYSTALS | AMORPHOUS SEDIMENTS | BACTERIA
RESULT | | | 1.0
REMARKS:
URINALYSIS
CHART COPY
BUSINESS OFFICE
NURSE'S COPY

Figure 16–4

TABLE 16–3

Common Tests Performed on Urine Specimens

Specimen	*Examination*	*Abbreviation*	*Normal*
Urine for:	Ammonia	NH_3	0.8 Gm.
	Catecholamines		80 mcg./24 hr.
	Culture & sensitivity	C & S	
	Hemoglobin	Hgb.	Negative
	Porphyrins		20 mcg.
	Urea		25
	Urobilinogen		2 mg.
	17-Hydroxycorticosteroids		5 mg./24 hr.
	17-Ketosteroids		15 mg./24 hr.

usually indicates the type of specimen necessary for a test when he/she writes the order.

Note: The tests shown in Table 16–3 are *urine chemistries, not routine urinalysis* (refer to section on chemistry below). When a 24-hour urine specimen is ordered, it may be the health unit coordinator's responsibility to obtain a container from the laboratory to be used for the collection of the specimen. The urine container may contain a special additive or be kept on ice to keep the urine from deteriorating during the collection period. Nursing will save all of the patient's urine for 24 hours and will then bring the container to the nurses' station. You will send the labeled container and the requisition you prepared when the original order was transcribed to the laboratory.

24-Hour Urines
*Aldosterone
Amylase
BUN
Calcium
*Catecholamines
*Coproporphyrins
*Cortisol
Creatinine
Estrogen
Follicle-stimulating hormone
Glucose

Heavy metals
***5 HIAA**
Hydroxy-proline
17-Hydroxycorticosteroids
17-Hydroxysteroids
17-Ketogenic steroids
17-Ketosteroids
LDH
***Metanephrine**
Oxalates
Phosphorous
***Porphyrins**
Porphobilinogen
Potassium
Pregnanetroil
Pregnanediol
Quantitative HCG
Sodium
Uric acid
Urine total protein
***Uroporphyrins**
***VMA**

***Specimens which require preservative.**

Chemistry

This laboratory division analyzes specimens of body fluids for chemical constituents. Blood and urine are the specimens most commonly collected for study in the chemistry division of the laboratory. However, chemistry tests may be performed on other body materials (e.g., vomitus or gastric—stomach—contents). Many tests of the same name can be done on either blood or urine. Therefore, the word **serum** will often be added to the order and will be your clue that the order is for blood rather than for urine.

Table 16–4 shows only a partial list of blood chemistry examinations. There are a vast number of chemistry exams the doctor may order. By studying the requisitions for chemistry supplied by the laboratory and by lists of chemistry exams your instructor may provide, you will grow in your knowledge of the types of chemistry examinations the doctor will order for his patients.

Because they are so commonly ordered, special mention is made of several blood chemistry orders:

- **Alkaline phosphatase**—many uses, but major purpose is to diagnose liver disease.
- **Electrolytes** (lytes)—The electrolytes help the body maintain a balance between acidity and alkalinity. This may be called an electrolyte panel and include Sodium (Na), Potassium (K), Chlorides (Cl), and Carbon Dioxide (CO_2).

These tests may be ordered separately.

- **Acid Phosphatase**—aids in diagnosis of cancer of the prostate gland.
- **Amylase**—aids in diagnosis of pancreatic disease, abdominal obstructions, diseases of salivary glands and ducts.

TABLE 16–4

Typical Blood Chemistry Examinations

Examination	Abbreviation	Normal Values
Acid Phosphatase	Acid P'tase	0–10 ng./ml.
Albumin	Alb.	3.5 Gm.–5.0 Gm./dl
Alkaline Phosphatase	Alk. P'tase	30 IU–90 IU/L
Amylase		30 IU–130 IU/L
Anti-Streptolysis Titration	asl	150 u./ml. serum
Bilirubin	Bili	0.5 mg.–1.2 mg./dl
Blood Urea Nitrogen	BUN	7 mg.–21 mg./dl
Calcium	Ca	8.6–10.7 mg./dl
Carbon Dioxide	CO_2	20 mEq–33 mEq/L
Chlorides	Cl	95 mEq–109 mEq/L
Cholesterol	chol.	150 mg.–300 mg./dl
Creatinine	creat.	0.7 mg.–1.3 mg./dl
Creatinine phosphokinase	CPK	F, 10 IU–100 IU/L M, 20 IU–140 IU/L
Electrolytes (See Na, K, Cl, and CO_2)	lytes	
Fasting Blood Sugar (also glucose)	FBS, BS	70 mg.–110 mg.dl
Glucose Tolerance Test	GTT	60–125 mg./dl
Lipase		0.2–1.5 U/ml.
Lithium		0.5–1.0 mEq/L
Lactic dehydrogenase	LDH	90 IU–200 IU/L
Non-Protein Nitrogen	NPN	20 mg.–35 mg./dl
Phosphorus	Phos	2.5 mg.–4.5 mg./dl
Potassium	K	3.4 mEq–5.0 mEq/L
Protein Bound Iodine	PBI	4.0–8.0 µg/dl
Serum Glutamic Oxaloacetic Transaminase or APT	SGOT	8 IU–36 IU/L
Serum Glutamic Pyruvic Transaminase or ALT	SGPT	2 IU–32 IU/L
Sodium	Na	135 mEq–145 mEq/L
T_3 Uptake		25%–35%
Total Proteins		5.9 Gm.–8.0 Gm./dl
Triglycerides		10–150 mg./dl
Uric Acid		F, 2.0 mg.–7.0 mg./dl M, 2.5 mg.–8.0 mg./dl

- **Bilirubin**—helps measure liver function.
- **Blood Urea Nitrogen** (BUN)—kidney function test.
- **Calcium**—one of essential ions of body; decrease called hypocalcemia occurs in alkalosis, celiac disease, sprue, hypoparathyroidism, and some kidney diseases; increase (hypercalcemia) found in acidosis, hyperparathyroidism, multiple myeloma, and some respiratory diseases.
- **Carbon dioxide (CO_2)**—measured in cases of suspected respiratory insufficiency; higher-than-normal concentration of CO_2 may indicate that gas exchange is inadequate.
- **Cardiac enzymes** (SGOT, LDH, and CPK)—When a patient has had a heart attack (myocardial infarction or MI), the enzymes found in the

cardiac muscle are elevated. These tests may also be ordered separately and may aid in the diagnosis of other disease conditions.

- **Chemistry screen (chem. screen) or SMA**—A special machine in the laboratory performs a number of tests on one sample of blood. An SMA 12 performs 12 tests; an SMA 20 performs 20 tests, etc.
- **Chlorides**—measured to help diagnose disorders in the maintenance of normal osmotic relationships, acid-base balance, and water balance of body; usually performed together with measurement of other ions of the blood.
- **Creatinine**—increased quantitites are found in advanced stages of renal (kidney) disease.
- **Lipase**—test for damage to the pancreas.
- **Lithium**—test to monitor the lithium dosage (a medication) in the treatment of manic-depressive psychosis (bipolar affective disorder).
- **Potassium (K^+)**—essential ion found in large concentrations in all cells; alterations in serum potassium levels may produce serious changes in body function, or even death.

  Marked decrease may cause cardiac arrhythmias and muscle weakness, causes include severe vomiting and diarrhea and chronic kidney disease.

  Marked increase also produces arrhythmias; there may also be lethargy and coma—causes include severe cell damage, adrenal cortical deficiency, and hypoventilation.
- **Serum Glutamic Oxaloacetic Transaminase (SGOT)**—elevated especially in liver disease.
- **Sodium (Na)**—the main cation of blood and extracellular fluid. Increased serum Na levels may be caused by markedly inadequate water intake or the administration of excessive amounts of Na.

  Decreased Na levels occur in diarrhea, heat exhaustion, Addison's disease, and certain kidney disorders.
- **T_3 Uptake, Thyroxine Index (free), T_3–T_4, T_4RIA**—tests for thyroid disease.
- **Uric acid**—usually performed to diagnose gout.

The Blood Sugar Tests

- **Blood sugar (BS or glucose)**—This determines the amount of sugar in the blood. Fasting Blood Sugar (FBS) determines the amount of sugar in the blood when the patient has not eaten for a period of time and so is done in the early A.M.
- **Glucose Tolerance Test (GTT)**—This test is done over several hours when the patient has been fasting. The patient is given a large amount of glucose to drink. Blood and urine specimens are taken to determine abnormalities in glucose metabolism.
- **Postprandial Blood Sugars (PP BS)**—This test is done to determine the patient's response to the intake of carbohydrates. It is most commonly ordered as a 2-hr PP BS, and the blood is drawn two hours after any meal. NOTE: The health unit coordinator will be expected to notify the laboratory when a patient has finished eating so that the laboratory may plan to draw the blood in two hours.

These tests are usually done to aid in the diagnosis of and monitoring of diabetes. Results of these tests may be included on the supplementary chart form often called the Diabetic Flow Sheet.

Results of the blood chemistry examinations (Fig. 16–5) will be sent to the unit to be filed on the patient's chart.

Sample Chemistry Requisitions. Many hospitals order laboratory tests by computer. If your hospital does not, requisitions similar to the ones pictured in Fig. 16–5 are used.

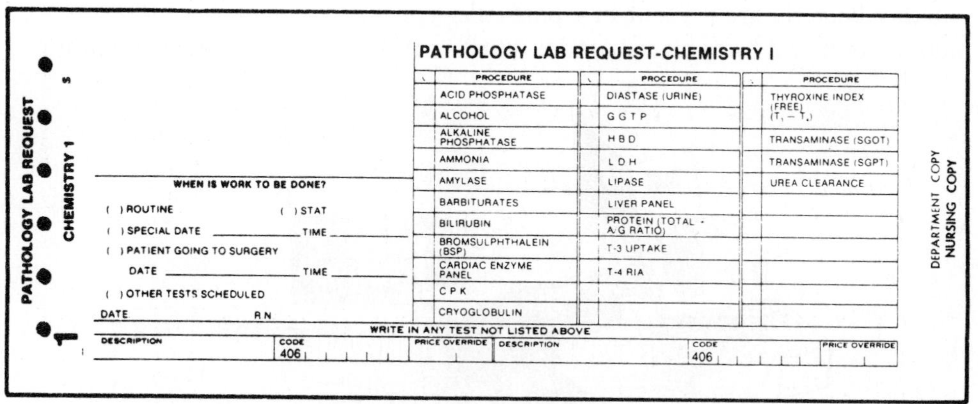

1 PATHOLOGY LAB REQUEST CHEMISTRY 1

PATHOLOGY LAB REQUEST-CHEMISTRY I

WHEN IS WORK TO BE DONE?

( ) ROUTINE ( ) STAT

( ) SPECIAL DATE ______ TIME ______

( ) PATIENT GOING TO SURGERY

DATE ______ TIME ______

( ) OTHER TESTS SCHEDULED

DATE R N

✓	PROCEDURE	✓	PROCEDURE	✓	PROCEDURE
	ACID PHOSPHATASE		DIASTASE (URINE)		THYROXINE INDEX (FREE) ($T_1 - T_4$)
	ALCOHOL		G G T P		
	ALKALINE PHOSPHATASE		H B D		TRANSAMINASE (SGOT)
	AMMONIA		L D H		TRANSAMINASE (SGPT)
	AMYLASE		LIPASE		UREA CLEARANCE
	BARBITURATES		LIVER PANEL		
	BILIRUBIN		PROTEIN (TOTAL - A/G RATIO)		
	BROMSULPHTHALEIN (BSP)		T-3 UPTAKE		
	CARDIAC ENZYME PANEL		T-4 RIA		
	C P K				
	CRYOGLOBULIN				

WRITE IN ANY TEST NOT LISTED ABOVE

DESCRIPTION	CODE	PRICE OVERRIDE	DESCRIPTION	CODE	PRICE OVERRIDE
	406			406	

DEPARTMENT COPY NURSING COPY

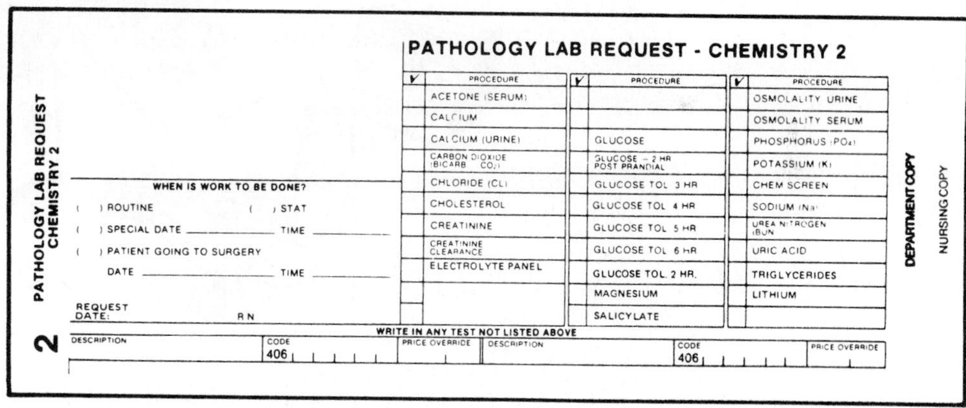

2 PATHOLOGY LAB REQUEST CHEMISTRY 2

PATHOLOGY LAB REQUEST - CHEMISTRY 2

WHEN IS WORK TO BE DONE?

( ) ROUTINE ( ) STAT

( ) SPECIAL DATE ______ TIME ______

( ) PATIENT GOING TO SURGERY

DATE ______ TIME ______

REQUEST DATE: R N

✓	PROCEDURE	✓	PROCEDURE	✓	PROCEDURE
	ACETONE (SERUM)				OSMOLALITY URINE
	CALCIUM				OSMOLALITY SERUM
	CALCIUM (URINE)		GLUCOSE		PHOSPHORUS (PO_4)
	CARBON DIOXIDE (BICARB CO_2)		GLUCOSE – 2 HR POST PRANDIAL		POTASSIUM (K)
	CHLORIDE (CL)		GLUCOSE TOL 3 HR		CHEM SCREEN
	CHOLESTEROL		GLUCOSE TOL 4 HR		SODIUM (Na)
	CREATININE		GLUCOSE TOL 5 HR		UREA NITROGEN (BUN)
	CREATININE CLEARANCE		GLUCOSE TOL 6 HR		URIC ACID
	ELECTROLYTE PANEL		GLUCOSE TOL. 2 HR.		TRIGLYCERIDES
			MAGNESIUM		LITHIUM
			SALICYLATE		

WRITE IN ANY TEST NOT LISTED ABOVE

DESCRIPTION	CODE	PRICE OVERRIDE	DESCRIPTION	CODE	PRICE OVERRIDE
	406			406	

DEPARTMENT COPY NURSING COPY

3

PATHOLOGY LAB REQUEST - CHEMISTRY 3

WHEN IS WORK TO BE DONE?

( ) ROUTINE ( ) STAT

( ) SPECIAL DATE ______ TIME ______

( ) PATIENT GOING TO SURGERY

DATE ______ TIME ______

( ) OTHER TESTS SCHEDULED

DATE R N

✓	PROCEDURE	✓	PROCEDURE	✓	PROCEDURE
	CATECHOLAMINES (Urine)		IMMUNO ELECTROPHORESIS		RENIN
	CORTISOL (PLASMA) Specify Time		IRON & IRON BINDING		SALICYLATE
			LDH ISOENZYMES		SEROTONIN (5-HIAA)
	DILANTIN		LEAD (Blood Urine)		THYROXINE BINDING GLOBULIN (TBG)
	DIGOXIN		LEUCINE AMINO PEPTIDASE		THYROID STIMULATING HORMONE (TSH)
	D-XYLOSE TOLERANCE		LIPID PROFILE		TRIGLYCERIDES
	ELECTROPHORESIS PROTEIN (SERUM)		LITHIUM		V.M.A. VANILLYL MANDELIC ACID
	ELECTROPHORESIS HEMOGLOBIN		MACROGLOBULIN (SIA WATER TEST)		VITAMIN A CAROTENE
	ESTRIOL (PLACENTA) URINE		MAGNESIUM		VITAMIN B-12
	FOLIC ACID (Folate)		ORINASE TOLERANCE		17 KETOSTEROIDS 24 HR URINE
	GENTAMYCIN		QUINIDINE		17 KETOGENIC STEROIDS 24 HR URINE

WRITE IN ANY TEST NOT LISTED ABOVE

DESCRIPTION	CODE	PRICE OVERRIDE	DESCRIPTION	CODE	PRICE OVERRIDE
	406			406	

LAB COPY NURSING COPY

Figure 16–5

Microbiology

This section is concerned primarily with tests designed to isolate and identify disease-causing microorganisms. These microorganisms may be present in a specimen of any type of material from the patient's body. The most common are blood, urine, sputum, and wound drainage but may also include stool, vaginal secretions, and others. (Fig. 16–6.)

Divisions within the microbiology department may include:

- **Bacteriology**—Bacteria found in body specimens are studied here. A frequent order for C&S is processed in this division.

The abbreviation C&S means culture and sensitivity. To determine whether bacteria are present in a particular specimen, a sample of the specimen is "cultured," or placed under sterile conditions on a special medium

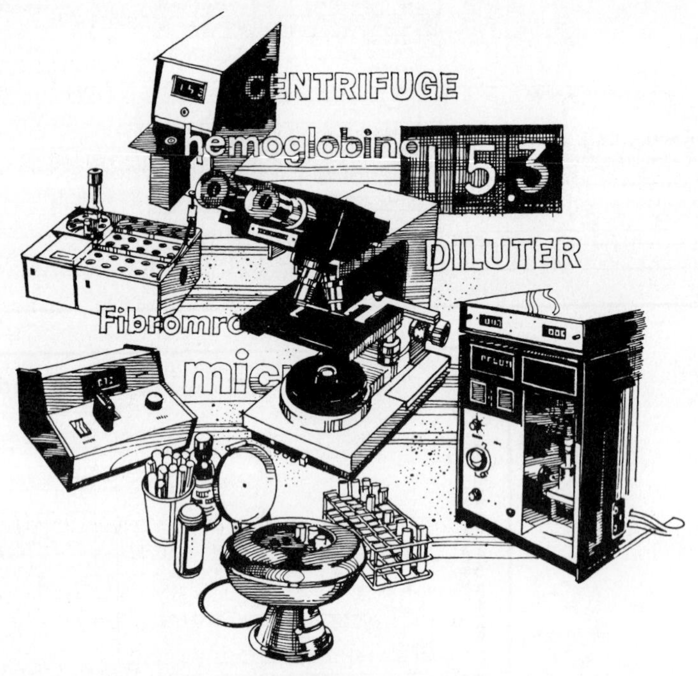

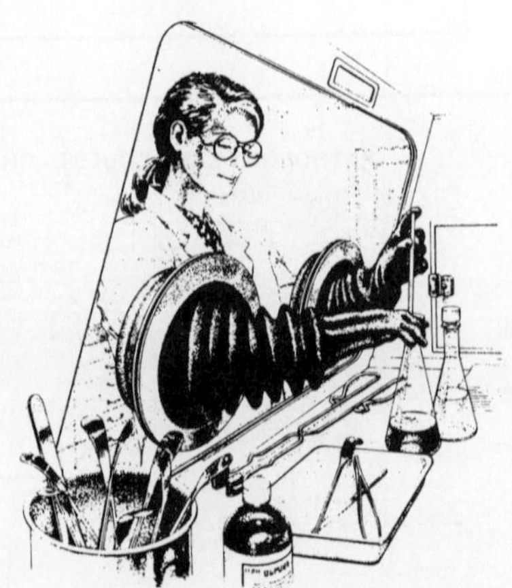

Figure 16–6

which bacteria require to grow. If certain bacteria are present in a specimen (and are therefore at work causing disease inside the patient), "sensitivity" tests are performed. In these tests, the growths of bacteria from the specimen are mixed with certain antibiotics. The bacteria will be destroyed by the particular antibiotics to which they are "sensitive." The doctor then knows which antibiotics to administer to cure the patient's bacterial infection.

The health unit coordinator should know that although a specimen for C&S may be *obtained* stat, the results will not be available immediately.

Blood Cultures

Multiple blood cultures must be ordered separately according to the number of times requested by the physician. For example:

- Order reads: Blood cultures × 2
  Enter two separate orders for blood cultures.
- Order reads: Blood cultures × 2, 15 minutes apart
  Enter two separate orders for blood cultures and type "15 minutes apart" in remarks.

Examples of orders for microbiology and serology are shown in Table 16–5.

- **Mycology**—analyzes specimens to identify fungi
- **Parasitology**—studies parasites, organisms that attach themselves to another organism and live off of that organism (e.g., helminths [worms] and the ova [eggs] of these parasites). Stool or fecal samples are studied here for ova and parasites (O&P).
- **Virology**—this division studies viruses.

Note: The health unit coordinator should know that specimens for microbiology should be taken to the laboratory immediately. Blood samples will be drawn by the laboratory; samples of urine, sputum, wound drainage, vaginal secretions, stool, and CSF will be obtained by the doctor or nurse and must be sent in the appropriate labeled container along with the requisition you prepared at the time the order was transcribed.

TABLE 16–5

Common Tests Related to Particular Body Materials

Specimen	*Examination*	*Abbreviation*
Stool for:	Culture & sensitivity	C&S
	Ova & parasites	O&P
Sputum for:	Culture & sensitivity	C&S
	Acid-Fast	
	Bacilli	C&S
	(For diagnosis of TB)	AFB
Cerebral Spinal Fluid CSF	Serology	CSF

Immunosuppressant Laboratory Tests. These are tests done to assess the effects of the body's diminished immune response as a result of disease (usually due to HIV).

Cytology

This department studies cells obtained from body tissues.

Pap smears, developed by Dr. Papanicolaou, can be performed on various types of specimens to determine the presence of cancer. The most common type of "Pap smear or test" is done from the cervix during a pelvic examination.

Biopsies, or pieces of body tissues, taken from the skin or from internal body organs are examined by cytology. Tissues removed in surgery are examined by this department.

Bone marrow aspirations, samples taken from the center of certain bones where red blood cells are produced, are obtained through a special procedure performed by the doctor. If the specimen is obtained from the breastbone, the procedure is called **sternal puncture.** This may be done on the nursing unit and sent to cytology for examination. Ascitic fluid (formed in the abdominal cavity and withdrawn by an abdominal **paracentesis**) or fluid formed in the chest cavity and withdrawn by **thoracentesis** by the doctor may be examined. (Fig. 16–7.)

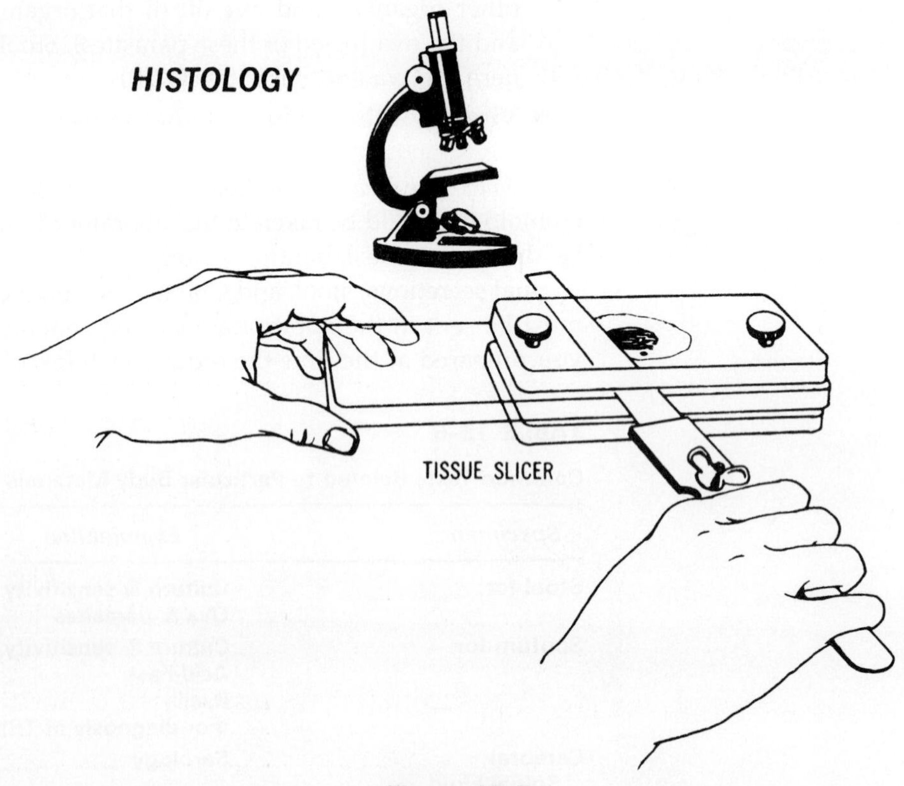

Figure 16–7

Serology

This division studies blood serum and some other body fluids such as cerebral spinal fluid (CSF). Tests for syphilis such as the VDRL and RPR are done in this division. (Fig. 16–8.)

Cerebral Spinal Fluid. Specimens of CSF are sometimes needed for laboratory analysis. A **lumbar puncture** (LP) is performed on the unit. A tray from central supply is requisitioned, and the doctor inserts a needle into the patient's lower spine below the level of the spinal cord. Fluid is withdrawn for laboratory analysis. An order for CSF might look this way:

> ***LP-Spinal fluid to lab for:***
> ***#1—Cells***
> ***#2—Protein***
> ***#3—Glucose***

The fluid removed is usually placed in vials labeled #1, #2, and #3; the doctor writes orders for tests for each vial number. You will note on your requisition which vial is for which test. The tests which may be ordered include:

- CSF examination
- Cell count
- Chloride
- Colloidal gold
- Glucose
- Protein
- VDRL

An example of a requisition for CSF sent from the lab and filed on the patient's chart is shown on the next page. (Fig. 16–9.)

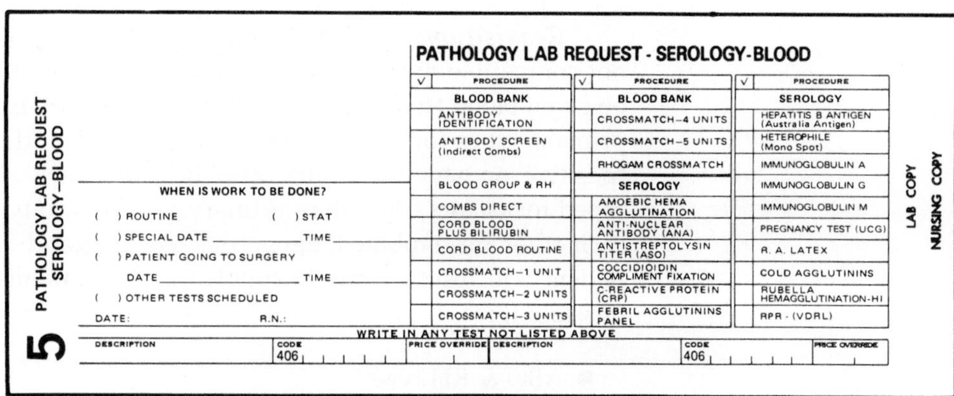

5 PATHOLOGY LAB REQUEST SEROLOGY–BLOOD

PATHOLOGY LAB REQUEST - SEROLOGY-BLOOD

√	PROCEDURE	√	PROCEDURE	√	PROCEDURE
	BLOOD BANK		**BLOOD BANK**		**SEROLOGY**
	ANTIBODY IDENTIFICATION		CROSSMATCH–4 UNITS		HEPATITIS B ANTIGEN (Australia Antigen)
	ANTIBODY SCREEN (Indirect Combs)		CROSSMATCH–5 UNITS		HETEROPHILE (Mono Spot)
			RHOGAM CROSSMATCH		IMMUNOGLOBULIN A
	BLOOD GROUP & RH		**SEROLOGY**		IMMUNOGLOBULIN G
	COMBS DIRECT		AMOEBIC HEMA AGGLUTINATION		IMMUNOGLOBULIN M
	CORD BLOOD PLUS BILIRUBIN		ANTI-NUCLEAR ANTIBODY (ANA)		PREGNANCY TEST (UCG)
	CORD BLOOD ROUTINE		ANTISTREPTOLYSIN TITER (ASO)		R. A. LATEX
	CROSSMATCH–1 UNIT		COCCIDIOIDIN COMPLIMENT FIXATION		COLD AGGLUTININS
	CROSSMATCH–2 UNITS		C-REACTIVE PROTEIN (CRP)		RUBELLA HEMAGGLUTINATION-HI
	CROSSMATCH–3 UNITS		FEBRIL AGGLUTININS PANEL		RPR - (VDRL)

WHEN IS WORK TO BE DONE?

( ) ROUTINE ( ) STAT

( ) SPECIAL DATE __________ TIME __________

( ) PATIENT GOING TO SURGERY

DATE __________ TIME __________

( ) OTHER TESTS SCHEDULED

DATE: R.N.:

WRITE IN ANY TEST NOT LISTED ABOVE

DESCRIPTION	CODE	PRICE OVERRIDE	DESCRIPTION	CODE	PRICE OVERRIDE
	406			406	

LAB COPY NURSING COPY

Figure 16–8

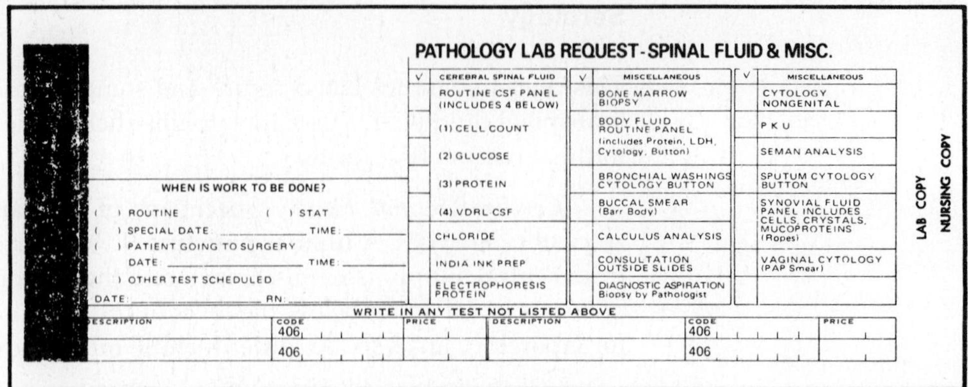

PATHOLOGY LAB REQUEST-SPINAL FLUID & MISC.

√	CEREBRAL SPINAL FLUID	√	MISCELLANEOUS	√	MISCELLANEOUS
	ROUTINE CSF PANEL (INCLUDES 4 BELOW)		BONE MARROW BIOPSY		CYTOLOGY NONGENITAL
	(1) CELL COUNT		BODY FLUID ROUTINE PANEL (includes Protein, LDH, Cytology, Button)		P K U
	(2) GLUCOSE				SEMAN ANALYSIS
	(3) PROTEIN		BRONCHIAL WASHINGS CYTOLOGY BUTTON		SPUTUM CYTOLOGY BUTTON
	(4) VDRL CSF		BUCCAL SMEAR (Barr Body)		SYNOVIAL FLUID PANEL INCLUDES CELLS, CRYSTALS, MUCOPROTEINS (Ropes)
	CHLORIDE		CALCULUS ANALYSIS		
	INDIA INK PREP		CONSULTATION OUTSIDE SLIDES		VAGINAL CYTOLOGY (PAP Smear)
	ELECTROPHORESIS PROTEIN		DIAGNOSTIC ASPIRATION Biopsy by Pathologist		

WHEN IS WORK TO BE DONE?

( ) ROUTINE ( ) STAT
( ) SPECIAL DATE ______ TIME: ______
( ) PATIENT GOING TO SURGERY
DATE: ______ TIME: ______
( ) OTHER TEST SCHEDULED
DATE: ______ RN: ______

LAB COPY NURSING COPY

WRITE IN ANY TEST NOT LISTED ABOVE

DESCRIPTION	CODE	PRICE	DESCRIPTION	CODE	PRICE
	406			406	
	406			406	

Figure 16–9

KEY IDEA: THE BLOOD BANK

Blood transfusions are given to replace blood loss or to correct an anemic condition.

A reserve stock of whole blood and plasma (the fluid portion of the blood) is ordinarily kept at the hospital's blood bank. The blood must be obtained from suitable donors (*homologous* blood)—that is, people free of disease and in good health. Blood is stored, for a specific length of time, under refrigeration for emergency use when major blood loss occurs, as during surgery or in cases of severe injury. *Autologous* blood is a patient's own blood deposited for later use.

The blood bank is usually a part of the laboratory. Responsibilities of the blood bank include:

- Scheduling donor appointments to maintain an adequate supply of various types of blood
- Collecting the blood from the donors and processing it for future use
- Performing blood tests
- Keeping records pertaining to blood donations and transfusions

Execution of Forms

If you work in a surgical unit, you will probably have frequent contact with the blood bank. The services of the blood bank, however, are often required by nonsurgical patients as well. The usual types of forms used in requesting the services of the blood bank are described on page 343. (Fig. 16–8.)

Requisitions for Blood Grouping. Because different types of blood are not compatible, it is necessary to type the blood of the patient so that he can be given blood from a compatible donor. (Fig. 16–10.) Human blood is of four primary types (or groups): **O, A, B,** and **AB.** Additional factors, such as Rh (positive or negative), must also be compatible. Blood must therefore be typed for factors other than primary type. If two types of blood not suited to each other are combined, dangerous reactions and sometimes the death of the patient will result. Some hospitals type all patients' blood routinely on admission. (Figs. 16–11 and 16–12.) Type and Crossmatch includes:

- ABO & RH type
- Antibody screen
- Units ordered

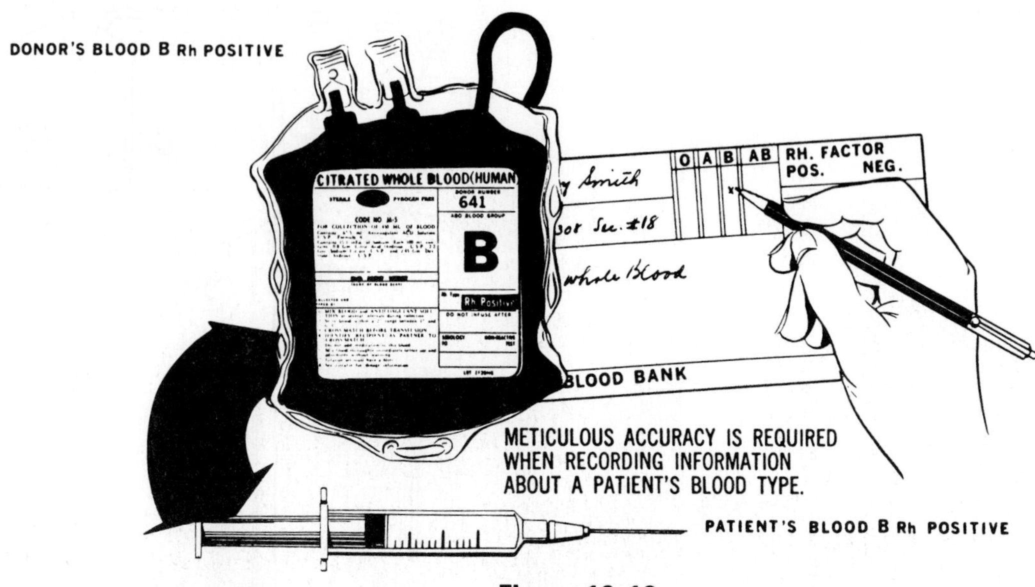

Figure 16–10

Requisition for Crossmatching. It is not sufficient, however, simply to give a patient blood of his own type. When it is expected that a patient will need a transfusion, a sample of his blood must actually be mixed with a sample from a potential donor, to ensure that the two bloods will definitely be compatible. This process is called **crossmatching.** It is always done before whole blood from any donor is given to any recipient. After the blood has been crossmatched, the suitable blood is carefully labeled and held in reserve for the patient. The physician will indicate how much blood may be needed. (Fig. 16–13.)

REQUISITION FOR BLOOD GROUPING

BLOOD GROUPING	CIRCLE TEST DESIRED	
Date	Diagnosis	
Room No.		Units
Name		Charge No.
Hospital No.		Date
Doctor		

Group	O A B AB	Rh Factor	Pos.	Neg.	Classification
Direct Coombs	Pos. Neg.	Phenotype:	HR	Kell	Duffy
Rh. Antibody Titre: Neg.			Pos.in Titre	1:	
Isosensitization:					
Remarks:					

Figure 16–11

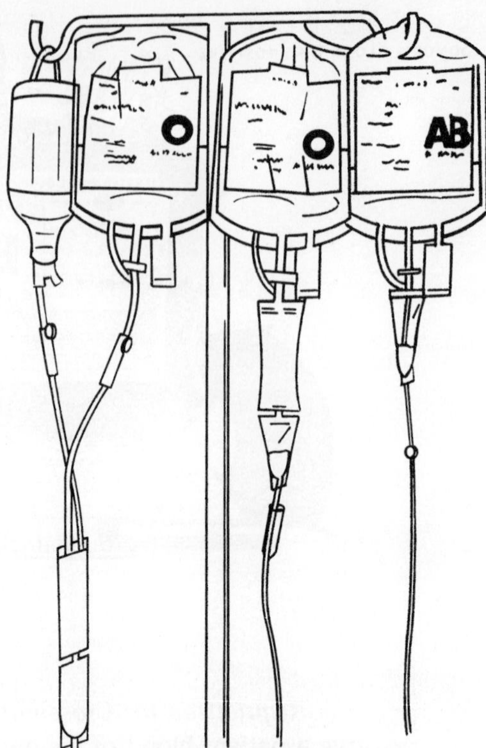

Figure 16–12

REQUISITION FOR CROSSMATCHING

BLOOD BANK—Crossmatch Request		Name ______
ONE UNIT ONLY ☐ Whole Blood ☐ Packaged Cells ☐ Fresh Blood (Specify Reason) ______ ______	Diagnosis ______ WHEN REQUIRED: Date ______ Time ______ am pm By ______ RN	Hospital No. ______ Room No. ______ Date ______ Doctor ______

	FOR LAB USE ONLY	
Patient:	Donor:	Reactions:
Group Rh	Donor No. Group Rh	
Compatible yes no Saline ☐ ☐ Protein ☐ ☐ Coombs ☐ ☐	VDRL:	Transfused by ______ Date ______ Time ______ am pm
	Report by Date	Type & Crossmatch ☐ Transfusion ☐ — Charge

Figure 16–13

Examples of doctor's orders for blood administration:

> *T & C 2 units WB (type and crossmatch units of whole blood)*
> *1 U PC now—(give one unit of packed cells immediately)*
> *Cryoprecipitates—1 unit*
> *2 U. FFP—(2 units fresh frozen plasma)*
> *Give 1 U PRCs—(1 unit packed red cells)*
> *Platelets, 2 units*

KEY IDEA: ORDERING TESTS

Health Unit Coordinator Responsibilities When Dealing with Orders for Laboratory Tests

Your greatest concern for laboratory tests should be for:

- Recognition of test names
- Correct spelling
- Abbreviations in common usage
- Knowledge of correct requisitions when applicable

Your primary concern with laboratory tests will be to correctly order. It will be especially important for you to learn what tests are performed by each laboratory division. Your instructor will teach you the procedures for ordering as they are performed in your hospital. In most hospitals you will not send requisitions for specimens to be obtained by nursing (which the patient must produce—urine, stool, sputum) until the specimen has been taken. Therefore, appropriate stamped requisitions must be kept in a designated place at the nurses' station. All specimens must have the time of collection, date, and initials or name of the nurse clearly marked on the laboratory specimen slip. In some cases, you may be expected to notify the laboratory by telephone of an emergency test or a test requiring that an appointment be made.

Many hospitals order laboratory tests by computer. You must be very accurate when performing this task.

Patient Preparations. Some laboratory tests will require special preparation of patients on the night before or morning of the test. The most common type of preparation for routine laboratory tests is to withhold food from the patient until the test has been performed. The designation may be "NPO," that is, nothing by mouth after a certain hour, or simply a "hold breakfast." It may be part of your work to compile lists of patients for whom tests make special preparations necessary. Your instructor will provide you with information on such tests as well as your duties in connection with the necessary preparations.

Receiving Telephone Reports. Often, when a laboratory test has been ordered stat., now, today, etc., the laboratory will telephone the results to the unit before sending them in written form. This may also occur if a result is abnormal and the laboratory wishes to bring it to the immediate attention of the doctor and nurse.

Always repeat laboratory results and write them down with the patient's name, date, time of day, and your signature. Tell the nurse and affix the telephone report to the front of the chart holder.

Computer Retrieval of Laboratory Results. If your computer is interfaced with the laboratory, it is possible to have retrieval of results as soon as the laboratory test is done. The laboratory will immediately generate a printout, so it is not necessary for you to call the laboratory or for them to call the unit. Laboratory results can be reviewed at any time using the computer.

Standard Precautions

Health Unit Coordinators should avoid handling a laboratory specimen container unless it is inside a protective container (such as a plastic bag) or unless gloves are worn.

RADIOLOGY

Rapid advances are occurring in the field of radiology. A new breed of imaging devices is enabling doctors to view organs at work and identify blockages and growths—all without surgery. (Fig. 16–14.)

X-rays were discovered by Wilhelm Konrad Roentgen, a German physicist, in 1895. They have since been renamed roentgen rays and serve as a diagnostic aid to visualize internal structures and organs. X-rays are high-energy electromagnetic waves that are invisible. They are able to penetrate solid materials because of a very short wavelength. They rely upon differences in density or thickness of various body structures to produce shadows on the radiographic film.

Contrast medium is used when the densities of two structures or organs that are next to each other are similar and can't be distinguished on the radiograph.

The simplest kind of radiographs are those that do not require preparation or use of a contrast medium.

Examples are:

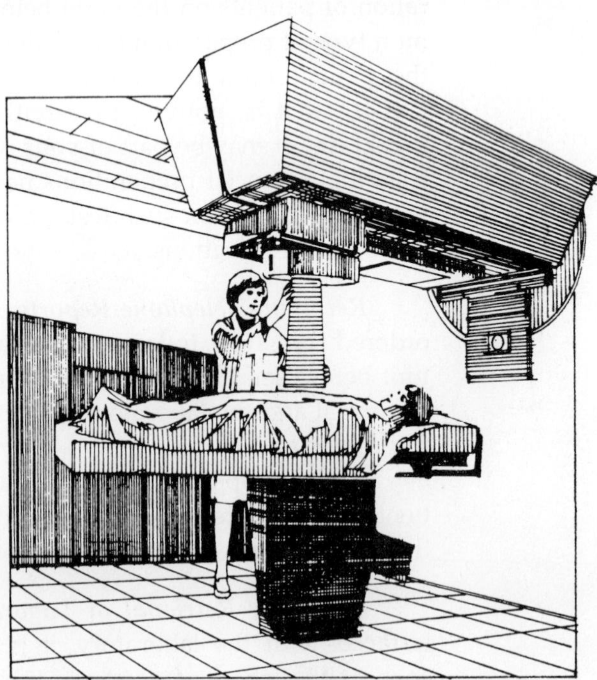

Figure 16–14

- Chest x-rays
- Extremity x-rays
- Skull x-rays
- Flat plates (shows bony structures, foreign bodies in tissue, or determines the position of other organs)
- Mammogram—uses low doses of x-rays to image the inside of the breast
- Xerogram—Utilizes paper instead of x-ray film to record pictures of soft body tissue.

Examples of orders for nonpreparation x-rays:

- Flat plate of abdomen in A.M.
- Chest x-ray on admission
- XR L-S spine tonight (x-ray lumbosacral spine)

Radiographs Requiring Preparation and the Use of Contrast Media

Many x-ray procedures of nonbony structures require the use of special "radiopaque" substances to increase the contrast in the film because there is so little difference in the density between some body parts and their surrounding organs or vessels. This substance is called **contrast medium** and, depending upon the x-ray procedure, is usually organic iodine or a barium preparation. Contrast medium may be swallowed, injected into a vessel, or inserted into the rectum. It has the ability to show up on the x-ray film, outline the organ, and indicate any abnormalities to the physician. (Fig. 16–15.)

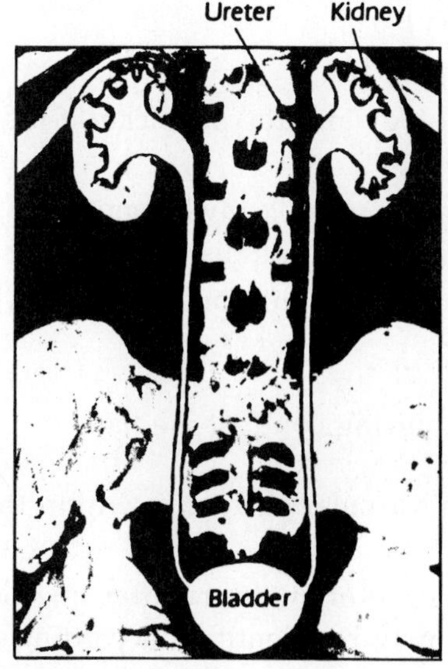

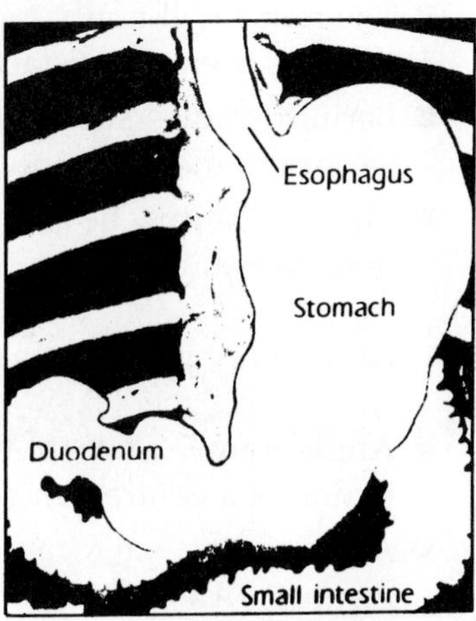

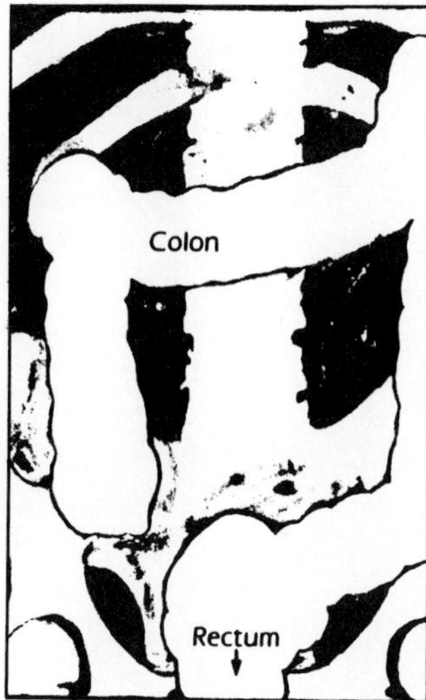

Figure 16–15

The following four radiographic studies are commonly ordered and require contrast media. The health unit coordinator must know that some of these radiographs cannot be done on the same day. Because this scheduling varies among hospitals, the proper sequence should be learned for ordering these radiographs in your hospital.

- **Intravenous pyelogram IVP**—the kidneys, ureters, and the bladder are outlined on the x-ray after an injection of radiopaque dye into the patient's veins.
- **Gallbladder series (GB Series)**—the gallbladder and its tubular connections to other body organs are outlined after radiopaque dye is taken by mouth and absorbed from the intestinal tract.
- **Gastrointestinal series (GI Series)**—the stomach and intestinal tract are outlined on the x-ray after a radiopaque substance called **barium** is swallowed by the patient.
- **Barium enema (BE)**—barium is given to the patient in enema form and the rectum and large intestine are outlined on the x-ray film.

Preparation of patients who are to receive radiographs utilizing contrast media usually begin the afternoon or evening before the procedure is to take place. Such preparations may include enemas, tablets, changes in diet, orders for NPO $\overline{p}$ midnight. Many hospitals utilize small cards or tickets on which are written the procedure to be followed in preparing the patient for each of the various special radiographic procedures. These preparation tickets are simply reminders to nursing as to what the preparation procedures will be. The tickets are placed in the patient's Kardex until the x-ray is completed.

Important Considerations

- Generally, the following studies may be ordered as outlined.
  - Gallbladder series and Upper GI
  - Gallbladder series and BE
  - Gallbladder series and IVP
  - IVP, Gallbladder series, and BE
- The nurse will notify radiology and the physician if the bowel preparation has been unsatisfactory.
- Barium studies should follow other x-rays, sonograms, or scans, since barium in the gastrointestinal tract can distort the other studies.
- The patient may be away from the unit for some time when undergoing these x-rays.

Other x-ray procedures requiring contrast media:

- **Angiogram**—x-rays of the vascular structures within the body after injection of a contrast medium.
- **Arteriogram**—an x-ray picture of an artery after injection of a contrast medium. An arteriogram may be identified according to the anatomic location (e.g., femoral arteriogram, carotid arteriogram, etc.).
- **Arthrogram**—an x-ray picture of an internal joint surface after injection of a contrast medium.

- **Bronchogram**—following the introduction of a contrast medium into the bronchi, an x-ray examination of the lungs and bronchial tree is made.
- **Cystogram**—a contrast medium is introduced into the bladder by x-ray personnel through a Foley catheter for the purpose of outlining the organ.
- **Esophagram (barium swallow)**—performed at the same time as an upper gastrointestinal x-ray study; the patient swallows the barium while the esophagus is studied by fluoroscopy and x-ray.
- **Hysterosalpingogram**—x-ray picture of the uterus and fallopian tubes made after injection of a contrast medium.
- **Lymphangiogram**—x-ray picture of the lymph channels and lymph nodes made after injection of a contrast medium.
- **Myelogram**—x-ray picture of the spinal cord after a contrast medium has been injected between the vertebrae into the spinal canal.
- **Pneumoencephalogram**—x-ray picture of the ventricles of the brain taken after injection of air into the spinal canal.
- **Sialogram**—an x-ray picture of the salivary ducts made after injection of a contrast medium.
- **T-tube cholangiogram**—a contrast medium is injected by x-ray personnel into a surgically placed T-tube, and the bile ducts are x-rayed.
- **Venogram**—x-ray picture of the veins made after injection of a contrast medium.
- **Ventriculogram**—x-ray picture of the cerebral ventricles taken after injection of a contrast medium.
- **Fluoroscopy**—a procedure which is used to observe the form and motion of internal structures of the body and to detect the presence of foreign bodies. The image, instead of being recorded on a film, is focused on a radiosensitive plate and can be studied "in action" by the doctor. A radiopaque medium is often used to outline the body parts. During the procedure radiographs can also be taken for further study and as a permanent record.
- **Computerized tomography or CT Scan**—A CT scan is a special kind of x-ray that produces three-dimensional pictures of a cross section of a part of the body. Developed in 1972, CT scans are able to detect some conditions that conventional x-rays cannot and are used for many diagnostic procedures, including head scans, which are used to detect tumors, blood clots, enlarged ventricles or openings in the brain, and other abnormalities of the brain structure and nerves or muscles of the eye. Body scans are used for many reasons and are especially important in diagnosing pancreatic disease, enlarged lymph nodes, back problems, and various types of cancer. (Fig. 16–16.)

  Patients may be NPO for 4–8 hours before the test if contrast medium is to be used. The test may be done with or without contrast medium and may be given orally or by injection immediately or after the first set of scans.

  The patient is placed in the scanner gantry (chamber) and the table will move. As the equipment scans, the patient hears a whirring sound of the motor.

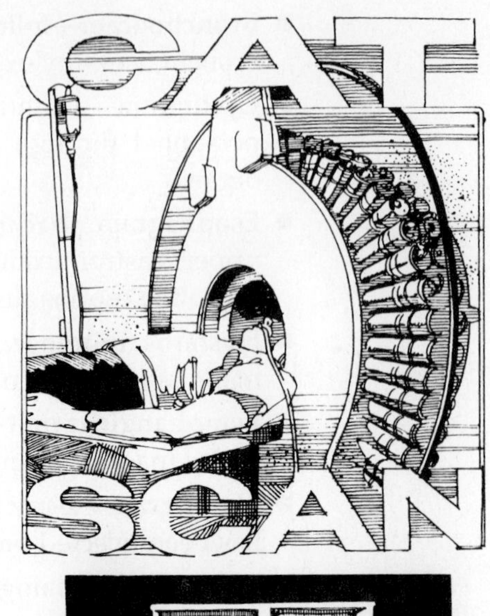

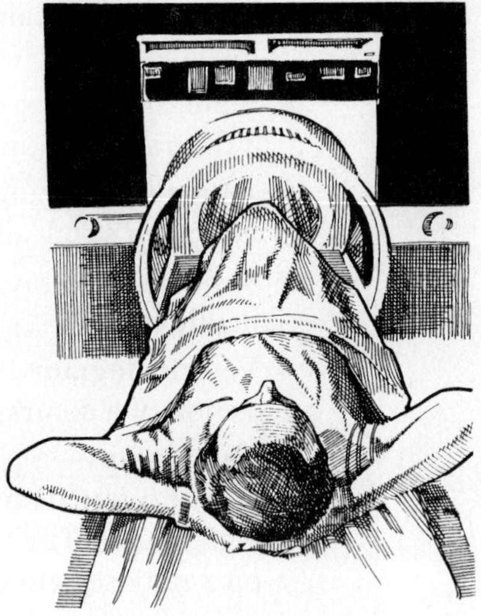

Figure 16–16

CT scans should always be done before barium studies. Because contrast medium may be given, a check will be made for allergies to seafood or iodine.

Ultrasound (Sonography). Ultrasound is not an x-ray. It is a procedure that uses sound waves at very high frequencies to produce images of internal body structures and organs. It can also image internal movements such as the heart beating or blood flowing through the veins as it measures and records the reflection of these pulsed or continuous high-frequency sound waves.

It is considered safe and painless because it doesn't involve the use of x-rays and has reduced the need for invasive procedures such as surgery and cardiac catheterization.

A transducer (transmitter and receiver), which is often hand held, is placed against the body and slowly moved over the area to be examined. As the sound waves pass through the skin into the body, they strike various organs and send echoes back to the transducer. The echoes differ based on the structures they strike and are separated and identified by the transducer.

The transducer then changes the sound waves into electrical energy and an image is formed on a TV screen which represents a cross section of the organ being studied. Films of the images are taken and the results are sent to the physician.

- Ultrasound is used widely in medicine and is particularly valuable for diagnosis during pregnancy.
- An ultrasound **Doppler** is useful in detecting diminished blood flow through the heart and arteries. Through a shift in the frequency of the sound waves the actual sound of the blood detects faulty valves and artery blockage.
- Patients having gallbladder scans are placed on a fat-free diet the day before and they are NPO after midnight before the procedure.
- Pelvic scans require a full bladder, and patients will have to drink several glasses of water and not void before the study.
- Barium studies should be done after ultrasonography.

Imaging

Magnetic Resonance Imaging (MRI) uses a huge electromagnet, a radiofrequency generator, and a computer to focus on hydrogen atoms in the body. When these atoms are subjected to a magnetic field, they arrange themselves in a line. When a radio frequency is aimed at the atoms, it changes the alignment of their nuclei, and when the radio frequency is turned off, the nuclei of the hydrogen atoms realign themselves and send out a small electrical signal. An image is formed from the returning signals or pulses showing a clearer image than ever seen by conventional x-ray or the CT scan. Patients will be questioned about the presence of metal plates, pins, etc., in the body; they will be asked if they have a metal splinter embedded in their eye; or they will be asked if they work with metal. Patients with pacemakers are excluded from this procedure.

Positron Emission Tomography (PET) is a procedure which uses radioactive substances, either inhaled or injected, that through combination of positively and negatively charged particles emit gamma rays. The PET detects the gamma rays and converts them into color-coded images that measure metabolism and how well the body is working. The PET technique studies blood flow and metabolism of the heart as well as various kinds of cancer and the biochemical activity of the brain.

Photon Emission Computed Tomography (SPECT) shows the blood flow by imaging trace amounts of radioisotopes.

Patient Positioning

The doctor often orders that the patient be placed in certain positions during x-ray to obtain the best view of the area being x-rayed.

When writing the x-ray order on the requisition, the health unit coordinator must be sure to transcribe the order exactly as written by the doctor. The doctor will always include R or L when a limb is to be x-rayed to indicate right or left.

Following is a list of positions for x-rays ordered most often:

- **AP view** (anterior-posterior)—the x-ray passes through the front and out the back of the body or body part
- **PA view** (posterior-anterior)—the x-ray passes through the back and out the front
- **Lateral view**—taken from the side
- **Oblique view**—the patient or limb is halfway on the side.

Portable x-rays. When a patient is unable to go to the Radiology Department, a portable x-ray is ordered. A mobile x-ray machine is taken to the patient's bedside. This is often not the procedure of choice because of the limitations in good patient positioning. The word portable must always be included when ordering.

KEY IDEA: NUCLEAR MEDICINE

This department uses radioactive materials called **radionuclides** that are injected into a vein or are ingested by the patient. These radioactive materials give off radiation in the form of gamma rays from the specific organ to be studied. These tests are often called **radioisotopic procedures.**

An instrument called a gamma scintillation camera images the concentration of the radioactive material and produces a picture called a **scan.**

Scans may be ordered of many body organs including the bones, brain, heart, kidneys, liver, lungs, pancreas, and spleen. They may be done to evaluate the performance of an organ such as a thyroid uptake and scan to help determine the presence of cancer.

The health unit coordinator should know that the patient will remain in Nuclear Medicine for at least an hour when a scan is ordered. (Fig. 16–17.)

KEY IDEA: RADIATION THERAPY

This division of radiology is highly specialized and utilizes radiotherapy to bombard malignant growths (cancer) with doses of radiation. The radiation is given in doses calculated to destroy malignant tissues without harming normal cells.

Usually a requisition form is utilized for the initial order, and the Radiation Therapy Department will arrange the subsequent visits and notify the nursing unit of that schedule. (Fig. 16–18.)

NUCLEAR MEDICINE REQUEST

NUCLEAR MEDICINE REQUEST

CLINICAL PROBLEM:

SPECIAL INSTRUCTIONS:

ROOM NO:

DATE & TIME TO BE PERFORMED:

REQUESTING PHYSICIAN:

TRANS: ☐ W/C ☐ STRETCHER ☐ PORTABLE ☐ OTHER

EXAM REQUESTED:

DO NOT WRITE BELOW THIS LINE

☐ ISOT THER HYPTHYR	☐ V–P LUNG SCAN
☐ THYROID UPTAKE	☐ RENOGRAM
☐ THYROID UPTAKE & SCAN	☐ RB–LIVER–FUNCTION
☐ B12–ABSORBT–TEST	☐ CISTERNOGRAM–STRT
☐ BONE SCAN	☐ CIST–FOLLOW UP
☐ BRAIN SCAN	☐ RENAL–SCAN
☐ LIVER SCAN	☐

DO NOT WRITE BELOW THIS LINE

DESCRIPTION	CODE	PRICE OVERRIDE
	416	
	416	
☐ NUCL—MED—MISC	416 7 8 9 9 6	

NEUCLEAR MEDICINE
NURSING COPY

Figure 16–17

RADIATION ONCOLOGY CHARGE SLIP

		HEYMAN FIELD PREP 4 APPLIC. ONLY	FOLLOW UP COMPREHENSIVE	
		HEYMAN MATERIAL PREP & MONITORING	HOSPITAL CARE BRIEF HISTORY	BRACHY. INTERSTIT PHYSICS
		RADIOACTIVE MAT. APPLICATORS, ETC.	HOSPITAL CARE INTERMED. HISTORY	BEAM BLOCKS
		INTERSTITIAL SIMPLE	HOSPITAL CARE COMP. HISTORY	COMPENSATOR
		INTERSTITIAL COMPLEX	HOSPITAL VISIT BRIEF	CONTOUR DEVICE
LOW VOLTAGE RT < 4 FIELDS	LA COMPLEX		HOSPITAL VISIT LIMITED	POSITION HOLDER
LOW VOLTAGE RT > 4 FIELDS	UNLISTED R.T.	OFFICE VISIT LIMITED	HOSPITAL VISIT INTERMEDIATE	CONT. RAD PHYSICS
BENIGN LESIONS	INTRACAVITARY SIMPLE	OFFICE VISIT INTERMEDIATE	HOSPITAL VISIT EXTENDED	TUMOR LOCAL SIMPLE
CO–60 SIMPLE	INTRACAVITARY COMPLEX	OFFICE VISIT COMPREHENSIVE		TUMOR LOCAL COMPLEX
L.A. SIMPLE	FIELD PREP AND APPLIC ONLY	FOLLOW UP LIMITED	DOSIMETRY SIMPLE	FILMS & TATOOS
LOW VOLTAGE RT COMPLEX	MATERIAL PREP AND MONITORING	FOLLOW UP INTERMEDIATE	DOSIMETRY COMPLEX	
CO–60 COMPLEX	HEYMAN PACKING	FOLLOW UP EXTENDED	BRACHY, INTRACAV PHYSICS	
		MISC.	CODE 415	PRICE OVERRIDE

DEPARTMENT COPY

Figure 16–18

Execution of Forms

The numbers and types of forms to be used in ordering procedures from Radiology will vary depending on the extent of use of computers, the size of the hospital, and the complexity of the radiological facilities. All hospitals do not provide all the services mentioned in this chapter; some will provide more. Your instructor will tell you about the services and method of ordering in your hospital or the hospitals in your community.

Health Unit Coordinator Responsibilities

- Order by computer or complete the proper requisition. If the addressograph plate does not include the patient's room number, be sure it is always written in. This is true of all requisitions. Radiology requires it so they will know where to go to pick up the patient.
- Many hospitals require that the health unit coordinator also telephones radiology with the order so that the x-ray may be scheduled in the appointment book in that department.
- Prepare the appropriate consent form as required by your facility.
- Most radiology requisitions have a space for the health unit coordinator to record the *clinical problem.* This is not always the same as the diagnosis and indicates the *reason* for the x-ray. For instance, a patient with a diagnosis of diabetes with an order for an IVP (intravenous pyelogram) may have a clinical problem such as urinary infection. If the doctor does not indicate the reason for the x-ray or the patient's clinical problem, you will often have to consult the nurse for this information. The routine chart form, called the progress notes, will often aid the nurse in making this decision. You would also communicate this information by computer.
- Communication to the nursing staff concerning patient preparation and communication to the Dietary Department regarding diet changes are prime responsibilities. Errors in any phase of patient preparation may affect the outcome of the x-ray and may result in additional costs and discomfort to the patient.

- On the day of the x-ray, the health unit coordinator must be aware of the time the patient leaves and when he returns so that postexamination procedures may be instituted or the regular regimen resumed.

CARDIOLOGY

The cardiology or cardiovascular department is responsible for many important tests and procedures within the hospital. Most hospitals also provide cardiac rehabilitation on an outpatient basis. Some of the important tests are:

- **Electrocardiogram (ECG)**—A mechanical tracing of the heart's action made by a special machine called an "electrocardiograph." The ECG is an important aid in the diagnosis and treatment of patients with heart disease. Electrocardiograms are usually taken at the patient's bedside with a portable unit. The routine 12-lead ECG examines the heart through 12 perspectives—a rhythm strip is 1 lead. (Figs. 16–19, 16–20, and 16–21.)
- **Echocardiogram**—A picture produced by sending sound waves through the body. A routine echocardiogram includes an *Echo M-Mode* which traces the activity and functioning of each chamber of the pericardium. *Echo-2-D* refers to a two-dimensional study and is performed with deeper ultrasound to show the valves and interior of the heart for diagnosis of abnormalities.
- **Phonocardiogram**—A study that shows a graphic representation of a patient's heart sounds and heart murmurs.
- **Treadmill stress test**—Records the patient's heart activity while the patient's blood pressure is monitored. The electrodes attached to his chest carry the electrical activity from the heart to a monitor in the form of a heart tracing. The angle of the slant on the treadmill walker and the rate of the walk is increased to the patient's tolerance. Certain changes in the tracing on the monitor are danger signals and the test will be discontinued. The treadmill stress test helps the physician determine the patient's tolerance to activity and aids in planning an appropriate exercise regimen. (Fig. 16–22.)
- **Holter monitor**—This is a small device that is worn by the patient on the nursing unit and provides a continuous ECG recording for a prescribed amount of time (often 12 to 24 hours) while the patient goes about his usual activities. Usually three leads (small buttons) are attached to the chest and wires are connected to the pack worn by the patient via a shoulder strap. A diary is kept by the patient during the time the Holter monitor is worn so that the physician may correlate abnormalities in the tracing with the activity of the patient at that time.
- **Cardiac monitors**—Continuous ECG tracings shown on an instrument called an oscilloscope or screen. In the critical or subintensive care units oscilloscopes are located at the nurses' station and in ICU and CCU at the patient's bedside as well. An ECG tracing on paper can be printed at will or will be printed automatically when abnormalities occur.

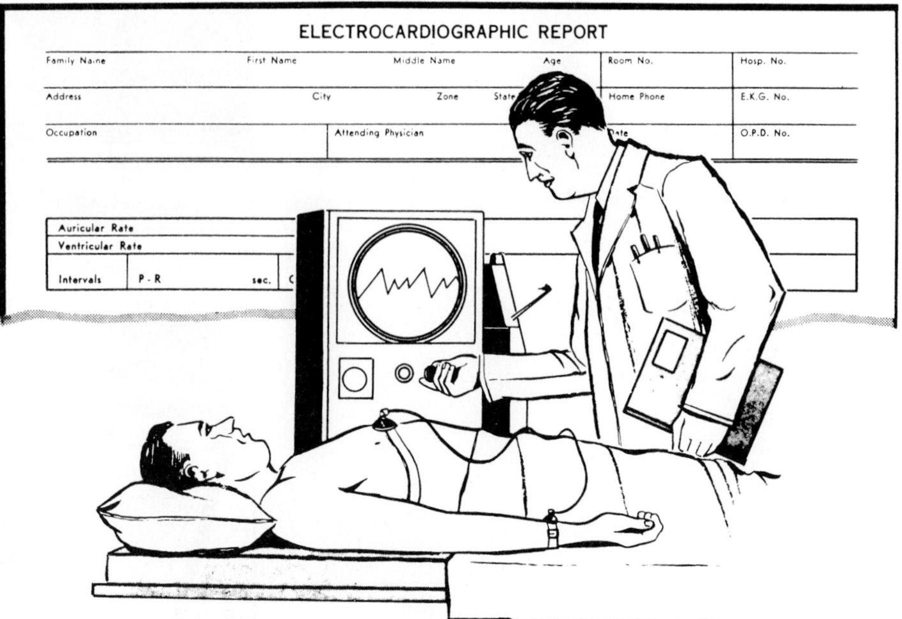

Figure 16–19

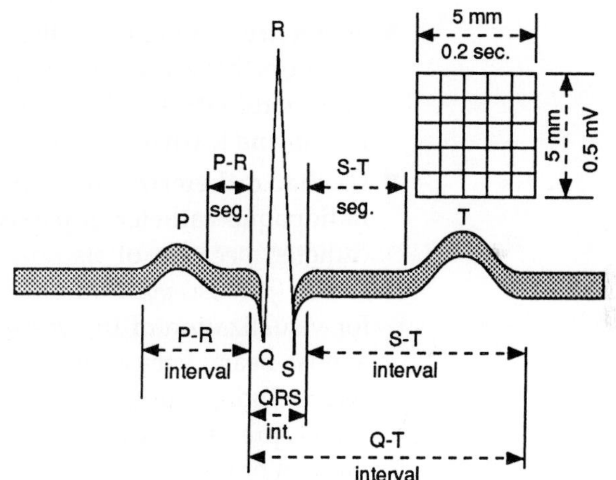

Figure 16–20

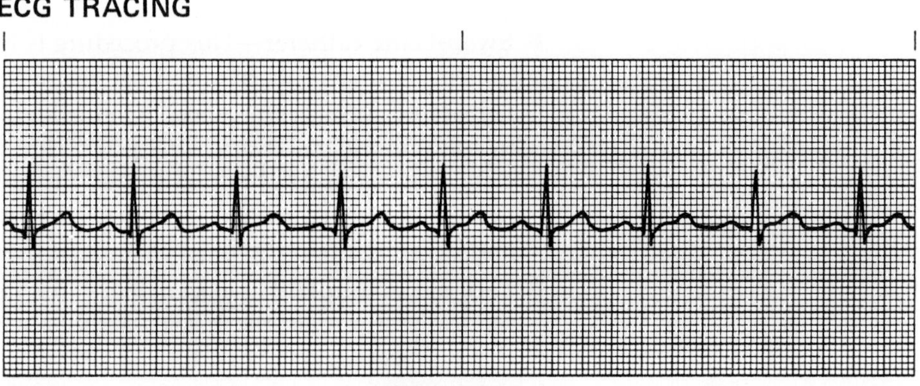

Figure 16–21

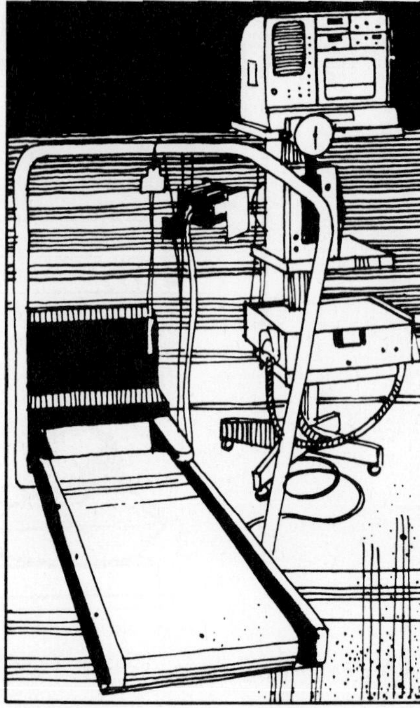

Figure 16–22

- **Telemetry**—Patients on the nursing unit may be connected to cardiac monitors that are viewed via oscilloscopes in the ICU/CCU units. Health unit coordinators in the units often receive special training in cardiac monitoring and learn to recognize common abnormalities in the ECG tracings.
- **Cardiac catheterization**—An invasive diagnostic procedure in which a radiopaque catheter is passed through a vein and into the heart. The catheter, because of its special coating, can be followed on a special screen *(flouroscopy)*. Samples of blood are taken and dye may be injected for visualization of the vessels. Cardiac catheterizations are done to diagnose heart diseases or defects. This is a serious procedure and orders will include a surgical consent, careful monitoring of the vital signs, IV fluids, pressure devices to the area if an artery was entered, and permission or restriction orders regarding diet and activity. This test is done in a cardiac catheterization lab or in radiology. (Fig. 16–23.)

Although not "done" by the cardiology department, the following procedures affect the heart:

- **Swan-Ganz catheter**—This procedure is highly specialized and is mentioned because of its frequent use in the critical care units. The catheter is inserted into a vein called the subclavian vein and through the heart to the pulmonary artery. This procedure is always done by the physician. The readings obtained by the Swan-Ganz help to show the function of the heart, measure the pressure within the circulatory system, and help maintain the fluid balance of the critically ill patient.
- **Pacemaker implants**—Pacemakers are mechanical devices that automatically stimulate the heart's activity when the heart is unable to do this on its own. (Fig. 16–24.)
- **Temporary pacemakers**—Connected by wires that lead from the patient's body to a control apparatus.

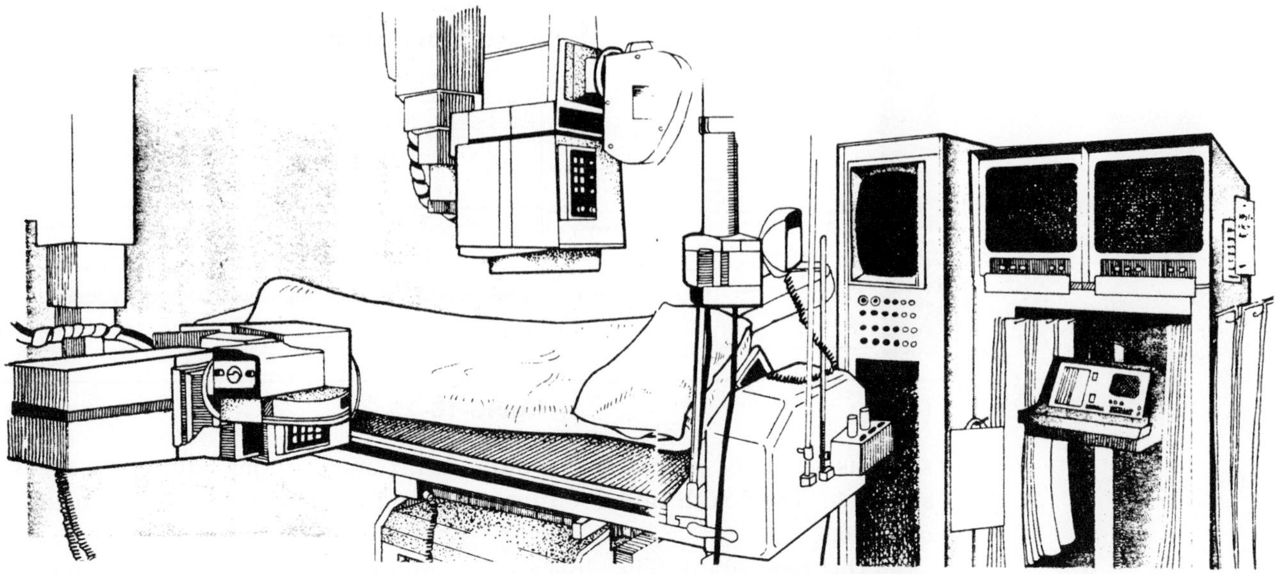

Figure 16–23

- **Permanent pacemakers**—Implanted under the muscle of the chest surgically. A catheter leads to the heart and stimulates heart activity.

By far the most common test the health unit coordinator will order through cardiology is the ECG. The ECG is ordered at least once on the majority of adult hospitalized patients.

Health Unit Coordinator Responsibilities

Cardiology requisitions usually ask for the clinical impression or reason for the ECG. Again, this may not be the admitting diagnosis, and the health unit coordinator must consult the nurse for this information.

Certain medications may affect the cardiologist's interpretation of the tracing. Many requisitions question medications the patient is receiving

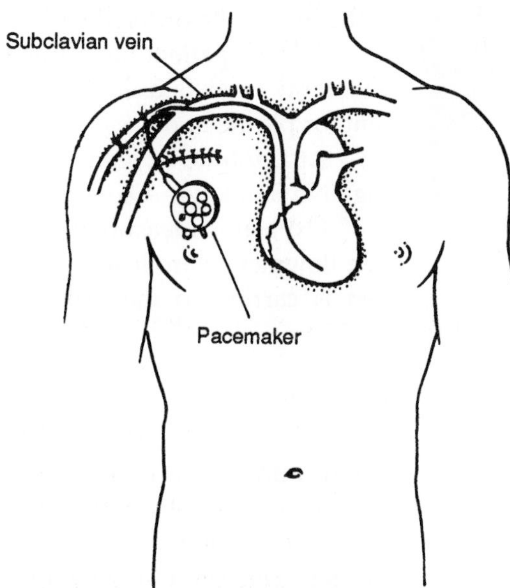

Figure 16–24

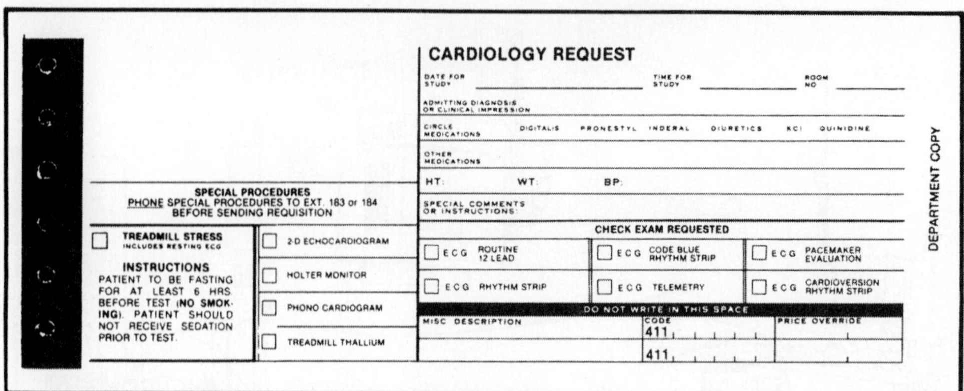

CARDIOLOGY REQUEST

DATE FOR STUDY ______ TIME FOR STUDY ______ ROOM NO ______

ADMITTING DIAGNOSIS OR CLINICAL IMPRESSION

CIRCLE MEDICATIONS DIGITALIS PRONESTYL INDERAL DIURETICS KCl QUINIDINE

OTHER MEDICATIONS

HT: WT: BP:

SPECIAL COMMENTS OR INSTRUCTIONS:

SPECIAL PROCEDURES
PHONE SPECIAL PROCEDURES TO EXT. 183 or 184 BEFORE SENDING REQUISITION

☐ TREADMILL STRESS INCLUDES RESTING ECG

INSTRUCTIONS
PATIENT TO BE FASTING FOR AT LEAST 6 HRS. BEFORE TEST (NO SMOKING). PATIENT SHOULD NOT RECEIVE SEDATION PRIOR TO TEST.

☐ 2-D ECHOCARDIOGRAM
☐ HOLTER MONITOR
☐ PHONO CARDIOGRAM
☐ TREADMILL THALLIUM

CHECK EXAM REQUESTED

☐ ECG ROUTINE 12 LEAD	☐ ECG CODE BLUE RHYTHM STRIP	☐ ECG PACEMAKER EVALUATION
☐ ECG RHYTHM STRIP	☐ ECG TELEMETRY	☐ ECG CARDIOVERSION RHYTHM STRIP

DO NOT WRITE IN THIS SPACE

MISC DESCRIPTION	CODE	PRICE OVERRIDE
	411	
	411	

DEPARTMENT COPY

Figure 16–25

such as digitalis preparations, other heart medications, diuretics, potassium, etc. The health unit coordinator should consult the nurse about these questions.

The requisition (Fig. 16–25) or computer may ask for the patient's height, weight, and blood pressure. The height and weight are taken on admission and in some cases, the weight is measured more frequently. The blood pressure is measured at regular intervals. The health unit coordinator will learn where to find this information.

RESPIRATORY THERAPY OR INHALATION THERAPY

KEY IDEA: ADMINISTERING OXYGEN

Oxygen and other gases are used in inhalation therapy as a treatment for pulmonary (lung) difficulties. Oxygen is essential to life. When given by artificial means it can be harmful if used incorrectly, and so it must be given as prescribed by the doctor. To monitor its effectiveness, special tests called arterial blood gases (ABGs) are often done. An oximeter measures the degree of oxygen saturation in the blood. Oxygen is most commonly administered to an adult by face mask or by nasal prongs. (Fig. 16–26.) Very occasionally a nasal catheter may be ordered.

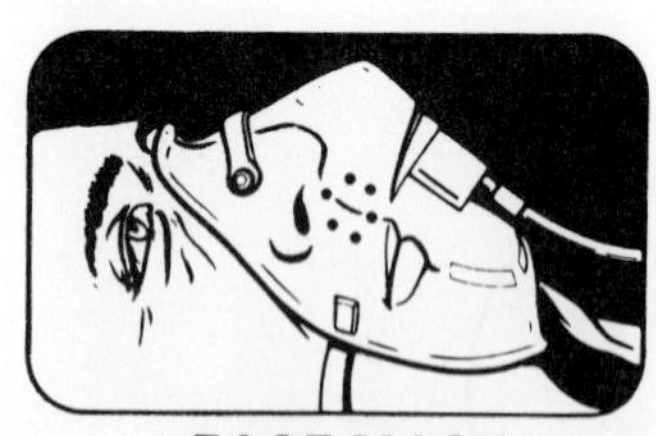

FACE MASK

Figure 16–26

When a patient has a tracheotomy a "T-tube" or surgically designed tracheotomy mask is used. Oxygen may be administered to children by isolette, tent, or plastic hood.

At any time oxygen is being used, a card will be hung on the door stating "No Smoking—Oxygen in use." (Fig. 16–27.)

Oxygen is measured in liters per minute (L/M) or by percentage. Oxygen flowmeters are inserted into wall outlets in the patient's room, and oxygen is carried to the flowmeter through a central delivery system. (Fig. 16–28.)

Nasal Cannulas

Nasal cannulas, or tubes, are used to give oxygen to a patient. The cannulas are inserted into the patient's nostrils. They are used when the patient needs extra oxygen, not when equipment must provide a patient's total supply of oxygen. The cannula, which is made of plastic, is a half-circle length of tub-

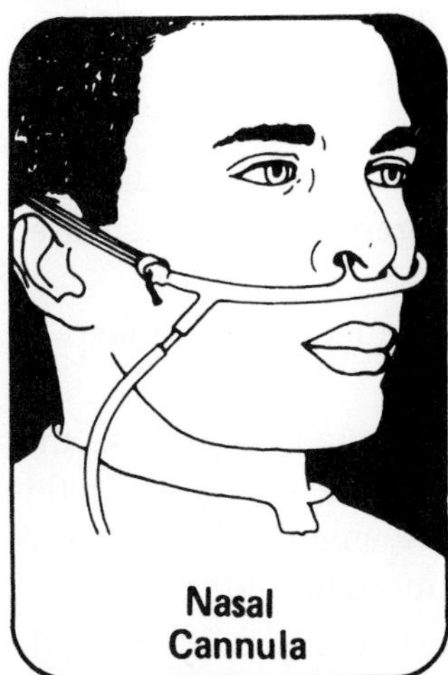

Figure 16–29

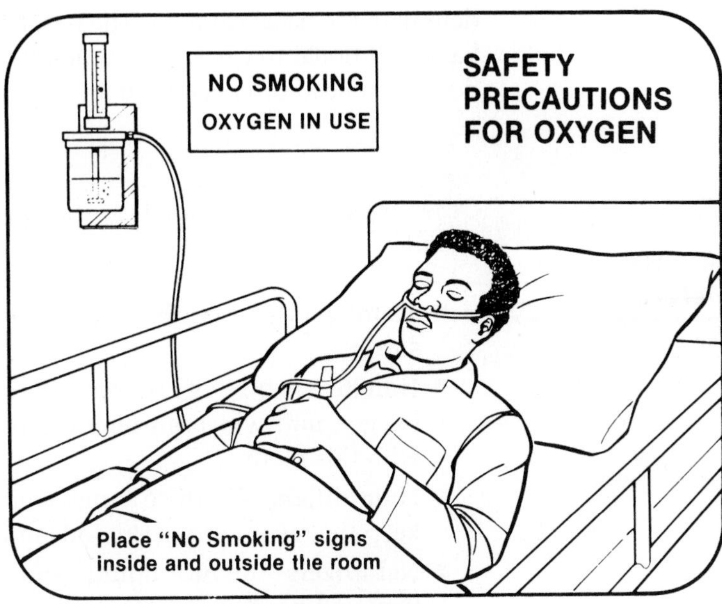
NO SMOKING
OXYGEN IN USE
SAFETY
PRECAUTIONS
FOR OXYGEN
Place "No Smoking" signs
inside and outside the room

Figure 16–27

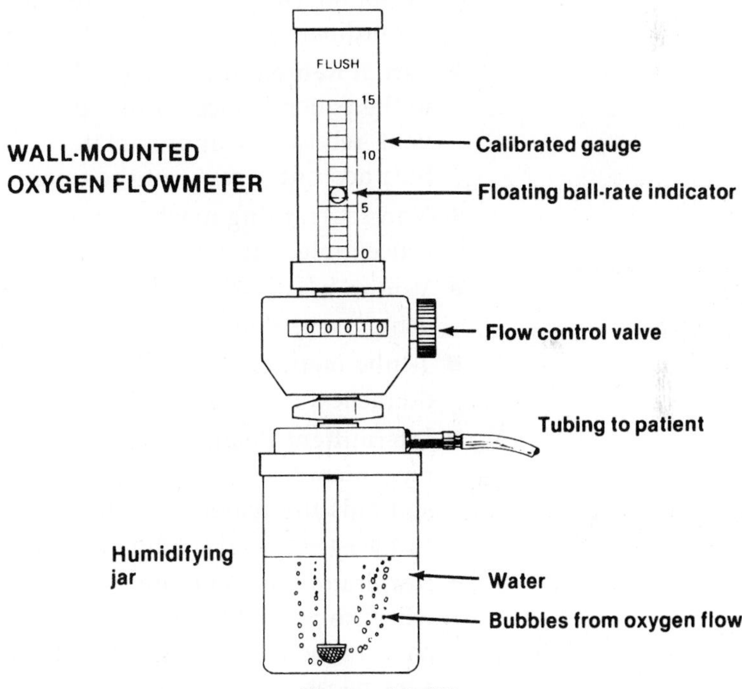

Figure 16–28

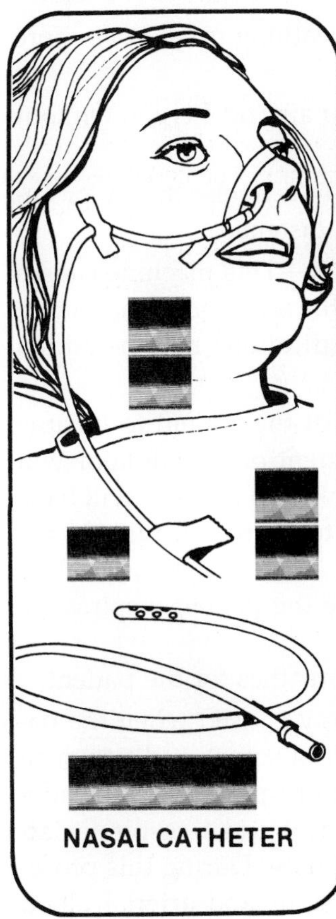

Figure 16–30

ing with two openings in the center. It fits about one-half inch into the patient's nostrils. Nasal cannulas are held in place by an elastic band around the patient's head and are connected to the source of oxygen by a length of plastic tubing. (Fig. 16–29.)

Nasal Catheter

The catheter (Fig. 16–30) is a piece of tubing that is longer than a cannula. It is inserted through the patient's nostril into the back of his mouth. The nasal catheter is a more effective but less comfortable way to give oxygen to the patient than the nasal cannula. The nasal catheter is used when the patient must have additional oxygen at all times. The nasal catheter is fastened to the patient's forehead or cheek with a piece of adhesive tape that holds it steady.

KEY IDEA: RESPIRATORY EQUIPMENT

Other equipment provided by the Respiratory Therapy Department may include:

- **Vaporizers**—Humidifying devices with a heating element to produce steam.
- **Isolette**—A type of crib that has controlled temperature, humidity, and oxygen into which an infant is placed. An **oxygen hood** is often used with this method.
- **Humidifiers**—Produce a mist which fills the patient's room and helps to keep the respiratory secretions moist.
- **Nebulizers**—Reduce liquids and medications to small droplets so that they will go deep into the respiratory tract. *Ultrasonic nebulizers* do this by sound vibrations. The droplets produced are smaller than those of the ordinary nebulizer and, therefore, provide more humidity.
- **Partial Rebreathing mask**—A mask with a reservoir bag is fitted tightly to the patient's face. With a prescribed flow of oxygen running, the patient rebreathes approximately 33% of the air which is expired or breathed out because of the reservoir bag.
- **Non-rebreathing mask**—Similar to partial rebreathing mask but a more concentrated supply of oxygen is delivered.
- **Venturi mask**—Maintains a constant mixture of air and oxygen without using a reservoir bag.
- **T-tube method**—This special tube is attached to a tracheostomy or endotracheal tube. The air is both warmed and moistened.
- **Intermittent Positive Pressure Breathing** (IPPB)—This machine causes the patient to breathe more deeply, helps open the small bronchial tubes, and aids the patient to cough up sputum. Medications may be added and are nebulized by the machine.
- **Respirators or Ventilators**—Machines that assist the patient to breathe when he is unable to do so on his own. A patient on a ventilator will have a tube in his trachea (intubation or endotracheal tube) or will have a tracheostomy. The respirator will be attached to the tube leading to the airway.

  Assist/control—With this setting, each time the patient inspires, he receives a machine breath.

  Control—With this setting, the respirator breathes for the patient.
- **Positive end expiratory pressure (PEEP)** therapy is used when the patient is in serious respiratory distress as a result of some condition such as shock, prematurity, surgery, trauma, etc., and respirations are inadequate. The patient is intubated (tube into trachea) and a respirator attached that cycles air through the endotracheal tube. During this procedure the patient is usually sedated and vital signs and arterial blood gases are monitored carefully.

- **Intermittent Mandatory Ventilator** (IMV)—The IMV gives the patient a set number of breaths at a set volume in addition to whatever spontaneous breaths he can generate. If the machine is set for 5 breaths a minute and 1000 cc TV (**tidal volume** or the amount of air exchanged during a normal breathing cycle), the patient will get 5 machine breaths at 1000 cc TV in addition to their own number of breaths. The order would read IMV_5 q1h.
- **Incentive Spirometer** (IS)—These devices are designed to cause the patient to breathe deeply. After surgery, they help the patient get rid of the anesthetic from the lungs. Patients are usually taught to use these bedside devices by the Respiratory Therapy Department before surgery.

KEY IDEA: OTHER FUNCTIONS OF RESPIRATORY THERAPY

- **Arterial Blood Gases** (ABGs)—ABG samples are drawn from a patient's artery by respiratory therapy and analyzed for their content of O_2 (oxygen), CO_2 (carbon dioxide), pH, PCO_2, PO_2, T_{40}, and percent of saturation.

  The doctor may order ABGs on R/A (room air) on when the patient is receiving oxygen as a treatment.

  Adjustments of the ventilator are made based on the results of the arterial blood gases.

Arterial Blood Gases

Gas	*Normal Values (at Sea Level)*
O_2 saturation	95%
PO_2	80–100 mm. Hg (mercury) partial pressure (room air)
PCO_2	38–42 mm. Hg partial pressure
HCO_3	24–28 mEq/L
pH	7.35–7.45

- **Chest physiotherapy** (CPT)—This procedure is done to loosen secretions. The respiratory therapist cups the back (produces percussion with the hands) while the patient is placed in a position with the head lower than feet. This is called **postural drainage.** Following CPT, the patient coughs and expectorates (spits out) secretions.
- **Suctioning**—Patients who are unable to cough and bring up their secretions or patients who are intubated or have tracheostomies may require tracheal suctioning. This is often done by respiratory therapy as well as by the licensed nurse. (Fig. 16–31.)
- **Pulmonary function tests**—analyze the state of the respiratory system through a variety of different measurements. These tests may be done with or without ABGs. (Fig. 16–32.)

KEY IDEA: EXECUTION OF FORMS

A patient requiring therapy from one of these departments will usually need a series of appointments. The health unit coordinator will generally be responsible for making the first appointment; later ones may be arranged by the therapist. You should be notified of all appointments so that you can keep a record of the times at which the patient will be receiving treatment.

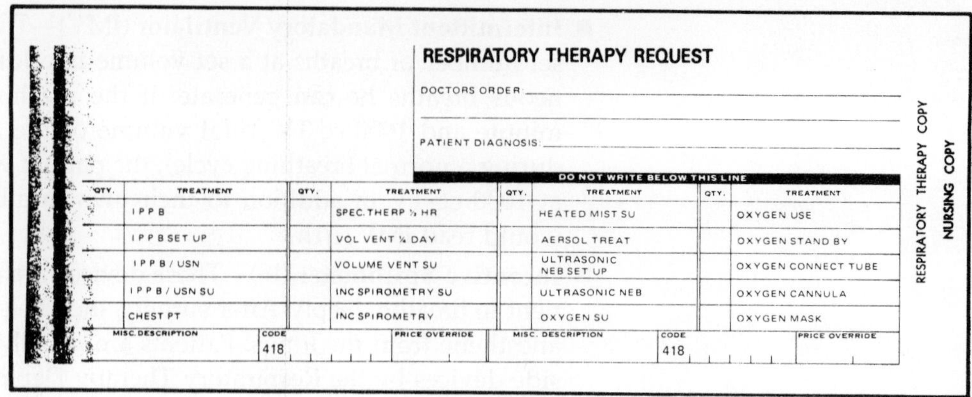

RESPIRATORY THERAPY REQUEST

DOCTORS ORDER

PATIENT DIAGNOSIS

DO NOT WRITE BELOW THIS LINE

QTY.	TREATMENT	QTY.	TREATMENT	QTY.	TREATMENT	QTY.	TREATMENT
	IPPB		SPEC.THERP ½ HR		HEATED MIST SU		OXYGEN USE
	IPPB SET UP		VOL VENT ¼ DAY		AERSOL TREAT		OXYGEN STAND BY
	IPPB / USN		VOLUME VENT SU		ULTRASONIC NEB SET UP		OXYGEN CONNECT TUBE
	IPPB / USN SU		INC SPIROMETRY SU		ULTRASONIC NEB		OXYGEN CANNULA
	CHEST PT		INC SPIROMETRY		OXYGEN SU		OXYGEN MASK

MISC DESCRIPTION	CODE	PRICE OVERRIDE	MISC. DESCRIPTION	CODE	PRICE OVERRIDE
	418			418	

RESPIRATORY THERAPY COPY
NURSING COPY

Figure 16–31

PULMONARY FUNCTION LAB REQUEST

PULMONARY FUNCTION LAB REQUEST

ROOM: ______ DATE: ______

R.N.: ______ ☐ PHONE REPORT

☐ COMPLETE PULMONARY FUNCTION TEST $\bar{c}$ A B G
☐ COMPLETE PULMONARY FUNCTION TEST w/o A B G
☐ FLOW VOLUME LOOP
☐ MEDICAL SCREEN (LOOP – SPIRO – PLETHYSMOGRAPHY)
☐ SPIRO B/A BRONK
☐ SPIRO SIMPLE
☐ PREOPERATIVE PULMONARY EVALUATION (SPIRO & A B G)
☐ ARTERIAL BLOOD GAS

ROOM AIR: ______ OXYGEN ______ LITERS

VENTILATOR: ______

SKIN TEST	
☐ BATTERY	☐ HISTOPLASMOSIS
☐ P P D	☐ CONTROL
☐ COCCIDOMYCOSIS	☐

DO NOT WRITE IN THIS BLOCK

		PRICE OVERRIDE
☐ O_2 ACID BASE MON	408 6 1 0 0 7	
☐	408	
☐ MISC.	408	

PULMONARY FUNCTION LAB
NURSING

Figure 16–32

When it is necessary that special equipment be brought from one of these departments to a patient's room, you may be expected to requisition it. When the patient no longer needs the equipment, you would call the department from which it came so that it can be returned.

Typical orders for inhalation therapy are shown below.

> ***Oxygen by nasal cannula at 6/L min.***
> ***Nasal O_2 at 8 liters/min. p.r.n.***
> ***IPPB with aerosol detergent 10 cc. q.i.d.***

PHYSICAL THERAPY

Orders for physical therapy treatments may be very general in nature if nursing personnel are to carry them out; they may be more specific and precise if qualified physical therapists are on hand or if special facilities are available. Examples of physical therapy orders under any of these circumstances are shown on the following page.

> ***Teach crutch-walking.***
> ***Measure for crutches and begin 2-point gait.***
> ***Whirlpool b.i.d.***
> ***Complete passive ROM (range of motion) exercises t.i.d.***
> ***Start patient on walker in A.M.***
> ***Begin ADL (aid to daily living) instruction.***

When an order is received for physical therapy, the health unit coordinator orders by computer or fills out the appropriate requisition and may telephone the department. Because the patient may require a series of treatments. Physical Therapy will then arrange the schedule of appointments based on the frequency of the treatment ordered by the doctor. (Figs. 16–33 and 16–34.)

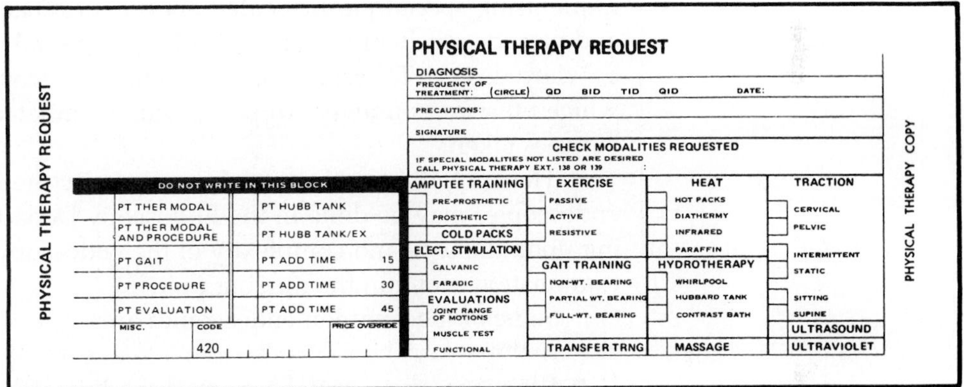

PHYSICAL THERAPY REQUEST

PHYSICAL THERAPY REQUEST

DIAGNOSIS

FREQUENCY OF TREATMENT: (CIRCLE) QD BID TID QID DATE:

PRECAUTIONS:

SIGNATURE

CHECK MODALITIES REQUESTED

IF SPECIAL MODALITIES NOT LISTED ARE DESIRED CALL PHYSICAL THERAPY EXT. 138 OR 139 :

DO NOT WRITE IN THIS BLOCK

PT THER MODAL		PT HUBB TANK	
PT THER MODAL AND PROCEDURE		PT HUBB TANK/EX	
PT GAIT		PT ADD TIME	15
PT PROCEDURE		PT ADD TIME	30
PT EVALUATION		PT ADD TIME	45
MISC.	CODE 420		PRICE OVERRIDE

AMPUTEE TRAINING	EXERCISE	HEAT	TRACTION
PRE-PROSTHETIC	PASSIVE	HOT PACKS	CERVICAL
PROSTHETIC	ACTIVE	DIATHERMY	PELVIC
COLD PACKS	RESISTIVE	INFRARED	
ELECT. STIMULATION		PARAFFIN	INTERMITTENT
GALVANIC	GAIT TRAINING	HYDROTHERAPY	STATIC
FARADIC	NON-WT. BEARING	WHIRLPOOL	
EVALUATIONS	PARTIAL WT. BEARING	HUBBARD TANK	SITTING
JOINT RANGE OF MOTIONS	FULL-WT. BEARING	CONTRAST BATH	SUPINE
MUSCLE TEST			ULTRASOUND
FUNCTIONAL	TRANSFER TRNG	MASSAGE	ULTRAVIOLET

PHYSICAL THERAPY COPY

Figure 16–33

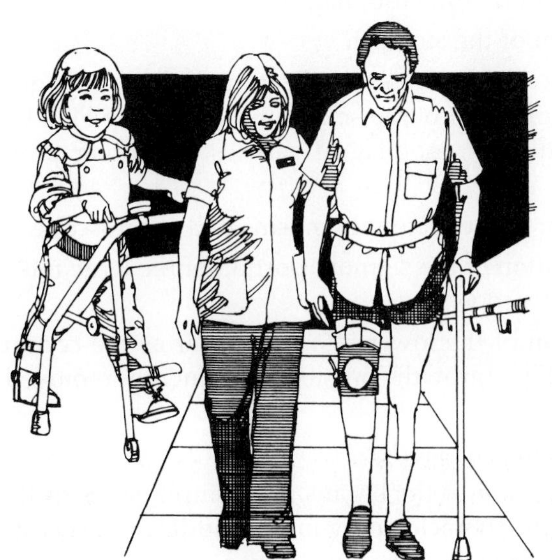

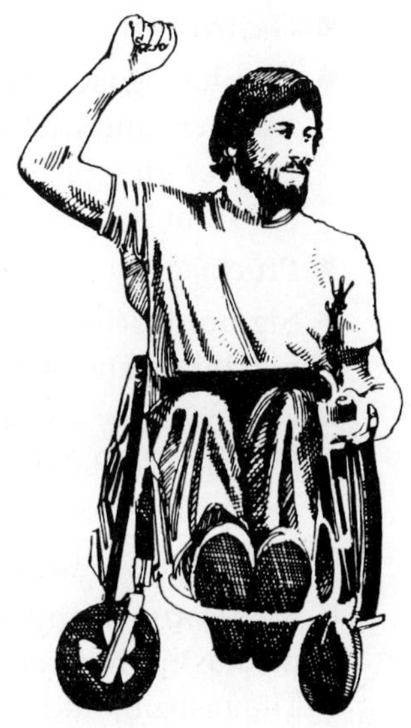

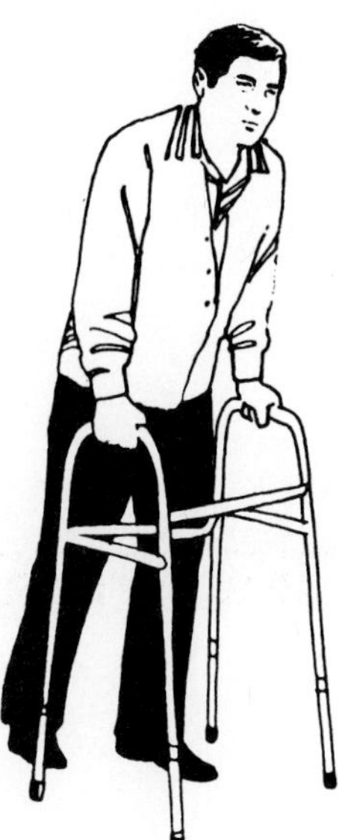

Figure 16–34

Occupational Therapy

Occupational therapy consists of directed activities, such as games and work projects. These activities aid in the treatment and rehabilitation of patients confined to the hospital. The program is adapted to suit the particular needs of each patient to provide him with the sort of diversion and skills that will best contribute to his physical and emotional progress. In this department, partially disabled patients learn to develop and explore new vocational possibilities. In many instances, the activities of the occupational therapy department are coordinated with those of the physical therapy department, so that each patient may develop his skills both at work and in recreation.

ENDOSCOPIES

An endoscopy is an examination of the body with the use of an instrument having a light source. Flexible fiberoptic endoscopy (FFE) describes a technique using special plastic-coated endoscopes that are easy to move around and provide excellent visualization. They can send magnified images that can be viewed on a TV screen or a camera. The scopes contain openings into which other instruments can be passed, air inflated, suction employed, and biopsies taken.

These are diagnostic procedures done by the doctor. In larger hospitals endoscopies may be done in the Endoscopy Department. In others (depending upon the type and complexity of the endoscopy) they may be done in an examination room on the nursing unit.

Some of the common endoscopies are:

- **Bronchoscopy**—visualization of the bronchi. FFE makes it possible to more completely view the bronchial tree than does the rigid bronchoscope.
- **Esophagoscopy**—visualization of the esophagus.
- **Gastroscopy**—visualization of the stomach.
- **Esophagogastroduodenoscopy (EGD)**—visualization of the esophagus, stomach, and duodenum (first part of the small intestine) using FFE. Ulcers, origins of bleeding, tumors, esophageal varicies, and other problems can be seen.
- **Proctoscopy**—visualization of the rectum by means of a proctoscope.
- **Sigmoidoscopy**—visualization of the sigmoid portion of the large intestine by means of a sigmoidoscope.
- **Colonoscopy**—visualization of the lower intestine as far as the cecum. Biopsies are taken and polyps (growths on stems) frequently removed. FFE is used for this procedure.
- **Cystoscopy**—visualization of the bladder.
- **Mediastinoscopy**—visualization of the organs and lymph nodes in the mediastinum (a portion of the thoracic cavity in the middle of the chest). The instrument is inserted through a small incision.

- **Laparaoscopy/Peritonoscopy**—visualization of the inside of the abdomen or peritoneum through a small incision in the abdomen.
- **Endoscopic retrograde cannulation of the papilla of Vater (ERCP)**—visualization of the pancreatic duct and biliary tree. Fluoroscopy is used, and if stones are seen they may be withdrawn using a basket adaptor following electrocauterization.
- **Arthroscopy**—visualization of the interior surface of a joint, most commonly the knee.

Endoscopies require a signed consent and most require some preparation prior to the procedure.

- Laxatives and enemas are ordered in preparation for examinations of the bowel.
- Because bleeding is possible, the nurse or doctor must determine if the patient is taking anticoagulants or aspirin, and prothrombin times (PT) and/or PTTs are often ordered.
- Prior to procedures in which the endoscope enters through the mouth, the patient will be NPO.
- Sedation is often given before the procedure.

When you receive an order for an endoscopy you will Kardex, requisition if necessary in your hospital, call the appropriate department, and if the procedure is to be done on the unit, check to see what equipment must be on hand. You will stamp an endoscopy consent (see pg. 368) if needed and prepare it for the nurse to obtain the patient's signature. You may communicate with the diet kitchen to "hold meals" until further notice.

Following the endoscopy, you will transcribe any postendoscopy orders written by the doctor.

The patient will be carefully monitored by the nursing staff. Possible complications include perforation and bleeding after biopsies or because of irritation of the mucosa. A patient who has undergone a procedure in which the scope has been passed through the mouth will not be allowed food or fluid until his/her gag reflex has returned (about two hours) because the throat was anesthetized.

ELECTROENCEPHALOGRAM (EEG)

Electroencephalography is the process of recording the brain-wave activity. Electrodes are attached to various places on the patient's head and a recording is made of the electrical activity within the brain. (Fig. 16–35.)

Prior to the test the patient should not have caffeine for 24 hours. The physician may withhold medications before the test. If the patient does take medication, the technician should be informed.

During the procedure, the patient remains quiet with the eyes closed. If being evaluated for seizure disorders, the patient will have been deprived of

MEMORIAL HOSPITAL

1. I, ______________________________, hereby request and authorize ______________________________, M.D. and such assistants as may participate with her/him for the following procedure (s): ______________________________
____

2. The nature and purpose of the procedure, the risks involved and the possibility of complications, possible perforation, hemorrhage, infection or drug reactions and even death, have been explained to my satisfaction by my Physician.

3. I consent to the administration of such sedatives and other medications as may be necessary or advisable by the Physician responsible for this service.

4. The hospital Pathologist is hereby authorized to use his/her discretion in disposition of any tissue or foreign body removed from my person during the above-named procedure(s).

5. I hereby authorize Memorial Hospital to undertake its appropriate hospital service and care necessary in conjunction with the procedure which I have asked my Physician and assistants to undertake in their efforts to alleviate my condition(s).

6. Permission is given to the above named hospital and the attending Physician to photograph or permit other persons to photograph during the surgical process as the Physician may deem necessary.

______________________________ ______________________________
Date **Signature of Patient**

______________________________ ______________________________
Time **(Witness)**

If patient is unable to sign or is a minor, complete the following:

(a) Patient is a minor of _____ years of age.

(b) Patient is unable to sign because ______________________________
____

I certify that I have informed the patient of the purpose, procedure, and potential risks and complications of the above mentioned endoscopic procedure(s).

____
Signature of Physician

MEMORIAL HOSPITAL

ENDOSCOPY CONSENT

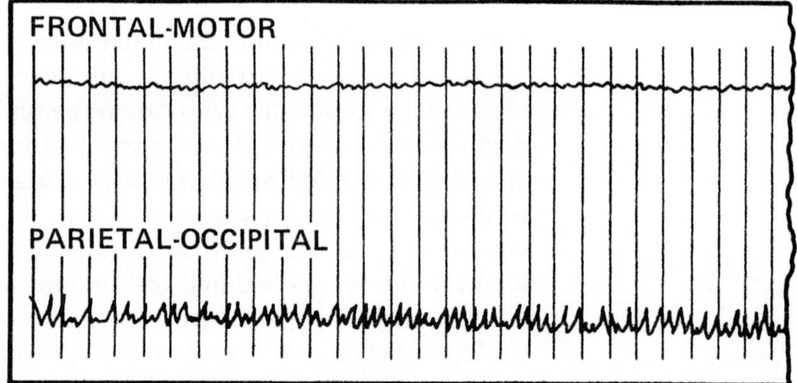

Figure 16–35

sleep, and then the EEG will be taken during sleep (which sometimes must be achieved by sedation). The procedure takes an hour or longer if the sleep study is done and does not cause pain.

The procedure is used to help diagnose seizure disorders and other brain abnormalities and is diagnostic for brain death. Your instructor will describe your hospital's method for ordering EEGs.

THE DIETARY DEPARTMENT

KEY IDEA: REGULAR AND SPECIAL DIETS

Eating properly is very important when you are healthy and feeling well. Good nourishment is even more important when a person is ill. The food service department or dietary department in your institution will be preparing a well-balanced diet of good nourishing meals for many different patients. This basic balanced diet is often called by different names:

- Normal diet
- Regular diet
- House diet
- Full diet

A well-balanced diet is one that contains a variety of foods from each of the four basic food groups at every meal.

The normal diet is sometimes changed to meet a patient's special nutritional needs. This modified diet is also known by several names:

- Special diet
- Restricted diet
- Modified diet
- Therapeutic diet

Therapeutic Diets

Therapeutic diets require the preparation of meals that differ from those regularly prepared for patients on the normal diet. (Table 16–6.) The special meals given to patients who cannot be on a normal diet are ordered by the doctor. They are worked out by the dietitian according to the patient's illness and what is needed for his recovery. These special meals help the doctor in treating a patient. For example, a man who has a disorder of his digestive system may be on a soft diet. A diabetic patient may be on a diet in which total calories are limited and the amounts of protein, fat, and carbohydrates are specified. A person with heart disease may be restricted to a low-salt (sodium) diet or a salt-free diet. The doctor may order changes in the normal diet for several reasons. These include:

- Changing the consistency of the patient's food, as in liquid or "soft" diets
- Changing the caloric intake, as in high- or low-calorie diets
- Changing the amounts of one or more nutrients, as in a high-protein, low-fat, or low-salt (sodium) diet
- Changing the amount of bulk, as in a low-residue diet
- Changing the seasonings in the patient's food, as in a bland diet
- Omitting foods to which the patient is allergic
- Changing the time and number of meals

TABLE 16–6

Types of Diets Given to Patients; What They Are and Why They Are Used

Type of Diet	*Description*	*Common Purpose*
Normal regular	Provides all essentials of good nourishment in normal forms	For patients who do not need special diets
Clear liquid (surgical/liquid)	Broth, tea, ginger ale, gelatin	Usually for patients who have had surgery or are very ill
Full liquid (medical liquid)	Broth, tea, coffee, ginger ale, gelatin, strained fruit juices, liquids, custard, junket, ice cream, sherbet, soft-cooked eggs	For those unable to chew or swallow solid food
Light or soft	Foods soft in consistency, no rich or strongly flavored foods that could cause distress	Final stage for postoperative patient before resuming regular diet
Soft (mechanical)	Same foods as on a normal diet, but chopped or strained	For patients who have difficulty in chewing or swallowing
Bland	Foods mild in flavor and easy to digest; omits spicy foods, alcohol, coffee, tea	Avoids irritation of the digestive tract, as with ulcer and colitis patients
Low residue	Foods low in bulk; omits foods difficult to digest	Spares the lower digestive tract, as with patients having rectal diseases

Whenever the word salt is used it means sodium, and when sodium is used it means salt. Therefore, when we refer to a salt-free diet we mean a sodium-free diet and when we refer to a low-sodium diet we mean a low-salt diet.

ADA or American Diabetic Association Diets

There are diets for diabetics which have been jointly agreed upon by The American Diabetes Association and The American Dietetic Association. Hospitals purchase booklets from the ADA which contain exchange lists for diabetics based on the number of calories and amounts of carbohydrates, proteins, and fats the physician prescribes.

The six exchange lists or groups are milk, vegetables, fruits, bread, meat, and fats. Foods in the same exchange list are interchangeable.

Tube Feedings

A tube feeding is the administration of nutritionally balanced liquefied foods through a tube inserted into the stomach or duodenum.

The physician will order the number of calories, the amount of fluid over 24 hours, and the frequency of the feedings. The dietitian will then prepare and blenderize the feedings, which will be sent to the nursing unit for administration.

Commercially prepared feedings may also be ordered. Ensure® is a brand name for a frequently ordered, lactose-free nutritional supplement

TABLE 16–6 (*Continued*)

Type of Diet	*Description*	*Common Purpose*
High calorie	Foods high in protein, minerals, and vitamins	For underweight or malnourished patients
Low calorie	Low in cream, butter, cereals, desserts, and fats	For patients who need to lose weight
Diabetic (see ADA)	Precise balance of carbohydrates, protein, and fats, devised according to the needs of individual patients	For diabetic patients; matches food intake with the insulin and nutritional requirements
High protein	Meals supplemented with high protein foods, such as meat, fish, cheese, milk, and eggs	Assists in the growth and repair of tissues wasted by disease
Low fat	Limited amounts of butter, cream, fats, and eggs	For patients who have difficulty digesting fats, as in gallbladder and liver disturbances
Low cholesterol	Low in eggs, whole milk, and meats	Helps regulate the amount of cholesterol in the blood
Low sodium (low salt)	Limited amount of foods containing sodium, no salt allowed on tray	For patients whose circulation would be impaired by fluid retention; patients with certain heart or kidney conditions

containing protein, carbohydrate, fat, vitamins, and minerals. Ensure Plus® is also available and has a higher caloric content.

KEY IDEA: A WELL-BALANCED DIET

The key to a healthy, well-balanced diet lies in eating a variety of foods and in not eating too much. The foods that are essential for keeping the body well are divided into four groups. Everybody needs the nutrients contained in all of the four groups. The number of servings and the size of portions will depend on the age, size, and activities of the individual. Following are the four basic food groups, along with suggestions for a good diet for the average person. Check your own eating habits to be sure you are eating a well-balanced diet. (Fig. 16–36.)

The Four Food Groups

1. **Dairy Products.** Milk or milk products are needed to supply protein, calcium, and other minerals, and to supply vitamins and carbohydrates. Every day a small child should have at least three to four 8-ounce glasses of milk. A teenager should have four or more glasses. An adult should have a glass or two daily, but pregnant women and nursing mothers need milk in greater quantity. Other forms of milk and milk products also acceptable include concentrated, evaporated, skim, and dry milk, yogurt, buttermilk, cream, and cheese.
2. **Vegetables and Fruits.** Four servings from this group are needed every day to supply an adequate amount of certain vitamins and minerals and to provide roughage. One of the servings should be from the citrus fruits—oranges, lemons, grapefruit—that are high in vitamin C. At least four meals a week should include a dark green or yellow vegetable for vitamin A.
3. **Meat and Meat Substitutes.** These include meat, fish, poultry, eggs, cheese, dried beans, peas, and nuts. Three servings daily from this group are recommended for a good diet. At least one serving should be meat, fish, or poultry. One serving might be an egg, a slice of cheese, or a small serving of split peas or baked beans.
4. **Breads, Cereals, and Potatoes.** Whole grain or enriched bread and cereals are necessary for the body's nutrition because they provide carbohydrates for energy. Six servings every day from this group are recommended.

KEY IDEA: WHAT ARE NUTRIENTS?

Food is able to give nourishment to the body because it contains various chemical substances called nutrients. Some 50 individual nutrients are needed to build the body. Many others are useful although they may not be required. Scientists also have discovered that nutrients work better together than alone. For instance, you may get enough calcium from milk but it is wasted if you do not get enough vitamin C or D from other foods to help the calcium develop the bones.

Many foods we eat contain combinations of various nutrients that are responsible for body functions. For example, whole-grain cereals are high in carbohydrates, but they also contain some protein, minerals, and vitamins.

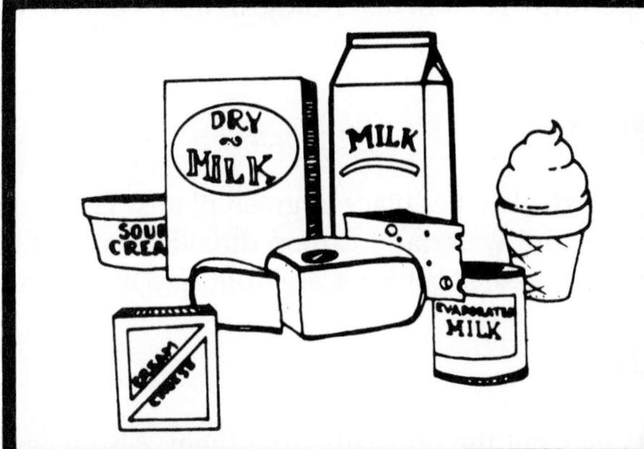

Group 1: Dairy Products

Milk

- 3 to 4 cups (Children)
- 4 or more cups (Teenagers)
- 2 or more cups (Adults)

Cheese, ice cream and other milk-made foods can be substituted for part of the milk requirement

Group 2: Vegetables and Fruit

- *4 or more servings*

Include dark green or deep yellow vegetables: citrus fruit or tomatoes

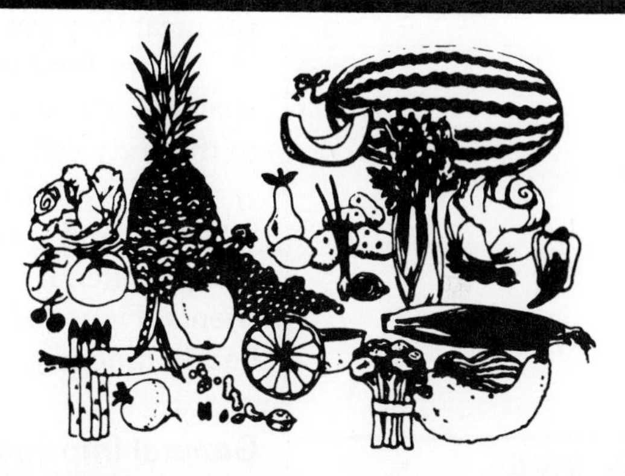

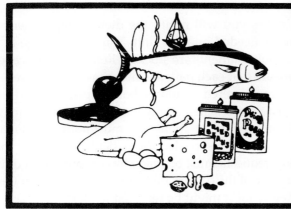

Group 3: Meat and Fish

- *3 servings*

Meats, fish, poultry, eggs or cheese, with dry beans, peas, nuts as alternates

Group 4: Breads, Cereals, and Potatoes

- *4 or more servings*

Enriched or whole grain. Added milk improves nutritional value

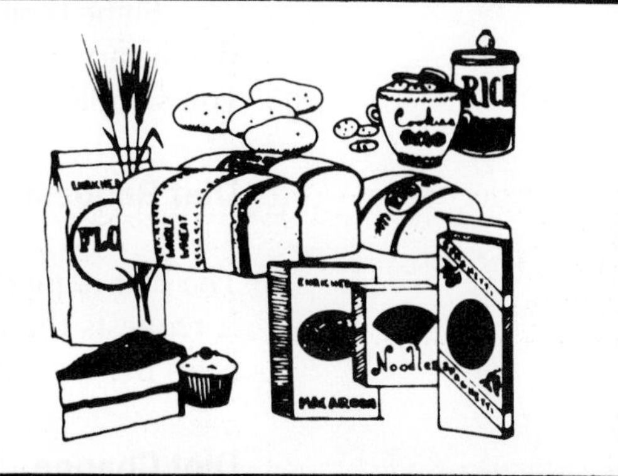

Figure 16–36 The Four Food Groups.

Foods help the body perform its functions only if they contain the right nutrients.

How Nutrients Are Made

The first step in making nutrients takes place in green plants. They take water and minerals from the soil, and water and carbon dioxide from the air. With the help of the sun's energy, these substances are built into nutrients.

How Nutrients Are Used

When people eat plants they get the nutrients from them. Also when people eat meat they get the nutrients animals have taken from green plants.

After food is eaten it enters the digestive tract where the nutrients are changed into simple forms. These simple forms then are carried by the blood to the body cells where the special functions of each are carried out.

There are six classes of nutrients: carbohydrates, fats, minerals, proteins, vitamins, and water. Because there are several kinds of each class of nutrients except water, it is clearer to speak of the classes instead of the individual nutrients. Figure 16–37 gives a brief description of each nutrient class and its bodily function.

KEY IDEA: EXECUTION OF FORMS

General Information

As a health unit coordinator, you will notify the dietary department of the number and kinds of meals needed on your unit. You may also see to it that supplies of supplemental nourishments are stocked. Remember, however, that your first concern is to ensure that each patient's meal has been ordered. Being overlooked when meals are delivered would be both depressing and uncomfortable for any patient. Therefore, when a newly admitted patient arrives, or when a dietary change is ordered for a patient, you must notify the dietary department in plenty of time to make sure that the patient will receive the next meal. Although all dietary requests must be made by computer or requisition, you may find it necessary to call the dietary department; telephone if there is a possibility that the written request might be received too late.

Some typical forms used by many hospitals for requisitioning food from the dietary department are included in this chapter. Your instructor will show you samples of the forms used in your hospitals.

Diet Request

The diet request form is filled out for each patient soon after he is admitted. It requests the kitchen to add a tray for him at the next meal and also indicates the type of diet he requires. (Fig. 16–38.)

Diet Change

Diet changes occur often in hospitals. Diets are canceled when a patient is discharged or expires. In all cases, dietary must be notified either by written notice or by computer. For example, a patient may have been on a normal

NUTRIENT CLASS	BODILY FUNCTIONS	FOOD SOURCES
CARBOHYDRATES 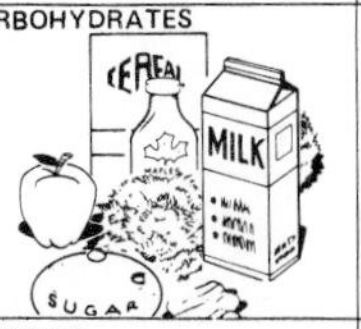	Provides work energy for body activities, and heat energy for maintenance of body temperature.	Cereal grains and their products (bread, breakfast cereals, macaroni products), potatoes, sugar, syrups, fruits, milk, vegetables, nuts
PROTEINS 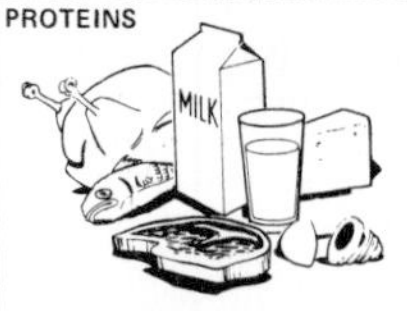	Build and renew body tissues; regulate body functions and supply energy. Complete proteins: maintain life and provide growth. Incomplete proteins: maintain life but do not provide for growth.	Complete proteins: Derived from animal foods – meat, milk, eggs, fish, cheese, poultry. Incomplete proteins: Derived from vegetable foods – soybeans, dry beans, peas, some nuts and whole-grain products.
FATS 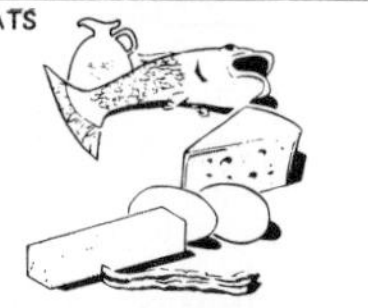	Give work energy for body activities and heat energy for maintenance of body temperature. Carrier of vitamins A and D, provide fatty acids necessary for growth and maintenance of body tissues.	Some foods are chiefly fat, such as lard, vegetable fats and oils, and butter. Many other foods contain smaller proportions of fats – nuts, meats, fish, poultry, cream, whole milk.
MINERALS Calcium 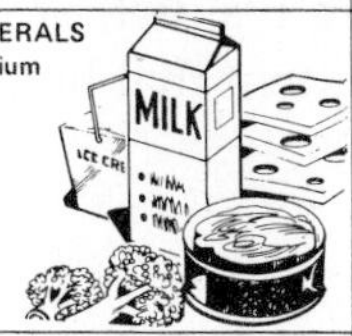	Builds and renews bones, teeth, and other tissues; regulates the activity of the muscles, heart. nerves; and controls the clotting of blood.	Milk and milk products, except butter; most dark green vegetables; canned salmon.
Phosphorus 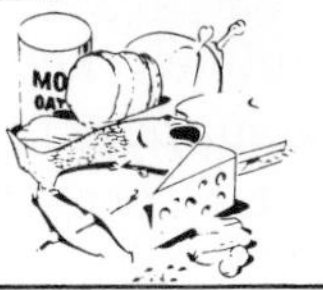	Associated with calcium in some functions needed to build and renew bones and teeth. Influences the oxidation of foods in the body cells; important in nerve tissue.	Widely distributed in foods; especially cheese, oat cereals, whole-wheat products, dry beans and peas, meat, fish, poultry, nuts.

NUTRIENT CLASS	BODILY FUNCTIONS	FOOD SOURCES
MINERALS (continued) Iron 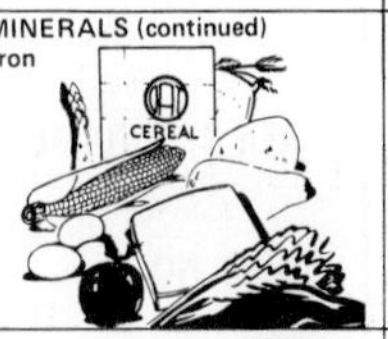	Builds and renews hemoglobin, the red pigment in blood which carries oxygen from the lungs to the cells.	Eggs, meat, especially liver and kidney; deep-yellow and dark green vegetables; potatoes, dried fruits, whole-grain products; enriched flour, bread, breakfast cereals.
Iodine 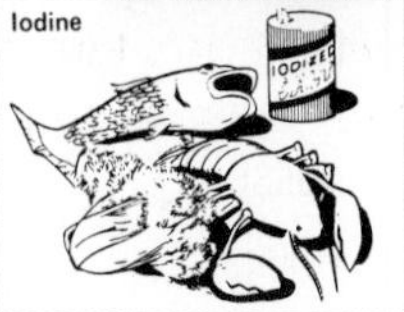	Enables the thyroid gland to perform its function of controling the rate at which foods are oxidized in the cells.	Fish (obtained from the sea), some plant-foods grown in soils containing iodine; table salt fortified with iodine (iodized).
VITAMINS A 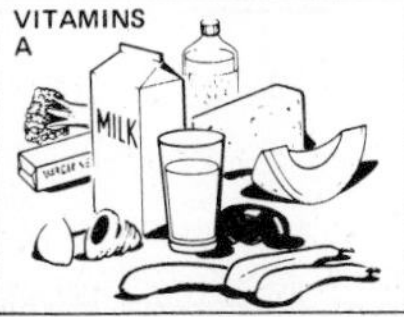	Necessary for normal functioning of the eyes, prevents night blindness. Ensures a healthy condition of the skin, hair, and mucous membranes. Maintains a state of resistance to infections of the eyes, mouth, and respiratory tract.	One form of Vitamin A is yelow and one form is colorless. Apricots, cantaloupe, milk, cheese, eggs, meat organs, (especially liver and kidney), fortified margarine, butter, fish-liver oils, dark green and deep yellow vegetables.
B Complex B_1 (Thiamine) 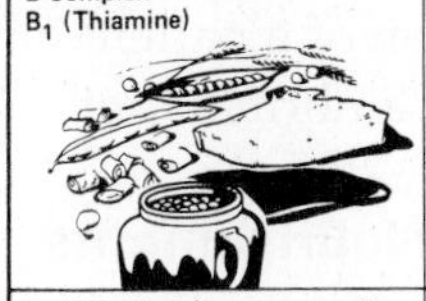	Maintains a healthy condition of the nerves. Fosters a good appetite. Helps the body cells use carbohydrates.	Whole-grain and enriched grain products; meats (especially pork, liver and kidney). dry beans and peas.
B_2 (Riboflavin) 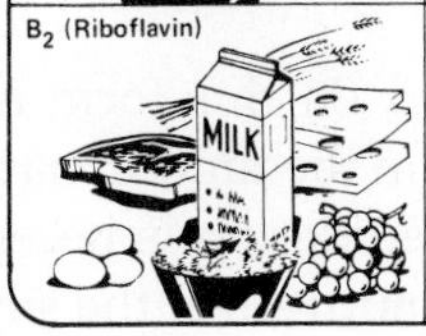	Keeps the skin, mouth, and eyes in a healthy condition. Acts with other nutrients to form enzymes and control oxidation in cells.	Milk, cheese, eggs, meat (especially liver and kidney), whole grain and enriched grain products, dark green vegetables.

NUTRIENT CLASS	BODILY FUNCTIONS	FOOD SOURCES
VITAMINS (Continued) Niacin 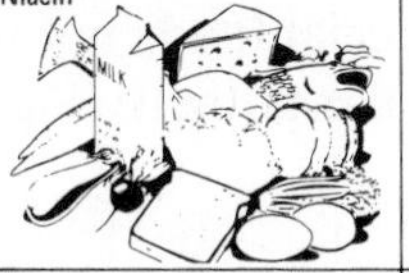	Influences the oxidation of carbohydrates and proteins in the body cells.	Liver, meat, fish, poultry, eggs, peanuts; dark green vegetables, whole-grain and enriched cereal products.
B_{12} 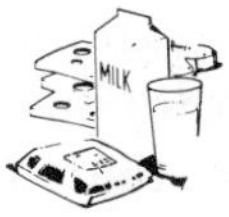	Regulates specific processes in digestion. Helps maintain normal functions of muscles, nerves, heart, blood – general body metabolism.	Liver, other organ meats, cheese, eggs, milk
C (Ascorbic Acid) 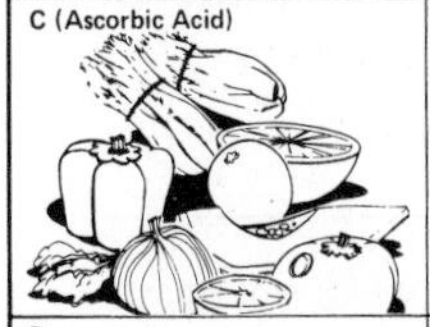	Acts as a cement between body cells, and helps them work together to carry out their special functions. Maintains a sound condition of bones, teeth, and gums. Not stored in the body.	Fresh, raw citrus fruits and vegetables – oranges, grapefruit, cantaloupe, strawberries, tomatoes, raw onions, cabbage, green and sweet red peppers, dark green vegetables.
D 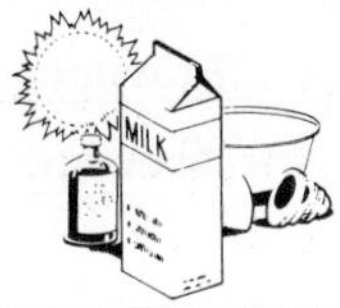	Enables the growing body to use calcium and phosphorus in a normal way to build bones and teeth.	Provided by Vitamin D fortification of certain foods, such as milk and margarine. Also fish-liver oils and eggs. Sunshine is also a source of Vitamin D.
WATER 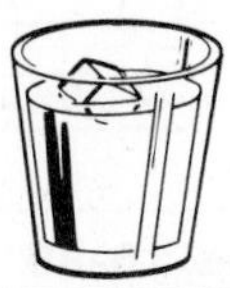	Regulates body processes. Aids in regulating body temperature. Carries nutrients to body cells and carries waste products away from them. Helps to lubricate joints. Water has no food value, although most water contains mineral elements. More immediately necessary to life than food – second only to oxygen.	Drinking water, and other beverages; all foods except those made up of a single nutrient, as sugar and some fats. Milk milk drinks, soups, vegetables, fruit juices. Ice cream, watermelon, strawberries, lettuce, tomatoes, cereals, other dry products.

Figure 16–37 How nutrients are used.

DIET CARD

PATIENT'S NAME George Thompson

ROOM NO. 437 FLOOR 2E

DIET Normal

NURSE DATE 11/20/XX

H.Brown HUC

Figure 16–38

diet before surgery, but after surgery he will need a postoperative diet, or the condition of a patient on a special diet may improve to the extent that he can resume a normal diet.

Stock Nourishments

Included on this form are all the standard nourishments routinely kept in supply in the unit. It may be your responsibility to check these supplies to see when reordering is necessary. In some hospitals, however, dietary personnel check and restock the supplies themselves.

Individual Patient Nourishments

This requisition is used to order special foods not included in the stock nourishments but required for a particular patient. (Fig. 16–39.)

Extra Meals for Guests

This requisition is used for ordering an extra meal so that a friend or family member may eat with a patient. This form must usually be made out in duplicate; one copy is sent to the kitchen, the other to the cashier so that the meal can be charged to the patient's account. (Fig. 16–40.)

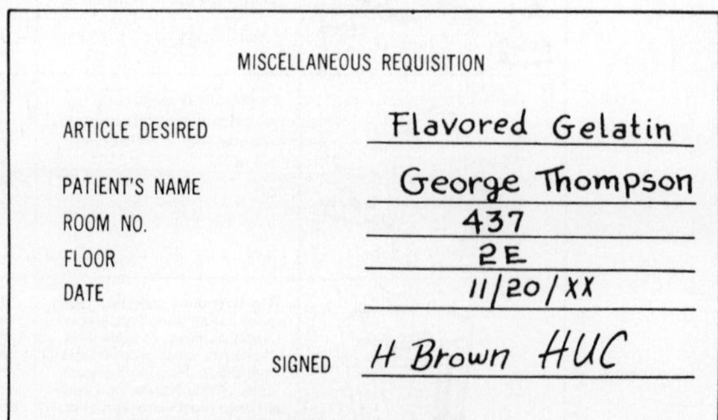

MISCELLANEOUS REQUISITION

ARTICLE DESIRED Flavored Gelatin

PATIENT'S NAME George Thompson

ROOM NO. 437

FLOOR 2E

DATE 11/20/XX

SIGNED H Brown HUC

Figure 16–39

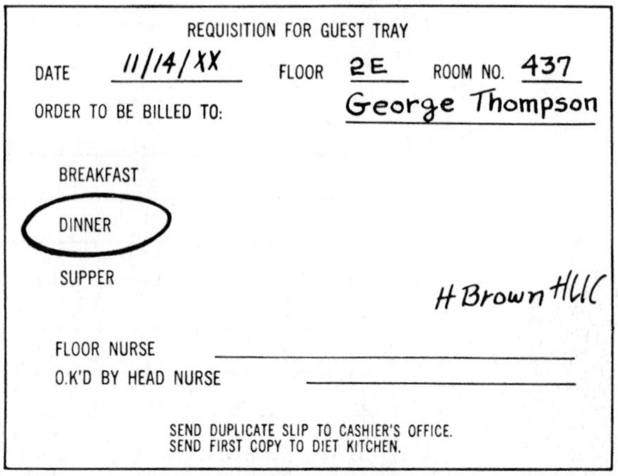

REQUISITION FOR GUEST TRAY

DATE 11/14/XX FLOOR 2E ROOM NO. 437

ORDER TO BE BILLED TO: George Thompson

BREAKFAST

DINNER

SUPPER

H Brown HUC

FLOOR NURSE ____________

O.K'D BY HEAD NURSE ____________

SEND DUPLICATE SLIP TO CASHIER'S OFFICE.
SEND FIRST COPY TO DIET KITCHEN.

Figure 16–40

LEARNING ACTIVITIES

LABORATORY

Complete the following:

1. The division of the laboratory which analyzes the blood for its basic physical properties is ____________.
2. The division which analyzes body fluids for chemical constituents is ____.
3. The section concerned primarily with tests designed to isolate and identify disease-causing microorganisms is ____________.
4. The division which studies cells obtained from body tissues is ________.
5. The urinalysis is often done by the ____________ division of the laboratory, although it is not a blood test.
6. A urinalysis consists of a ____________, ____________, and ____________ examination of the urine.
7. Urine specimens are obtained by ____________, not by the laboratory.
8. When you receive an order for a Ua (urinalysis), what will you do?
9. How would you handle an order for a 24° urine?
10. List some of the responsibilities of the blood bank.
    (a) ____________
    (b) ____________

(c) ______________________________

(d) ______________________________

11. What is the purpose of crossmatching?

____

____

____

12. What is the purpose of blood typing?

____

____

____

13. Your greatest concern for laboratory tests should be for:

(a) ______________________________

(b) ______________________________

(c) ______________________________

(d) ______________________________

14. How would you handle a telephone laboratory report?

____

____

____

____

Match the name of the hematology test or abbreviation in column A with the definition in column B.

Column A	*Column B*
(a) ESR	____ Measurement of the time it takes a fingerstick wound to cease bleeding
(b) Hct	____ Examination of the different kinds of WBCs
(c) LE cell Prep	____ Count of immature red blood cells
(d) APTT	____ Measures hemoglobin—the oxygen-carrying portion of the blood
(e) Bleeding time	____ Measurements reported as MCH, MCHC, and MCV
(f) Hgb	____ Diagnostic study for lupus erythematosus
(g) Reticulocytes	____ Determines rate at which RBCs settle out of liquid portion of blood; used to determine progress of inflammatory diseases
(h) RBC Indices	____ A coagulation study
(i) Differential	____ Measurement of the volume percentage of erythrocytes in whole blood

Match column A with column B in regard to chemistry studies.

Column A	*Column B*
(a) Uric acid	____ Determines amount of sugar in the blood stream after the patient has fasted
(b) GTT	____ Used in diagnosis of metastatic carcinoma of prostate gland
(c) Creatinine	

(d) BUN
(e) Acid phosphatase
(f) Na, K, Cl, CO_2
(g) FBS
(h) SGOT, LDH, CPK
(i) Bilirubin
(j) SMA_{12-20}
(k) PP BS

____ Chem screen
____ Measures liver function
____ Electrolytes
____ Measures blood sugar *after* eating
____ *Blood* test for kidney function
____ Cardiac enzymes
____ Used principally to diagnose gout
____ Done over several hours to measure glucose in urine and blood
____ Increased quantities are found in advanced stages of kidney disease

Matching

Column A

(a) Biopsy
(b) Postprandial
(c) Cytology
(d) Differential
(e) Erythrocyte
(f) Mycology
(g) Paracentesis
(h) Serology
(i) Lumbar puncture
(j) Sternal puncture
(k) Electrolytes
(l) Virology

Column B

____ The study of viruses and the diseases caused by them
____ The removal of cerebral spinal fluid from the spinal canal
____ Those body substances that help maintain a balance between acidity and alkalinity
____ Tissue removed from a living body for examination
____ The study of fungi that cause disease
____ Removal of bone marrow from the breastbone cavity for diagnostic purposes
____ After eating
____ The study of blood serum for diseases such as syphilis
____ Identification of the type of WBCs found in the blood
____ The study of cells
____ The puncture and drainage of a body cavity
____ Red blood cell

Multiple Choice

1. A culture and sensitivity would be performed by which laboratory division?
   (a) Hematology
   (b) Biochemistry
   (c) Serology
   (d) Bacteriology
2. Histology means:
   (a) Study of blood
   (b) Study of cells
   (c) Study of tissues
   (d) Study of bacteria

3. A routine CBC would *not* include which of the following:
   (a) RBCs
   (b) WBCs
   (c) Platelets
   (d) Potassium
4. The greatest precautions for preventing contamination of urine may be taken by obtaining which kind of specimen?
   (a) Clean catch
   (b) Catheterized
   (c) Voided
   (d) Mid-stream
5. Lymphocytes are a type of:
   (a) Erythrocyte
   (b) Platelet
   (c) Reticulocyte
   (d) Leukocyte
6. An abnormal formation of fluid in the abdominal cavity is called:
   (a) CSF
   (b) Guaiac
   (c) Ascites
   (d) Urea

RADIOLOGY

Complete the following:

1. The three major divisions of radiology are:
   (a) ____________________
   (b) ____________________
   (c) ____________________
2. Preparations of patients who are to receive x-rays utilizing contrast media may include:
   (a) ____________________
   (b) ____________________
   (c) ____________________
   (d) ____________________
3. Why do many hospitals require that the health unit coordinator also telephone radiology with the order in addition to sending a requisition?
   ____
   ____
   ____
4. Why do many radiology requisitions have a space for the health unit coordinator to record the clinical problem? ____________________
   ____
   ____

5. Why must the health unit coordinator be aware of the time the patient leaves for radiology and when he returns? ______________________

____

____

6. Give the abbreviation and meaning of each of the following x-rays.

	Abbreviation	*Meaning*
(a) barium enema	________	________
(b) gastrointestinal series	________	________
(c) gallbladder series	________	________
(d) intravenous pyelogram	________	________

7. A barium enema, gastrointestinal series, gallbladder series, and intravenous pyelogram must be done ______________________

____

Match the terms in column A with the definitions in column B.

Column A	*Column B*
(a) Thermogram	____ Substances introduced into the body which permit the radiologist to distinguish between different body densities
(b) Ultrasound	____ Photograph of body surface temperature based on infrared radiation given off by body
(c) Xerogram	____ X-ray of vascular structures
(d) Tomogram	____ X-ray of salivary ducts
(e) Contrast media	____ Technique that utilizes xerox paper instead of x-ray film to record pictures of soft body tissue
(f) Angiogram	____ The visible observation of internal structures "in action"
(g) Myelogram	____ Process of recording echoes of sound waves striking body tissues of different densities
(h) Scan	____ X-ray of arteries
(i) Arteriogram	____ X-ray that studies selected levels of body
(j) Fluoroscopy	____ X-ray of spinal cord after injection of contrast medium into spinal canal
(k) Sialogram	____ Picture produced by concentration of radionuclides in specific organ

8. Define the following:
   (a) PEEP ______________________
   (b) Doppler ______________________
   (c) MRI ______________________
   (d) FFE ______________________
   (e) EGD ______________________

CARDIOLOGY

Complete the following:

1. The most common test the health unit coordinator will order through cardiology is the ______________________.

2. The ECG or EKG is usually taken in the patient's room/in the department?
______

3. Types of medications which may need to be included in the cardiology requisition are:
   (a) ______
   (b) ______
   (c) ______
   (d) ______

4. Other information frequently requested on the cardiology requisition includes:
   (a) ______
   (b) ______
   (c) ______
   (d) ______

Match the terms in column A with the definitions in column B.

Column A	*Column B*
(a) Treadmill stress test	____ Small portable device worn by patient which provides a continuous ECG recording while the patient goes about usual activities
(b) Echocardiogram	____ Tracing of electrical activity of heart
(c) Holter monitor	____ Usually taken to establish regularity of heartbeat on one lead
(d) Swan-Ganz catheter	____ Catheter inserted by physician into pulmonary artery to measure pressure in circulatory system
(e) Cardiac pacemaker	____ Measures heart's ability to tolerate increased activity
(f) Electrocardiogram	____ Produced by sending sound waves through the body
(g) Rhythm strip	____ Mechanical device to stimulate heart activity

RESPIRATORY OR INHALATION THERAPY

Complete the following:

1. Oxygen is measured in ______ or ______.
2. Oxygen is administered in several different ways:
   (a) ______
   (b) ______
   (c) ______
   (d) ______
3. What is a common method of letting others know, as a safety precaution, that oxygen is in use?
______
______
______

4. Machines that assist the patient to breathe when he is unable to do so on his own are called ______ or ______.
5. IPPB is the abbreviation for ______.
6. The machine which gives the patient a set number of breaths at a set volume in addition to whatever spontaneous breaths he can generate is the ______.
7. Patients are usually taught to use these bedside devices before surgery: ______
8. Percussion of the back to loosen secretions is called: ______
9. Tests which measure the state of the respiratory system are called ______ tests.
10. Samples drawn from arteries and analyzed by respiratory therapy are called ______.
11. Interpret the following orders:
   (a) O_2 @ 6L/M ______
   (b) IPPB q.i.d. ______
   (c) IMV_2 q1h ______
   (d) ABGs on R/A ______
   (e) CPT q.i.d. ______
12. A patient requiring treatment from inhalation therapy will usually need a series of ______.

PHYSICAL THERAPY

Complete the following:

1. Physical therapy includes the use of
   (a) ______
   (b) ______
   (c) ______
   (d) ______
   (e) ______
   (f) ______
   (g) ______
2. The physical therapy department will ordinarily have equipment such as
   (a) ______
   (b) ______
   (c) ______
   (d) ______
   (e) ______
   (f) ______
3. Through instruction and supervised practice, trained physical therapists help patients ______
   ______.

OCCUPATIONAL THERAPY

1. Describe your understanding of the purpose of occupational therapy.
____
____
____
____
____
____

ENDOSCOPIES

Complete the following:

1. An endoscopy is ______________________________
______________________________.
2. Endo means ______________________________.
3. -scopy means ______________________________.
4. Most endoscopies require a signed ______________________________ and some require ______________________ prior to the procedure.
5. A patient who has undergone an examination of the upper gastrointestinal tract will not be fed until ______________________________.

Match the following:

Column A		*Column B*
(a) Esophagoscopy	____	Visualization of the bronchi through the mouth
(b) Sigmoidoscopy	____	Visualization of the stomach
(c) Gastroscopy	____	Visualization of the sigmoid portion of the large intestine through the anus
(d) Proctoscopy	____	Visualization of the esophagus through the mouth
(e) Bronchoscopy	____	Visualization of the rectum

ELECTROENCEPHALOGRAPHY

Complete the following:

1. The abbreviation for electroencephalogram is ______________________.
2. An electroencephalogram is a ______________________________
______________________________.

DIETARY

1. Label each of the pictures in Fig. 16–41 with the number of the food groups listed here that it represents:
   Group 1: Dairy Products
   Group 2: Vegetables and Fruit
   Group 3: Meat and Fish
   Group 4: Breads, Cereals, and Potatoes
2. Beside each food listed below write the *LETTER* or letters of the food group, listed below, to which it belongs:

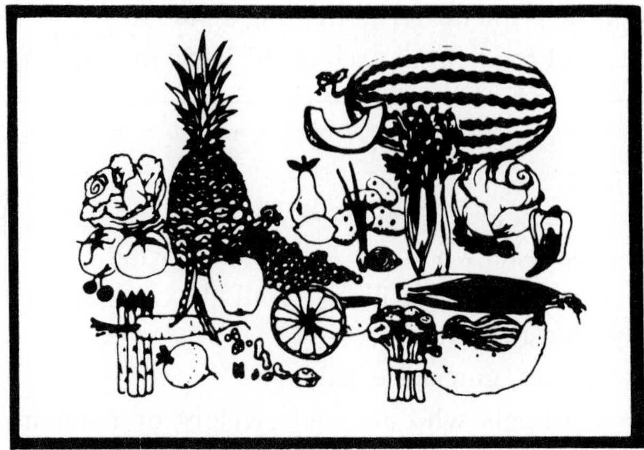

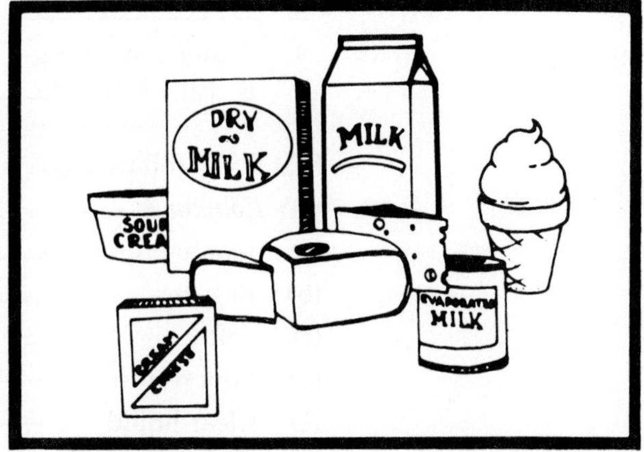

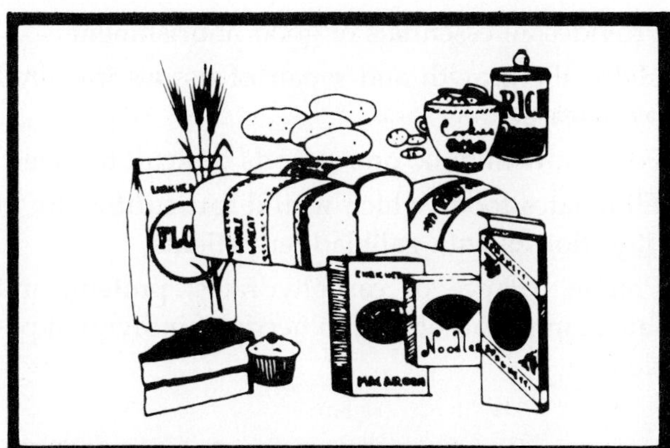

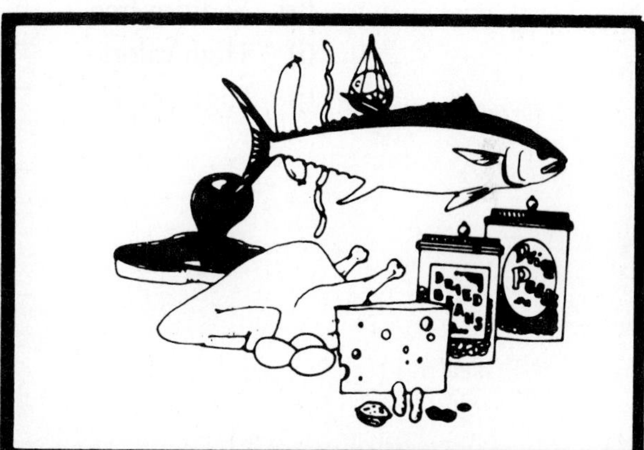

Figure 16–41

D—Dairy Products
V&F—Vegetables and Fruits
M—Meat and Meat Substitutes
B—Breads, Cereals, and Potatoes

1. Peas ______
2. Onions ______
3. Milk ______
4. Macaroni ______
5. Broccoli ______
6. Rice ______
7. Bread ______
8. Dried beans ______
9. Yogurt ______
10. Cake ______
11. Nuts ______
12. Carrots ______
13. Potatoes ______
14. Cheese ______

Fill in the blanks:

1. Various chemical substances which give nourishment to the body are called ______.
2. The process of taking food into the body to maintain life is referred to as ______.

3. ____________________ diets help the doctor in treating a patient.
4. A diet containing a variety of foods from each of the basic food groups is called a ________________-________________ ________________.

Match the following:

Column A		Column B
(a) Bland	____	For patients who have difficulty chewing
(b) Regular	____	For patients whose illness would be compounded by fluid retention
(c) Soft	____	Broth, tea, ginger ale, jello
(d) Low residue	____	For patients who are underweight or malnourished
(e) Clear liquid	____	Series of diets mild in flavor and easy to digest; omits spicy foods
(f) Low fat	____	Provides all essentials of good nourishment
(g) Diabetic	____	Helps the growth and repair of tissues impaired by disease
(h) Sodium free	____	Foods low in bulk; omits foods difficult to digest
(i) High calorie	____	Eliminates foods which would cause difficulty in digestion as with gallbladder patients
(j) High protein	____	Precise balance of carbohydrates, protein, and fats planned according to needs of individual patient

CHAPTER 17
Health Unit Coordinator Procedures

OBJECTIVES

When you complete this chapter, you will be able to discuss the health unit coordinator's responsibilities as they relate to the following hospital procedures:

- Admissions
- Transfers
- Discharges
- Deaths
- The Surgical Patient

ADMISSIONS

A patient coming into a hospital is often frightened and uncomfortable. He may or may not be seriously ill or in pain. This is a time when the health unit coordinator is very important to the patient. Being pleasant and courteous will make the patient's arrival easier for him. A nice welcome will create a favorable impression.

Introduce yourself. Learn the patient's name and use it often. Remember that the way you speak and behave will have a lot to do with the patient's impression of the institution. Smile, be friendly. Do not appear to be rushed or busy with other things.

As you efficiently perform your tasks as a health unit coordinator, you can do much to facilitate a smoother transition for patients as they begin their stay in your hospital. (Fig. 17–1.)

There are two types of patient admissions:

1. Routine admissions which have been planned in advance
2. Emergency admissions which are unplanned and are due to a sudden illness or accident

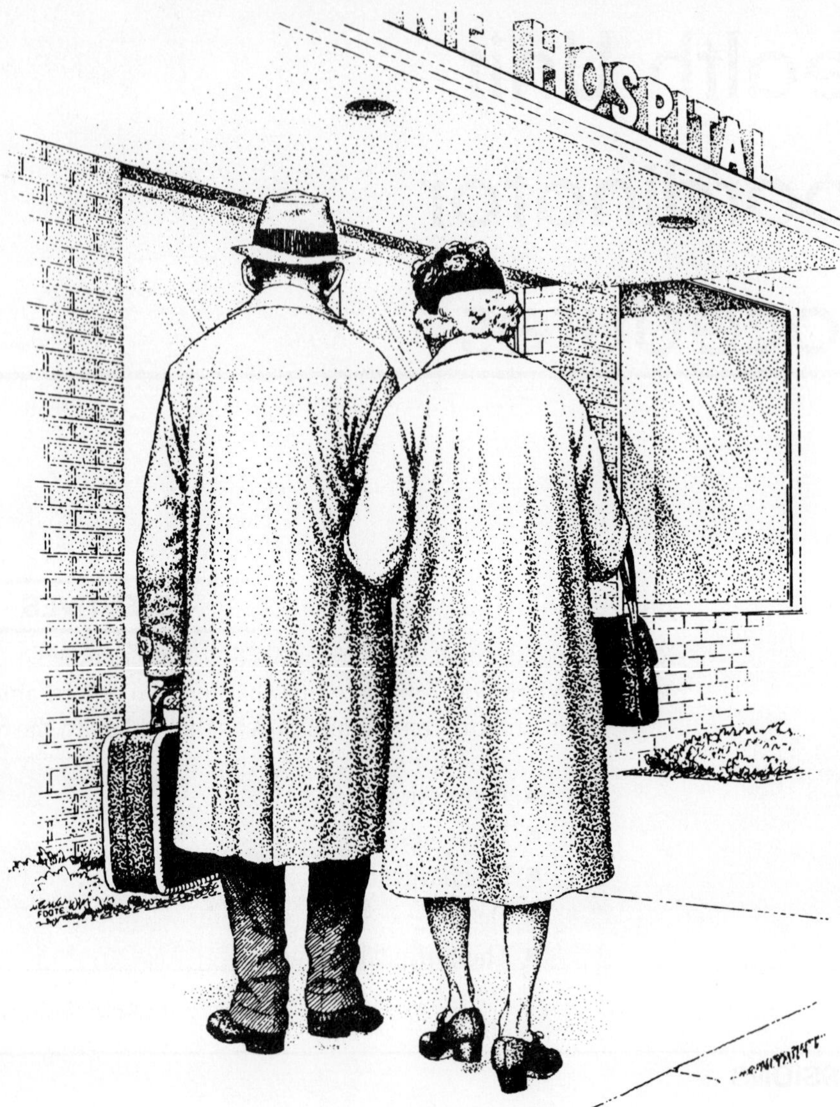

Figure 17–1

KEY IDEA: ROUTINE ADMISSIONS

Appointments for routine admissions are arranged by the patient's doctor. Admissions of service patients are arranged by the clinic with the admissions office. A census of all empty beds is kept in the admissions office.

Patients entering for routine admission must be processed through the admitting office before they are escorted to their rooms.

- The summary or face sheet, discussed in Chapter 11, is filled out by admitting office personnel and the "release of liability" clause is signed by the patient at the same time. Patients are given the Patient's Rights form and Advance Directive to sign.
- The admitting office assigns a unit number to the patient which will be used to identify all records kept on the patient while he is in the hospital.

PATIENT IDENTIFICATION

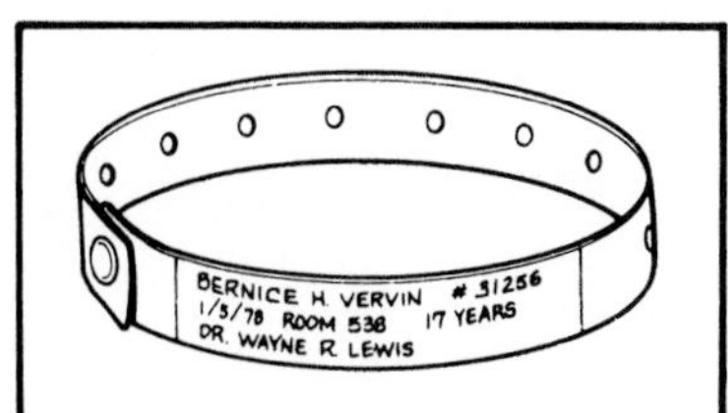

Figure 17–2

- The patient's name, unit number, and other identifying information will be transferred to an addressograph plate or imprinter card, which will be used by nursing personnel to stamp identification information on requisitions and chart forms.
- In most hospitals, the admitting office also makes out the patient's identification bracelet. This bracelet, usually made of plastic with a thin cardboard insert, is attached to the patient's wrist and must not be removed during hospitalization. (Fig. 17–2.)

Sometimes patients will have completed their routine laboratory tests, such as chest x-rays and blood tests, which may be required on admission (preadmission testing or PAT), before they are escorted to the nursing unit.

When these preliminary procedures have been completed, the patient is ready to be taken to his room.

- A volunteer or an escort aide usually helps the patient by carrying his luggage and directing him to the correct nursing unit. Family members often accompany the patient at this time.
- Some routine admission patients may walk to the nursing unit; most, however, including elderly or disabled patients, are transported to the nursing unit in wheelchairs or by gurney.

The escort may leave the patient in his assigned room and notify the health unit coordinator or he may bring the patient to the nurses' station and introduce him to the health unit coordinator. In either instance, the escort will leave the summary or face sheet and the addressograph plate with the health unit coordinator.

KEY IDEA: EMERGENCY ADMISSIONS

The admitting procedure for emergency patients is usually different from that for routine admissions. (Fig. 17–3.)

- Emergency patients are usually admitted through the emergency department where immediate examinations take place.
- Emergency treatment may be initiated in the emergency room. If possible, identification information is requested from the patient.
- The admitting office must be notified so that they may assign a bed to the patient. Ordinarily, the admitting personnel do not see the patient at this time but they may come to the emergency room to complete the ad-

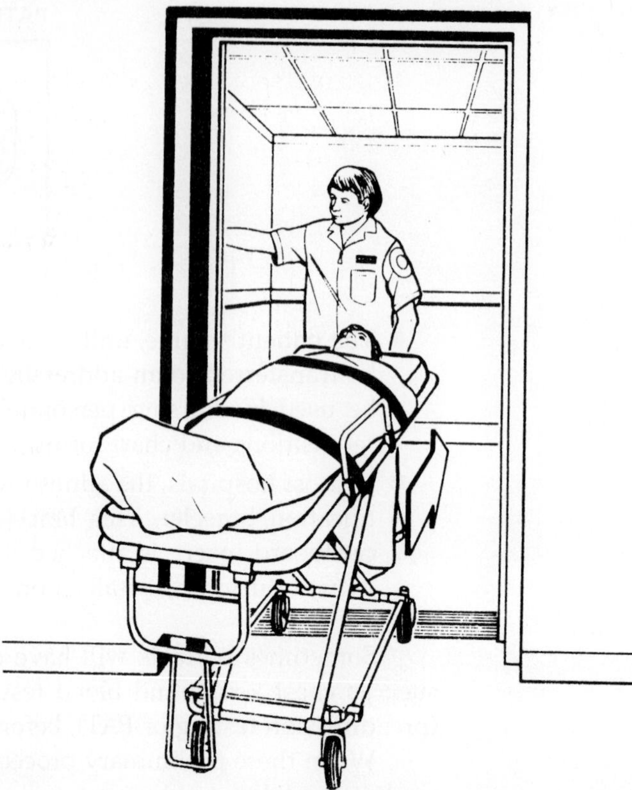

Figure 17-3

mission or may request that a member of the patient's family come to the admitting office as soon as possible.

- As soon as possible, the emergency patient and his belongings are transferred to the nursing unit, usually by stretcher.
- Emergency admission patients are always taken directly to their rooms.
- Emergency patients may be admitted at any time of the day or night. The emergency patient or his representative must sign Conditions of Admissions or Release of Liability Form. As with a routine admission, the Admitting Department will assign a unit number, prepare a face or summary sheet, and imprinter or addressograph plate and, if not made in the ER, an identification bracelet. The health unit coordinator should be familiar with the ER record so he/she will know which diagnostic tests and treatment were instituted there.

KEY IDEA: ADMISSIONS AND HEALTH UNIT COORDINATOR RESPONSIBILITIES

Your clerical duties with respect to a newly admitted patient are less likely to vary than your receptionist duties. Since you are primarily responsible for attending the desk at all times, you will generally give directions to the new patient and answer his questions only when it is impossible for someone else to do so. At the desk, however, you will be entirely responsible for getting the new patient's records in order. Listed below are the admitting procedures in which you may be expected to participate.

Clerical Duties

- Preparing the new chart by stamping all chart forms with the patient's identification plate and assembling them in the proper order.
- Locating old charts on the patient by calling the medical record room and requesting that the charts be sent to the nursing unit.
- Making available a valuables envelope and valuables control sheet if the patient wishes to have money and other items locked in the hospital safe. Figure 17–4 shows a valuables control sheet and Figure 17–5 a valuables envelope receipt.
- Entering TPR, blood pressure, weight, and other pertinent information on the patient's graphic chart.
- Entering the patient's name in the TPR book, on the day's census report, and on other pertinent records.
- Transcribing all doctor's orders written on the new patient.
- If admitting still needs to see the patient, contact them as soon as possible. Figure 17–6 (pg. 394) shows a computer-generated notice to admitting.

Receptionist Duties

In a particular hospital, some of these duties may be the responsibility of nursing personnel. Learn the duties you will be expected to carry out. In general, receptionist duties will include the following:

- Greeting the patient at the nurses' station, introducing yourself, and welcoming the patient to the hospital.
- Notifying a member of the nursing staff that the patient has arrived on the floor and is awaiting admission instructions.
- Directing or guiding the new patient to his room and introducing him to his roommates, if any.
- Checking the application or actually applying the patient's identification bracelet.
- Notifying the intern, resident, or attending doctor who will be responsible for completing the new patient's medical history and physical examination.

Orienting the patient to hospital personnel and routines are responsibilities that the nurse usually carries out. However, those that you may assist with include providing information about:

- Hospital smoking and noise control regulations
- Hours and regulations concerning meals and visitors
- Regulations concerning use of day room and isolation unit
- Policies concerning radio and television rental
- The head nurse's name and introductions to other nursing staff members (Fig. 17–7, pg. 395.)

PATIENT BELONGINGS RECORD

TRANSFERRED TO: ______ FROM: ______
ADMITTED TO: ______ FROM: ______

CLOTHING NONE ______ SENT HOME WITH: ______
JEWELRY NONE ______ RELATIONSHIP: ______
DATE: ______ TIME: ______

	DESCRIPTION COLOR	WITH PT	SENT HOME
BELT			
BLOUSE			
BRA			
COAT			
DRESS			
HAT			
JACKET			
NIGHTGOWN			
PANTIES			
PANTS			
PAJAMAS			
ROBE			
SCARF			
SHIRT			
SHOES			
SKIRT			
SLACKS			
SLIP			
SLIPPERS			
SOCKS			
STOCKINGS			
SWEATER			
TIE			
T – SHIRT			
UNDERSHORTS			
MISC.			

MEDICATIONS:	LIST BY NAME	TO PHARM	SENT HOME

	DESCRIPTION COLOR	WITH PT	SENT HOME
BRACELET			
EARRINGS			
NECKLACE			
RING			
WATCH			
RAZOR			
DRYER			
RADIO			
OTHER			

		WITH PT	SENT HOME
PROSTHESIS	NONE ______		
DENTURES:			
UPPER ______	FULL ______ PARTIAL ______		
LOWER ______	FULL ______ PARTIAL ______		
HEARING AID	LT ___ RT ___		
GLASSES			
CONTACTS			
WIG / HAIRPIECE			
AMBULATORY AID: TYPE			
OTHER			

MISCELLANEOUS	TO SAFE	WITH PT	SENT HOME
CREDIT CARDS			
KEYS			
PURSE			
WALLET			
SUITCASE			
INSURANCE / MEDICARE CARD			
OTHER			

CASH ______

SAFE ENVELOPE # ______ AMOUNT $ ______

AMOUNT WITH PATIENT $ ______

THIS IS A CORRECT LISTING OF MY BELONGINGS AND THEIR DISPOSITION.

PT. OR RESP. PARTY ______

WITNESS ______

CHART COPY White - PATIENT COPY Yellow

Figure 17–4

No. 00012

VALUABLES ENVELOPE

CONTENTS

	TOTAL NUMBER OF ITEMS

This envelope MUST be signed by the depositor. Valuables will be surrendered ONLY to the person whose signature appears below.

Signature of Depositor ______________________________

Signature of Custodian ______________________________

Date ______________________

NOTE: The hospital is not responsible for items which you retain in your possession.

- -

RECEIPT No. 00012

Signature of Depositor ______________________________

Signature of Custodian ______________________________

Date ______________________

Figure 17–5

MEMORIAL HOSPITAL
****
S P E C I A L
MAIL MAN MESSAGE
REGARDING THIS PATIENT'S
CONFIDENTIAL ADMITTING INFORMATION
****

PATIENT: EXAMPLE, IMANOTHER — AGE: 20 SEX: F DOB: 12/12/1977

MED REC NUMBER: 000000000 — ADMITTING MD: FINEDOCTOR, MARY

PATIENT NUMBER: 0000000 — NURSING UNIT: M ROOM/BED: M202

SOC SEC NUMBER: 00000000000 — FC: SP ADMIT DATE: 04/21/9X

ADMIT DX: BRONCHITIS — CURRENT DX: pneumonia

ENTRY DEPARTMENT NO: 077
ENTRY DEPT. MNEUMONIC: XXX

TO ADMITTING - ADMITTING INFO FORM

ADMITTING CLERK MAY COME & SEE PATIENT NOW

FAMILY IS HERE TO INTERPRET

SENT BY: SUSIE SECRETARY
PH/EXT#: 1212

ORDER NO. 716
ORDER DATE: 05/30/9X
ORDER TIME: 16:09
ENTERED BY: — PATTERN NO:

Figure 17–6

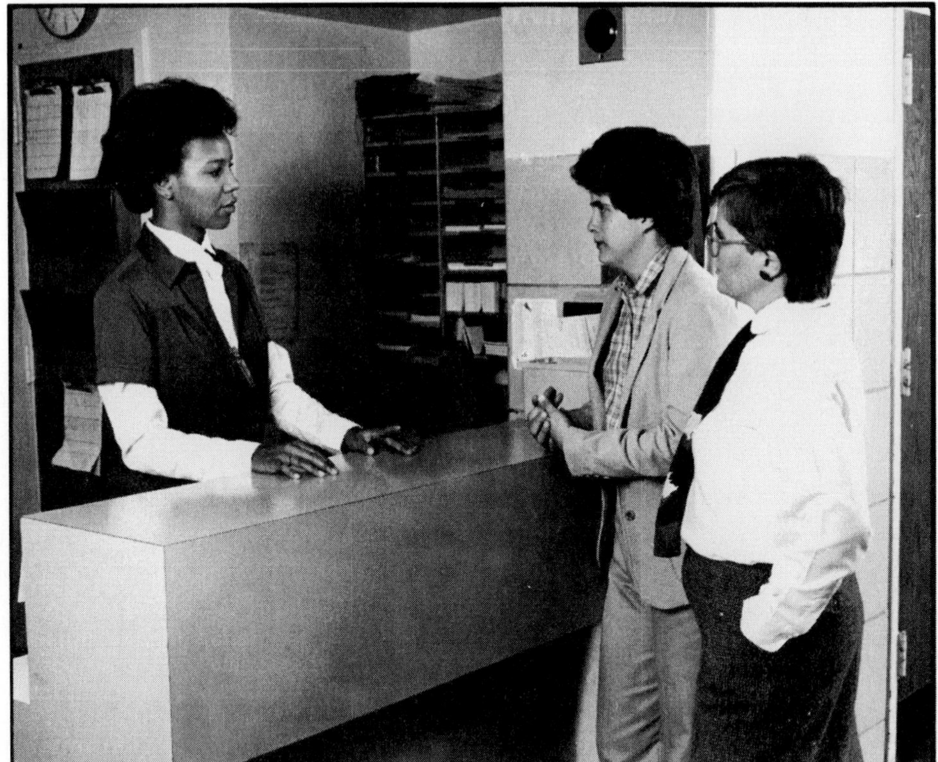

Figure 17–7

ADMISSION ORDERS

KEY IDEA: TYPES OF ADMISSION ORDERS

In most hospitals, nothing beyond the routine admission procedure is permitted to be done for the patient until the doctor has written the admission orders. These orders include all the general instructions pertaining to the patient's care. In most cases, you will find at least one order from each of the following categories.

DOCTOR'S ADMISSION ORDERS

- Diet
- Activity
- Diagnostic Tests
- Treatment
- Medications

Diet

Every patient must have a dietary regimen, whether it be a regular diet, a therapeutic diet, or a complete restriction on his intake (as when emergency surgery is anticipated).

Activity

All patients ordinarily have orders written to indicate the amount of activity they are allowed. In some hospitals, doctors may not be required to write an order if their patients are permitted movement "ad lib," that is, without restriction.

Diagnostic Tests

Most hospital admissions must have at least two diagnostic tests: a CBC and a urinalysis. These and other tests must be ordered by the doctor. Other common admission diagnostic tests are ECGs and chest x-rays.

Treatments

Except in cases where the patient has been admitted to the hospital only for diagnostic reasons, some treatment will probably be started to make him more comfortable or to improve his condition.

Medications

Admission orders usually include an order for medications. In some cases, the doctor may simply continue a medication the patient has been taking at home. In others, new medications intended to treat his condition will be ordered. Sleeping medications (sedatives) are often ordered p.r.n., as many people find it difficult to sleep in the hospital.

A sample of orders written at admission are as follows:

Complete bedrest.
Low Na Diet.
Routine CBC & UA.
Serum electrolytes.
ESR & SGOT.
Stat. ECG.
Digitoxin 0.2 mg. p.o. q.d.
Meperidine 75 mg. IM q4n p.r.n. for chest pain.
Secobarbital sodium gr. i $\overline{ss}$ h.s. p.o. p.r.n.
VS q2h Call Dr. Green for P > 120 or < 60.

KEY IDEA: ROUTINE ORDERS

Some physicians have their orders printed because they routinely order many of the same things for different patients. The doctor will then add or delete as necessary to meet the needs of the individual patient. These orders are called *routine orders* and are usually kept in the nursing unit and may be put into effect when the patient arrives. Changes or additional orders will be given by the doctor by telephone or written when he visits the patient. Routine orders (and all orders) must be signed by the doctor.

KEY IDEA: MEDICAL SHORT STAY OR LESS THAN 24-HOUR ADMISSIONS

The purpose of Medical Short Stay is to provide treatment on a short-term basis to patients who would otherwise be admitted to the hospital. Patients cannot remain in the MSSU for more than 23 hours 59 minutes and patients who, after 12 hours are still in the MSSU, must be evaluated by the physician. If the patient requires hospital admission, those orders must be written.

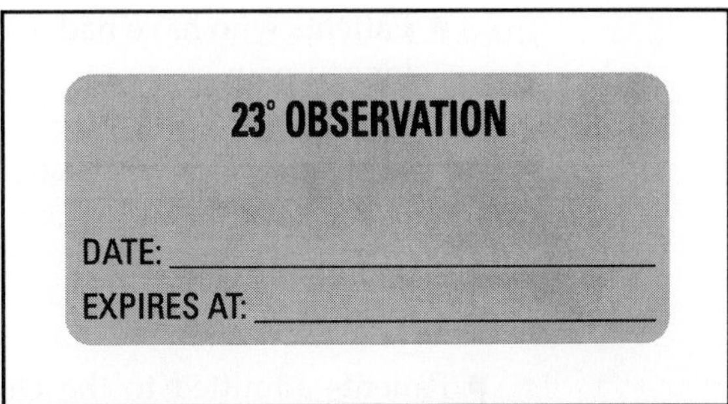

- Medical Records: All patients in the MSSU require a medical record, which includes physician's orders for treatment, a history and a physical, and criteria for discharge, signed by the physician.
- Scheduling: Patients requiring specialized procedures are prescheduled through the designated scheduling office such as Out-Patient Admitting. Those admitted through the Emergency Room may be registered through that department, depending upon hospital policy.

The following is an example of common criteria for admission to the Medical Short Stay Unit:

- Diabetes Mellitus
  - Blood sugar should be below 600.
  - No evidence of significant ketoacidosis (bicarbonate greater than 20).
- Congestive Heart Failure
  - Illness should be chronic rather than acute.
  - Require modest diuretic efforts and not complex cardiac drugs.
  - A response to treatment should be expected within 8 to 12 hours.
- Acute Bronchitis
  - Patient should have symptoms capable of response to brief treatment with respiratory therapy techniques, and chest x-ray should show no acute disease.
- Pneumonia
  - Acute pneumonias not requiring IV therapy, rather two courses IM therapy wherein a response is expected within 12 hours.
  - A diagnosis of pulmonary embolus is not considered.
  - Blood gases should be near normal values.
- Asthma
  - Patient should be without severe bronchospasm.
  - Patient should be without serious hypoxemia or CO_2 retention.

- Gastroenteritis
  - Patient should not have GI bleeding.
  - Patient should have no serious abdominal pain.
- Dehydration
  - Patients who are considered to be responsive to brief IV therapy.
- ASC Patients
  - Patients who have had a surgical procedure and are experiencing prolonged pain.
- Surgical work up
  - Patients requiring extensive testing prior to a surgical procedure.

Categories of Patients

- Patients admitted to the Unit for antibiotic, chemotherapy, and blood transfusion will be Category I. The procedure shall be prescheduled.
- Patients admitted for stabilization shall be Category II.
- Patients admitted for special procedures shall be Category III. The procedures are prescheduled.

Patients Not Eligible for MSSU

- Patients requiring intensive care or special equipment.
  - Cardiovascular monitoring.
  - Suctioning of airways.
- The patient who is unconscious, who demonstrates a deteriorating sensorium.
- Suspected MI/chest pain.
- Unstable angina/chest pain.
- Life-threatening arrhythmias.
- Suspected pulmonary embolus.
- GI bleeders.
- Vaginal bleeders.
- Possible ectopic pregnancies.
- Quadriplegics.
- Patients who require a Heparin infusion.
- Patients requiring isolation for infectious disease.
- Patients being observed for a seizure disorder.
- Patients suffering from symptoms of alcohol or drug withdrawal, or patients requiring psychiatric disposition.
- Patients less than 13 years old.
- Patients who need hospital admission.
- Patients scheduled for surgery.
- Patients who require a sitter.
- Patients who require Social Service disposition.

Transcription

At the end of this chapter sample admission orders have been provided. Use the symbols and methods you have been taught to transcribe each order.

TRANSFER OF PATIENTS

After patients have been admitted to a bed in a hospital unit, it may become necessary to transfer them elsewhere. Some transfers take place within the same nursing unit: the patient simply changes rooms. Other transfers may be between floors. The best time of day for a patient transfer is usually in the afternoon. This is because most patient care has been completed, patients have been discharged, and rooms are clean and ready to receive transfer patients. Whenever a doctor orders a patient transferred, the admitting office must be notified so that the census records can be corrected. (Fig. 17–8.) Another type of transfer is between hospitals, which will be discussed last.

KEY IDEA: TRANSFERS TO OTHER ROOMS

Transfer of a patient to another room in the same nursing unit may be made for the following reasons:

- A patient may have been admitted to a ward room because there were no private rooms available. Once a private room becomes vacant, however, he may be transferred.
- A patient may be asked to be transferred from a private room to a semiprivate room.
- A patient wishes to be with a smoker or a nonsmoker (although more and more hospitals are strictly forbidding smoking in the facility).
- The age or condition of another patient in the room may warrant the transfer to a more appropriate room.
- A patient may develop a postoperative wound infection and require transfer to an isolation unit on the same floor.

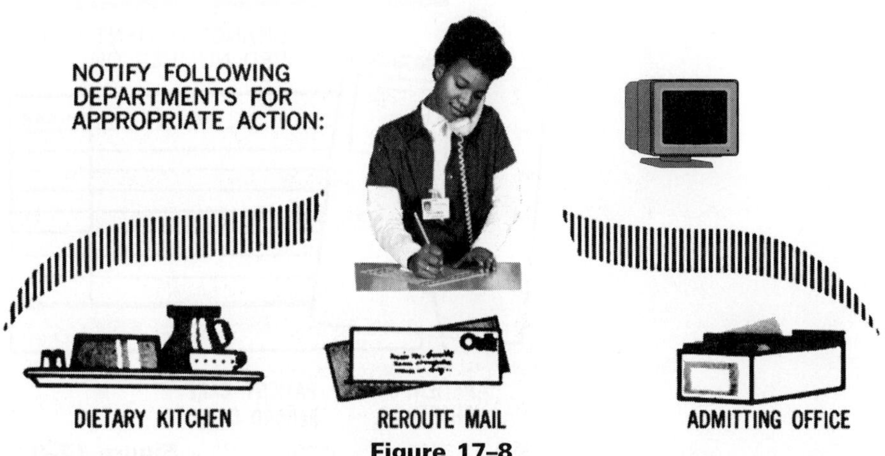
NOTIFY FOLLOWING DEPARTMENTS FOR APPROPRIATE ACTION:
DIETARY KITCHEN
REROUTE MAIL
ADMITTING OFFICE
Figure 17–8

Your duties in connection with transfers of patients to other rooms will be to make sure that the patient's records are kept in order and that their new locations are properly registered wherever necessary.

- The change in the patient's room and bed number must be made.
  - On the chart holder
  - On his Kardex, which must then be replaced in its holder in the newly designated place
  - On all of the patient's medicine tickets in current use
  - In the TPR book, if one is used in your hospital.
  - Any other forms, such as the diet sheet which contains the patient's name and room number, must also be changed.
- Take care to redirect the patient's visitors and mail to his new location in the unit. It is very important that a visitor not enter the room and simply find the patient gone! (Fig. 17–9.)

KEY IDEA: TRANSFERS TO OTHER UNITS

Patients are transferred to other nursing units because of a change in their condition and a change in the level of care that is required. For example, a patient's condition may worsen and he/she is transferred to the critical care unit, or it may improve and he/she is transferred to a less intensive level of care. When a patient is transferred, all orders cancel and must be reviewed and renewed.

Figure 17–10 shows a computer-generated patient transfer document. This document is often many pages long.

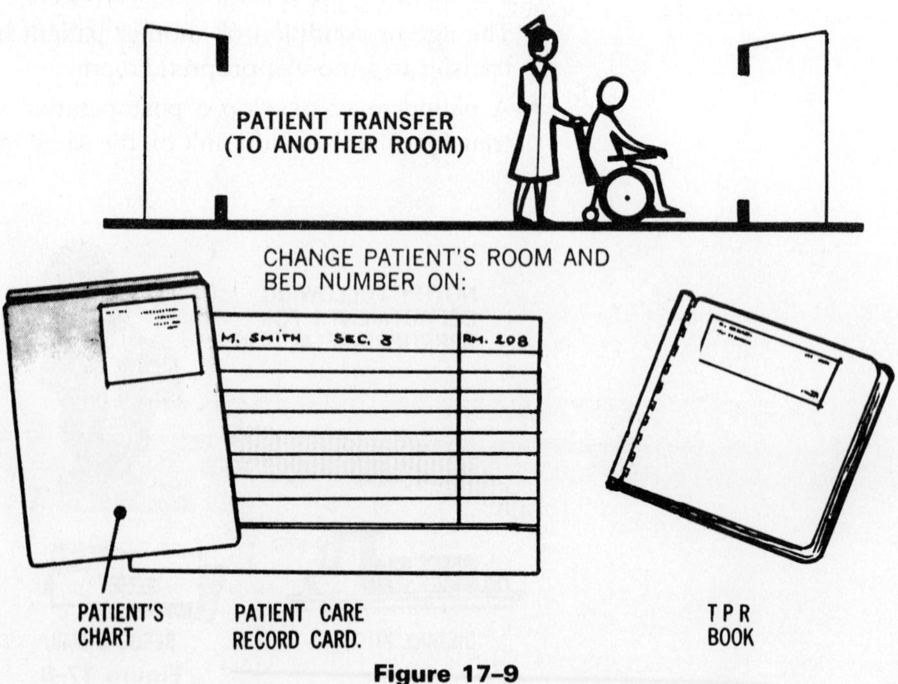

Figure 17–9

```
********** PATIENT TRANSFER DOCUMENT **********
_______________________________________________________________________________
 THIS IS A PERMANENT CHART DOCUMENT.  PLEASE PLACE IN CHART.  FAX TO PHARMACY
_______________________________________________________________________________
05/30/9X 16:49                                                        Page: 1

4MS  00000  EXAMPLE, IMA
F  60   DOB: 111737                   Pt. No: 100053677        Allergies:
64    150                             MR  No: 0000000000        PCN
Admit Date:  11/19/58 0000            Admit:  GOODDOCTOR JOHN   ASA
Isol:      Diab:                                                CODEINE
                                      Cons:   VERYFINE, MARY
_______________________________________________________________________________
  TRANSFER PATIENT:
                           ______ STAT
                           ______ WHEN BED AVAILABLE
                           ______ IN A.M.
                           ______ SPECIFY

              TO:
                           ______ CRITICAL CARE UNIT
                           ______ MEDICAL/SURGICAL UNIT
                           ______ TRANSITIONAL CARE UNIT
                           ______ BEHAVIORAL MEDICINE UNIT
                           ______ MATERNAL/CHILD HEALTH UNIT

ADMIT DX:     BRONCHITIS
CURRENT DX:   PNEUMONIA
              ARDS
UPDATE CURRENT DX AS FOLLOWS: ______________________________________

ATTENDING MD:  GOODDOCTOR, JOHN
UPDATE ATTENDING MD AS FOLLOWS:_____________________________________
_______________________________________________________________________________

    ALL PATIENT ORDERS HAVE BEEN REVIEWED BY THE PHYSICIAN SIGNED BELOW.
      ORDERS ARE TO BE REORDERED UNLESS INDICATED TO BE DISCONTINUED.

      ----- Laboratory ------------------------------    CONTINUE    D/C
  483 053097 URINE, CREATININE RANDOM

             COLLECT BY NURSE

                 ROUTINE                                  ______    ______
_______________________________________________________________________________
  717 053097 TYPE & SCREEN

             COLLECT BY LAB

                 ROUTINE                                  ______    ______
_______________________________________________________________________________


                               CONT.
```

Figure 17–10

KEY IDEA: RECEIVING TRANSFER PATIENTS

When a patient is transferred from another floor to your nursing unit, you will be responsible for many tasks similar to those carried out in connection with admission.

- When you expect a transfer patient, check with the responsible nursing personnel to make sure the new room is ready for the patient.
- When the patient arrives on the floor, you will be given his medical records and new identification plate.
- Place the chart in the proper chart holder.
- Change all necessary information (floor number, room number, bed number) on the Kardex and file it properly.
- Change the room and bed number on all the medication tickets and file them in the ticket holder according to the time of administration of the medication. You may need help from a nurse with this or other tasks; you should feel free to seek assistance if words or orders seem unfamiliar.
- Add the patient's name to your TPR book, diet sheet, and any other appropriate unit record.
- Make sure that the staff member responsible has oriented the patient to his new hospital environment. (Fig. 17–11.)

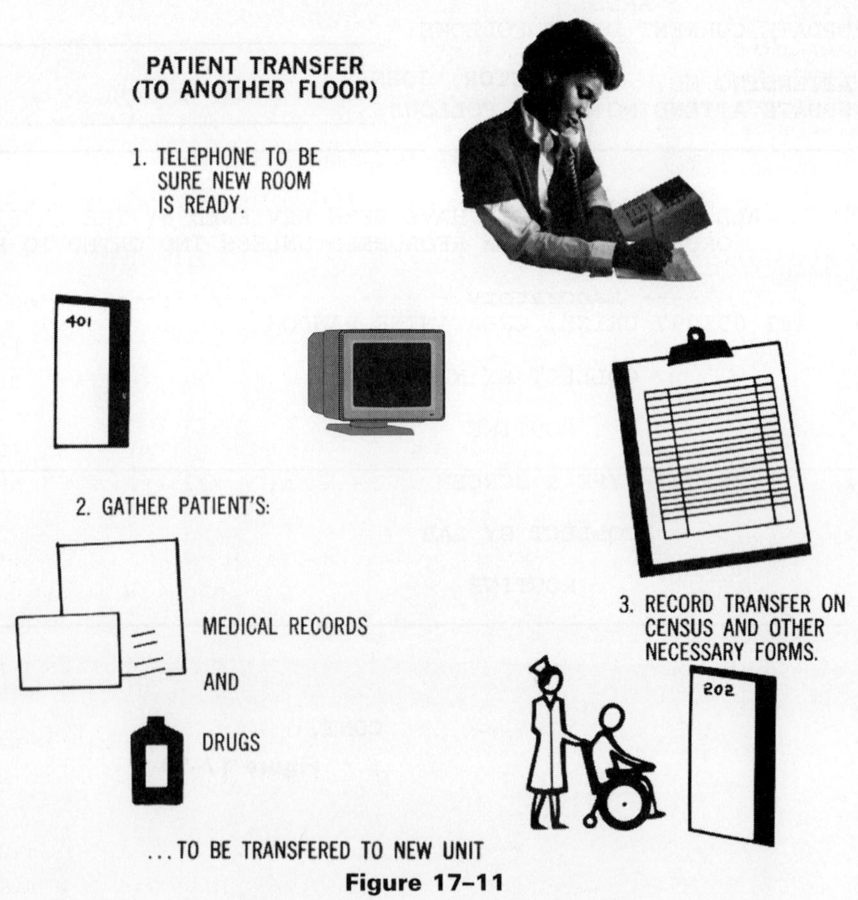

PATIENT TRANSFER
(TO ANOTHER FLOOR)
1. TELEPHONE TO BE SURE NEW ROOM IS READY.
401
2. GATHER PATIENT'S:
MEDICAL RECORDS
AND
DRUGS
3. RECORD TRANSFER ON CENSUS AND OTHER NECESSARY FORMS.
202
...TO BE TRANSFERED TO NEW UNIT

Figure 17–11

A patient who has been transferred, and his family, may be unnecessarily anxious about such a change because they do not fully understand the reasons for it. They may have become accustomed to the original hospital unit and might be apprehensive about the new one. In any direct meeting you may have with the patient or his visitors, be as reassuring and friendly as possible.

KEY IDEA: TRANSFER TO ANOTHER HOSPITAL

Sometimes a patient must be transferred from one hospital to another. This may be at the patient's request or it may be for another reason. Figures 17–12 and 17–13 show examples of forms used for this purpose. The patient in other respects is treated as a discharge.

DISCHARGE OF PATIENTS

Patients are normally discharged to their homes after correction of the medical condition for which they were admitted. Sometimes, however, additional care is needed and the patient is discharged to another medical institution with special facilities such as a nursing home. (Fig. 17–14, pg. 406.)

KEY IDEA: DISCHARGE PROCEDURES

The following outline of patient discharge procedures will give you an understanding of how your own duties fit into the entire patient discharge process.

- An order to discharge a patient must be written by the physician on the doctor's order sheet.
- In most hospitals, patients to be discharged must leave by a certain time in the morning so that their rooms can be cleaned and prepared for new patients.
- The patient may need a follow-up appointment with his private physician or with the clinic if he is a service patient.
- The nurse performs all ordered treatments a final time before the patient is discharged, and checks to see that the patient thoroughly understands the doctor's instructions about such matters as diet, medications, or further treatment. He or she must also write a final discharge note on the nurses' notes.
- The patient/significant other has received discharge education (Fig. 17–15, pg. 407) and the patient discharge record is completed (Fig. 17–16, pg. 408).
- Another department, such as social services or discharge planning, has seen the patient.
- Members of the nursing staff help the patient prepare for discharge by assembling his belongings and, if necessary, helping him dress. Valuables are returned.
- When the patient is ready to leave he must be accompanied by a friend or relative. Any exceptions require written permission from the doctor.

________ **Patient Request for Transfer**
Initials

This is to certify that ______________________________,
Name of Patient

a patient who has received services in this hospital, is being transferred at the request of the patient (or the patient's legal representative).

I acknowledge that I have been informed of the risk and consequences potentially involved in the transfer, the possible benefits of continuing treatment at this hospital, and the alternatives (if any) to the transfer I am requesting. I hereby release the attending physician, any other physicians involved in the patient's care, the hospital and its agents and employees, from all responsibility for any ill effects which may result from the transfer.

________ **Patient Transfer Acknowledgement**
Initials

I understand that I have a right to receive medical screening, examination, and evaluation by a physician, or appropriate personnel, without regard to my ability to pay, prior to any transfer from this hospital and that I have a right to be informed of the reasons for any transfer. I acknowledge that I have received medical screening examination, and evaluation by a physician, or other appropriate personnel, and that I have been informed of the following reasons for my transfer.

________ **Authorization to Release Medical Records**
Initials

Physician Certification

I ____, the undersigned physician, have examined and evaluated
Name of Physician

____. Based on this examination, the information available to me at the time, and the reasonable risks and benefits to the patient, I have concluded for the reasons which follow that the medical benefits reasonably expected from the provision of emergency treatment at another facility outweigh the increased risks to the patient's medical condition involved in the transfer process.

Please explain: ____
____

________	________	X ________	X ________
Date	**Time**	**E D Physician**	**Other Physician (if applicable)**
________	________	X ________	________
Date	**Time**	**Patient**	**Relationship if signed by other than patient**
________	________	X ________	
Date	**Time**	**Witness**	

ADDRESSOGRAPH

MEMORIAL HOSPITAL

PATIENT TRANSFER

White – Receiving Facility **Canary** – Medical Records **Pink** – Nursing Unit

Figure 17–12

ACUTE INTERHOSPITAL PATIENT TRANSFER FORM

PATIENT:____________________ DATE:__________

ADDRESS:____________________ TIME OF DISCHARGE:__________

____________________ D.O.B.__________ AGE:__________

DIAGNOSIS:____________________

PATIENT'S CONDITION AT TIME OF TRANSFER: ❐ Stable ❐ Unstable ❐ Critical ❐ Serious

❐ Fair ❐ Satisfactory ❐ Other:__________

REASON FOR TRANSFER:____________________

____

ADDITIONAL COMMENTS:____________________

PHYSICIAN ORDERING TRANSFER:____________________

HOSPITAL ACCEPTING PATIENT:____________________

PHYSICIAN ACCEPTING PATIENT:____________________

DETAILS OF PHYSICIAN TO PHYSICIAN CONTACT:____________________

NAME OF RESPONSIBLE PARTY/FAMILY:____________________

TRANSPORT MODE: ❐ Ambulance ❐ BLS ❐ ALS ❐ Paramedic ❐ Taxi ❐ Private

❐ Other:____________________ Transport Service:__________

Accompanied by:____________________

VITAL SIGNS ON TRANSFER: Time:____:____ P____ R____ BP____ /____

I.V. PATIENT: Solution__________ Amount Remaining__________ Amount Given__________

RECORDS ACCOMPANYING PATIENT: ❐ PATIENT TRANSFER FORM ❐ WRITTEN TRANSFER

ORDERS (medication, fluids, etc.) ❐ X-RAYS (___originals___copies) ❐ EKG ❐ ED

HOSPITAL ADMIT FORM/CHART

LAB RESULTS____________________

OTHER____________________

PERSONAL EFFECTS____________________

NAME AND SIGNATURE OF PHYSICIAN:____________________

NAME AND SIGNATURE OF NURSE:____________________

REPORT IS COMPLETE: (Signature)____________________

MEMORIAL HOSPITAL ACUTE INTERHOSPITAL PATIENT TRANSFER FORM	Addressograph

Figure 17–13

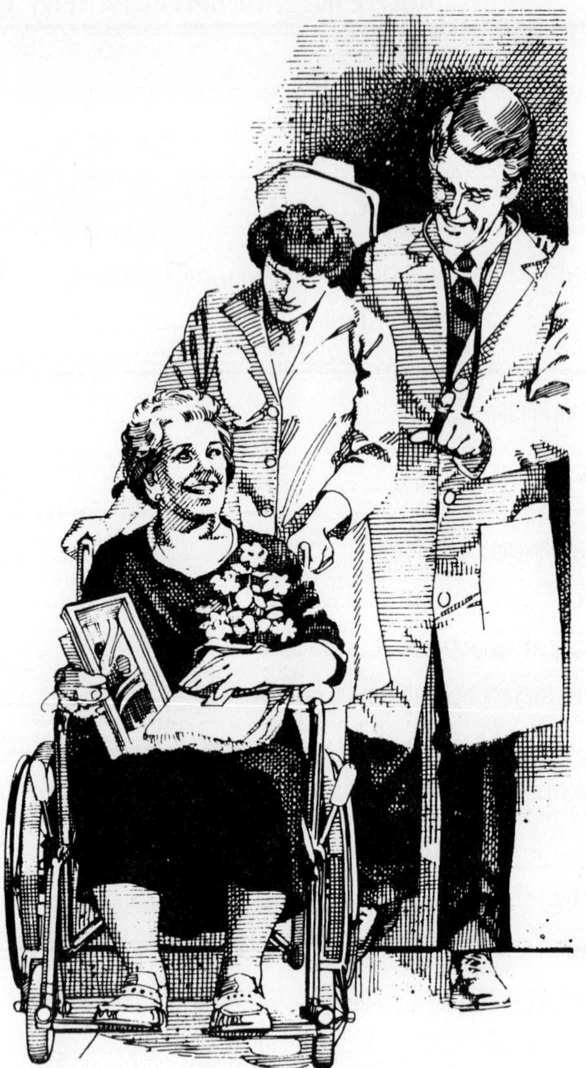

Figure 17–14

After the patient is discharged, the following procedures must be completed:

1. The diet kitchen must be notified so meals are not sent to the floor for that patient.
2. Other departments such as admitting and the laboratory may be notified. If medications that have been charged to the patient remain on the nursing unit, they must be returned to the pharmacy so the patient's account can be credited.
3. The physician must complete the discharge summary on the summary sheet.
4. The order of the chart forms must be rearranged when the patient is discharged and the reassembled chart must be delivered to the medical records room where it will be filed.

PATIENT/SIGNIFICANT OTHER EDUCATION LOG

PRIMARY DX:

OTHER MEDICAL PROBLEMS/DX:

FAMILY/SIGNIFICANT OTHERS	1 -	2 -

PHYSICAL/COGNITIVE DEFICIT/LIMITATION:

SPECIAL LEARNING NEEDS/REQUESTS:

DISCHARGE PLANNING FOLLOW-UP/RESOURCES:

EDUCATION TOPIC	INSTRUCTION GIVEN	DEMONSTRATION GIVEN	VERBALIZES KNOWLEDGE	DEMONSTRATES SKILLS	NEEDS COMPLETE REINFORCEMENT	RESOURCES USED COMMENTS
Safe and effective use of medication.	PT/SO:	PT/SO:	PT/SO:	PT/SO:	PT/SO:	
	DATE/INITIALS:	DATE/INITIALS:	DATE/INTITALS:	DATE/INITIALS:	DATE/INITIALS:	
Safe and effective use of medical equipment.	PT/SO:	PT/SO:	PT/SO:	PT/SO:	PT/SO:	
	DATE/INITIALS:	DATE/INITIALS:	DATE/INITIALS:	DATE/INITIALS:	DATE/INITIALS:	
Potential drug/food interactions.	PT/SO:	PT/SO:	PT/SO:	PT/SO:	PT/SO:	
	DATE/INITIALS:	DATE/INITIALS:	DATE/INITIALS:	DATE/INITIALS:	DATE/INITIALS:	
Dietary consult on modified diets.	PT/SO:	PT/SO:	PT/SO:	PT/SO:	PT/SO:	
	DATE/INITIALS:	DATE/INITIALS:	DATE/INITIALS:	DATE/INITIALS:	DATE/INITIALS:	
Rehabilitation techniques to facilitate independence in ADL's.	PT/SO:	PT/SO:	PT/SO:	PT/SO:	PT/SO:	
	DATE/INITIALS:	DATE/INITIALS:	DATE/INITIALS:	DATE/INITIALS:	DATE/INITIALS:	
	PT/SO:	PT/SO:	PT/SO:	PT/SO:	PT/SO:	
	DATE/INITIALS:	DATE/INITIALS:	DATE/INITIALS:	DATE/INITIALS:	DATE/INITIALS:	
	PT/SO:	PT/SO:	PT/SO:	PT/SO:	PT/SO:	
	DATE/INITIALS:	DATE/INITIALS:	DATE/INITIALS:	DATE/INITIALS:	DATE/INITIALS:	
	PT/SO:	PT/SO:	PT/SO:	PT/SO:	PT/SO:	
	DATE/INITIALS:	DATE/INITIALS:	DATE/INITIALS:	DATE/INITIALS:	DATE/INITIALS:	
	PT/SO:	PT/SO:	PT/SO:	PT/SO:	PT/SO:	
	DATE/INITIALS:	DATE/INITIALS:	DATE/INITIALS:	DATE/INITIALS:	DATE/INITIALS:	
	PT/SO:	PT/SO:	PT/SO:	PT/SO:	PT/SO:	
	DATE/INITIALS:	DATE/INITIALS:	DATE/INITIALS:	DATE/INITIALS:	DATE/INITIALS:	

SIGNATURE:	INITIALS:	DISCIPLINE:	ADDRESSOGRAPH
PT/SIGNIFICANT OTHER EDUCATION LOG			

Figure 17–15

NURSING DISCHARGE SUMMARY

Dismissed by M.D. ☐ Yes ☐ No ☐ Released ☐ AMA Release Signed

☐ Ambulatory ☐ Wheelchair ☐ Ambulance Accompanied by ______

Discharge to: ☐ Home ☐ SNF ☐ Other ______

Vital Signs: T ____ P ____ R ____ B/P ______

Afebrile for 24 hrs. (< 99.6) ______ Temp. Above 99.6 ______ M.D. Notified ______

Mental Status: ☐ Alert ☐ Oriented ☐ Cooperative ☐ Confused ☐ Other ______

COMPLIANCE	YES	NO	COMMENTS
Understands physical condition			
Willing to comply with regimen			
States understanding of instructions			

SELF CARE:	INDEPEND	ASSIST	DEP	SELF CARE:	INDEPEND	ASSIST	DEP
Ambulatory				Dressing			
Turns self in bed				Transfer to W.C.			
Personal Hygiene				Other			

CONDITION OF SKIN	YES	NO	LOCATION/DESCRIPTION
Bruises			
Rashes			
Reddened Areas			
Pressure Ulcer			
Wound/Incision			

IMPAIRMENT	YES	NO	LOCATION/DESCRIPTION
Speech			
Hearing			
Vision			
Paralysis			
Contracture			

Bladder: ☐ Continent ☐ Incontinent ☐ Catheter Type: ______ ☐ Other ______

Bowel: ☐ Continent ☐ Incontinent ☐ Ostomy ☐ Other ______

Date ____/____/____ Time ______ Nurse Signature:

PATIENT DISCHARGE INSTRUCTIONS

DISCHARGE MEDICINES AND MEDICATION INSTRUCTIONS:

POST-DISCHARGE INSTRUCTIONS: (i.e. Diet, Activity, Equipment, Physical Therapy, Respiratory Therapy, Pharmacy, Support Group)

Office Appointment: Doctor______ return to the office in____days / week. Please call______for an appointment.

DISCHARGE PLANNING

EQUIPMENT ______ COMPANY ______ Telephone (   ) ______

HOME HEALTH CARE ______ Telephone (   ) ______

OTHER ______ Telephone (   ) ______

AUTHORIZATION: I acknowledge that the above information has been explained to me. I have had the opportunity to clarify any questions. I have received a copy of these instructions.

SIGNATURE

PATIENT / FAMILY SIGNATURE ______ RELATIONSHIP ______ DATE ______

PATIENT DISCHARGE RECORD

SC W46 (2/94) WHITE - CHART Canary - Patient Pink - Physician

Figure 17–16

KEY IDEA: DISCHARGE AND HEALTH UNIT COORDINATOR RESPONSIBILITIES

Following is a list of instructions to guide you in discharging patients:

- Make sure that a written order for discharge is included on the doctor's order sheet.
- Check with the patient to make certain that he knows the time by which he must leave the hospital in order to avoid additional expense, that he has someone coming to accompany him home, and that he has a follow-up appointment.
- If the patient does not have anyone to accompany him from the hospital, you may have to notify his doctor to write a taxi permission order.
- If the person is a service patient, you will be responsible for calling the clinic by telephone for a follow-up appointment and writing up an appointment slip to give the patient.
- If the person is a private patient, you may need to call his doctor or the doctor's office to arrange for a follow-up appointment.
- If the patient needs special diet instructions, you may need to call the diet kitchen to arrange for a dietitian to come up to the floor and explain the instructions.
- If patients in your hospital do not routinely stop at the business office on their way out of the hospital, find out which patients must do so before leaving, according to the procedure in use at your hospital.
- Check to see what valuables are returned to the patient.
- If the patient is a "police case," permission for discharge home must be obtained from the local police department.
- Notify the diet kitchen of the patient's discharge.
- Add the patient's name to your daily census records as a discharge.
- Record the discharge of the patient in the discharge and transfer book if one is used.
- Rearrange the chart forms in proper sequence for discharge. Remove and discard all blank forms and send the chart to the medical record room.
- In many hospitals, a written notice of discharge must be sent to other departments, such as the admitting and business offices. The instructor will explain the regulations in use in your hospital.

When you have completed your training course, you will also be responsible for transcribing the discharge orders written by the doctor and returning medications to the pharmacy for credit, as necessary. (Fig. 17–17.)

KEY IDEA: DISCHARGE TO ANOTHER FACILITY

Patients are not always discharged directly to their homes. The Joint Commission on Accreditation of Health Care Organizations (JCAHO) requires that accredited hospitals that accept Medicare patients review the condition of all patients who remain in the hospital longer than a certain prescribed amount of time. A JCAHO accredited hospital must have a Utilization Review Committee for this purpose.

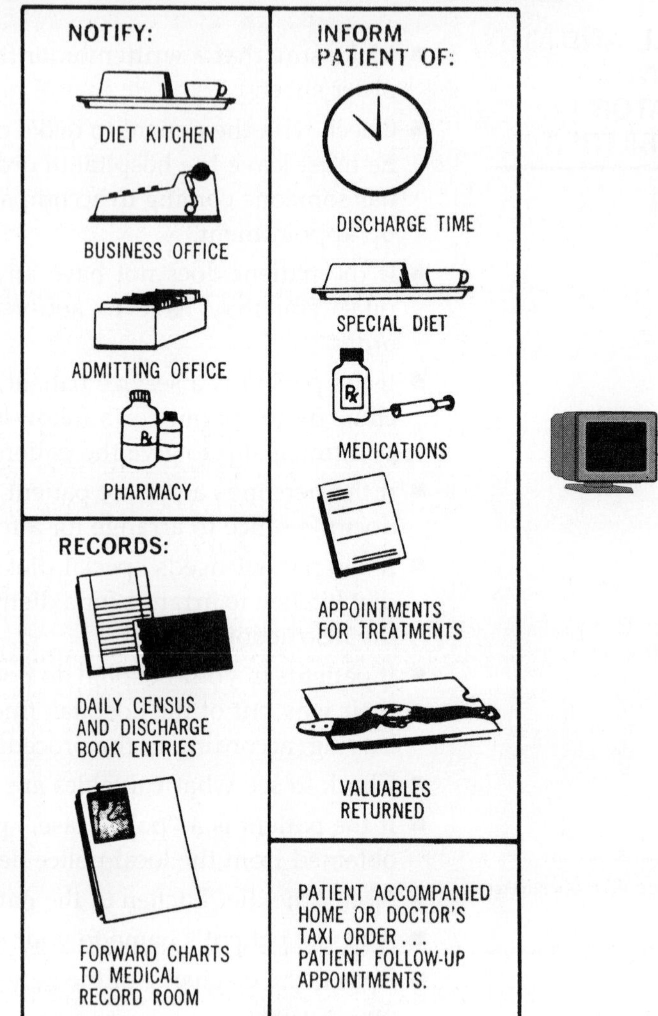

Figure 17–17

When the committee deems that a patient no longer requires "acute nursing care," the doctor is asked to transfer the patient to an extended care facility (ECF). An ECF is also called a convalescent or nursing home.

The discharge of a patient to an ECF is similar to a routine discharge except that:

- The bed patient will likely require transportation to the new facility by ambulance.
- A special form for interhospital transfer will be required. This form will often be partially completed by the health unit coordinator and partially by nursing. Photocopies of the patient's chart are made by medical records and placed in an envelope to be sent with the ambulance attendant or the family to the new facility.

The procedure for routine discharge is then completed by the health unit coordinator.

KEY IDEA: DISCHARGE AGAINST MEDICAL ADVICE (AMA)

On occasion, a patient will decide that he does not want to remain in the hospital, even though his doctor feels that he is not yet well enough to go home. The patient may believe that the doctors and nurses are not helping him to get better. He may think he is well enough to go home despite the doctor's opinion, or he may simply be tired and depressed by a lengthy hospitalization. Whatever his reasons, you can encourage him to stay, but you cannot prevent him from leaving, if he wants to go.

If this situation should arise, steps must be taken to protect the hospital and its personnel from liability in case of serious medical consequences arising from premature discharge. As a health unit coordinator you have certain responsibilities to the patient who insists on leaving the hospital against the advice of his doctor.

- First, notify the nurse in charge who will ask you to call the patient's attending physician, or the chief resident, if the person is a service patient. In most hospitals, you would also notify the nursing service office.
- A special release form must be signed by the patient or, if he is unable to sign, by the next of kin. The signature must be obtained before witnesses.
- Once this release is signed and the patient and/or family are fully aware of the possible consequences of premature discharge, your responsibilities and duties are the same as for any routine discharge.

DISCHARGE ORDERS

KEY IDEA: TYPES OF DISCHARGE ORDERS

If the patient has fully recovered and needs little or no follow-up care or detailed home instruction, the doctor may write simple discharge orders on the day of discharge, for example:

> ***Discharge home in P.M.***
> ***Make 6-week follow-up clinic appointment.***

Ordinarily, however, discharge orders are written prior to the actual day of discharge and include more details. Orders from the following categories are usually included.

Discharge

The doctor must always state in writing that the patient is to be discharged and must include the date and time of day. The order may also specify where the patient is to be discharged and by what means (e.g., he may be discharged to his home or to a nursing home; he may be leaving by ambulance or by taxi).

Medications

In some hospitals, the pharmacy provides the patient with medications he must continue to take at home. If this is the case, the doctor will write an order for the medications, and they must be requisitioned from the pharmacy.

Follow-up Appointments

Many patients are discharged from the hospital to convalesce at home. Ordinarily, every patient who has been hospitalized is advised to continue under a doctor's care until recovery is complete. Most doctors will write discharge orders for follow-up appointments which include the date or time the patient is expected to see him or visit the clinic.

Special Instructions

Many patients must be taught to perform simple tasks related to their illnesses which they will carry out at home. Some patients will be taught to change dressings on draining wounds. Others may require special diet instructions. Diabetics must often learn to test their own urine or blood for glucose and to give their own insulin injections. This instruction is the responsibility of the patient educator who is usually a nurse.

Other Discharge Orders

Discharge orders that do not fall into any of the categories already discussed may include:

Disposable-type enema on A.M. of discharge, if pt. has not defecated during previous 24 hours.
Change dressing before discharge.
Notify brother of impending discharge.
Send pt. home c̄ elastic stockings in place.

KEY IDEA: TRANSCRIPTION

Transcribe the group of discharge orders shown below.

Discharge home Tuesday A.M.
Teach urine testing prior to discharge.
Have dietitian discuss diabetic diet c̄ pt. and wife.
To diabetic follow-up clinic in 4 weeks.
Instruct pt. in care of leg ulcer.
Order Colace tab. $\dot{\bar{\text{i}}}$ p.o. q.d. h.s.
Order Multivitamins tabs. $\ddot{\bar{\text{ii}}}$ p.o. a.m.

PATIENT DEATHS

Some patients who enter a health care institution are terminally ill, that is, dying. Sometimes death is sudden or unexpected. More often it is not. Nursing's first responsibility is to help make the patient as comfortable as possible. Their second responsibility is to assist in meeting the emotional needs of the patient and his family.

The most important single fact to remember about the dying patient is that he is just as important as the patient who is going to recover. It is the goal of the health care team to help a human being to end his life in peace, comfort, and dignity. Everyone must die. Surely we would all prefer to die in reassuring and comfortable surroundings.

In the presence of death, there are certain attitudes your hospital expects of you—toward yourself, the dying patient, and his family. Try to adopt these attitudes with sympathy and tact.

- First, try hard to avoid becoming emotionally involved in deaths and medical tragedies. To show sympathy and quiet understanding for the misfortunes of others at such a time is praiseworthy, but to identify yourself with a dying patient will prevent you from extending the warmth and understanding necessary at such times.
- Second, you must never forget that most people fear the uncertainty of death. You must learn to accept the patient regardless of his reactions or his possible unreasonableness to you or other members of the staff. Never categorize patients as "good" or "bad." Simply try to appreciate the difficulties they face and learn to accept their behavior.
- Finally, you must respect the feelings of the patient's family when they come to visit the patient. Under the pressure of helplessness and anxiety, these visitors may not always act reasonably. Accept their behavior and try to help them through a difficult period.

When it is known that death is approaching, the dying patient's family may want to spend a lot of time with him. This is usually permitted as much as possible. Be as helpful to them as you can. You might suggest that they have a cup of coffee. Tell them where the coffee shop is. Also, learn the policy in your institution of serving meals to visitors. You may be able to arrange for trays to be delivered to the patient's family at mealtimes. If this is not allowed, tell the visitors where they can find the cafeteria or a nearby restaurant. Make sure the visitors know the location of the restrooms, lounge, telephones, and chapel.

KEY IDEA: SIGNS OF APPROACHING DEATH

Death comes in different ways. It may come quite suddenly after a patient has seemed to be recovering. Or it may come after a long period during which there has been a steady decline of body functions. Death also may result from complications during convalescence. Here are some signs showing that death may be near:

- Blood circulation slows down. The patient's hands and feet are cold to the touch.
- If the patient is conscious, he may complain that he is cold.
- The patient's face may become pale because of decreased circulation.
- His eyes may be staring blankly into space. There may be no eye movement when the nurse's hand moves across his line of vision.
- The patient may perspire heavily, even though his body is cold.
- The patient loses muscle tone, and his body becomes limp. His jaw may drop, and his mouth may stay partly open.
- Respirations may become slower and more difficult.
- Mucus collecting in the patient's throat and bronchial tubes may cause a sound that is sometimes called the "death rattle."
- The pulse often is rapid, but it becomes weak and irregular.
- Just before death, respiration stops and the pulse gets very faint. The nurse may not be able to feel the patient's pulse at all.
- Contrary to popular belief, a dying person is rarely in great pain. As the patient's condition gets worse, less blood may be flowing to the brain. Therefore, the patient may feel little or no pain.

In some health care institutions, the head nurse or team leader confirms that a patient has no pulse or has stopped breathing and she can call a "code." Code Blue, Cardiac Arrest, or whatever name is used for the code in your institution, is an emergency announcement to the entire staff. As previously discussed, a preassigned team will come to help the patient. Only when the team fails to keep the patient alive is the patient declared to be dead by a physician.

After a patient's death, his body still is treated with respect and is given gentle care. If family members are present, they usually wait outside the room until the doctor has finished his examination. The patient's family will probably be allowed to view the body if they wish.

Sometimes the family is not present when the patient dies. In this case, the nurse calls the doctor and tells him the family is not there. Either the doctor or the nurse then notifies the family and finds out whether they wish to view the body before it is sent to the morgue. If so, the body stays in the room until the family arrives.

When the family is present, they may be given the patient's personal belongings which they sign for. These items are checked against the clothing list to be sure that everything is accounted for. You will learn the procedure in your health care institution for taking care of the deceased patient's clothes. If the members of the family do not wish to view the body, the nurse will then proceed with the postmortem care.

KEY IDEA: POSTMORTEM PROCEDURE

Although, as a health unit coordinator, you will have no direct responsibility for postmortem procedures, it will help you to be familiar with them. After the patient has been pronounced dead, nursing personnel carry out postmortem (after death) care.

- The body must be cleaned, the eyes and jaw closed, and the limbs positioned in good body alignment. If members of the family are present, they are often allowed to view the body at this time.
- Following this, the limbs are carefully tied together and the body is carefully wrapped in a large sheet, called a shroud. Policies will differ somewhat on this procedure.

The body is then placed on a special stretcher. It is covered with a sheet and removed to the morgue. It is stored in a large refrigerator there until the family has made funeral arrangements with a mortician. The mortician, having obtained proper authorization, removes the body from hospital premises.

KEY IDEA: PATIENT DEATHS AND HEALTH UNIT COORDINATOR RESPONSIBILITIES

As a health unit coordinator, your duties at the time of a patient's death will be primarily clerical, although you may often be asked to make necessary telephone calls. Below are some of the responsibilities you may be assigned:

- You may be asked to locate, by paging or by telephone, the patient's doctor for certification of death.
- You may be expected to notify the nursing service office, the reception or information desk, and sometimes the business office and admitting office. This may be done by telephone, computer, or in writing.
- For situations in which the deceased patient's family cannot be reached by telephone by the doctor or nurse, your hospital will have regulations specifying who should be notified to contact the family. In small communities, this responsibility is often given to the police department.
- The death certificate is usually processed for the physician's completion and signature by the admitting office or the medical records department. You may be asked to expedite this form by taking a copy from the file upon request.
- You must have a stamped autopsy consent form ready if it is to be used.
- You may be required to requisition a shroud pack for use in wrapping the body.
- You may be asked to prepare identification tags to be used on the body in several places and in the morgue.
- You may be responsible for collecting and identifying the patient's personal belongings, and sending them to a designated hospital area, if the family is not at hand.
- You must add the patient's name to the daily census record as a death and record the proper information in summary records, such as a discharge and transfer book.
- Finally, you will be required to assemble the patient's chart records in discharge sequence and send them to the medical records room. The patient's name should be deleted from all current hospital records in use on the unit. Any other procedures associated with a routine discharge,

such as returning medications to the pharmacy for credit, are also carried out if they apply to the deceased patient's situation.

KEY IDEA: CERTIFICATION OF DEATH

This can take place only after examination by a physician. The death certificate is signed by the doctor, and permission to perform an autopsy is usually requested from the family.

Autopsies

Autopsies are dissections of the corpse. They are performed to determine the extent of disease and the cause of death. They cannot be done routinely without the permission of the family. The signed permission of the next of kin is

AUTHORIZATION FOR AUTOPSY

TO: PATHOLOGIST, MEMORIAL HOSPITAL DATED: ________ 19 ___

I certify that I am the ______________________
(Relationship)

of ______________ deceased, and have the right to control the disposition of the remains of said decedent. I hereby authorize you, together with your assistants, to perform an autopsy and complete post mortem examination on the body of such deceased, including the taking of photographs, and the removal of such structures or organs as you may deem necessary for special study or for therapeutic or scientific uses as provided in the health and safety code.

I also authorize the pathologist to have present at the examination such person or persons as he may deem proper.

I also authorize any cemetery authority, licensed funeral director or licensed hospital, having custody of such remains, through its authorized personnel, to permit or assist in such autopsy and examination including the transportation of the remains by any such cemetery authority or funeral director to and from the hospital or other place as may be arranged by you for such autopsy and examination.

WITNESS: ______________ SIGNED ______________

WITNESS: ______________ SIGNED ______________

The nurse is instructed to list the names of the physicians to whom reports are to be sent. These are physicians who have attended the patient on present or previous admission.

ATTENDING PHYSICIAN ______________ M.D.

SURGICAL CONSULTANT ______________ M.D.

MEDICAL CONSULTANT ______________ M.D.

UROLOGIC CONSULTANT ______________ M.D.

OTHER PHYSICIANS WHO ATTENDED THE DECEASED ______________ M.D.

______________ M.D.

INSTRUCTIONS:

1. The autopsy permission is to be completed in duplicate and witnessed.
2. Both copies of autopsy premission, with hospital chart, are brought to the pathologist's office.
3. Notify the pathologist and he will arrange the time of the post mortem examination.
4. When the post mortem exam is completed, the pathology office will notify nursing supervisor when the remains may be released to the mortician.

Figure 17–18

(Complete this in duplicate—one for the mortician)

AUTHORITY FOR RELEASE OF REMAINS

PART I: MEMORIAL HOSPITAL

Release Remains of ______

To Mortician ______ Address ______

______

Date ______ Signed ______

Relationship ______

PART II: RECEIVED FROM MEMORIAL HOSPITAL THE PERSONAL EFFECTS LISTED BELOW:

______ ______

______ ______

______ ______

______ ______

______ ______

______ ______

Date ______ Signed ______

Witness ______

PART III: REMAINS RECEIVED:

Date ______ Mortuary ______

Signed ______

INFORMATION FOR MORTICIAN

Date of Death ______ Hour ______

Attending Physician ______

Address ______

Telephone Number ______

Figure 17–19

given in a special chart form called the autopsy consent. (Figs. 17–18 and 17–19.)

Coroner's Cases

In coroner's cases, hospital personnel are not allowed to approach the family for autopsy authorization; the responsibility for conducting the autopsy lies with the coroner. Usually, the local, county, or state government will have regulations defining coroner's cases. For example, cases of deaths occurring within 24 hours after hospitalization, or of victims of suspected poisoning, or of apparently accidental deaths may be considered coroner's cases in your locality.

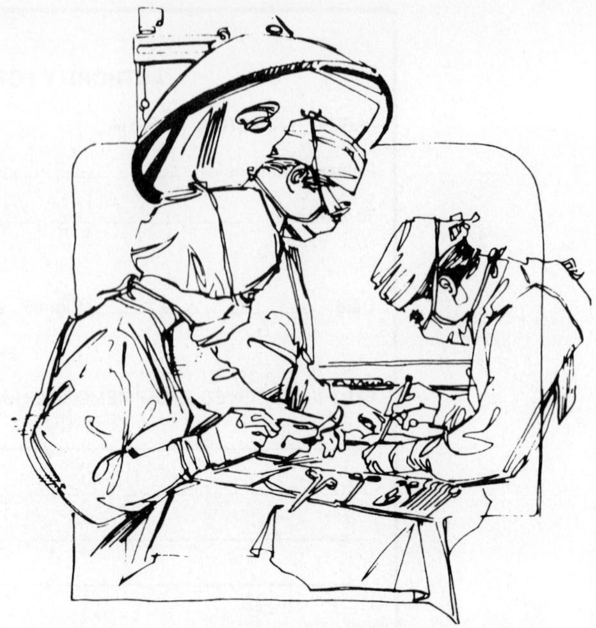

Figure 17–20

SURGICAL ORDERS

Surgical patients require an operation because of illness or injury. (Fig. 17–20.) Surgical patients can be divided into three groups:

1. **Preoperative** . . . before the operation.
2. **Intraoperative** . . . those in the process of having an operation.
3. **Postoperative** . . . after the operation.

KEY IDEA: TYPES OF SURGERY

Surgery may be divided into several categories:

- Optional (Elective)—done totally at the patient's request.
- Required—must be performed within a certain time frame (usually no more than two weeks).
- Urgent—needs surgery within one to two days.
- Emergency—immediate intervention is necessary.

Surgery may also be performed on an out-patient or in-patient basis.

Outpatient (Ambulatory) Surgery

Outpatient surgery provides care for patients scheduled for selected diagnostic procedures, surgical intervention, and other specified treatment modalities of an elective nature. Patients are not admitted overnight. It is designed for the type of surgery which is of short duration, where risk and probability of complications are low, and recovery period is minimal. (Fig. 17–21.)

Figure 17–22 shows an example of an outpatient surgery record.

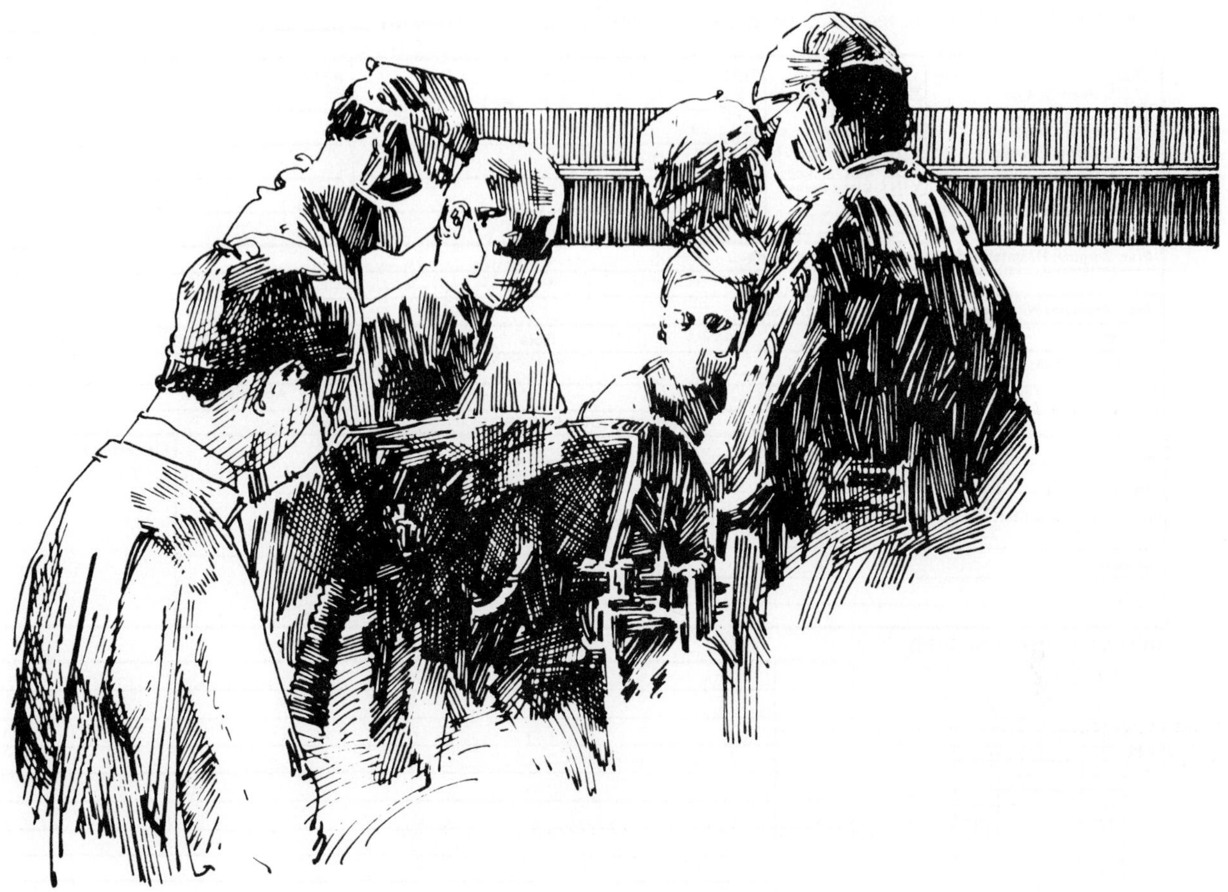

Figure 17–21

The following is a list of surgeries and procedures that might be scheduled on an outpatient basis:

PROCEDURES

- Gynecological
  - Bartholin Cystectomy
  - Dilation and Curettage
  - Examination under Anesthesia
  - Hymenotomy
  - Laparoscopy, Diagnostic
  - Laparoscopy with Tubal Ligation
  - Removal of I.U.D.
- **Neurosurgical**
  - Carpal Tunnel
  - Alcohol Injection of Nerve and Coagulation of Nerves for Control of Pain
  - Intercostal Neurectomy
  - Excision of Neuroma
  - Morton's Neuroma
- **Orthopedic**
  - (Without Use of Image Intensifier)
  - Closed Reduction—Fracture
  - Ganglion
  - Removal of Orthopedic Appliance (e.g. screws, Steinman pins)
  - Tenotomy, Hand or Foot
  - Excision of Foreign Body
  - Exostosis, Excision (Small)
  - Release of Tendon Sheath

ADMITTING RECORD Rm. No. ____ DATE ____ TIME ____ Procedure ____

Nickname ____
Y N Heart Disease
Y N Lung Disease
Y N Liver Disease
Y N Kidney Disease
Y N Diabetes/ Hypoglycemia
Y N Bleeding
Y N G.I. Disease
Y N ↑ B.P.
Height ____
Weight ____

Y N Dentures
Y N Contact Lenses
Y N Jewelry
Y N Smoke
Y N Cough/Sob
Y N Mot. Sickness Dizzy Faint

TEMP. ____ P. ____ R. ____ B.P. ____
N.P.O. ____ Hct. ____ U/A ____
RIDE ____
DRUGS ____
When Drugs Taken Last:

Allergies ____
C of A ____ H & P ____

Prev. Surgery, Hospitalizations and / or Same Procedure:

Prev. Problems With Medication and / or Same Procedure:

I.V. Sol. Size Site Rate Patent ☐ DSG ☐ HEP. LOC ☐

MEDICATIONS:

Admitted By

PROCEDURE RECORD

Procedure ____
Doctor ____
Procedure Time:—Start ____ Finish ____ Total ____
Diagnosis:
Nurse: ____ R.N.

Dressings

Supplies Used

Medications

RECOVERY ROOM RECORD

TIME

280 260 240 220 200 180 160 140 120 100 80 60 40 20 15 10 5

Total Recovery Rm Time ____

Start ____ Finish ____

Time Of Discharge ____ BY: ____

REMARKS AND TREATMENTS

P.O. Intake:	Voided:	I.V. Intake:

OUTPATIENT PROCEDURES
NURSING ASSESSMENT

Figure 17–22

- Debridement, Irrigation, and Closure (Small)
- Hand Surgery

- **Plastic Surgery**
  - Augmentation Mammoplasty
  - Dermabrasion
  - Otoplasty
  - Skin Graft
  - Face Lift
  - Face Lift with Blepharoplasty

- Blepharoplasty
  - Scar Revisions
  - Rhinoplasty and Septoplasty
  - Excision of Skin Tumors (Small)
- **Urological**
  - Circumcision
  - Dorsal Slit
  - Meatomy
  - Prostate Biopsy (Needle)
  - Urethral Dilation
  - Cystoscopy
  - Retrograde
  - TUR (M.D. Discretion—Minor)
- **Dental**
  - Peridontal
  - Extractions
  - Impacted Wisdom Teeth, Removal
- **Ear, Nose, and Throat**
  - Antral Puncture
  - Arch Bars, Removal
  - Closed Reduction, Nose or Zygoma
  - Inferior Turbinates Fracture
  - Myringotomy
  - Nasal Polypectomy
  - Septal Reconstruction, Submucous Resection
  - Adenoidectomy
- **Endoscopy**
  - Bronchoscopy
  - Cystoscopy
  - Cystoscopy and Retrograde
  - Esophogoscopy
- **Eye**
  - Cataract
  - Muscle Surgery
  - Chalazion
  - Discission
  - Plastic Surgery of the Eyelids
  - Eye Examination under General Anesthesia
  - Lacrimal Duct Probing
  - Pterygium
  - Insertion of Glass Tube into Lacrimal Duct
  - Laser Beam
- **General Surgery**
  - Breast Biopsy (Only)
  - Removal of Foreign Body
  - Hernioplasty
  - Node Biopsy
  - Muscle Biopsy
  - Soft Tissue Tumors
  - Scalene Node Biopsy
  - Umbilical Hernia
  - Rectal Polypectomy
  - Excision of Sebaceous Cyst
  - Excision of Skin Lesions
  - Evacuation of Hematoma
  - Liver Biopsy—Menghini Needle

The health unit coordinator working in Outpatient Surgery will be responsible for many of the clerical and receptionist duties described on the pages that follow. However, because the patient does not stay overnight (unless a change of condition warrants admission to the hospital), certain procedures will be modified based on hospital policy.

Below is a list of responsibilities of a Same Day or Outpatient Surgery health unit coordinator.

1. Keeps office in order and well supplied.
2. Greets physicians, offers assistance, and calls nurse in charge/nurse manager when needed.
3. Is aware of physicians and other personnel on the floor.

4. Answers telephone promptly and courteously. Gives name, position, and location. Relays messages promptly and accurately.
5. Relays telephone calls concerning patient's condition and physician's orders to the nurse in charge.
6. Answers patient's and visitor's questions promptly and courteously.
7. Handles communications daily and during emergencies.
8. Assists RN in obtaining central and pharmacy supplies and maintenance repairs.
9. Operates the computer.
10. Enters surgery, recovery, and special nursing procedures data in patient operative log.
11. Completes monthly utilization reports and distributes to medical records, surgery, utilization, and finance departments.
12. Collects scheduling slips from operating room and enters into Outpatient Surgery scheduling book.
13. Calls each patient for preadmitting information and instructions, and verifies time of surgery.
14. Arranges with patient when to come in for laboratory work, ECG, and x-rays.
15. Performs admitting functions to gather all pertinent information prior to or upon patient's arrival.
16. Obtains proper signatures on all necessary consents and explains consents to the patient. (Does not explain procedure.)
17. Records complete and accurate information for each admission and registration, obtaining copies of third-party payor information as necessary.
18. Obtains copies of insurance card/cards and insurance forms for chart.
19. Prepares patient charts.
20. Coordinates services of Outpatient Surgery Department and Business Office under supervision of admitting supervisor and charge nurse/nurse manager of Outpatient Surgery.
21. Schedules special nursing procedures under supervision of charge nurse/nurse manager.
22. Disassembles patient's charts for medical records after discharge.
23. Assists with counting, batching, charging, and delivery to data processing.
24. Performs other duties as assigned.

KEY IDEA: PREOPERATIVE PREPARATION

The nursing staff will prepare patients physically and emotionally for the impending surgery. Nursing personnel will shave and clean the operative area, regulate the patient's diet, administer enemas as necessary, and carry out any other preoperative doctor's orders.

The health unit coordinator will be responsible for seeing that certain clerical duties have been carried out and for assembling the chart forms in the proper order.

Preoperative Checklist

The purpose of the preoperative checklist is to assure that all necessary tasks and information are complete before the patient goes to surgery. This checklist is sent to the operating room on the chart.

Two categories of activities generally will require checking:

1. Tasks pertaining to the patient's chart forms and records, to be performed by the health unit coordinator.
2. Tasks pertaining to the preparation of the patient, performed by nursing personnel.

Nursing Responsibilities

The following procedures must be certified as having been completed by appropriate nursing personnel:

- Recording the time of the surgical prep of the operative area; when the enemas were completed, and by whom.
- Confirmation that the patient's TPR and BP were taken on the morning of surgery. If these values are not within the normal range, indicating possible disease, the surgery may have to be canceled. The health unit coordinator may be responsible for recording these values on the graphic chart.
- Noting the time, dosage, and name of the preoperative medications given. The anesthesiologist will then be able to coordinate the anesthesia with the medications given to achieve the optimum state of unconsciousness.
- Recording the time and amount of the patient's final voiding before transport to the operating room.
- Verifying the patient's identification number on the identification band on his/her wrist.
- Removal of the patient's dentures (sometimes not done until arrival in OR), jewelry, hairpins, nail polish, lipstick, and all prostheses prior to transport to the operating room.
- Having the patient properly dressed in hospital gown or other clothing, as required in your hospital.

Note: Special items may be required for patients with particular disease conditions or preoperative needs.

Health Unit Coordinator Responsibilities

The health unit coordinator must be sure that the following records are completed and included in the chart:

- The preoperative checklist (Fig. 17–23).
- The operative consent must be signed by the patient (or another person responsible for the patient according to the regulations of your hospital) (Fig. 17–24).

DATE	YES	NO	N/A	COMMENTS	UNIT RN INITIAL	HR RN INITIAL
Patient ID Band Checked						
Nickname						
Allergies				List:		
Allergy Band						

PATIENT CHART / CHART FORMS	YES	NO	N/A	COMMENTS	UNIT RN INITIAL	HR RN INITIAL
Face Sheet						
Conditions of Admission / Advance DIrect Form						
History & Physical						
Surgical Consent						
Anesthesia Consent				❑ Dr. Orders ❑ Signed ❑ Witnessed		
Anesthesia Questionnaire						
Sterilization / Observation / Photo Consent						

LAB / CLINICAL REPORTS	YES	NO	N/A	ON CHART	ABNORMAL REPORT CALLED TO DR/OR TIME	UNIT RN INITIAL	HR RN INITIAL
Tests Done							
Chest X-Ray							
EKG							
CBC							
LYTES							
UA							
Other: Nuclear Medicine Test within 24 hours				(If yes - contact Nuc. Med.)			

TYPE / X MATCH	AUTOLOGOUS DONATION	DESIGNATED DONATION	RED CROSS DONATION	TOTAL	UNIT RN INITIAL	HR RN INITIAL
No. Units Donated			N/A			
No. Units X Match						

BELONGINGS	YES	NO	N/A	COMMENTS	DISPOSITION	UNIT RN INITIAL	HR RN INITIAL
Dental Appliances				❑ Upper ❑ Lower			
Prosthesis				Type:			
Glasses / Contacts							
Jewelry				Type:			
Hearing Aides							
Other:				Type:			

MISCELLANEOUS

NPO SINCE	LAST VOID	PRE-OP TEACHING ❑ DONE	VISITORS WAITING

IV Started @__________. Size #__________ gauge ❑ LR1000cc ❑D5W__________cc. Site:

❑ Patent ❑ Opsite ❑ Pump set ❑ Secondary Set ❑ Ext. Set ❑ 1% Xylocaine__________cc. infiltrate

❑ Alka Seltzer TT tabs in 30cc/H_2O po @__________ Versed__________ mg IVP @__________

Comments____________________

NURSE SIGNATURE & TITLE	NURSE SIGNATURE & TITLE	TO O.R. @

PRE-OP CHECKLIST

Figure 17–23

AUTHORIZATION FOR AND CONSENT TO SURGERY OR SPECIAL DIAGNOSTIC OR THERAPEUTIC PROCEDURES

To ______________________
Name of Patient

Your admitting physician is ______________________, M.D.

Your surgeon is ______________________, M.D.

1. The hospital maintains personnel and facilities to assist your physicians and surgeons in their performance of various surgical operations and other special diagnostic and therapeutic procedures. These surgical operations and special diagnostic or therapeutic procedures all may involve calculated risks of complications, injury or even death, from both known and unknown causes and no warranty or guarantee has been made as to result or cure. Except in a case of emergency or exceptional circumstances, these operations and procedures are therefore not performed upon patients unless and until the patient has had an opportunity to discuss them with his physician. Each patient has the right to consent or refuse any proposed operation or special procedure (based upon the description or explanation received).
2. Your physicians and surgeons have determined that the operations or special procedures listed below may be beneficial in the diagnosis or treatment of your condition. Upon your authorization and consent, such operations or special procedures will be performed for you by your physicians and surgeons and/or by other physicians and surgeons selected by them. The persons in attendance for the purpose of administering anesthesia or performing other specialized professional services, such as radiology, pathology and the like, are not the agents, servants or employees of the hospital or your physician or surgeon, but are independent contractors performing specialized services on your behalf and, as such, are your agents, servants or employees. Any tissue or member severed in any operation will be disposed of in the discretion of the pathologist, except ______________________
3. Your signature below the operations or special procedures listed below constitutes your acknowledgment (i) that you have read and agreed to the foregoing (ii) that the operations or special procedures have been adequately explained to you by your attending physicians or surgeons and that you have all of the information that you desire, and (iii) that you authorize and consent to the performance of the operations or special procedures.

Operation or Procedure

____

SIGNATURE ______________ DATE ________ TIME ________
Patient

SIGNATURE ______________ DATE ________ TIME ________
Witness

(If patient is a minor or unable to sign, complete the following):

Patient is a minor, or is unable to sign, because ______________________

______________ Father ______________ Guardian

______________ Mother ______________ Other Person and Relationship

Figure 17–24

- A preanesthesia questionaire and consent for anesthesia (Figs. 17–25 and 17–26).
- An anesthesia record (Fig. 17–27, pg. 428).
- A sterilization consent must also be signed if the surgery will render the patient unable to reproduce (Fig. 17–28, pg. 429).
- History and physical records, completed and recorded by the physician responsible. These are required before surgery. Short forms are usually available for patients hospitalized under 24 to 48 hours.
- Preoperative laboratory results posted on the clinical pathology record. Preoperative patients routinely have a blood count and urinalysis done

ANESTHESIA QUESTIONNAIRE Name__________ Ht.______ Wt. ______

1. Please list all medications taken in last ten days (including aspirin):
2. Are you allergic to any medication, iodine, soap, latex, rubber products, or tape? What adverse reaction did you have?
3. Please check (✔) if you have had the following:

❑ High blood pressure	❑ Asthma or wheezing	❑ Nuclear Medicine test within 24 hours
❑ Chest pains or angina	❑ Emphysema or chronic bronchitis	❑ Diabetes
❑ Heart attack	❑ Cough up phlegm daily	❑ Thyroid problems
❑ Palpitations	❑ Recent cold or flu	❑ Kidney problems
❑ Heart failure	❑ Polio	❑ Heavy Bleeding
❑ Heart murmur	❑ Seizures or convulsions	❑ Prednisone or steroid in last 6 months
❑ Rheumatic fever	❑ Fainting spells	❑ Hepatitis
❑ Other heart disease	❑ Strokes	❑ Peptic ulcer disease
❑ Shortness of breath	❑ Weakness on one side of body	❑ Hiatal hernia or reflux
❑ Ankle swelling	❑ Temporary blindness, in an eye	❑ Other significant illness ______

4. Do you smoke? ❑ No ❑ How much______ When did you quit? ______
5. What is your alcohol use? ❑ Never ❑ Occasional ❑ Few times a week ❑ Daily
6. Is it possible that you are pregnant? ....❑ Yes ❑ No When was your last menstrual period? ______
7. Is your ability to exercise limited? ....❑ Yes ❑ No Explain ______
8. Has any relative had problems with anesthesia?....❑ Yes ❑ No
9. Do you have ....❑ Dentures ❑ Loose teeth ❑ Capped or bonded teeth ❑ Contact lenses
10. Do you have any problems with neck mobility or have you ever been told you have an abnormal airway? ❑ Yes ❑ No
11. Please list your previous operations:

Year	Operation	Type of Anesthesia (general, spinal, local)	Complications

12. This form has been filled out by ______

PREANESTHESIA QUESTIONNAIRE

Figure 17–25

CONSENT FOR ANESTHESIA

Although anesthesia is very safe, there are certain inherent risks every time anesthesia is administered. The medicines used for anesthesia may affect the cardiovascular system to lower blood pressure, may cause breathing problems, may cause allergic reations, and may directly cause injury to any of the organs of the body. There is the potential for very serious complications that even result in brain damage and/or death. Serious complications are very infrequent, and occur much less than 1% of the time in the general population.

Additional Risks Include the Following:

GENERAL ANESTHESIA:

Frequent (more than 1% occurrence): nausea and vomiting, sore throat, brief disorientation

Rare (less than 1% occurrence): damage to teeth, awareness under anesthesia, damage to peripheral nerves, damage to major organs (including brain, heart, lungs, liver, kidneys)

REGIONAL ANESTHESIA:

Frequent (more than 1% occurrence): bruising, minor pain and discomfort, residual sensation, need for general anesthesia, headache

Rare (less than 1% occurrence): damage to nerves and/or blood vessels, infection, convulsions, damage to major organs (including brain, heart, lungs, liver, kidneys)

I have read this and acknowledge that I understand that I am to have anesthesia to relieve pain during my surgical procedure and that this administration of anesthesia carries risk to life and limb. I understand that these risks stated above are not meant to be a complete list, and that other unexpected complications may occur. I have had the opportunity to have all of my questions answered by an anesthesiologist.

Date	Time	Patient/Parent/Guardian/Conservator
Date	Time	Witness

CONSENT FOR ANESTHESIA

Figure 17-26

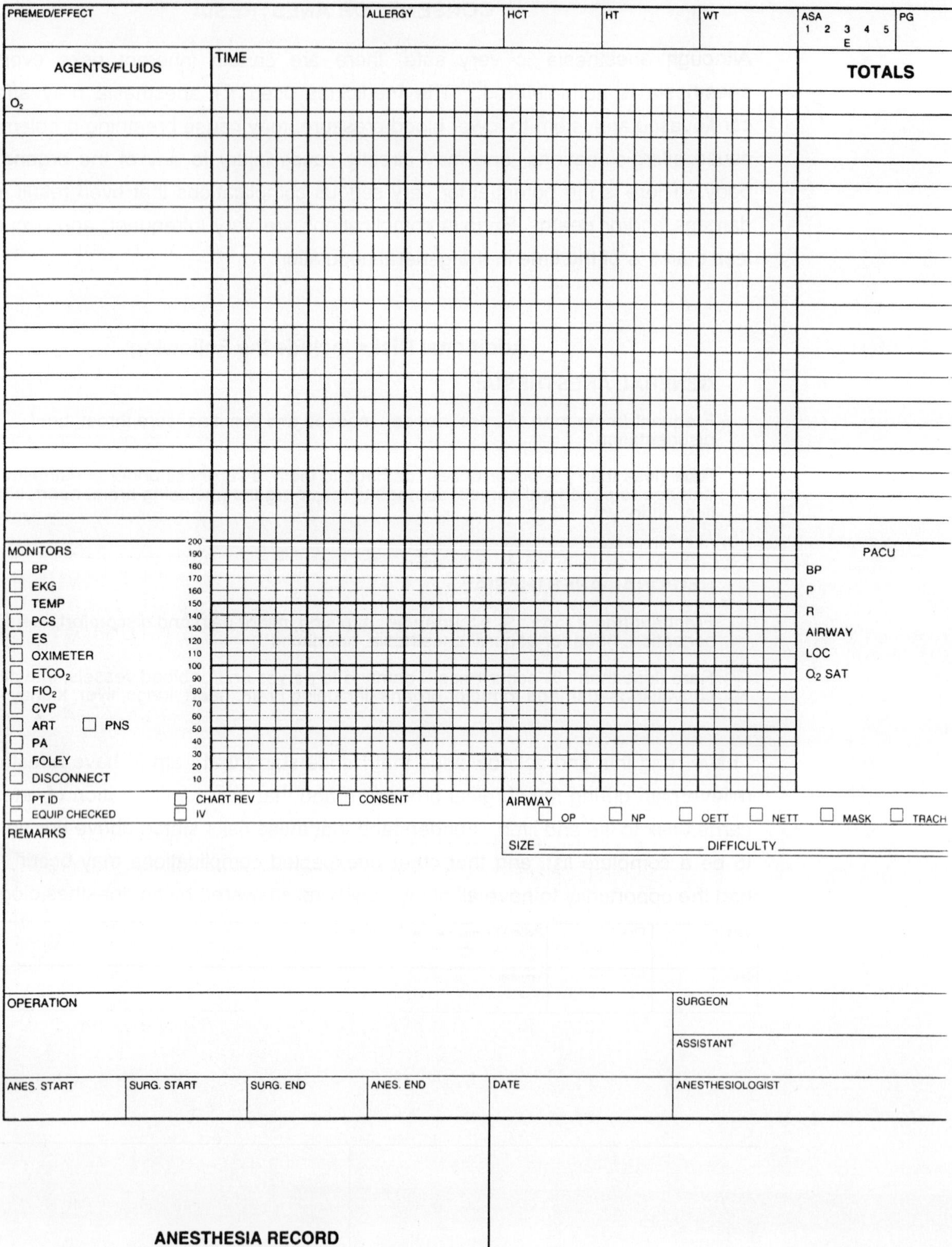

PREMED/EFFECT | ALLERGY | HCT | HT | WT | ASA 1 2 3 4 5 E | PG

AGENTS/FLUIDS | TIME | TOTALS

O_2

200 190 180 170 160 150 140 130 120 110 100 90 80 70 60 50 40 30 20 10

MONITORS
- ☐ BP
- ☐ EKG
- ☐ TEMP
- ☐ PCS
- ☐ ES
- ☐ OXIMETER
- ☐ $ETCO_2$
- ☐ FIO_2
- ☐ CVP
- ☐ ART ☐ PNS
- ☐ PA
- ☐ FOLEY
- ☐ DISCONNECT

PACU
BP
P
R
AIRWAY
LOC
O_2 SAT

☐ PT ID ☐ CHART REV ☐ CONSENT
☐ EQUIP CHECKED ☐ IV

AIRWAY ☐ OP ☐ NP ☐ OETT ☐ NETT ☐ MASK ☐ TRACH

REMARKS

SIZE ____________ DIFFICULTY ____________

OPERATION | SURGEON
 | ASSISTANT

ANES. START | SURG. START | SURG. END | ANES. END | DATE | ANESTHESIOLOGIST

ANESTHESIA RECORD

Figure 17–27

MEMORIAL HOSPITAL
STERILIZATION PERMIT

Date ____________ Hour ________.M.

I hereby authorize and direct Doctor ________________________________
and assistants of his choice to perform the following operation upon me at the above named hospital: ____ and to do any other procedure that his (their) judgment may dictate during the above operation. It has been explained to me that I may (or will probably) be sterile as a result of this operation but no such result has been warranted. I understand that the word "sterility" means that I may be unable to conceive or bear children and in giving my consent to the operation have in mind the possibility (probability) of such a result. I absolve said doctor, his assistants and the hospital from all responsibility for my present condition or any condition that may result from said operation.

Signed ________________________

Signature Witnessed:

By ____________________________ By ____________________________

I have read the foregoing matter and, as the spouse of the above named patient, do hereby join in authorizing the performance of the surgery under the terms set forth and consented to above.

Signed ________________________

Signature Witnessed:

By ____________________________ By ____________________________

Figure 17–28

prior to surgery. There will be policies regarding the recency of CBC and UA tests. Usually they will be valid for no longer than 48 hours. If any patient has evidence of anemia or a bladder infection, these conditions must be corrected prior to surgery. If not, they could cause serious complications during or after surgery.

- Any other tests done preoperatively, such as ECGs and x-rays.
- Other preoperative forms (e.g., preanesthesia form) as required by your hospital.
- Blank chart forms to be used in the operating room and recovery room, such as the anesthesia record and intake and output sheets.
- The patient's imprinter plate for use on forms in the operating room and recovery room.

PREOPERATIVE ORDERS

KEY IDEA: TYPES OF PREOPERATIVE ORDERS

Orders for a patient prior to surgery vary not only according to the operation to be performed, but also according to the preferences of each surgeon. Ordinarily, preoperative orders will include one order from each of the following categories. (Fig. 17–29.)

Enema

Many preoperative patients receive an enema. The type of enema ordered will depend upon the operation to be performed. Cleaning out the bowel prior to surgery serves two purposes:

1. The patient is less likely to contaminate the operating field with feces when his rectal sphincter relaxes under anesthesia.
2. A bowel distended with feces will block the surgeon's view once he enters the abdominal cavity.

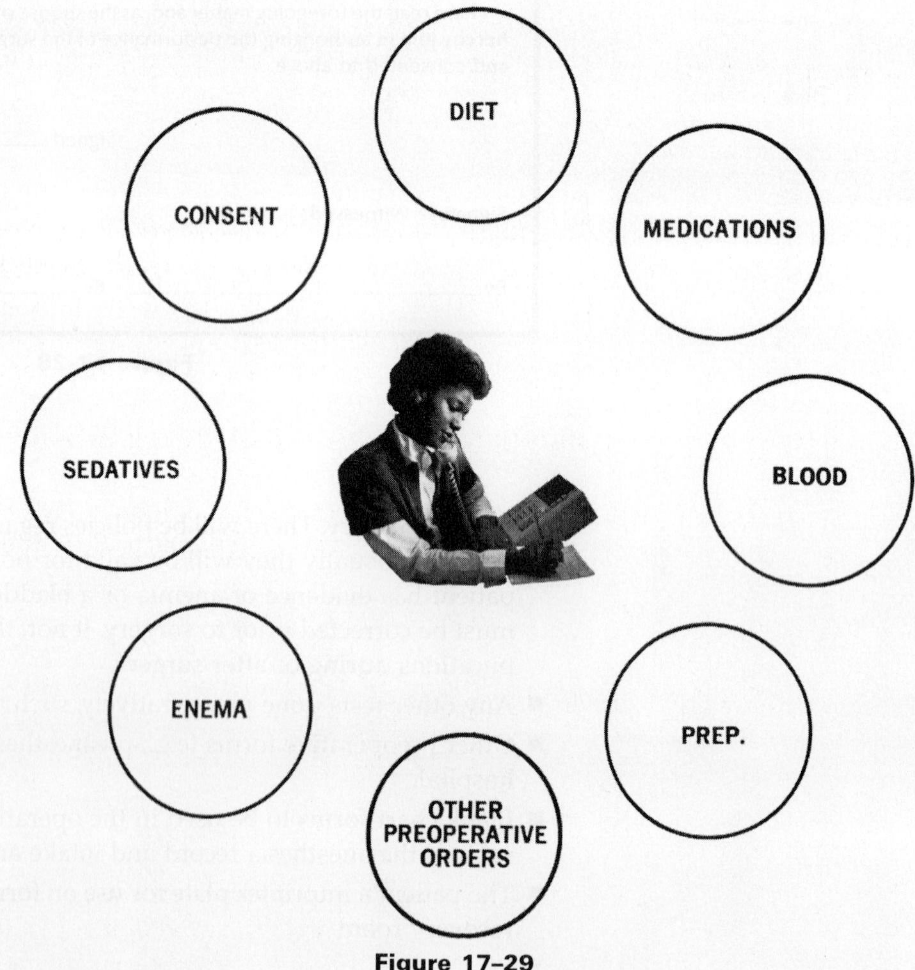

Figure 17–29

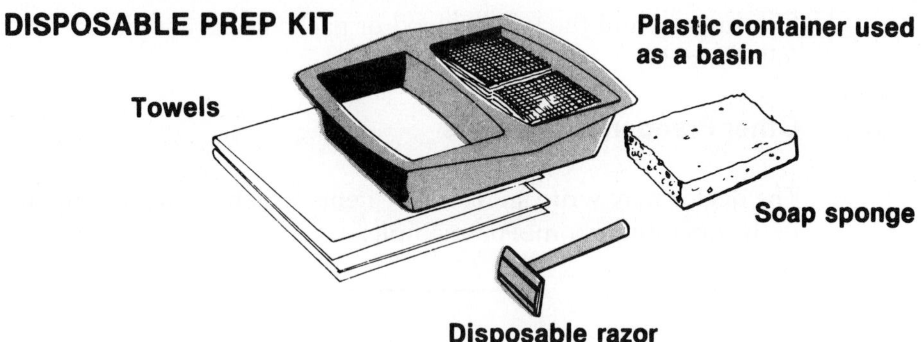

Figure 17–30

Prep

The area where the surgical incision will be made must be shaved and cleaned before surgery. The shave and scrub is called a surgical "prep." (Fig. 17–30.)

The purpose of this preparation is to clean the skin and reduce the possibility of the spread of microorganisms from the skin into the operative incision.

Diet

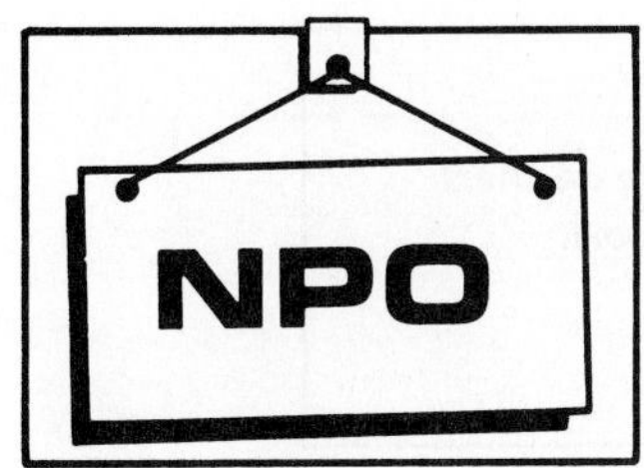

Figure 17–31

If the patient does not have an empty stomach, he may vomit during and after surgery as a reaction to the anesthesia. Therefore, he is usually made NPO at midnight on the day of surgery. (Fig. 17–31.) If surgery is to be performed on the lower GI system, the patient's diet may be modified for two to three days before the operation.

Consent

All patients must have an operative consent signed before the operation may take place. If the patient is underage or unable to sign, the next of kin or another person responsible for the patient must do so.

The doctor may obtain the patient's written consent himself; if not, he writes an order to that effect and relies on the nursing staff to carry out the order.

Sleeping Medication (Sedatives and Hypnotics)

Most doctors order sleeping medications for their patients preoperatively, to reduce their anxiety and to help them sleep well the night before surgery.

Preoperative Medications

Shortly before the patient is taken to the operating room, he is given injections to help him relax. In many hospitals, these medications are ordered by the anesthesiologist rather than the surgeon.

Blood Replacement

Most patients scheduled for major surgery should have blood reserved for them in the blood bank. Their blood must be typed and crossmatched with blood units available in the blood bank. This is usually done the evening before surgery, and the whole blood or packed cells are placed "on call" for the following day.

Other Preoperative Orders

The doctor may write an order for items which are to accompany the patient to the operating room. For example:

> ***To OR c̄ skull x-rays.***
> ***To OR c̄ 1 vial regular insulin***

The doctor may also order that certain miscellaneous duties be performed the morning of surgery. For example:

Figure 17–32 shows an example of preprinted preoperative anesthesia orders. The physician will check those which apply, and they are transcribed in the usual manner.

> ***Phone lab for results of CBC and UA. Include on chart.***
> ***Start IV 500 cc. 5% D/W prior to OR transport.***
> ***Give one unit whole blood tonight.***

KEY IDEA: TRANSCRIPTION

Below is a sample group of preoperative orders. Transcribe these on a separate sheet of paper. Practice using the symbols and abbreviations you have been taught.

> ***Have operative consent signed.***
> ***SS enema tonight and at 6 A.M.***
> ***Abdominal-perineal prep c̄ 5 min. antiseptic scrub.***
> ***NPO p̄ midnight.***
> ***Type and x-match 3 units whole blood. Give one tonight and place 2 on-call for 8 A.M.***
> ***Sodium pentobarbital 200 mg. p.o. h.s.***
> ***Catheterize pt. prior to giving preop meds.***
> ***Preop meds. by order of Dr. Jones.***
> ***Pt. to OR c̄ pelvic x-rays.***

POSTOPERATIVE ORDERS

Most patients are taken to the recovery room (RR or PACU) immediately following surgery. They remain in the recovery room until they begin to recover from the effects of anesthesia. When it is felt that the patient may safely

1. **TESTS:**
   - ☐ EKG
   - ☐ CHEST X-RAY
   - ☐ PULMONARY FUNCTION SCREEN
   - ☐ OTHER______________
   - ☐ CBC
   - ☐ UA
   - ☐ SMA - 7
   - ☐ ELECTROLYTES

2. **DIET**
   - ☐ NPO p 2400
   - ☐ CLEAR LIQUIDS (NO JELLO, NO SOUP) UNTIL____________

3. **START IV** ☐ OPS ☐ HOLDING ROOM ☐ FLOOR
   - ☐ Extension Set
   - ☐ 1000 D 5 1/2 N.S. @ ____________ cc/hr
   - ☐ 500 D 5 W @ ____________ cc/hr
   - ☐ 1000 R L @ ____________ cc/hr
   - ☐ 1000 D 5 Isolyte S @______________ cc/hr
   - ☐ OTHER__________________
   - ☐ LIDOCAINE 1% plain intradermal infiltrate for IV start

4. **MEDICATIONS**
   - ☐ Daily meds c̄ sip of H_2O in a.m. pre-op

   SLEEP
   - ☐ NEMBUTAL 100 mgm p.o. H.S. M.R. x _______ prn
   - ☐ DALMANE 15 mgm p.o. H.S. M.R. x _______ prn
   - ☐ DALMANE 30 mgm p.o. H.S. M.R. x _______ prn
   - ☐ HALCION .25 mgm p.o. H.S. M.R. x _______ prn
   - ☐ OTHER_________________

   PRE-OP
   - ☐ LEAVE DENTURES IN PLACE
   - ☐ NO PRE-OP MEDICATION
   - ☐ ALKA SELTZER COLD TABS II c̄ 30 cc H_2O 1/2 - 1 h. pre-op
   - ☐ VALIUM ______ mgm. ☐ IV ☐ P.O. @ ______
   - ☐ DROPERIDOL ______ mgm I.M. @ ______
   - ☐ MORPHINE ______ mgm I.M. @ ______
   - ☐ FENTANYL ______ mgm. ☐ IV ☐ I.M. @ ______
   - ☐ DEMEROL ______ mgm I.M. @ ______
   - ☐ VISTARIL ______ mgm ☐ p.o. ☐ I.M. @ ______
   - ☐ ATIVAN ______ mgm ☐ p.o. ☐ I.M. @ ______
   - ☐ ATROPINE ______ mgm I.M. @ ______
   - ☐ SCOPOLAMINE ______ mgm I.M. @ ______
   - ☐ ROBINUL ______ mgm I.M. @ ______
   - ☐ VERSED ______ mgm ☐ IV ☐ I.M. @ ______
   - ☐ OTHER____________

5. **ADDITIONAL PRE-OP ORDERS** ____

Nurse's Signature	Date	Time	Transcriber	M.D. Signature

PRE-OPERATIVE ANESTHESIA ORDERS

Figure 17–32

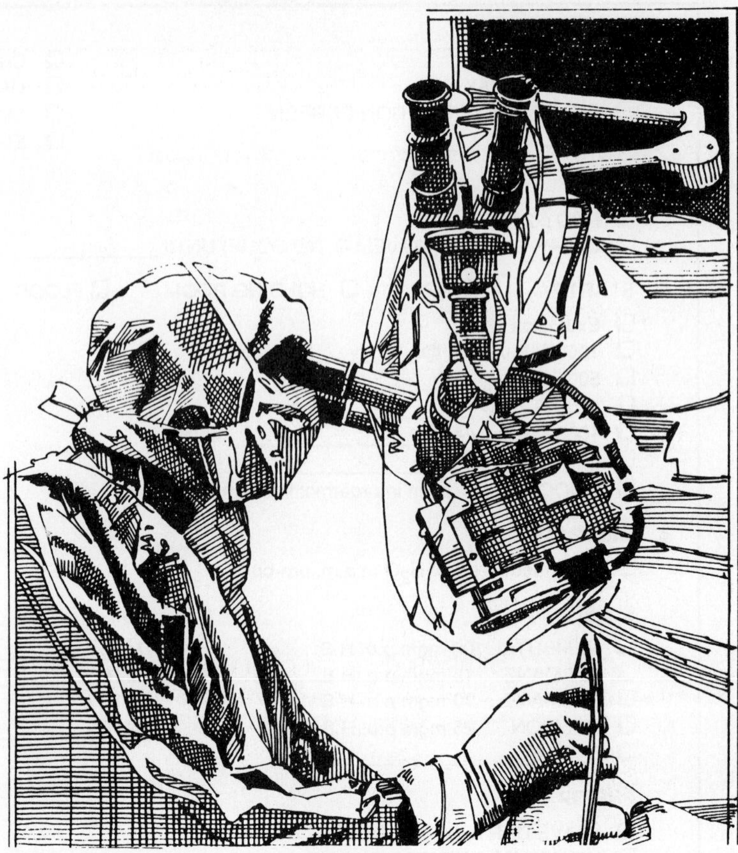

Figure 17–33

return to the floor (nursing unit), the recovery room staff will bring the patient, by gurney, back to his room.

KEY IDEA: TYPES OF POSTOPERATIVE ORDERS

Surgery usually affects a patient's hospitalization more than any other single event.

- Following surgery, his diet and activity orders usually change.
- Treatments and medications given before the operation may no longer be necessary.
- The postoperative patient usually requires special care for a period of hours or days following surgery, and new orders for this care must be written.

Postoperative orders vary according to the operation performed. Following surgery, all preoperative orders written **on a patient are automatically canceled.** The postoperative orders must be rewritten by the time the patient is transferred to the recovery room, so that the nurses there will know what must be done for the patient. The health unit coordinator should be familiar with this type of order so that he/she will know if new orders were instituted in the recovery room. Figure 17–34 shows an example of postanesthesia orders for PACU and the floor. Postoperative orders usually include most of the following categories.

POST ANESTHESIA CARE UNIT

1. MEDICATIONS:
   - ☐ Fentanyl 25 mcg. IV q5 min. x ______doses prn pain
   - ☐ Fentanyl 50 mcg. IV q5 min. x ______doses prn pain
   - ☐ Morphine_______mgm. IV q5 min. x ______doses prn pain
   - ☐ Demerol_______mgm. IV q5 min. x ______doses prn pain
   - ☐ Droperidol_______mgm. IV prn nausea M.R. x ______
   - ☐ Compazine ☐ 1.25 mgm. IV prn nausea M.R. x ______
     ☐ 2.5 mgm. IV prn nausea M.R. x ______
   - ☐ Atropine mgm. IV prn pulse below_______and notify anesthesiologist M.R. x ______prn
   - ☐ Narcan 0.1 mgm. IV prn respiratory depression M.R. x ______and notify anesthesiologist.
2. ADDITIONAL ORDERS:
   OXYGEN
   - ☐ Mask ☐ Nasal Prongs______LPM ☐ Mist_______% ☐ Pulse Oximeter
   - ☐ Warm Air Therapy for Temp ↓ 96F.

   ____
   ____
   ____
   ____
3. DISCHARGE FROM PACU TO: ☐ Ward ☐ DOU ☐ ICU ☐ Same day Surgery ☐ Extended Care
   - ☐ Time ______
   - ☐ PACU Score of ______
   - ☐ Block sensory level of ______
   - ☐ Return of motor function ______
   - ☐ DC EPIDURAL
4. ☐ Discharge home in care of responsible party when V.S.S., awake, comfortable, takes P.O. fluids with minimal nausea/vomiting, voids, sits up and walks with assistance and instructed how to contact Anesthesiologist if necessary through hospital operator.
   - ☐ DC I.V. BEFORE DISCHARGE

Nurse's Signature	Date	Time

POST ANESTHESIA ORDER FOR FLOOR

____
____
____
____

Nurse's Signature	Date	Time	Transcriber	M.D. Signature

MEMORIAL HOSPITAL

POST ANESTHESIA ORDERS

Figure 17–34

Postoperative Orders

- ***Diet***
- ***Activity***
- ***Intravenous feeding (IV)***
- ***Vital signs***
- ***Wound and dressing***
- ***Medications***
- ***Tubes and catheters***
- ***Intake and output***
- ***Special equipment***

Diet

A diet order of some kind is generally indicated. A patient with minor surgery may have few, if any, restrictions. For example:

Diet as tolerated.
Regular diet; serve dinner.
Resume low Na diet as tolerated.

A patient with major surgery usually is fed intravenously for a day or two. However, reference to diet may be made. For example:

NPO
Ice chips as tolerated.
Sips of tap water as pt. desires.

Activity

A patient's activity is almost always limited after surgery. Limitations may be insignificant in the case of minor surgery. For example:

OOB ad. lib. $\bar{p}$ pt. awake.
OOB tonight as tolerated.

When certain major surgery has been performed, far stricter regulations apply. The patient is usually confined to bed entirely until the following morning, when orders for progressive ambulation are written. Some activity orders concern the surgical procedure performed. For example:

Pt. to be kept flat in bed for 24 hrs.
Elevate right arm at all times.

IVs

An intravenous infusion is begun on almost every adult patient who has surgery. Moreover, some anesthetics are given intravenously; their administration is often simplified if an IV is running. Most physicians also consider it wise to have an IV running during surgery, in case of an emergency. The type of surgery and the patient's postoperative condition largely determine the type of IV order to be written. For example:

Finish current IV; then discontinue.
Hang 1 bottle 500 cc. D/W after current IV finishes; then discontinue.
Keep IV open with 1000 cc 5% D/W till 8 A.M.
1000 cc. 5% D/W follow $\bar{c}$ 500 cc. 5% D/S to run till morning.
Finish blood, then hang 1000 cc. NS $\bar{c}$ 2 million U. aqueous penicillin added.

As the last order shows, postoperative IV orders may contain orders for medication. Antibiotics to combat possible infection and vitamins to help rebuild the body after surgery are some of the most common medications given in connection with IVs.

Vital Signs

Accurate records of the blood pressure, pulse, and respirations are extremely important during the immediate postoperative period. A rising pulse, increased respirations, and falling blood pressure may indicate the onset of shock. Shock can occur after surgery from excessive or continuing blood loss or as a reaction to the anesthetic used. Since these two situations can occur in any postoperative patient, vital signs are generally taken every 15 minutes in the recovery room. The physician will usually write orders pertaining to the VS to be carried out after the patient has been returned to his own hospital unit. For example:

VS q15min. ×4, q1h ×4, q4h, then q.d.
VS q15min. until stable.

Wound and Dressing

After surgery, there is often the possibility that the patient will bleed internally. Hemorrhage usually takes place near the wound site, so a frequent check of the dressing for blood may assist in early detection. Physicians often order continuous observation for signs of bleeding. For example:

> ***Check dressing q15min. for bleeding.***
> ***Call Dr. Green if bleeding excessive.***

Medications

After all surgery, except the most minor, a physician will ordinarily write a p.r.n. order for the relief of pain. For treatment or prevention of postoperative nausea and vomiting, an order for an *antiemetic* drug might be written. In cases of potential infection, the doctor will usually order *antibiotics* postoperatively. Other medications may be ordered, but these types are ordered most often. Examples are:

> ***Meperidine 75 mg. IM q4h p.r.n.***
> ***Codeine gr. $\dot{\bar{\text{i}}}$ (H) q3h p.r.n.***
> ***Prochlorperazine 5 mg. IM q4h p.r.n.***
> ***Streptomycin 0.5 Gm. IM b.i.d.***

Tubes and Catheters

Many patients leave the operating room with tubes or a catheter in place. Observation and care of tubes or catheters require a written order, for example:

> ***Foley catheter to gravity drainage. Irrigate q4h c̄ 10 cc NSS.***
> ***Wound catheter to Hemovac.***
> ***Levine tube to suction. Irrigate q4h.***

Intake and Output

Postoperative records of I & O are kept on almost every patient subjected to major surgery, primarily because fluid balance is easily upset by surgery. The doctor must know when to add fluids or withhold them to attain fluid balance. A record of output is also important, because urinary retention is a common complication following certain types of surgery. Examples of orders associated with these difficulties are:

Strict I & O for 3 days.
Check voiding q8h.
Cath pt. q8h p.r.n. if unable to void
If pt. has not voided by 4 A.M., call Dr. White for cath. order.

Special Equipment

Sometimes patients require the postoperative use of special equipment. A patient with a spinal fusion may need a bedboard; a patient recovering from chest surgery may require chest tubes; a postoperative prostatectomy patient will sometimes require a special apparatus for irrigating the bladder with distilled water or a saline solution called a "Murphy drip." Pneumatic and elastic stockings are ordered on patients following a variety of surgical procedures. Examples of orders of this type are:

Bedboard.
Murphy drip at gtts. 10/min.

KEY IDEA: TRANSCRIPTION

A group of typical postoperative orders are shown below. Transcribe them for practice in the manner indicated previously in the chapter.

NPO
Complete bedrest.
VS q15 min. until stable. Then q2h × 12 hrs.
Check bleeding q15 min.
Wound catheter to suction. Measure and empty q4h.
I & O
Cath pt. at 8 P.M. if unable to void.
Elastic stockings toes to knees. Remove q.d., wash and dry legs, then replace stockings.
Meperidine 50 mg IM q3h p.r.n.
1000 cc 5% D/W c̄ 4,000,000 U aqueous penicillin to run until 12 Mn.; then keep open c̄ 500 cc 5% D/S.

LEARNING ACTIVITIES

1. Explain how you would greet a patient being admitted to your unit.
2. What are the two types of patient admissions?
   (a)
   (b)
3. What is the MSSU?
4. When the patient is admitted, what forms or items will come to the unit from the admitting department?
   (a)
   (b)
   (c)
5. In your words, explain how you would admit a patient to a nursing unit.
6. Orders for new admissions will usually include the following categories.
   (a)
   (b)
   (c)
   (d)
   (e)
7. The two most commonly ordered diagnostic tests are:
   (a)
   (b)
8. What are "routine orders"?

9. Why might a patient be transferred to another room?
   (a) ______
   (b) ______
   (c) ______
   (d) ______

10. Why might a patient be transferred to another unit?
    ______

11. Explain your duties when a patient is transferred to another room.
    ______

    To another unit. ______

12. Describe your responsibilities when a patient is discharged.
    ______

13. What does it mean when a patient leaves the hospital AMA?
    ______

14. In the presence of death, there are certain attitudes the hospital expects of you. List at least three.
    (a) ______
    (b) ______
    (c) ______

15. List some of your clerical and communication duties at the time of a patient's death.
 (a) ______
 (b) ______
 (c) ______
 (d) ______
 (e) ______
 (f) ______
 (g) ______
 (h) ______
 (i) ______
16. Surgery may be ______ or ______ in nature.
17. Surgical patients can be divided into three groups. They are:
 (a) ______
 (b) ______
 (c) ______
18. Preoperatively, two categories of activities generally will require checking:
 (a) ______
 (b) ______
19. List the records that may be included in the preoperative chart.
 (a) ______
 (b) ______
 (c) ______
 (d) ______
 (e) ______
 (f) ______
 (g) ______
 (h) ______
20. Preoperative orders frequently include orders for:
 (a) ______
 (b) ______
 (c) ______
 (d) ______
 (e) ______
 (f) ______
 (g) ______
21. Before surgery an ______ must be signed.
22. Preoperatively, which two laboratory tests must be current according to hospital policy?
 (a) ______
 (b) ______

SAMPLE HEALTH UNIT COORDINATOR PROCEDURES

1. ADMITTING
   Use the information below and the forms provided by your instructor to admit the following patients.
   (a) Joseph P. Anyone
   Rm. 123
   Admitting M.D.—James Stevens, M.D.
   Diagnosis—Congestive heart failure.
   Age—78
   Unit #—68754
   (b) Clara Fied
   Rm. 765
   Admitting M.D.—Laila Morgan, M.D.
   Diagnosis—C.O.P.D.
   Age—82
   Unit #—98123
2. TRANSFER
   Use the information below and the forms provided by your instructor to transfer the following patients.
   (a) Transfer Mr. Anyone to Rm. 124 on the same floor.
   Transfer Mr. Anyone to I.C.U.
   (b) Transfer Mrs. Fied to Riversweet Convalescent Hospital today.
3. DISCHARGE
   Use your hospital's forms and procedures to discharge Mr. Anyone. (Following I.C.U. he returned to your floor, room 124. He has improved and is going home today.)
4. DEATHS
   Use the forms and procedures required by your hospital and complete this exercise.

   Mr. John C. Over was admitted to your floor three days ago. His condition became worse and this morning he expired. He was pronounced dead by his physician, Tod Matthew, M.D., at 8:03 A.M. His diagnosis was acute myocardial infarction and he was in room 888. His wife was with him at the time of his death and has taken home all of his belongings. He is not a coroner's case. He is to go to Drake's Mortuary. There is no autopsy.
5. SURGICAL PATIENTS
   Using the forms and procedures required by your hospital, set up the following patients for surgery:

   Ryan A. Cox
   Rm. 794
   Diagnosis—acute appendicitis
   Surgery—appendectomy
   Date of surgery—use tomorrow's date
   Age—22
   Surgeon—Velma Blade, M.D.
   Allergies—Penicillin

Kathleen Doyle
Rm. 8921
Diagnosis—uterine fibroids
Surgery—hysterectomy
Date of surgery—use tomorrow's date
Age—39
Surgeon—Calvin Cutter, M.D.
Allergies—none

Kardexing

Use the Kardexes provided in Figure 17–35, or ones given to you by your instructor.

DATE	X-RAY AND OTHER	DATE	LAB

RESPIRATORY	

DATE		DAILY LAB

HEIGHT: WEIGHT:	CODE STATUS:
DIET	DISCHARGE PLANNING/REHAB:
FORCE FLUIDS	
TUBE FEEDING	
TEST DIET	
	ALLERGIES:
I & O	
ACTIVITY	
DATE LAST BM	RELATIVE PHONE #

DATE	SURGICAL OR SPECIAL PROCEDURES

Figure 17–35

DATE	MEDS - ROUTINE	DOSE	RT	FREQ	RO

DATE	FREQ	BOTTLES	IVs	DO

DATE	MEDS - PRN	DOSE	RT.	FREQ.	RO

DATE	FREQ	MEDS	DO

DATE	MEDS - ONE TIME	DOSE	RT.	FREQ.	RO

DATE	TREATMENTS

SURGICAL PROCEDURE DATE: AGE SEX CONSULTING M.D.

DIAGNOSIS: ADMITTING M.D.

ROOM # NAME: ADMIT DATE TRANSFER DATE

Figure 17–35 ***(Continued)***

DATE	X-RAY AND OTHER	DATE	LAB

RESPIRATORY			DAILY LAB
HEIGHT: WEIGHT:	CODE STATUS:		

		DATE	SURGICAL OR SPECIAL PROCEDURES
DIET	DISCHARGE PLANNING/REHAB:		
FORCE FLUIDS			
TUBE FEEDING			
TEST DIET			
	ALLERGIES:		
I & O			
ACTIVITY			
DATE LAST BM	RELATIVE PHONE #		

Figure 17–35 *(Continued)*

DATE	MEDS - ROUTINE	DOSE	RT	FREQ	RO

DATE	FREQ	BOTTLES	IV'S	DO

DATE	FREQ	MEDS	DO

DATE	MEDS - PRN	DOSE	RT.	FREQ.	RO

DATE	TREATMENTS

DATE	MEDS - ONE TIME	DOSE	RT.	FREQ.	RO

SURGICAL PROCEDURE DATE: AGE SEX CONSULTING M.D.

DIAGNOSIS: ADMITTING M.D.

ROOM # NAME: ADMIT DATE TRANSFER DATE

Figure 17–35 ***(Continued)***

DATE	X-RAY AND OTHER

RESPIRATORY	
HEIGHT: WEIGHT:	CODE STATUS:
DIET	DISCHARGE PLANNING/REHAB:
FORCE FLUIDS	
TUBE FEEDING	
TEST DIET	
	ALLERGIES:
I & O	
ACTIVITY	
DATE LAST BM	RELATIVE PHONE #

DATE	LAB	
		DAILY LAB

DATE	SURGICAL OR SPECIAL PROCEDURES

Figure 17–35 (*Continued*)

DATE	MEDS - ROUTINE	DOSE	RT	FREQ	RO

DATE	MEDS - PRN	DOSE	RT.	FREQ.	RO

DATE	MEDS - ONE TIME	DOSE	RT.	FREQ.	RO

DATE	FREQ	BOTTLES	IV'S	DO

DATE	FREQ	MEDS	DO

DATE	TREATMENTS

SURGICAL PROCEDURE DATE: AGE SEX CONSULTING M.D.

DIAGNOSIS: ADMITTING M.D.

ROOM # NAME: ADMIT DATE TRANSFER DATE

Figure 17–35 ***(Continued)***

DATE	X-RAY AND OTHER	DATE	LAB

RESPIRATORY

DAILY LAB

HEIGHT: WEIGHT:

CODE STATUS:

DIET

DISCHARGE PLANNING/REHAB:

DATE	SURGICAL OR SPECIAL PROCEDURES

FORCE FLUIDS

TUBE FEEDING

TEST DIET

ALLERGIES:

I & O

ACTIVITY

DATE LAST BM

RELATIVE PHONE #

Figure 17–35 *(Continued)*

DATE	MEDS - ROUTINE	DOSE	RT	FREQ	RO

DATE	FREQ	BOTTLES	IV'S	DO

DATE	FREQ	MEDS	DO

DATE	MEDS - PRN	DOSE	RT.	FREQ.	RO

DATE	TREATMENTS

DATE	MEDS - ONE TIME	DOSE	RT.	FREQ.	RO

SURGICAL PROCEDURE DATE: AGE	SEX	CONSULTING M.D.
DIAGNOSIS:		ADMITTING M.D.
ROOM # NAME:		ADMIT DATE TRANSFER DATE

Figure 17–35 ***(Continued)***

CHAPTER 18
Review

Now that you have completed your health unit coordinator training course, consider all that you have accomplished. Throughout this program, you have been taught skills, attitudes, and information necessary to perform your duties.

- You have learned to answer the telephone and intercom; how to receive and give instructions to patients and visitors; and you have learned the proper attitudes you should have toward all the people you meet in your work.
- You have studied the routine of the hospital, the duties of its staff, and the variety of services offered by its departments. You have recognized the important role you play in helping the hospital run efficiently to give each patient the best of care.
- You have learned how to handle charts and have become familiar with patient care records.
- You have learned how to transcribe doctor's orders so that the patients receive the treatments and care that have been prescribed for them at the correct time and exactly as the doctor intended.
- You have learned the importance of accuracy, promptness, and attention to detail in carrying out your tasks.

These points, then, must be kept in mind as you assume your full responsibilities as a health unit coordinator.

REVIEWING FOR YOUR EXAMINATION

For effective and meaninful review of your course work, you will find it helpful to follow a few simple recommendations.

KEY IDEA: GETTING READY

- Choose a time when you are not likely to be disturbed. It is difficult to organize your thoughts when you are subject to constant interruptions.

- Find a quiet place for study. Be sure that you have a good light and a flat surface (a table, desk, or counter top) on which you can spread your materials.
- Assemble all the equipment you will need. This will include your health unit coordinator manual, pencils, and some scratch paper.
- Sit up straight. Bad posture causes fatigue. Your mind will be more alert and your attention span longer if your body is not too relaxed.

KEY IDEA: HOW TO REVIEW

Your review should have three primary objectives:

1. To refresh your memory about all the material you have studied during the course.
2. To help you relate the specific tasks you have learned to your total job.
3. To identify any subject areas about which you may still be confused or unsure of yourself.

Everyone has his own method of reviewing, and what works well for one person may not work at all for another. Here are some further suggestions that may be helpful.

- Begin by jotting down the titles of each of the chapters in your manual. Look over the list and try to recall the main points of each chapter.
- Turn to the first chapter and scan it quickly, noting especially the main headings. If you have already underlined the most important points, read them over. Also, reread any notes you may have taken in class.
- Proceed in this way through the remaining chapters. Copy out any lists of detailed procedures (such as chart order) as an aid in your review.
- Write down any points about which you are still unsure so that you can discuss them with your instructor before the examination.
- There are certain things which you absolutely must *know.* If you have not already memorized them, start now. Some of these are:
  - Abbreviations for times of administration for medications and your hospital's time schedule.
  - The hospital's regulations regarding visitors, patients, and personnel.
  - Correct chart order.
  - The appropriate hospital department to which you must send each requisition.
  - The seven steps of the transcription procedure and their application.
- There are many other abbreviations and symbols with which you are expected to be familiar. These include, for example, abbreviations for treatments, diet, diagnostic examinations, dosages, and routes of administration. Review these lists carefully.

As you prepare for your final examination, prepare yourself for the NAHUC national certification examination. If you will not be taking this until after your final, be sure to save your notes and plan to review again before the examination.

The NAHUC national certification examination is offered in May in testing sites nationwide. It is a comprehensive examination designed to test your skills as a health unit coordinator and give you recognition as an educated member of the health team in this emerging health occupation. For information on the NAHUC examination, contact NAHUC.

Your final examination will cover all the material you have studied in this course. The examination will give you an opportunity to demonstrate the knowledge you have acquired, the skills you have learned, and your readiness to assume the full responsibilities of a health unit coordinator.

HEALTH UNIT COORDINATOR CERTIFICATION EXAMINATION CONTENT OUTLINE

Students should note that this is a *sample* content outline and should request the most current information before sitting for the examination. The new examination content outline is based on the results of a 1996 health unit coordinator job analysis conducted by NAHUC. The percentage of questions in each area was statistically determined by the number of knowledge statements associated with those areas.

Clinical Training Plan: Health Unit Coordinator (pages 456-462) contains a list of skills the health unit coordinator should possess. If you are a student, your instructor may wish you to use this training plan to document your learning during your externship.

If you are already employed as a health unit coordinator, you may wish to use this skill list to review what you already know, and that which you need to learn.

NAHUC Outline
(Based on 1996 Job Analysis)

	Percentage
I. Coordination of the Health Unit	**48%**
A. Operations	
1. Supplies and services management	
2. Information management: patient record, unit staff, organization	
B. Communications	
1. Equipment	
2. Skills	
C. Orientation and training personnel	
D. Safety	
II. Confidentiality and Patient Rights	**10%**
III. Critical Thinking	**6%**
A. Problem identification and resources	
B. Prioritization and decision making	
IV. Order Transcription	**31%**
A. Process	
B. Classifications: Diagnostics, Dietary, Nursing, Pharmacy, Therapy, Misc.	
C. Medical terms, abbreviations, and symbols	
V. Professional Development	**5%**

(Courtesy of NAHUC.)
Note: Content and percent of emphasis may change.

Clinical Training Plan: Health Unit Coordinator

Student: ____________ **Semester:** ____________

*Tasks	Est. Time Needed	On-Site Trainer Signature	Date of Competency	Actual Time
ORIENTATION				
Shows knowledge of:				
Hospital environment				
Nursing Service Dept.				
Working Environment				
Daily routine				
COMMUNICATIONS				
Uses computer				
Uses the telephone				
Pages				
Records and delivers messages				
Operates the intercom				
PATIENTS AND VISITORS				
Greets new patients				
Handles patient requests				
Delivers patients' gifts, mail, etc.				
Receives and directs visitors				
EMERGENCIES				
Shows knowledge of emergency procedures				
Knows locations of fire alarms & extinguishers				
Shows knowledge of safety procedures				
Knows emergency telephone numbers & codes (e.g., cardiac arrest, etc.)				
Reports hazards				
Reports fires				
Shows knowledge of incident report forms				
Reports medical emergencies				
Shows ability to carry out HUC responsibilities by keeping telephone lines free & remaining alert and responsive to supervisor's directions				
CLERICAL RESPONSIBILITIES—General				
Keeps the nurses' station neat				
Handles mail				
Maintains files and supplies				
Posts bulletin board notices				
Helps fill out routine forms				

Clinical Training Plan: Health Unit Coordinator *(Continued)*
Student: ______________ Semester: ______________

***Tasks**	***Est. Time Needed***	***On-Site Trainer Signature***	***Date of Competency***	***Actual Time***
THE PATIENT'S CHART				
Is able to assemble patients' charts				
Shows knowledge of routine & supplemental chart forms				
Keeps track of charts: records, removals, and replacements				
Does routine chart checks				
Demonstrates understanding of chart as legal document that must be in ink, legible, current, & signed as prescribed by hospital				
CHARTING RESPONSIBILITIES				
Enters information on graphic sheet as applicable to hospital				
Keeps chart forms in standard sequential order				
PATIENT-CENTERED ACTIVITIES				
Admitting Patients:				
Makes up new chart				
Enters name on all records				
Notifies nurse of admission				
Checks for signature on release of liability				
Makes note of allergies				
Adds proper supplemental chart forms				
Shows knowledge of all prescribed HUC admitting procedures				
Makes patient appointments for treatments and examinations				
Makes appointments for consultations				
Surgery Patients:				
Prepares preoperative chart forms and checklists				
Checks for current CBC & Ua				
Makes sure all ordered tests on chart				
Checks for history & physical				
Checks for allergies				
Checks chart for completeness				

Clinical Training Plan: Health Unit Coordinator *(Continued)*
Student: ____________ Semester: ____________

**Tasks*	*Est. Time Needed*	*On-Site Trainer Signature*	*Date of Compe-tency*	*Actual Time*
Shows ability to follow all prescribed HUC pre-op procedures				
Transferring Patients:				
Redirects patients' mail and visitors				
Records patient transfers				
Notifies appropriate departments				
Redirects all incoming test results				
Notifies housekeeping				
Receiving Transfer Patients:				
Receives patients' medical records & identification plates				
Makes changes on all necessary records				
Notifies all appropriate departments				
Discharging Patients:				
Checks discharge orders				
Makes follow-up appointments				
Checks with business office				
Returns valuables to patients				
Notifies diet kitchen & other depts. as prescribed				
Records discharges in daily census records				
Notifies housekeeping				
Rearranges chart forms				
Records discharges on all records as prescribed				
Returns medications to pharmacy				
Discharging Patients against Medical Advice				
Notifies attending physician at nurse's direction				
Notifies patient's family at nurse's direction				
Uses appropriate forms & procedures				
Patient Deaths				
Locates patient's doctor for certification if applicable				
Notifies nursing service office, reception desk, business office and/or admitting office, & any other dept. as prescribed by hospital				

Clinical Training Plan: Health Unit Coordinator *(Continued)*
Student: ______________ Semester: ______________

**Tasks*	*Est. Time Needed*	*On-Site Trainer Signature*	*Date of Compe-tency*	*Actual Time*
Procures autopsy consent form				
Requisitions shroud pack				
Prepares identification tags				
Collects patient's personal belongings and/or knows procedure for placement in hospital until claimed by family				
Adds patient's name to daily census record as an expiration				
Assembles patient's chart records in proper sequence				
Sends patient's chart records to medical records room				
Shows knowledge of all forms utilized				
Maintains professional and helpful attitude				
WORKING WITH THE DIETARY DEPARTMENT				
Notifies dietary department of number and kinds of meals needed on the unit by utilizing prescribed procedures				
Checks and orders stocks of supplemental nourishments				
Requisitions meals				
Notifies diet department of changes				
Requisitions individual patient nourishments				
Requisitions guest trays				
WORKING WITH THE LABORATORIES				
Prepares requisition forms for laboratory tests/orders by computer				
Transcribes orders directly from doctor's order sheet				
Notifies the laboratory of emergency tests or appointments to be made				
Cancels patient meals				
Compiles lists of patients scheduled for tests				
Compiles lists of patients needing special preparations				

Clinical Training Plan: Health Unit Coordinator ***(Continued)***
Student: ______________________ **Semester:** ______________________

**Tasks*	*Est. Time Needed*	*On-Site Trainer Signature*	*Date of Competency*	*Actual Time*
WORKING WITH OTHER HOSPITAL DEPARTMENTS				
(e.g., X-ray, Inhalation Therapy, Cardiopulmonary, Physical Therapy, Housekeeping, Environmental Services, Engineering)				
Prepares requisitions/ orders by computer				
Makes appointments				
Telephones "stat" orders				
Contacts departments for repairs or supplies				
Sends requisitions to blood bank				
Sends requisitions to business office				
TRANSCRIPTION OF ORDERS				
Recognizes that a "doctor's order" needs transcription				
After doctor's order sheet stamped with identification plates sends copies to appropriate departments				
Requisitions all equipment & services needed				
Transfers orders to special records & forms; shows understanding of Kardex				
Writes transcription symbols to show that the order is being processed				
Has transcribed orders checked and initialed by nurse				
Transcribing Medication Orders				
Recognizes the need for transcription from "doctor's order"				
After doctor's order sheet is stamped with identification plates, sends copies to appropriate departments				
Requisitions equipment and services				
Transfers orders to special forms; shows understanding of Kardex				
Writes transcription symbols to indicate order is in process				
Checks transcribed order with nurse				

Clinical Training Plan: Health Unit Coordinator ***(Continued)***
Student: ______________ **Semester:** ______________

***Tasks**	**Est. Time Needed**	**On-Site Trainer Signature**	**Date of Competency**	**Actual Time**
Cancels medication orders Transcribes renewal orders Transcribes single-dose and stat orders *Transcribing Treatment Orders* Transcribes standing orders Transcribes stat and single-time orders Transcribes cancellations and changes in orders *Transcribing Miscellaneous Orders* Can properly transcribe: Diet orders Activity orders Diagnostic test orders Permission, restrictions Consultations Critical condition list Other orders: transfers, deaths, blood bank, isolation *Common Order Groups* Can demonstrate ability to transcribe: Admission orders Preoperative orders Postoperative orders Discharge orders				

**Note:* Utilization of Medical Terminology to be integrated into practical experience.

This is to certify that ______________ has successfully performed the skills listed under the direct supervision of the designated on-site trainer and/or the instructor of record.

Date of completion of entire training plan: ______________

Comments:

______________ ______________

On-Site Trainer Student

______________ ______________

Instructor Date

Student: In the spaces below list additional tasks included in this occupation in your hospital, but not listed in the preceding pages. This page will be especially useful when you are assigned to special areas of the hospital such as ICU, Mental Health, Obstetrics, etc. Please show number of hours spent on additional tasks performed.

Additional Tasks Performed	**Hours**	**Date**

CHAPTER 19
Order Transcription Practice

There are 49 sets of authentic physician's orders in this section. Sets 1 to 12 are examples of preprinted doctor's orders. Practice transcribing these first and you will build your skills using orders that are easy to read.

Sets 13 to 18 are real handwritten orders. An answer key is included below each set.

Sets 19 to 49 offer a variety of actual orders to give you further practice with different writing styles.

Transcribe the following orders for Sets 1 through 49. Use the computer or your hospital's Kardexes and requisitions if possible. A sample Kardex is included at the end of Chapter 17.

PHYSICIAN'S ORDER SHEET

APPROVED EQUIVALENTS MAY BE DISPENSED UNLESS CHECKED HERE ☐

DATE & TIME	ORDERS	PATIENT NAME
	1. Admit.	
	2. Bedrest—May feed self, read.	
	3. Bedside commode prn BM c̄ full assistance 1–2x/day.	
	4. TPR & BP/qid.	
	5. I & O	
	6. Low salt diet.	
	7. Maalox 30 cc q 2h while awake.	
	8. Valium 5 mg p.o. q 8 hrs.	
	9. Valium 5–10 mg p.o. additional h.s. prn sleep.	

TIME NOTED | NURSE'S SIGNATURE | DOCTOR'S SIGNATURE | ☐ TO BE DISCHARGED

EQUIVALENTS MAY BE UNLESS CHECKED HERE ☐

DATE & TIME	ORDERS
	10. Surfak i̇ daily.
	11. MOM 30 cc prn constipation.
	12. Demerol 75 mg-100 mg IM q 2–4 hrs. PRN chest pain.
	13. O_2 6L/min, Nasal prn chest pain or dyspnea.
	14. EKG, CPK, SGOT, HBD, SGPT tomorrow.
	15. Bilirubin, alk ptase, ceph floc tomorrow.
	16. IV keep open c̄ D5W.

Set 1

			1. Pentobarb 100 mg. IM (or PO) hs.
			2. Oil retention enema followed by ss enema for impaction.
			3. Vital signs & temp q.i.d.
			4. I & O
			5. Up to bathroom c̄ help PRN.
			6. Demerol 25–50 mgm IM q 3h prn.
			7. CBC, Ua, Na, K, BUN now.
			8. IV's 5% D/1/2 N saline (add K+ 30 mEq/1000) 100 cc's/hr.
			9. NPO

Set 2

APPROVED EQUIVALENTS MAY BE DISPENSED UNLESS CHECKED HERE ☐			DATE & TIME	ORDERS	PATIENT NAME
				1. Transfer to the Rehabilitation Unit.	
				2. Rehabilitation Evaluation: P.T., O.T., Speech Therapy	
				and Social Worker.	
				3. B.I.D. P.T., gait and exercise.	
				4. B.I.D. O.T., ADL, ROM, strengthening and coordination exercises.	
				5. Vital signs q. shift.	
				6. May have shampoo.	
				7. Diet as follows: 1000 mg Na - 1800 cal.	
				8. See medication orders on separate Physician's Order Sheet.	

Set 3

DATE & TIME	ORDERS	PATIENT NAME

APPROVED EQUIVALENTS MAY BE DISPENSED UNLESS CHECKED HERE ☐

ROUTINE BED REST ORDERS

1. Foot board attached to bed.
2. Knee length antiembolism stockings.
3. Push feet against foot board ten times hourly.
4. Ascriptin 2 B.I.D. if not allergic to aspirin.
5. Vitamin C 500 MGS Q.I.D.
6. Bathroom privileges or bedside commode for bowel movements.
7. Overhead frame with trapeze.
8. Semi-Fowler's for position of comfort.

TIME NOTED | NURSE'S SIGNATURE | DOCTOR'S SIGNATURE | ☐ TO BE DISCHARGED

APPROVED EQUIVALENTS MAY BE DISPENSED UNLESS CHECKED HERE ☐

DATE & TIME

9. Sheepskin or air mattress.
10. Bran cereal daily.
11. Metamucil 1 oz. daily in juice.
12. Surfak 1 cap. T.I.D.
13. Enema, Laxative, or suppository of choice PRN.
14. 4000 CC'S oral fluid each 24 hrs.
15. Shampoo PRN.

TIME NOTED | NURSE'S SIGNATURE | DOCTOR'S SIGNATURE | ☐ TO BE DISCHARGED

APPROVED EQUIVALENTS MAY BE DISPENSED UNLESS CHECKED HERE ☐

DATE & TIME

16. Incentive spirometry hourly while awake, 10 breaths, VT ten times patients' body weight to be supervised by respiratory therapist twice daily.

TIME NOTED | NURSE'S SIGNATURE | DOCTOR'S SIGNATURE | ☐ TO BE DISCHARGED

		DATE & TIME	
			10. Surfak i̇ daily.
			11. MOM 30 cc prn constipation.
			12. Demerol 75 mg-100 mg IM q 2–4 hrs. PRN chest pain.
			13. O_2 6L/min, Nasal prn chest pain or dyspnea.
			14. EKG, CPK, SGOT, HBD, SGPT tomorrow.
			15. Bilirubin, alk ptase, ceph floc tomorrow.
			16. IV keep open c̄ D5W.

Set 5

PHYSICIAN'S ORDER SHEET

	DATE & TIME	ORDERS	PATIENT NAME
APPROVED EQUIVALENTS MAY BE DISPENSED UNLESS CHECKED HERE ☐		1. T & C 3 UPC for surgery.	
		2. Transfuse 3 UWB—each over 3 period.	
		3. DSW @ 100 cc/h.	
		4. Consent: Reconstruction ® carotid artery.	
		5. Prep neck.	
		6. Dalmane 30 mgm po HS prn sleep.	
		7. Teds	
		8. Ampicillin 250 mgm po QID.	
		9. Pre-Op Meds.	
	TIME NOTED	NURSE'S SIGNATURE / DOCTOR'S SIGNATURE	☐ TO BE DISCHARGED
APPROVED EQUIVALENTS MAY BE DISPENSED UNLESS CHECKED HERE ☐	DATE & TIME	Demerol 50 mgm IM i pre-op or on-call.	
		Vistaril 25 mgm IM i pre-op or on call.	
		Valium 5 mgm po i pre-op or on-call.	
		10. Pt to void immediately before leaving for surgery.	
		11. NPO p̄ midnight.	
	TIME NOTED	NURSE'S SIGNATURE / DOCTOR'S SIGNATURE	☐ TO BE DISCHARGED
APPROVED EQUIVALENTS MAY BE DISPENSED UNLESS CHECKED HERE ☐	DATE & TIME		
	TIME NOTED	NURSE'S SIGNATURE / DOCTOR'S SIGNATURE	☐ TO BE DISCHARGED

Set 6

1. TESTS:

☐ EKG
☐ CHEST X–RAY
☐ PULMONARY FUNCTION SCREEN
☐ OTHER ______________

☐ CBC
☐ UA
☐ SMA – 7
☐ ELECTROLYTES

2. DIET

☑ NPO p 2400
☐ CLEAR LIQUIDS UNTIL ________

3. START IV ☑ OPS ☐ HOLDING ROOM ☐ FLOOR

☐ Extension Set
☐ 1000 D 5 ½ N.S. @ ________ cc/hr
☐ 500 D 5 W @ ________ cc/hr
☑ 1000 R L @ TKO cc/hr
☐ 1000 D 5 Isolyte S @ __________ cc/hr
☐ OTHER ______________

4. MEDICATIONS

☐ Daily meds c̄ sip of H_2O in a.m. pre-op

SLEEP

☐ NEMBUTAL 100 mgm p.o. H.S. M.R. x ______ prn
☐ DALMANE 15 mgm p.o. H.S. M.R. x ______ prn
☐ DALMANE 30 mgm p.o. H.S. M.R. x ______ prn
☐ HALCION .25 mgm p.o. H.S. M.R. x ______ prn
☐ OTHER ______________

PRE – OP

☐ LEAVE DENTURES IN PLACE
☐ NO PRE–OP MEDICATION
☑ ALKA SELTZER GOLD TABS ii c̄ 30 cc H20 ½ - 1 h. pre - op
☐ VALIUM ______ mgm. ☐IV ☐P.O. @ ______
☐ DROPERIDOL ______ mgm I.M. @ ______
☐ MORPHINE ______ mgm I.M. @ ______
☐ FENTANYL ______ mgm. ☐IV ☐I.M.@ ______
☐ DEMEROL ______ mgm I.M. @ ______
☐ VISTARIL ______ mgm ☐p.o. ☐I.M. @ ______
☐ ATIVAN ______ mgm ☐p.o. ☐I.M. @ ______
☐ ATROPINE ______ mgm I.M. @ ______
☐ SCOPOLAMINE ______ mgm I.M. @ ______
☐ ROBINUL ______ mgm I.M. @ ______
☒ VERSED 2-4 mgm ☒IV ☐IM@ on call
☐ OTHER ______

5. ADDITIONAL PRE–OP ORDERS ______________________________

Nurse's Signature	Date	Time	Transcriber		

PRE – OPERATIVE ANESTHESIA ORDERS

PHYSICIAN'S ORDER SHEET

DATE & TIME	ORDERS	PATIENT NAME
	PRE-OPERATIVE ORDERS FOR COLOSTOMY CLOSURE:	
	1. Laboratory: CBC, U/A, Lytes, Creatinine, Glucose,	
	2. Chest X-Ray.	
	3. Plain abdominal film.	
	4. EKG—to be read by patient's internist.	
	5. Dulcolax, two (2) tabs on admission; repeat in the A.M.	
	6. Fleet enemas through both colostomy stomas on admission.	
TIME NOTED	NURSE'S SIGNATURE / DOCTOR'S SIGNATURE	☐ TO BE DISCHARGED
DATE & TIME	7. Cleansing enemas rectally the night of admission.	
	8. Fleet enema at bedside for physicians to administer.	
	9. Minimum residue diet on admission.	
	10. Change to clear liquid diet the morning after admission.	
	11. Ambulate prn.	
	12. Consent for colostomy closure.	
	13. Prep for possible laparotomy.	
	14. Dalmane, 30 mg., po, @ hs, prn sleep.	
	15. D.S.S., 250 mg, p.o., bid.	
TIME NOTED	NURSE'S SIGNATURE / DOCTOR'S SIGNATURE	☐ TO BE DISCHARGED
DATE & TIME	16. Petrogalar, one (1) ounce, p.o., bid.	
	17. Routine colostomy care.	
	18. Other medications:	
TIME NOTED	NURSE'S SIGNATURE / DOCTOR'S SIGNATURE	☐ TO BE DISCHARGED

☐ APPROVED EQUIVALENTS MAY BE DISPENSED UNLESS CHECKED HERE

☐ APPROVED EQUIVALENTS MAY BE DISPENSED UNLESS CHECKED HERE

☐ APPROVED EQUIVALENTS MAY BE DISPENSED UNLESS CHECKED HERE

PHYSICIAN'S ORDER SHEET

DATE & TIME	ORDERS	PATIENT NAME
	PRE-OPERATIVE ORDERS	
	Patient Name: Date:	
	1. Type of surgery:	
	Date:	
	Time:	
	2. Anesthesia:	
	3. Operation permit to be obtained.	
	4. Notify O.R. & Anesthesia Department.	
	5. NPO after midnight:	
TIME NOTED	NURSE'S SIGNATURE DOCTOR'S SIGNATURE	☐ TO BE DISCHARGED
DATE & TIME	6. Upon rising in the morning of surgery, patient must wash face	
	with Phisohex, void urine, and have a bowel movement.	
	7. Chloroptic Ophthalmic Solution	
	1 drop to ______ q 1 hr. upon rising in the morning of	
	surgery.	
	8. Pre-Operative Medication	
	______ mgm Demerol I.M. 1 hr. pre-operative (time ______)	
	______ mgm Valium P.O. 1 hr. pre-operative (time ______)	
	9. Pre-Operative Antibiotics	
TIME NOTED	NURSE'S SIGNATURE DOCTOR'S SIGNATURE	☐ TO BE DISCHARGED
DATE & TIME	______ mgm Ampicillin I.M. 1 hr. pre-operative (time ______)	
	10. Void urine immediately before patient leaves for O.R.	
	11. Diamox 250 mgm ______ tab P.O. 1 hr. pre-operative (time ______)	
	12. Special Medications:	
TIME NOTED	NURSE'S SIGNATURE DOCTOR'S SIGNATURE	☐ TO BE DISCHARGED

☐ APPROVED EQUIVALENTS MAY BE DISPENSED UNLESS CHECKED HERE

☐ APPROVED EQUIVALENTS MAY BE DISPENSED UNLESS CHECKED HERE

☐ APPROVED EQUIVALENTS MAY BE DISPENSED UNLESS CHECKED HERE

Set 9

PHYSICIAN'S ORDER SHEET

DATE & TIME | ORDERS | PATIENT NAME

APPROVED EQUIVALENTS MAY BE DISPENSED UNLESS CHECKED HERE ☐

ADMITTING ORDERS: PRE-OP COLON SURGERY

1. Clear liquid diet with gum drops.
2. Dulcolax tabs ii on admission, repeat in A.M.
3. D.S.S. 250 mg po BID.
4. Petrogalar 1 oz. po q hs.
5. CBC, Lytes, Creatinine, Glucose, U/A.
6. EKG—to be read by patient's internist.
7. CXR.

TIME NOTED | NURSE'S SIGNATURE | DOCTOR'S SIGNATURE | ☐ TO BE DISCHARGED

APPROVED EQUIVALENTS MAY BE DISPENSED UNLESS CHECKED HERE ☐

DATE & TIME

8. SMA-12 in A.M.
9. T & C __________ u. pc. for surgery.
10. May shower.
11. Ambulatory.
12. Routine vital signs.
13. Abdominal prep.
14. Cleansing enema on eve. prior to surgery.
15. Consent for:

TIME NOTED | NURSE'S SIGNATURE | DOCTOR'S SIGNATURE | ☐ TO BE DISCHARGED

APPROVED EQUIVALENTS MAY BE DISPENSED UNLESS CHECKED HERE ☐

DATE & TIME

16. Dalmane 30 mg po @ hs PRN.

TIME NOTED | NURSE'S SIGNATURE | DOCTOR'S SIGNATURE | ☐ TO BE DISCHARGED

PHYSICIAN'S ORDER SHEET

			DATE & TIME	ORDERS	PATIENT NAME
APPROVED EQUIVALENTS MAY BE DISPENSED UNLESS CHECKED HERE ☐				POST-OPERATIVE ORDERS FOR:	
				1. Vital signs until stable.	
				2. Bed rest. head up.	
				3. May be up to bathroom with assist only.	
				4. Progress to regular diet as tolerated.	
				5. Chloral hydrate 0.5 gm h.s. PRN for sleep	
				repeat × 1 PRN.	
				6. Compazine 5 mgm I.M. q 4 hr. PRN for nausea.	
			TIME NOTED	NURSE'S SIGNATURE DOCTOR'S SIGNATURE	☐ TO BE DISCHARGED
APPROVED EQUIVALENTS MAY BE DISPENSED UNLESS CHECKED HERE ☐			DATE & TIME	7. Milk of Magnesia 30cc PRN for laxative.	
				8. Empirin with codeine #3 tabs ii q 4 hr.	
				PRN for pain.	
				9. Place eye medications at bedside tray, especially note	
				those from O.R.	
				10. Continue previous medications as follows:	
			TIME NOTED	NURSE'S SIGNATURE DOCTOR'S SIGNATURE	☐ TO BE DISCHARGED
APPROVED EQUIVALENTS MAY BE DISPENSED UNLESS CHECKED HERE ☐			DATE & TIME		
			TIME NOTED	NURSE'S SIGNATURE DOCTOR'S SIGNATURE	☐ TO BE DISCHARGED

POST—OP PACU ORDERS

1. MEDICATIONS:

- ☒ Fentanyl 25 mcg. IV q5 min. x 4 doses prn pain
- ☐ Fentanyl 50 mcg. IV q5 min. x ______ doses prn pain
- ☐ Morphine ______ mgm IV q 5 min x ______ doses prn pain
- ☐ Compazine ☒ 1.25 mgm. IV prn nausea M.R.X.- 0
- ☒ Inapsine ☐ 2.5 mgm. IV prn nausea M.R.X. ______
- ☐ Atropine 0.2 mgm. IV prn pulse below ______ and notify anesthesiologist M.R. x ______ prn
- ☒ OTHER Pulse Oximetry
  ABG's 1200

2. ADDITIONAL ORDERS:
OXYGEN
☐ Mask ☐ Nasal Prongs ______ LPM ☒ Mist 40 %

Verapamil 2.5mg IV } in PAR stat
Digoxin 0.25 mg IV }
Call Dr. [redacted] for ICU orders

3. DISCHARGE:

To ☐ Ward ☐ DOU ☒ ICU ☐ Home
☒ Time 1300
☒ PACU Score of ______
☐ Block sensory level of ______
☐ Return of motor function

4. POST — OP ANESTHESIA ORDERS FOR FLOOR

O2 mist 40% ABGs in AM
Suction airway q 2 hr + prn poor cough
CXR in AM
Pulse Oximetry

ANOTHER BRAND OF DRUG IDENTICAL IN FORM AND CONTENT MAY BE DISPENSED UNLESS

Date	Time	R.N.	Date	Time	M.D.

ANOTHER BRAND OF DRUG IDENTICAL IN FORM AND CONTENT MAY BE DISPENSED UNLESS CHECKED. ☐

Date	Time	R.N.	Date	Time	M.D.

Admit–Definitive Observation Unit
Diagnosis–Rule out right hip fracture
Slipped left hip replacement
Condition–Guarded
Vitals–every 2–4 hrs. to every 4 hrs.
Diet–Regular
Ensure when necessary three times a day—240 cc
Activity–Immobility right hip. Bedrest.
Allergy–None
Medications–Tylenol $\overline{\text{ii}}$ p.o. q 4 hrs.
Ascriptin $\overline{\text{ii}}$ p.o. q 6 hrs.
Demerol 25 mg } IV q 3° prn pain
Vistaril 25 mg }
MVI $\overline{\text{ii}}$ p.o. q A.M.
IV D5½ NS at 50 cc/hr. $\bar{c}$ 20 KCI
Deep breathing & foot flexion q 1 hr.
Eggcrate mattress

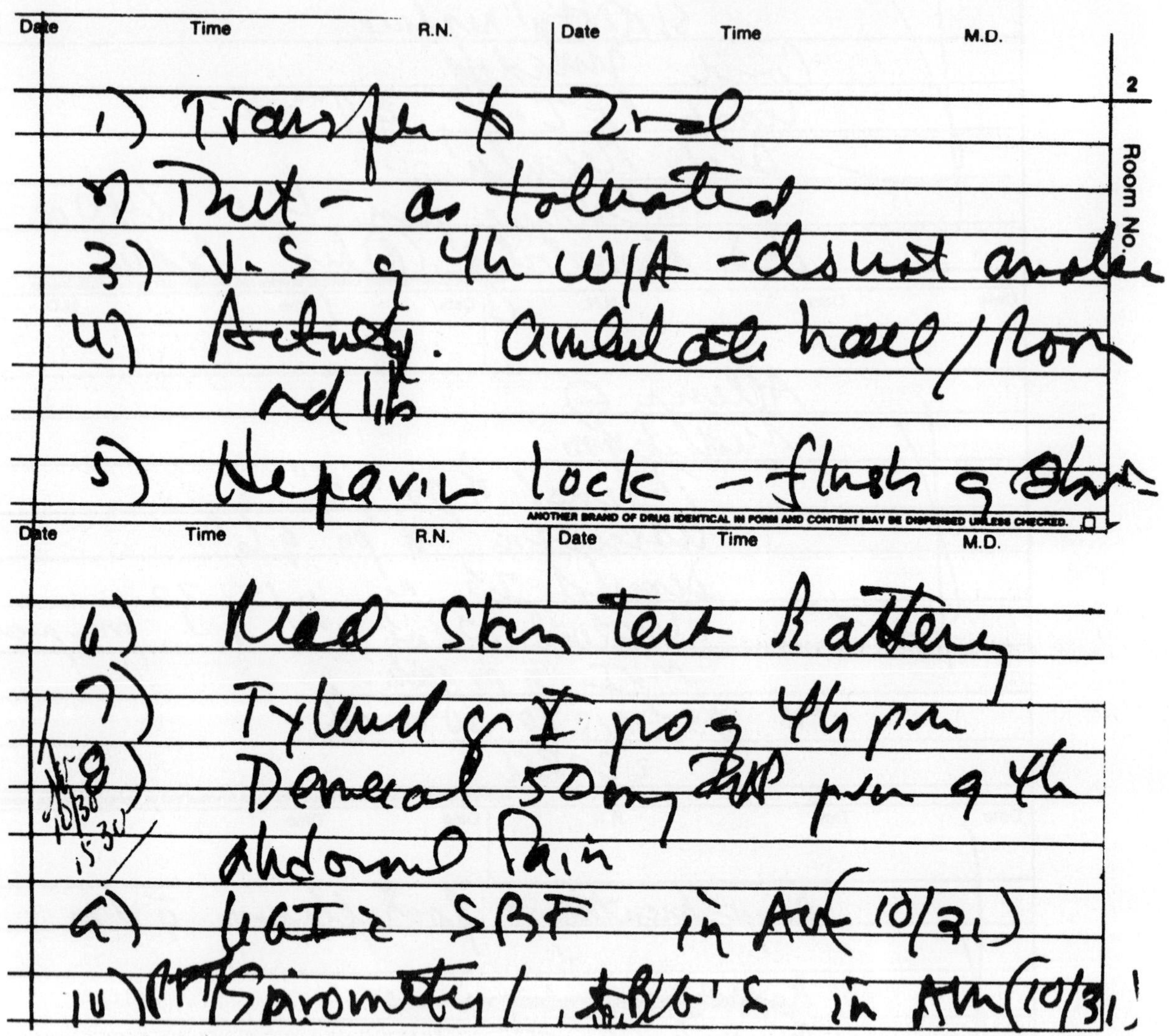

1) Transfer to 2nd (floor)
2) Diet as tolerated
3) Vital signs every 4 hrs. while awake—do not awake
4) Activity - Ambulate hall/room ad lib.
5) Heparin lock - flush every 8 hrs.
6) Read skin test battery
7) Tylenol grain 10 p.o. every 4 hrs. prn
8) Demerol 50 mg prn q4h abdominal pain
9) Upper gastrointestinal series, small bowel film in A.M.
10) Pulmonary function tests/spirometry/arterial blood gases in A.M.

ANOTHER BRAND OF DRUG IDENTICAL IN FORM AND CONTENT MAY BE DISPENSED UNLESS CHECKED. ☐

Date	Time	R.N.	Date	Time	M.D.

1) Nasal oxygen 2 L prn
2) Soft diet
3) Foley
4) out of bed invalid chair twice a day
5) right hip on pillows—heel off bed. May turn to either side.
6) Ancef Gm $\dot{\bar{\text{i}}}$ intravenous piggyback every 8 hrs.
7) Bactrim DS $\dot{\bar{\text{i}}}$ p.o. BID
8) Morphine Sulphate 1–3 mg IV q3° prn pain

Set 15

Change IV orders:

Continue current L DSW $\bar{c}$ 40 KCI/L at 85 cc/hr.

Next L D5NS $\bar{c}$ 40 KCI @ 85/hr.

Then D5½ $\bar{c}$ 40 KCI/L at 85/hr. continuous

Lytes in A.M.

Set 16

ANOTHER BRAND OF DRUG IDENTICAL IN FORM AND CONTENT MAY BE DISPENSED UNLESS CHECKED.

Date	Time	R.N.	Date	Time	M.D.

Tagamet 300 mg IM q 6h
NPO
Chart I&O
Sodium luminal gr. $\ddot{\text{ii}}$ Ⓗ prn sleep
Hematocrit & hemoglobin at 6 A.M.
Continuous gastric suction

Set 17

Physical Therapy consult c̄ patient c̄ ruptured disc L5-S1 - c̄ nerve root S1
Sponge baths & shampoo
Cont. bedside commode
Zantac 150mg po BID
D/C IV
↑ Percocet to ii tabs po q 3 Hrs prn pain
K-pad to (L) buttock & low back

Physical Therapy consult with patient with ruptured disc - lumbar 5 - sacral 1 with nerve root S_1
Sponge baths and shampoo
Continue bedside commode
Zantac 150 mg p.o. B.I.D.
Discontinue IV
Increase Percocet to 2 tablets p.o. every 3 hrs. prn pain
K-pad to left buttock and low back

Set 18

① Admit → R/O acute [illegible].
② NPO
③ VS q 8h
④ CBC c̄ diff. @ 1300 STAT

ANOTHER BRAND OF DRUG IDENTICAL IN FORM AND CONTENT MAY BE DISPENSED UNLESS CHECKED. ☐

Date	Time	R.N.	Date	Time	M.D.

⑤ IV: D5 ½NS + 20 mEq KCl/l @ 150cc/h.
⑥ Ambulate ad lib.

Set 19

1) Sign Consent → exploratory laparotomy c̄ appendectomy

2) Mefoxin 1 gm IV now

11/3/87 1300

ANOTHER BRAND OF DRUG IDENTICAL IN FORM AND CONTENT MAY BE DISPENSED UNLESS CHECKED. ☐

Date Time R.N. Date Time M.D.

3) Demerol 75 mg IM now.

Set 20

Post op appendectomy

1) RR → 2nd

2) VS q 8h

ANOTHER BRAND OF DRUG IDENTICAL IN FORM AND CONTENT MAY BE DISPENSED UNLESS CHECKED. ☐

Date Time R.N. Date Time M.D.

3) NPO

4) IV D5 ½ NS + 20 mEq KCl/l @ 150 cc/h.

5) Mefoxin 1 gm IV q 6h due @1900

6) TCDB q 2 h while awake

7) leg exercises

ANOTHER BRAND OF DRUG IDENTICAL IN FORM AND CONTENT MAY BE DISPENSED UNLESS CHECKED. ☐

Date Time R.N. Date Time M.D.

8) Ambulate tid

9) St. cath. q 8h prn.

Set 21

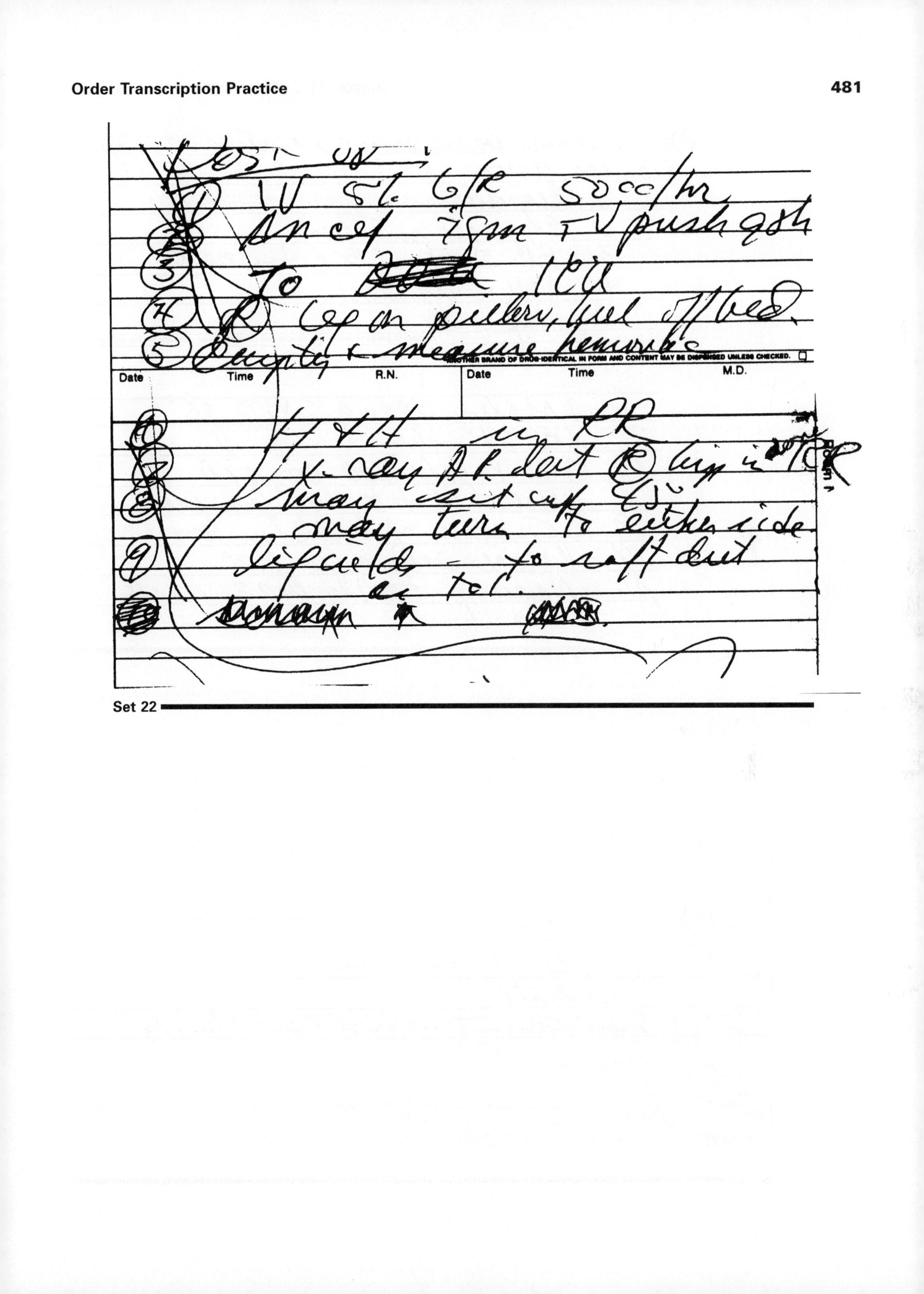

ANOTHER BRAND OF DRUG IDENTICAL IN FORM AND CONTENT MAY BE DISPENSED UNLESS CHECKED. ☐

Date	Time	R.N.	Date	Time	M.D.

Dx: Severe Back pain c̄ sciatica + slipped lumbar disc.

1. Reg diet
2. Eggcrate mattress
3. BR strict – BSC for BM only
4. Pelvic Tx 20#
5. Heplock

ANOTHER BRAND OF DRUG IDENTICAL IN FORM AND CONTENT MAY BE DISPENSED UNLESS CHECKED. ☐

Time	R.N.	Date	Time	M.D.

6. Robaxin 500mg IVPB q8° for 24° then
7. Oral Robaxin 750 po qid
8. Percocet i tab q3° prn pain
9. CT scan of back in AM. LS spine
10. Colace 200mg po q12°
11. Naprosyn 500mg BID c̄ meals

Set 23

(1) UGI today

(2) Triple lumen cath. @ bedside

(3) Sign consent → insertion triple lumen catheter

(4) Hold KCl in IV for now.

ANOTHER BRAND OF DRUG IDE

Date	Time	R.N.	Date

CHART

(5) SMA-14 today

Set 24

① IV- D5½NS c̄ 20mEq KCl at 125cc/hr.
② Digoxin 0.25mg 2hrs p̄ dose given in d/c
③ Verapamil 5mg IVP q 4° prn SVT > 150/min
Maximum of 4 doses in 24°
Call Dr. [redacted] if rate remains > 150
p̄ one dose of Verapamil
④ M.S. 1-3mg IV q 3° prn pain
⑤ H+H at 1500
⑥ CPK X3 per ICU protocol - starting now

ANOTHER BRAND OF DRUG IDENTICAL IN FORM AND CONTENT MAY BE DISPENSED UNLESS CHECKED. ☐

Date	Time	R.N.	Date	Time	M.D.

⑦ K at 1800
⑧ CBC and SMA 7 in AM
⑨ EKG in AM

Set 25

CBC
UA
SMA 14
ABG
EGG
Chest X-ray
1+1 z ceinc
Stat

ANOTHER BRAND OF DRUG IDENTICAL IN FORM AND CONTENT MAY BE DISPENSED UNLESS CHECKED. ☐

Set 26

Digoxin 0.25mg po now given
D/C O2 mist
Nasal prong O2 @ 2l/min - observe for desaturation
on pulse oximeter - increase O2 to 3 or 4l
prn SaO2 ↓ 92%

ANOTHER BRAND OF DRUG IDENTICAL IN FORM AND CONTENT MAY BE DISPENSED UNLESS CHECKED.

Set 27

Type + X match blood 2 units

Give one unit blood now + repeat H+H @ 4PM + 7AM

ANOTHER BRAND OF DRUG IDENTICAL IN FORM AND CONTENT MAY BE DISPENSED UNLESS CHECKED.

Time R.N. Date Time

digoxin .25 mg (2) q day

5% D/W c̄ 40 mEq KCl @ 85 cc/hour

Set 28

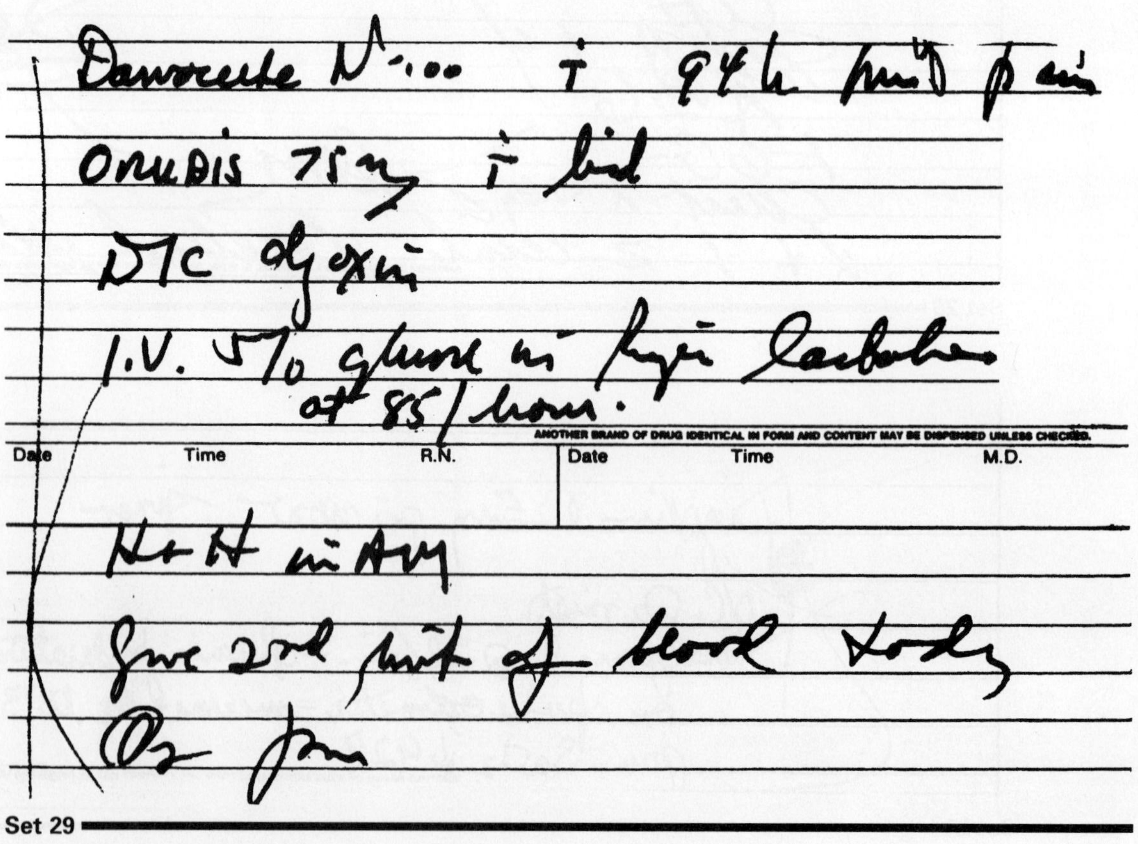

Darvocet N-100 i q4h prn for pain

ORUDIS 75 mg i bid

D/C digoxin

I.V. 5% glucose in Ringer lactate at 85/hour.

ANOTHER BRAND OF DRUG IDENTICAL IN FORM AND CONTENT MAY BE DISPENSED UNLESS CHECKED.

Date Time R.N. Date Time M.D.

H+H in AM

Give 2nd unit of blood today

O2 prn

Set 29

Zantac 150 mg bid

H & H in AM / BUN/Cr / lytes also

40 mg Depomedrol 1cc
40 u ACTH 1cc] i.m.

Give Darvocet N-100 i q4h prn pain

Use IV M.S. only if absolutely necessary

Compazine 5mg i q4h prn nausea

ANOTHER BRAND OF DRUG IDENTICAL IN FORM AND CONTENT MAY BE DISPENSED UN...

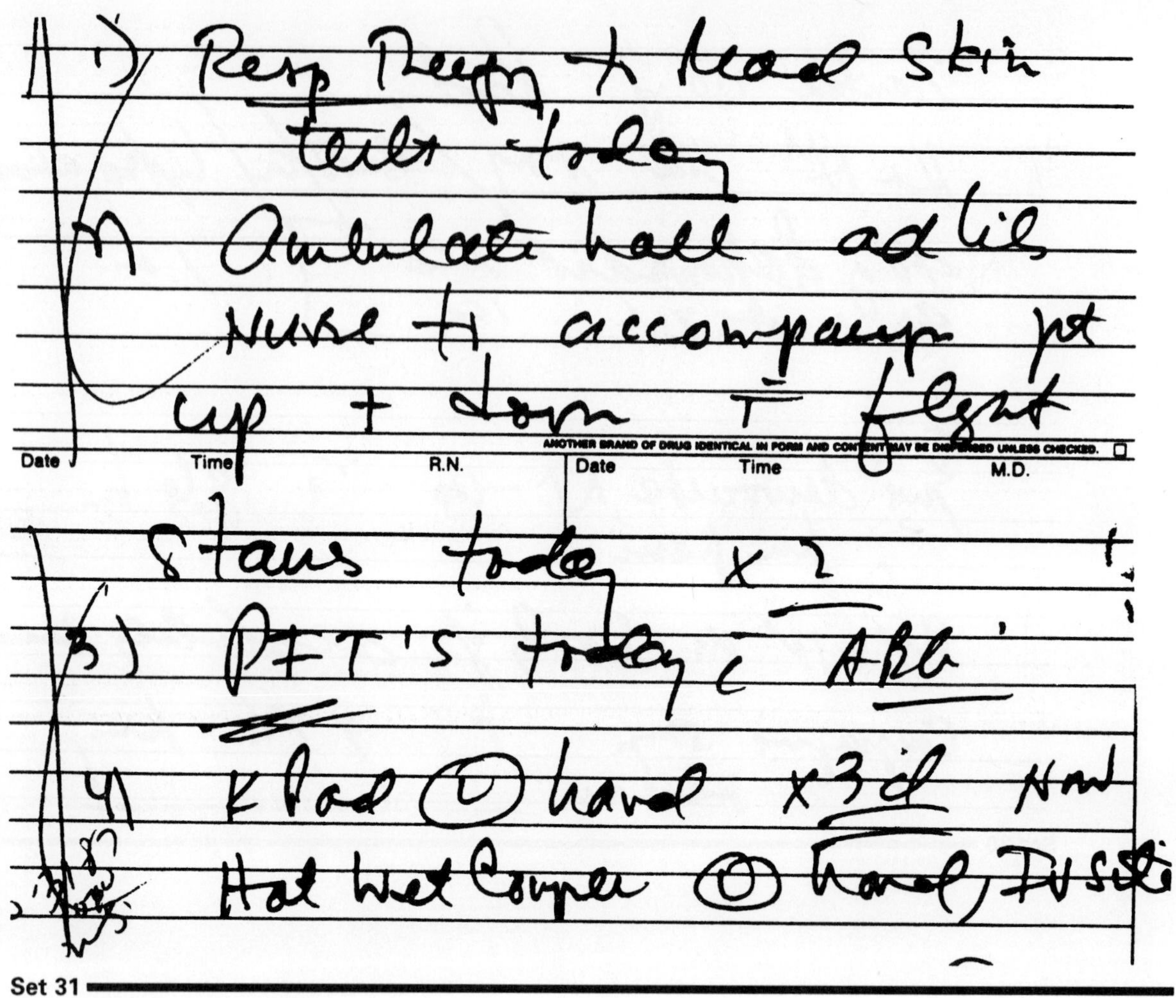
1) Resp Therapy & Mead Skin tests today

2) Ambulate hall ad lib. Nurse to accompany pt up + down 1 flight

Date Time R.N.

ANOTHER BRAND OF DRUG IDENTICAL IN FORM AND CONTENT MAY BE DISPENSED UNLESS CHECKED. ☐

Date Time M.D.

stairs today x 2

3) PFT's today c ABG

4) K pad (L) hand x 3d Now

Hot Wet Compress (L) hand, IV site

Set 31

11) Halcion 0.5mg po q HS prn

12) MOM 30cc po QD prn

13) Lomotil T q 6h prn diarrhea

4) ambulate in hall
BRP c Amb prn

5) D/C Cefoxitin after 2 post
Biopsy dose

1) Abdominal CT Scan and chest CT ~~today~~ called

No EZ cat

~~2)~~ CBC daily
3) ~~Amylase~~ ~~today~~ PAP

ANOTHER BRAND OF DRUG IDENTICAL IN FORM AND CONTENT MAY BE DISPENSED UNLESS CHECKED.

Date Time R.N. Date Time M.D.

4) ESR in AM 10/29

5) EKG in AM (10/29)

6) Obtain all charts called on Floor

7) CEA titer ~~today~~ called

8) Skin test Battery: PPD, Cocci, mumps ~~today~~ called

CONTENT MAY BE DISPENSED UNLESS CHECKED

Set 33

1) Obtain consent for colonoscopy c̄ poss Bx for 8:31 AM

Set 34

For Colonoscopy in am
Begin go-lytely colonic lavage 4L as prep per NG tube over 2-3 hrs.

Set 35

2) Diet. — Regular
No Caffeine. No Alcohol
3) V.S q 4h w/A
4) IV — D5NS at 100 cc/hr
5) Activity — ambulate BR ē Assist as needed — ~~Act OOB ad lib~~

ANOTHER BRAND OF DRUG IDENTICAL IN FORM AND CONTENT MAY BE DISPENSED UNLESS CHECKED. ☐

Date	Time	R.N.	Date	Time	M.D.

6) Nystatin Oral Suspension — 5 cc swish + swallow QID — pt may use own — pt. has his own
7) Hycodan 5 mg ii tab po q HS — may repeat i q 4h prn cough
8) Ativan 2 mg po q HS

ANOTHER BRAND OF DRUG IDENTICAL IN FORM AND CONTENT MAY BE DISPENSED UNLESS CHECKED. ☐

Date	Time	R.N.	Date	Time	M.D.

9) Pepcid 20 mg po BID
10) Digoxin 0.25 mg po QD
11) Tylenol gr X po q 4h prn pain
12) ~~Imodium 2 mg po q 4h prn diarrhea~~
13) IPPB ē NS q 4h w/A
14) ABG on Room Air Now
15) Urinalysis — Now

ANOTHER BRAND OF DRUG IDENTICAL IN FORM AND CONTENT MAY BE DISPENSED UNLESS CHECKED. ☐

Date	Time	R.N.	Date	Time	M.D.

16) NPO after Midnight tonight
17) Septra DS i tab po BID
18) Blood culture X3 — 5 min apart

4) Dietician to see pt today

5) Ensure Plus ī can TID

6) Obtain copy of pt's EKG from outpatient record of 11/4

ANOTHER BRAND OF DRUG IDENTICAL IN FORM AND CONTENT MAY BE DISPENSED UNLESS CHECKED. ☐

Date	Time	R.N.	Date	Time	M.D.

7) Demerol 75 mg } IM or Vistaril 50 mg

Call to Radiology for Thoracentesis — may repeat q 4h prn chest pain

ANOTHER BRAND OF DRUG IDENTICAL IN FORM AND CONTENT MAY BE DISPENSED UNLESS CHECKED. ☐

Date	Time	R.N.	Date	Time	M.D.

8) Chest x-ray in AM (11/6)

~~9) May D/C IV if stable~~

11/5 1345 9) May D/C IV after Thoracentesis if pt stable

incision care to abd + ® axilla incisions as done at home, BID – clean incisions c̄ hydrogen peroxide + apply new bandaide
send culture tubes to radiology c̄ pt + have thoracentesis fluid sent to lab for aerobic + anaerobic organisms

Set 38

NPH insulin 20 units SQ now
Call me c̄ AM glucose when available – notified
Glucose at 1600 STAT

ANOTHER BRAND OF DRUG IDENTICAL IN FORM AND CONTENT MAY BE DISPENSED UNLESS CHECKED. ☐

Time	R.N.	Date	Time	M.D.

Call me c̄ results
Ait OOB for meals + [illegible] in [illegible] – [illegible]
P.T [illegible] in [illegible]
EKG in AM (11/3)
H/H, SMA-7 in AM (11/3)
Increase Heparin to 1000 u/hr

ANOTHER BRAND OF DRUG IDENTICAL IN FORM AND CONTENT MAY BE DISPENSED UNLESS CHECKED. ☐

Time	R.N.	Date	Time	M.D.

Daily PTT in AM's

Set 39

1. D/C Robaxin
2. Soma 350 mg po qid
3. Prednisone 60 mg po today
   40 mg po 11/8
   20 mg po 11/9
   10 mg po 11/10 & 11/11 then D/C
4. For acute severe back pain or spasm give Demerol 50 c̄ Vistaril 50 mg I.M. q3hrs prn.

ANOTHER BRAND OF DRUG IDENTICAL IN FORM AND CONTENT MAY BE DISPENSED UNLESS CHECKED. ☐

Set 40

1) Lopressor 5 mg I.V. P.B. q 6 hr
   Hold for SBP < 110
   Cont until pt can take PO Lopressor
   25 mg PO q 12 h
2) Add 30 mEq/L of KCl to I.V.
   a) Reduce I.V. to 75 cc/h
3) Piggy back Plasmanate at 50 cc/hr for total of 1000 cc then D.C & resume I.V. at 100 cc/hr.

ANOTHER BRAND OF DRUG IDENTICAL IN FORM AND CONTENT MAY BE DISPENSED UNLESS CHECKED. ☐

Date	Time	R.N.	Date	Time	M.D.

Set 41

1) DC Compazine
2) Torecan 10 mg PO or IM q 4h prn N/V
3) Valium 2–10 mg IV or po q 2 hr prn acute agitation
4) Increase I.V. to 125 cc/h
5) Tagamet — called

Set 42

Room No.

D/S, Q4H W/A

St. cath if no void by midnight → Q10H prn thereafter.

P.T.: isometrics & bed mobility

Set 43

T & C wife's 1 unit of whole blood & transfuse today

Set 44

Post op Prosthesis precautions at all times

I.V. Lopressor per Dr. [redacted] until pt tol P.O. 50mg QD

Pillows between knees at all times

May turn to R or supine only

IV Ancef 1 Gm Q8H IVPB x 24 hours

I.V. 1000cc D5½NS @ 100cc/hr

Surg liq. to Reg diet post nausea

ANOTHER BRAND OF DRUG IDENTICAL IN FORM AND CONTENT MAY BE DISPENSED UNLESS CHECKED. ☐

Date Time R.N. Date Time M.D.

X-rays: AP & cross table lat. R Hip.

Compazine 10mg IM or PR QID prn

Pneumatic hose/booties both LEs AK length

Halcion 0.25mg QHS prn; MR x 1.

Vasotec 10mg QD

H&H & lytes in AM

ANOTHER BRAND OF DRUG IDENTICAL IN FORM AND CONTENT MAY BE DISPENSED UNLESS CHECKED. ☐

Date Time

H&H QD x3.

Set 45

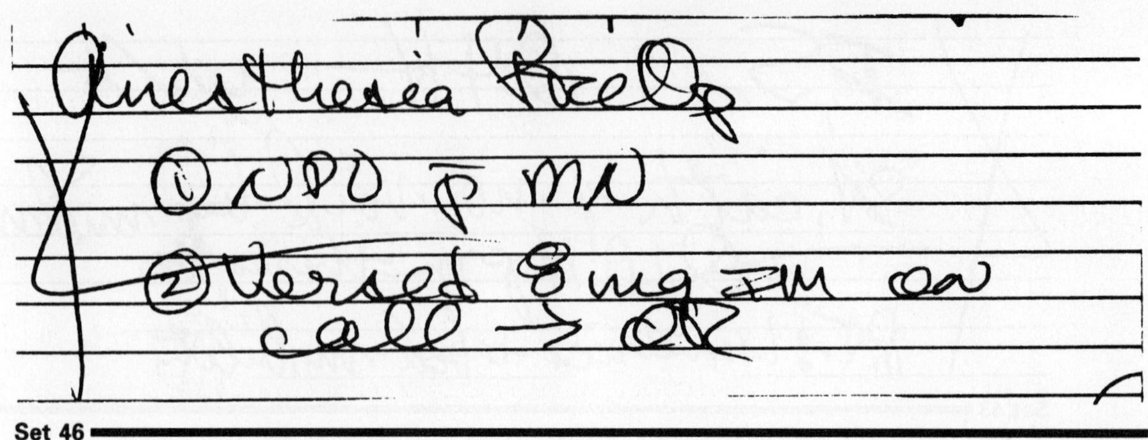
Anesthesia Orders
1) NPO p̄ MN
2) Versed 8 mg IM on call → OR

Set 46

1) NPO midnight
2) Consent for laparoscopy vs. laparotomy / bronchoscopy
3) void on call to surg

Pneumatic Hose leg on
Call to Surgery called + po Asp
EKG 12

Set 47

1) RR → floor
2) V.S. Q15 min til stable then Q 2 hrs x 4 then Q 8 hrs.
3) NPO
4) IV's D5 1/2 NS + 20 mEq KCl/L ✓ at 100 cc QH
5) Collect all post bronch sputum for cytology.

ANOTHER BRAND OF DRUG IDENTICAL IN FORM AND CONTENT MAY BE DISPENSED UNLESS CHECKED. ☐

Date	Time	R.N.	Date	Time	M.D.

6) Pneumatic boots Done
7) EKG in RR ✓ done
8) Demerol 50-75 mg IM Q 2 hrs prn pain
9) Pentobarb 100mg IM HS ✓ prn sleep
10) Torecan 10mg IM Q 6 hrs ✓ prn nausea.

Set 48

1) Clear liq as tol. If tol diet may D/C IV
2) Amb as tol c̄ help
3) Harris flush now & prn.

Set 49

Bibliography

BADASCH, SHIRLEY, and CHESEBRO, DOREEN, ***Introduction to Health Occupations*** (4th ed.). Upper Saddle River, NJ: Brady, 1997.

BARBER, LINDA, ***Being a Medical Admissions Clerk.*** Upper Saddle River, N.J.: Brady, 1994.

BENTLY MCDANIEL, JAN, and ORANGE COUNTY APIC. ***New Guidelines for Isolation Precautions in Hospitals,*** 1996.

BLACKBURN, ELSA, ***Health Unit Coordinator.*** Upper Saddle River, N.J.: Brady, 1991.

BORTON, DOROTHY, *Isolation Precautions.* ***Nursing 1997,*** January 1997, pp. 49–51.

BRUST, DONNA, and FOSTER, JOYCE, ***From Nursing Assistant to Patient Care Technician.*** Philadelphia: W. B. Saunders Co., 1997.

CHABNER, DAVI-ELLEN, ***The Language of Medicine*** (5th ed.). Philadelphia: W. B. Saunders Co., 1996.

Code-it-Right. Salt Lake City: Medicode, Inc., 1996.

DAMJANOV, IVAN, ***Pathology for the Health-Related Professions.*** Philadelphia: W. B. Saunders Co., 1996.

GARBER, DEBRA, ***Introduction to Clinical Allied Healthcare.*** Orange, Calif.: Career Publishing, Inc., 1996.

HARTSHORN, JEANETTE, SOLE, MARY LOU, and LAMBORN, MARILYN, ***Introduction to Critical Care Nursing*** (2d ed.). Philadelphia, W. B. Saunders Co., 1997.

HODGSON, BARBARA, KIZIOR, ROBERT, and KINGDON, RUTH, ***Nurse's Drug Handbook 1997.*** Philadelphia: W. B. Saunders Co., 1997.

KARCH, AMY, ***1997 Lippincott's Nursing Drug Guide.*** Philadelphia: Lippincott, 1997.

LAFLEUR-BROOKS, MYRNA, ***Health Unit Coordinating*** (3d ed.). Philadelphia: W. B. Saunders Co., 1993.

MARSHALL, JACQUELYN, ***Being a Medical Clerical Worker.*** Upper Saddle River, N.J.: Brady, 1990.

MARTINI, FREDERIC, ***Fundamentals of Anatomy and Physiology.*** Upper Saddle River, N.J.: Prentice Hall, 1989.

MCMILLER, KATHRYN, ***Being a Medical Records Clerk.*** Upper Saddle River, N.J.: Brady, 1992.

Miller-Keane Encyclopedia and Dictionary of Medicine, Nursing, and Allied Health (6th ed.). Philadelphia: W. B. Saunders Co., 1997.

POZGAR, GEORGE, ***Legal Aspects of Health Care Administration*** (6th ed.). Gaithersburg: Aspen Publishers, Inc., 1996.

Taber's Cyclopedic Medical Dictionary (18th ed.). Philadelphia: F. A. Davis Co., 1997.

WOLGIN, FRANCIE, ***Being a Nursing Assistant*** (7th ed.). Upper Saddle River, N.J.: Brady, 1997.

Index